ACSM's
Foundations of Strength Training and Conditioning

ACSM's
Foundations of Strength Training and Conditioning

NICHOLAS RATAMESS Jr, PHD, CSCS*D, FNSCA
Department of Health and Exercise Science
The College of New Jersey
Ewing, NJ

AMERICAN COLLEGE of SPORTS MEDICINE®
w w w . a c s m . o r g

 Wolters Kluwer | Lippincott Williams & Wilkins
Health
Philadelphia · Baltimore · New York · London
Buenos Aires · Hong Kong · Sydney · Tokyo

Acquisitions Editor: Emily Lupash
Product Manager: Andrea M. Klingler
Vendor Manager: Kevin Johnson
Marketing Manager: Allison Powell
Design Coordinator: Doug Smock
Production Service: SPi Global

Library of Congress Cataloging-in-Publication Data
Ratamess, Nicholas A.
    ACSM's foundations of strength training and conditioning / Nicholas Ratamess.
        p. ; cm.
    Foundations of strength training and conditioning
    Includes bibliographical references.
    ISBN 978-0-7817-8267-8
    1. Exercise—Physiological aspects. 2. Physical fitness. 3. Weight training. I. American College of Sports Medicine. II. Title. III. Title: Foundations of strength training and conditioning.
    [DNLM: 1. Physical Fitness. 2. Resistance Training. QT 255]
    QP301.R36   2011
    613.7—dc23

                                                                    2011015912

To purchase additional copies of this book, call our customer service department at (800) 638-3030 or fax orders to (301) 223-2320. International customers should call (301) 223-2300.

Visit Lippincott Williams & Wilkins on the Internet: at LWW.com. Lippincott Williams & Wilkins customer service representatives are available from 8:30 am to 6 pm, EST.

10 9 8 7 6

This book is dedicated to my wife, Alison; my children, Jessica, Vinnie, and Nicole; and my parents, Nick and Veronica, for their love and support.

Preface

Optimizing sports performance through improved athleticism has long been a primary goal among athletes, coaches, and practitioners. Although athleticism is improved substantially by participating in sports via regular practice and competition, most recognize that maximizing athletic performance can only be attained by combining sport participation with an effective strength training and conditioning program. The field of strength training and conditioning has grown immensely over the past 20 years. As a result, the number of practitioners, educators, and students in strength and conditioning–related careers and academic programs has dramatically increased. Greater scientific study, practical recommendations, and dissemination of knowledge to practitioners are needed to meet the needs of a growing field. *ACSM's Foundations of Strength Training and Conditioning* provides a review of scientific and practical information and presents the information in a logical manner. It bridges the gap between scientific study and professional practice and is aimed at coaches, athletes, personal trainers, fitness instructors, and students preparing for a career in a strength training and conditioning–related field.

ORGANIZATION

The primary objectives of *ACSM's Foundations of Strength Training and Conditioning* are to provide the most pertinent and up-to-date information regarding the training and testing of athletes and a foundation in basic physiology and kinesiology. The book is organized into four basic sections: (1) historical and strength and conditioning field–related foundations; (2) basic biomechanics and physiology; (3) flexibility, sprint, plyometric, balance, agility, aerobic, and resistance training program design and exercise prescription; and (4) testing and evaluation. Chapter 1 provides some historical and field-related information. It is important for strength and conditioning students and professionals to have a basic understanding of its history. Chapters 2 through 8 provide the reader with basic information in human biomechanics and physiology. A foundation in human movement and physiology is paramount for the strength and conditioning professional to understand proper movement and the acute responses and subsequent adaptations that affect human performance. Chapter 9 discusses key strength and conditioning principles that form the basic template of any training program prescribed to athletes. Chapters 10 through 16 provide up-to-date information for improving athletic performance. Training recommendations and several exercise prescription examples are provided to help guide the reader through the program design process. Chapter 17 discusses the importance of training periodization when designing long-term training programs for athletes. Chapter 18 provides current information regarding the testing and evaluation of human performance. In addition, norms are provided for key fitness components and test results. Although there is not a specific nutrition chapter, pertinent nutritional information is discussed throughout in several chapters where appropriate.

FEATURES

Various learning tools have been incorporated into each chapter to help facilitate learning and comprehension. **Interpreting Research** boxes draw attention to important research findings and explain their application to strength and conditioning practice. **Myths and Misconceptions** debunk common myths and clarify widespread misconceptions. **Case Studies** throughout the chapters present real-world scenarios. Using the skills and knowledge gained from the text, these case studies require the reader to evaluate the issues and devise effective solutions. **Sidebars** amplify important concepts presented within the chapters. Finally, **Review Questions** at the end of each chapter assess the reader's grasp of key concepts.

ADDITIONAL RESOURCES

ACSM's Foundations of Strength Training and Conditioning includes additional resources for both instructors and students that are available on the book's companion Web site at http://thepoint.lww.com/ACSMS&C.

INSTRUCTORS

- Image Bank
- PowerPoint Lecture Outlines
- Brownstone Test Generator
- WebCT/Blackboard/Angel Cartridge

STUDENTS

- Videos
- Animations

In addition, purchasers of the text can access the searchable Full Text through the book's Web site. See the front inside cover of this text for more details and include the passcode to gain access to the Web site.

Nick Ratamess

User's Guide

ACSM's *Foundations of Strength Training and Conditioning* was created and developed to provide a review of scientific and practical information, bridging the gap between scientific study and professional practice. Written for coaches, athletes, personal trainers, fitness instructors, and students preparing for a career in a strength training and conditioning-related field, this text helps link greater scientific study, practical recommendations, and dissemination of knowledge to meet the needs of this growing field. Please take a few moments to look through this User's Guide, which will introduce you to the tools and features that will enhance your learning experience.

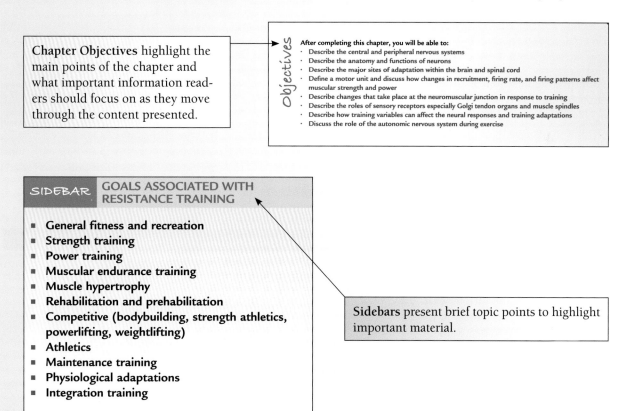

Chapter Objectives highlight the main points of the chapter and what important information readers should focus on as they move through the content presented.

Objectives

After completing this chapter, you will be able to:
- Describe the central and peripheral nervous systems
- Describe the anatomy and functions of neurons
- Describe the major sites of adaptation within the brain and spinal cord
- Define a motor unit and discuss how changes in recruitment, firing rate, and firing patterns affect muscular strength and power
- Describe changes that take place at the neuromuscular junction in response to training
- Describe the roles of sensory receptors especially Golgi tendon organs and muscle spindles
- Describe how training variables can affect the neural responses and training adaptations
- Discuss the role of the autonomic nervous system during exercise

SIDEBAR · **GOALS ASSOCIATED WITH RESISTANCE TRAINING**

- General fitness and recreation
- Strength training
- Power training
- Muscular endurance training
- Muscle hypertrophy
- Rehabilitation and prehabilitation
- Competitive (bodybuilding, strength athletics, powerlifting, weightlifting)
- Athletics
- Maintenance training
- Physiological adaptations
- Integration training

Sidebars present brief topic points to highlight important material.

Case Study 1.1

Terry, a NCAA Division II junior collegiate football player (linebacker), engaged in an off-season S&C program. Although he has lifted weights in the past, Terry did not take RT seriously until this past off-season training period because he was third string on the depth chart as a sophomore and now wanted to compete for a starting position in his junior season. After a rigorous off-season where Terry and his partner trained 4 days per week with weights plus 1–2 days of plyometrics, Terry went through the team's preseason testing battery. His 1RM bench press increased from 250 to 295 lb, squat increased from 315 to 400 lb, power clean increased from 205 to 260 lb, vertical jump increased from 25 to

Case Studies throughout the chapters present real-world scenarios. Using the skills and knowledge gained from the text, these case studies require the reader to evaluate the issues and devise effective solutions.

Myths & Misconceptions

Resistance Training will Make One "Muscle Bound," Slower, and Reduce Performance

Throughout the history of S&C several myths and misconceptions developed and several remain in existence today despite scientific evidence pointing to the contrary. It remains a mystery why certain myths continue to perpetuate; however, it is clear that the S&C professionals need to do their best to dispel these myths whenever possible. One myth is the creation of the muscle-bound individual via RT. This muscle-bound phenomenon is thought to reduce movement mobility, speed, and performance. This myth dates back more than 100 years to the Strongman Era. The reality is that RT enhances virtually all components of fitness and increases athletic performance (1,2,13). An exception exists in that if one always trains with slow velocities and gains a large amount of mass, it is theoretically possible to become slower. However, specificity of RT tell

Myths and Misconceptions boxes debunk popular myths and clarify widespread misconceptions about strength and conditioning.

Interpreting Research

Bench Press Performance and the SSC

Wilson GJ, Elliott BC, Wood GA. The effect on performance of imposing a delay during a stretch-shorten cycle movement. *Med Sci Sports Exerc.* 1991;23:364–370.

Wilson et al. (37) examined bench press performance under four conditions: (a) a regular "touch and go" bench press (RBP), (b) a bench press with a short pause (SPBP) of ~0.6 seconds, a bench press with a lo pause (LPBP) of 1.27 seconds, and a purely CON bench press (PCBP) initiated from the bottom starting position. A continuum was found where maximal bench press strength was greatest with RBP (~143.1 kg followed by SPBP (~137.3 kg), LPBP (~132.9 kg), and PCBP (125.0 kg). Ground reaction force patterns were similar (Fig. 2.3). These data showed that strength performance was maximized with high SSC activ (no pause) and decreased in proportion to pause length. Purely CON actions resulted in the lowest stren values. The take-home message for S&C professionals is that maximal strength performance is observed with no pause, and training, in part, should be centered on maximizing SSC activity. However, some athl (powerlifters) benefit from including a pause between ECC and CON actions at various points in trainin because competition necessitates it.

Interpreting Research boxes draw attention to important research findings and explain their application to strength and conditioning practice.

Exercises

Exercise boxes provide step-by-step instruction for various exercises, along with photos of the proper positioning and movement. With these exercise boxes can be found **Caution! boxes**, which provide warning and reminders about important things to remember while doing the specific exercise. **Variations** of the exercise described are also provided.

BENT-OVER BARBELL ROW
Rating: B

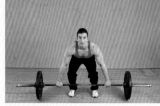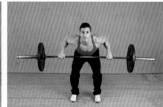

- Athlete stands with feet shoulder width apart and knees flexed.
- Bar is grasped from the floor with a closed, pronated grip wider than shoulder width while the back is flat, chest out, shoulders retracted, head is tilted forward, elbows are fully extended, and torso is flexed forward 10–30 degrees above horizontal.
- Athlete should remain flexed forward throughout the exercise.
- Bar is pulled upward (using back muscles mostly and not the elbow flexors) touching the upper abdomen.
- The elbows are pointed up with a rigid torso and the back should remain hyperextended (straight) throughout the movement.
- Bar is lowered with control until elbows are fully extended.

! *CAUTION! Standing too upright greatly limits ROM and muscle development. A common mistake is to see this exercise performed with the athlete maintaining nearly an upright posture.*

OTHER VARIATIONS AND SIMILAR EXERCISES Reverse-grip bent-over row, bent-over DB row (with various grip positions), BB bench row, T-bar row, Smith machine row, rows with keg, mastiff bar, or sand bag, one-arm DB/core ball/band/tubing row, one-arm cable row, DB/KB row (single leg for balance), renegade row with DB or KB, one-arm bench row, and inverted row (BW with bar or TRX and feet elevated on bench/SB or placed on the floor, pronated or supinated grip).

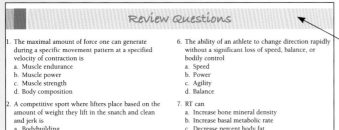

Review Questions

1. The maximal amount of force one can generate during a specific movement pattern at a specified velocity of contraction is
   a. Muscle endurance
   b. Muscle power
   c. Muscle strength
   d. Body composition

2. A competitive sport where lifters place based on the amount of weight they lift in the snatch and clean and jerk is
   a. Bodybuilding
   b. Weightlifting

6. The ability of an athlete to change direction rapidly without a significant loss of speed, balance, or bodily control
   a. Speed
   b. Power
   c. Agility
   d. Balance

7. RT can
   a. Increase bone mineral density
   b. Increase basal metabolic rate
   c. Decrease percent body fat
   d. All of the above

> At the end of each chapter, an extensive list of **Review Questions** provide students with a chance to apply what they've learned and assess their knowledge through multiple choice and true/false questions.

Summary Points

✔ Skeletal muscles produce greater force during ECC actions, followed by ISOM and CON actions.

✔ A relationship between muscle length and force exists where muscles are strongest near resting sarcomere lengths (where the optimal number of myofilament cross-bridges are formed) but weaken as the muscle shortens. At longer lengths, passive elements become more engaged and enhance muscle force production.

✔ When maximal intensity contractions are used, greatest muscle force is produced at slow velocities whereas less force is produced at fast velocities.

✔ Muscle architectural changes, *e.g.*, in a pennate muscle's angle of pennation and/or fascicle length, take place during training that enhances muscular strength.

✔ Strength and speed performance is based, in part, upon stature, leverage, and mechanical advantage, *e.g.*, the ratio of the moment arm of force to the moment arm of resistance.

✔ Torque production changes throughout joint ROM. An ascending-descending curve is seen with single-joint movements, an ascending curve is seen with pushing movements, and descending curves are seen with pulling movements.

✔ Friction is a critical component to force production and stability.

✔ The development of intra-abdominal pressure is important for relieving spinal stress during lifting.

✔ Various lifting accessories have been developed that can reduce the risk of injury but also can significantly enhance lifting performance.

> **Summary Points** provide a checklist of the important concepts discussed in each chapter for a quick review.

> High-quality, four-color illustrations and photos throughout the text help to draw attention to important concepts in a visually stimulating and intriguing manner. They help to clarify the text and are particularly helpful for visual learners.

enormous. He was well known for his feud with Bob Hoffman, books and publications (*Your Physique*, *Muscle Power*, later *Muscle and Fitness and Flex*), coining of training terms and principles, promotion of bodybuilding training and events (the Mr. and Ms. Olympia), and equipment and nutrition supplement manufacturing. Although *Muscle Beach*, Santa Monica, CA, was a popular sport, recreational,

Reinhoudt, Ed Coan, Dr. Fred Hatfield, Louie Simmo Anthony Clark, Ted Arcidi, Tamara Grimwood-Rainwa and Becca Swanson to name a few.

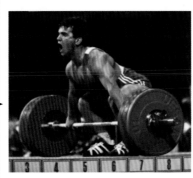

■ **FIGURE 1-7.** Naim Suleymanoglu.

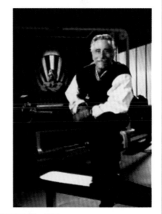

■ **FIGURE 1-8.** Joe Weider.

STUDENT RESOURCES

Inside the front cover of your textbook, you'll find your personal access code. Use it to log on to http://thePoint. lww.com/ACSMS&C—the companion Web site for this textbook. On the Web site, you can access various supplemental materials available to help enhance and further your learning. These assets include an interactive quiz bank and animations and videos, as well as the fully searchable online text. Adopting instructors have access to an image bank and test generator.

Reviewers

Brent A. Alvar, PhD, CSCS*D, FNSCA
Faculty-Sport Performance Director
Exercise Science
Chandler Gilbert Community College
Chandler, Arizona

Ken Anderson, MPE
Coordinator, Bachelor of Physical Education &
  Coaching
Department of Sport Science
Douglas College
New Westminster, British Columbia, Canada

Scott W. Arnett, PhD, CSCS,*D
Assistant Professor
Kinesiology, Recreation, and Sport
Western Kentucky University
Bowling Green, Kentucky

Ron Cox, PhD
Department of Physical Education, Health & Sport
Miami University
Oxford, Ohio

Eric Dugan, PhD
Boise State University
Boise, Idaho

Michael Hartman, PhD, CSCS*D
Professor of Exercise Science
Department of Kinesiology
Texas Wesleyan University
Fort Worth, Texas

Robert Hess, MS, ATC, STS
Associate Professor of Health
Wellness Department
Community College of Baltimore County Catonsville
Baltimore, Maryland

Gary Hunter, PhD, FACSM
Department of HPER
University of Alabama-Birmingham
School of Education
Birmingham, Alabama

Alexander Koch, PhD
Truman State University
Kirksville, Missouri

William Kraemer, PhD, FACSM
Department of Kinesiology
Human Performance Lab
The University of Connecticut
Storrs, Connecticut

G. Barry Legh, MSPE, DipEd
Senior Instructor
School of Human Kinetics
University of British Columbia
Vancouver, British Columbia, Canada

Jerry Mayhew, PhD
HES Division
Truman State University
Kirksville, Missouri

Robert Ryan, MA, ATC, CSCS
Director, Athletic Training Education Program
Department of Kinesiology
Mesa State College
Grand Junction, Colorado

Brian K. Schilling, PhD, CSCS
Associate Professor
Exercise Neuromechanics Laboratory Director,
  Institutional Review Board Chair
Department of Health and Sport Sciences
University of Memphis
Memphis, Tennessee

David Tomchuk, MS, ATC, LAT, CSCS
Clinical Education Coordinator/Assistant Professor
Missouri Valley College
School of Nursing & Health Sciences
Marshall, Missouri

N. Travis Triplett, PhD
HLES Department
Appalachian State University
Boone, North Carolina

Heather E. Webb, PhD, ATC, LAT
Assistant Professor
Department of Kinesiology
Mississippi State University
Starkville, Mississippi

Acknowledgments

I would like to thank the American College of Sports Medicine for giving me the opportunity and support to write this book and D. Mark Robertson for his assistance in project development. Special thanks go out to the staff at Lippincott Williams & Wilkins for their support and assistance with this book, especially Acquisitions Editor Emily Lupash for her project insight and direction, Product Manager Andrea Klingler for all of her guidance and editorial assistance, and Brett MacNaughton and Mark Lozier for their outstanding work during the photo shoot. I want to thank my colleagues Drs. William Kraemer, Jay Hoffman, Avery Faigenbaum, and Jie Kang for their valuable feedback on the book. Lastly, I want to thank Lisa Curtin for her assistance during manuscript preparation and Jaclyn Levowsky, Christina Rzeszutko, Jaishon Scott, Nicholas Gambino, Ryan Ross, Cameron Richardson, Joseph Rosenberg, and Kavan Latham for their assistance in demonstrating several exercises portrayed in this book.

Contents

Part One

Foundations

Introduction to Strength Training and Conditioning

Objectives

After completing this chapter, you will be able to:

- Define basic strength and conditioning terms
- Understand a brief history of strength training and conditioning from its early origins to modern times
- Describe common goals associated with resistance training
- Describe the benefits of strength training and conditioning
- Describe health- and skill-related components of fitness
- Describe competitive forms of resistance training
- Discuss the strength and conditioning profession in terms of preparation, proficiencies, and duties/responsibilities

WHAT IS STRENGTH TRAINING AND CONDITIONING?

Strength training and conditioning (S&C) is a term that has been adapted to include several modalities of exercise. Strength training via **resistance training** (RT) serves as the core, and other modalities of exercises are included depending on the needs of the athlete. For example, an S&C program for strength and power athletes would include **weight training** but also **plyometrics**, **sprint/agility training**, **flexibility** exercises, and **aerobic training** (in addition to the rigors of practice and competition). For an individual exercising for general fitness, weight training would be included in addition to flexibility and cardiovascular training. Multiple modalities of training enhance several health- and skill-related components of muscular fitness. Thus, integration of multiple modalities of training is critical to optimizing total conditioning.

The importance of a high-quality S&C program cannot be overemphasized. From an athletic standpoint, improving and establishing good motor skill technique is critical but can only take an athlete to a certain level of achievement. Many times, it is the health- and skill-related components of fitness that separate athletic talent. Elite athletes possess greater strength, power, speed, and jumping ability compared to athletes of lesser rank (10). A recent analysis of National Football League (NFL) drafted players versus nondrafted players showed that the drafted players had faster 40-yd dash times, vertical jump height, pro-agility shuttle times, and 3-cone drill times compared to nondrafted players eligible for the draft

(17). A study by Garstecki et al. (9) compared Division I and Division II National Collegiate Athletic Association (NCAA) football players and showed that Division I athletes had greater one-repetition maximum (1RM) bench press, squat, power clean, vertical jump height, fat-free mass, lower percent body, and faster 40-yd dash times than Division II athletes. Fleisig et al. (7) compared high school, collegiate, and professional baseball pitchers and showed that the professional pitchers had greater muscle strength, shoulder, and elbow throwing velocities compared to lesser-skilled pitchers. Thus, there is a relationship between an athlete's status and several components of physical conditioning.

Case Study 1.1

Terry, a NCAA Division II junior collegiate football player (linebacker), engaged in an off-season S&C program. Although he has lifted weights in the past, Terry did not take RT seriously until this past off-season training period because he was third string on the depth chart as a sophomore and now wanted to compete for a starting position in his junior season. After a rigorous off-season where Terry and his partner trained 4 days per week with weights plus 1–2 days of plyometrics, Terry went through the team's preseason testing battery. His 1RM bench press increased from 250 to 295 lb, squat increased from 315 to 400 lb, power clean increased from 205 to 260 lb, vertical jump increased from 25 to

28 in, and 40-yd dash time decreased from 4.92 to 4.81 seconds. During preseason practice, Terry noticed his performance on the field had improved. As a result of Terry's hard work in the weight room, he earned a starting position on the school's football team.

Question for Consideration: **How much of Terry's recent success would you attribute to his off-season training program?**

BRIEF HISTORY OF STRENGTH TRAINING AND CONDITIONING

A brief examination of the history of S&C is important for any practitioner (5,20,21). Knowledge of prominent individuals, eras, events, and training practices is critical to understanding the field. In fact, some important training concepts currently popular are not new; rather, they were used in the past, fell out of popularity, and have resurfaced. One may state that study of the past may be important in preparation of future S&C trends. Nevertheless, it is certainly fascinating to examine this facet of our history.

EARLY ORIGINS

Feats of muscular strength and evidence of some type of RT date back several thousands of years to ancient times. Walls of ancient Egyptian tombs circa 2500 B.C. displayed artwork depicting strength contests of various types. In Ireland circa 1800 B.C., weight-throwing contests were held that involved explosive strength and power. A strong military was also desired in many areas because warfare was common. This was seen in China where strength tests were being used for military purposes circa 1122–255 B.C.

Perhaps more familiar were the accolades of the ancient Greeks circa sixth century B.C. The ancient Greeks were well known for their pursuit of excellence in physical education and sport. Although the city of Athens valued the aesthetic sides of physical education, Sparta's main objective was to have a strong, powerful army. Men and women were required to be in shape. Boys were sent to military school ~6–7 years of age and were trained rigorously in gymnastics, running, jumping, javelin and discus throwing, swimming, and hunting. Women were not required to leave home but were trained rigorously as well. In addition, sports were popular as the Olympic Games (consisting of events such as foot races, discus and javelin throwing, long jump [with weights], wrestling, boxing, pankration, equestrian, and pentathlon) initiated circa 776 B.C., and many individuals trained at gymnasiums to enhance physical performance. Perhaps

the best-known Greek strongman was *Milo of Crotona*. Milo was a 5-time wrestling champion and a 22-time strength champion. He has been credited with the first use of progressive overload during RT. It was reported that Milo carried a young calf across his shoulders every day until the animal was fully grown and ultimately carried the 4-year-old heifer the length (~200 m) of the Stadium at Olympia. In addition, the ancient Greeks were well known for lifting heavy stones. In fact, one of the earliest bodybuilding events was thought to occur in Sparta. Spartan men were judged on their physiques and punished if found to be lacking adequate development. Strength training for military purposes was continued by the armies of the Roman Empire. After the fall of the Roman Empire, religious opposition to training predominated for the next 1,000 years and not much progress was made during this time.

CONNECTIONS WITH SCIENCE AND MEDICINE

Throughout early times a relationship existed between the medical/scientific communities and fascination with muscular strength and development. The famous Greek physician *Galen* (129–199 A.D.) was thought to be one of the first medical doctors to recommend RT. He promoted the use of handheld weights as he worked extensively with gladiators at the time. Large strides from the scientific community in the development of strength training came during the Renaissance. It was suggested that the famous French writer *Michel de Montaigne* described the benefits of strength training with reference to his father. German educator *Joachim Camerarius* (circa 1544) wrote about weight training and how it could lead to improved health and performance. Appreciation for the human body (and adaptations to RT) was gained by advances in human anatomy. The landmark text of *Andreas Vesalius* (1514–1564) *De Humani Corporis Fabrica* and several works of *Bernard Siegfried Albinus* (1697–1770) emphasizing the musculoskeletal system vastly increased the understanding of human anatomy and, to some degree, awareness of changes associated with physical exercise.

NINETEENTH-CENTURY ADVANCES

The 1800s were a time in our history where S&C gained increased popularity. Strides in physical education were made. Nationalistic influences were seen where prominent physical educators (from Germany and Sweden) trained several students who brought their ideas and philosophies to the Unites States. These philosophies were adopted and modified by several American educators. Some programs were rigorous and comprised mostly of gymnastics exercises, and others were modified and included other modalities such as manual resistance exercise, calisthenics, flexibility exercises, games/sports, and dance. Interestingly, the use of resistance equipment such as ropes, medicine balls (whose variations have been used since the times of the ancient Greeks), dumbbells, clubs, and other implements could be seen in the curricula. A very influential individual at the time was *Dudley Sargent* (1849–1924), a Harvard-trained medical doctor (Fig. 1.1). He invented several exercise machines and developed methods to assess muscular strength and performance (Sargent vertical jump test).

Perhaps one of the most early influential time periods during the mid-1800s to the early 1900s was known as the Era of the Strongmen. This was a time where great feats of strength performance led to the realization of the potential for improving strength and appearance. In Europe and North America, various individuals promoted their muscular strength for entertainment and commercial purposes. Interestingly, many of these strong men brought to light extraordinary strength performances. However, some were responsible to some extent for some RT myths that perpetuated. Although a discussion of many of these strength legends is beyond the scope of this chapter, several pioneering strength athletes need to be recognized. *George Barker Windship*, a Harvard-trained medical doctor, toured North America performing feats of strength including what he termed the *Health Lift* (a partial range of motion [ROM] dead lift). Canadian strongman *Louis Cyr* (1863–1912) (Fig. 1.2) was a large (~300 lb) individual who possessed phenomenal strength including a 4,337-lb back lift and a famous horse pull demonstration. However, members of the anti-weight training community pointed to Cyr stating that weight training could lead to excessive bulk, slowness, and make

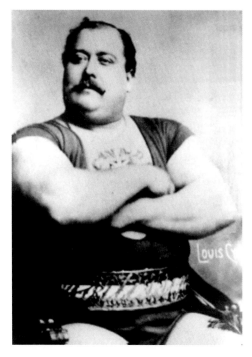

FIGURE 1.2. Louis Cyr.

an individual "muscle bound." *Louis Uni* (1862–1928), The Great Apollon, was a French circus strongman who performed amazing feats of strength (one-arm snatch with 80–90 kg, juggling with 20-kg weights) and was known to train with what today would be akin to thick bars. *Ludwig Durlacher* (1844–1924), also known as Professor Attila, was a German strongman with incredible core strength who had claimed to invent, adapt, or modify several pieces of training equipment including the Roman Chair. Perhaps his greatest attribute was his ability to train other strongmen. *George Hackenschmidt* (1877–1968), also known as The Russian Lion (Fig. 1.3), was a wrestling champion and strongman who later laid claim to inventing the Hack Squat. *Henry "Milo" Steinborn* (1894–1989) was a renowned wrestler and strongman who set the prototype for the modern-day Olympic-style barbell with revolving ends. *Sigmund Klein* (1902–1987), a strongman from Germany who immigrated to the United States, was known for amazing strength, an excellent physique, and for writing articles on weight training. *Thomas Inch* (1881–1963), known as "Britain's Strongest Youth," was most renowned for being the only man at that time capable of lifting a 3+-in-grip, 173-lb dumbbell overhead from the ground with one arm, which today is commonly known as the Thomas Inch Replica Dumbbell and is used by several strength competitors in training. Lastly, *Eugen Sandow* (1867–1925) (Fig. 1.4) was a German strongman who moved to England and performed incredible feats of strength. However, he was renowned for his fabulous physique and is immortalized on the trophy awarded to the winner of the Mr. Olympia bodybuilding contest each year.

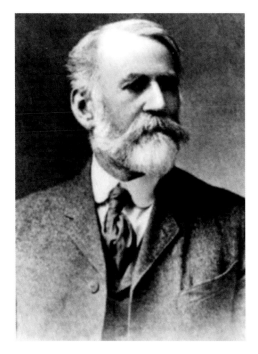

FIGURE 1.1. Dudley Sargent.

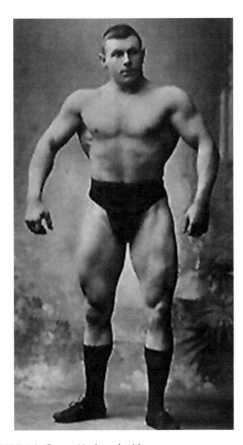

■ **FIGURE 1.3.** George Hackenschmidt.

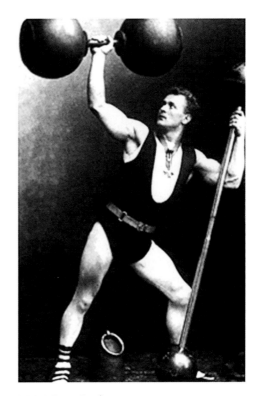

■ **FIGURE 1.4.** Eugen Sandow.

TWENTIETH-CENTURY ADVANCES

The early to mid-1900s were times marked by change. Myths and misconceptions associated with RT began to escalate, and despite the fact that strongmen were touring, a number of individuals known for their strength accomplishments became market driven. Although they had all attained their strength and size through weight training methods, they began to market other forms of RT equipment as alternatives that claimed to increase strength without becoming muscle bound. Although many individuals contributed to alternative forms of RT (cable devices, isometrics, etc.), the most popular was Angelo Siciliano. *Angelo Siciliano* (1892–1972), better known as Charles Atlas (Fig. 1.5), became known as the "world's most perfectly developed man who began as a 97-lb weakling." His landmark advertisements were well known where if one followed his course then he or she could transcend into a strong, well-developed individual.

Myths & Misconceptions

Resistance Training will Make One "Muscle Bound," Slower, and Reduce Performance

Throughout the history of S&C several myths and misconceptions developed and several remain in existence today despite scientific evidence pointing to the contrary. It remains a mystery why certain myths continue to perpetuate; however, it is clear that the S&C professionals need to do their best to dispel these myths whenever possible. One myth is the creation of the muscle-bound individual via RT. This muscle-bound phenomenon is thought to reduce movement mobility, speed, and performance. This myth dates back more than 100 years to the Strongman Era. The reality is that RT enhances virtually all components of fitness and increases athletic performance (1,2,13). An exception exists in that if one always trains with slow velocities and gains a large amount of mass, it is theoretically possible to become slower. However, specificity of RT tells us that moderate-to-fast lifting velocities can increase speed and performance. The majority of strength/power athletes currently resistance train and few have shown signs of slowing down. Thus, proper program design is critical to increasing speed and performance, and RT will enhance performance when performed properly.

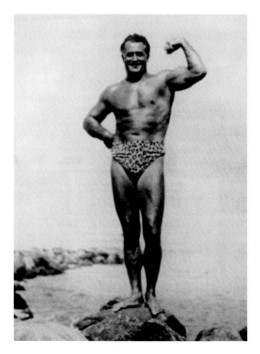

FIGURE 1.5. Charles Atlas.

His training philosophy was known as *Dynamic Tension* and consisted of 12 lessons of resistance exercises (body weight, isometrics) that could be performed anywhere for 15 minutes a day. Several million people have read his material to this day and/or incorporated some facet of his training advice, evidence of his marketing genius in the 1920s.

It was around this time when some early weight training magazines, books, and courses were published predominantly by well-known strongmen or lifting practitioners. In 1899, the first issue of the landmark magazine *Physical Culture* (which was a common term to describe the promotion of muscular growth, strength, and health through exercise at the turn of the century) was published by Bernarr McFadden. Around this time another magazine called *Health and Strength* was published by Hopton Hadley. In 1902 a magazine called *Strength Magazine* was published by Alan Calvert (which later became the popular *Strength and Health* magazine published by Bob Hoffman in the 1930s). The long-time running magazine *Iron Man* began circulation in 1936 by Peary and Mabel Rader. Several popular weight training books/courses were published at the time including *Sandow's System of Physical Training* (1894) and *Strength and How to Obtain It* (1897) by Eugen Sandow; *The Way to Live in Health and Physical Fitness* (1908) by George Hackenschmidt; *Milo Barbell Courses* (1902) by Alan Calvert; *The Development of Muscle Power* (1906) and *The Textbook of Weight-Lifting* (1910) by Arthur Saxon; *Muscle Building* (1924) and *Secrets of Strength* (1925) by Earle Liederman; *Muscle Building and Physical Culture* (1927) by George Jowett; *Physical* *Training Simplified — The Complete Science of Muscular Development* (1930) by Mark Berry; and *The Rader Master Bodybuilding and Weight Gaining System* (1946) by Peary Rader. Therefore, RT literature became popular during this time and continued to rise in popularity until present day.

COMPETITIVE LIFTING SPORTS

Competitive lifting sports began in the late 1800s with Olympic weightlifting rising to the forefront. The first weightlifting championship was held in 1891 and weightlifting first entered the Olympic Games in 1896. At first, the lifts contested were the one- and two-hand overhead lifts, with no weight classes. Weightlifting returned to the Olympic Games in 1904 after a brief hiatus. By 1920, the snatch, clean and press, and clean and jerk were the competitive lifts; eventually the clean and press was discontinued in 1972 due to difficulty in judging the lift. The sport of Olympic weightlifting (or just weightlifting) was largely popularized in the United States by legendary strength pioneer Bob Hoffman (Fig. 1.6). *Bob Hoffman (1898–1985)* was known as the "Father of American Weightlifting." He formed the world famous York Lifting Club (as Hoffman had purchased Milo Barbell Co. in 1935 and formed the York Barbell Company). Hoffman's accolades were enormous as he published magazines, wrote several books, manufactured nutrition supplements, and helped make the United States a weightlifting powerhouse through the mid-1950s. Although weightlifting was his passion, Hoffman showed some interest in other lifting sports and was instrumental in encouraging athletes to incorporate weight training in their conditioning programs. After the 1950s, other countries such

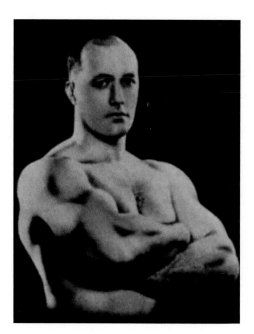

FIGURE 1.6. Bob Hoffman.

as the Soviet Union, Turkey, Greece, and China emerged in the sport of weightlifting. Some notable legendary weightlifters during this period include Tommy Kono, Vasily Alexeev, Imre Foldi, Norbert Schemansky, Ken Patera, Naim Suleymanoglu (Pocket Hercules; Fig. 1.7), Paul Anderson, and Andrei Chermerkin to name a few.

The next major lifting sport to develop from weight-lifting was bodybuilding. Although interest in physique training was seen throughout history, bodybuilding competition, as we know it, can be traced back to the early 1900s. The first organized competition dates back to Britain in 1901 and was facilitated by Eugen Sandow. In 1903, the first bodybuilding ("Physical Culture") competition was held in Madison Square Garden, NY. However, bodybuilding did not stand alone in competition. That is, athletes who competed in bodybuilding had to compete in weightlifting first. Bodybuilding grew in popularity during the 1930s and 1940s as some notable athletes brought some recognition by successfully competing in Mr. America competitions, *e.g.*, John Grimek, Clancy Ross, Steve Reeves, etc. However, the 1940s marked a historical time period due to a large extent of the work of Joe and Ben Weider. The Weiders sought more respect for bodybuilders and subsequently formed the International Federation of Body Builders (to rival the Amateur Athletic Union which dominated lifting sports). Joe Weider's (Fig. 1.8) status in bodybuilding was truly legendary and is a major reason why bodybuilding is so popular in the United States today. His accolades were enormous. He was well known for his feud with Bob Hoffman, books and publications (*Your Physique*, *Muscle Power*, later *Muscle and Fitness and Flex*), coining of training terms and principles, promotion of bodybuilding training and events (the Mr. and Ms. Olympia), and equipment and nutrition supplement manufacturing. Although *Muscle Beach*, Santa Monica, CA, was a popular sport, recreational,

and bodybuilding venue from 1934 to 1958, the mecca for bodybuilding later became Venice Beach, CA. Many notable and prominent bodybuilders were seen from the 1950s on but some very influential individuals included Joe Gold, Jack LaLanne, Reg Park, Bill Pearl, Larry Scott, Arnold Schwarzenegger, Lou Ferrigno, Franco Colombu, Lee Haney, Rachel McLish, Cori Everson, Dorian Yates, Lenda Murray, Ronnie Coleman, and Jay Cutler.

Powerlifting evolved during the late 1950s. It was initially referred to as the *odd lift* competition because it did not include the Olympic lifts but was composed of the squat, bench press, and deadlift exercises. Although critics of powerlifting claimed that it lacked image, the sport began to increase in popularity during the early 1960s. During its first ~15 years, more than 68 powerlifting records were set. The first US championships were held in 1964 in York, PA, the first world championships were held in 1971, the first US women's championship was held in 1978, and the first women's world championship was contested in 1980. In 1972, the International Powerlifting Federation was formed (with Bob Crist president and Bob Hoffman treasurer) and thereafter other organizations were formed. In the 1980s, the major magazine *Powerlifting USA* began publication and powerlifters became noted for using specialized apparel that substantially enhanced lifting performance, *e.g.*, bench press shirts, squat suits and briefs, and so on. Through the years, the United States has dominated international powerlifting competitions. Some notable powerlifters include Larry Pacifico, Vince Anello, Don Reinhoudt, Ed Coan, Dr. Fred Hatfield, Louie Simmons, Anthony Clark, Ted Arcidi, Tamara Grimwood-Rainwater, and Becca Swanson.

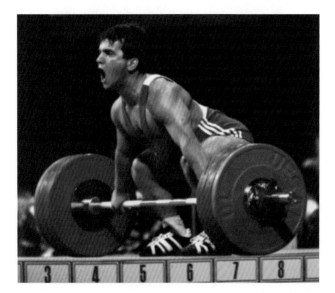

FIGURE 1.7. Naim Suleymanoglu.

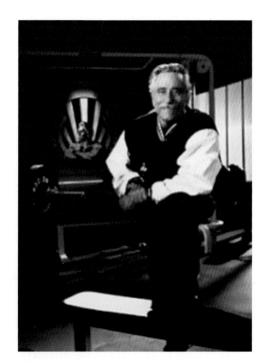

FIGURE 1.8. Joe Weider.

The last competitive lifting sport to develop was strength competitions. Strength competitions consisted of approximately six to eight events. Modern-day strength competitions began in 1977 with the World's Strongest Man competition. This annual competition is very popular and since then many other strength competitions have evolved. Strength competitions initially began with athletes of different backgrounds. For example, Olympic weightlifters, bodybuilders, NFL football players, arm wrestling champions, powerlifters, and professional wrestlers competed amongst each other. In modern-day competitions, hybrid athletes dominate the sport. That is, athletes with various backgrounds train specifically for these events. Some notable competitors included Bruce Wilhelm, Bill Kazmaier, Jon Pall Sigmarsson, Magnus ver Magnusson, Jouko Ahola, Magnus Samuelsson, Jill Mills, and Mariusz Pudzianowski. Interestingly, events and training practices of strength athletes have increased in popularity to where other groups of athletes have integrated these training modalities.

Weight training for other nonlifting sports was something that was originally not widely accepted because of myths and misconceptions associated with RT. Among the first sports to accept RT was track and field throwing in the 1950s. One prominent supporter of RT was four-time Olympic discus gold medal winner, *Al Oerter*. At this time, Bob Hoffman promoted weight training for athletes and encouraged some boxers to train, but very few other athletes followed. American football players helped pave the way in the 1960s and 1970s when the first full-time strength coaches were hired in the late 1960s. In the 1970s mostly strength and power athletes began RT. A key development in the field was the formation of the National Strength and Conditioning Association (NSCA) that began widespread recommendations of RT and was instrumental in dispelling myths and demonstrating benefits both practically and scientifically. From the 1980s on, most athletes and coaches have recommended RT to some extent for all sports.

STRENGTH AND CONDITIONING TODAY

Currently, RT is a modality of exercise recommended for virtually everyone because it has been shown to enhance health, well-being, and performance in clinical, fitness, and athletic populations (2,13). There has been a large increase in the scientific study of RT since the 1970s (as only small magnitudes of studies were conducted between the mid-1940s through the 1960s). Thus, we have seen a dramatic change not only in the perception of RT but also in the total magnitude of individuals who actively participate in RT. Contributing to the increased popularity of RT has been its adoption into general exercise programming by major health organizations including the American College of Sports Medicine (ACSM). In the ACSM's 1998 position stand, "The recommended quantity and quality of exercise for developing and maintaining cardiorespiratory and muscular fitness, and flexibility in healthy adults," the initial standard was set for a RT program with the performance of one set of 8–12 repetitions for 8–10 exercises, including one exercise for all major muscle groups; and 10–15 repetitions for older and more frail persons (1). This initial program has been shown to be effective in previously untrained individuals for improving muscular fitness during the first 3–4 months of training. The ACSM in 2002 (2) then extended these recommendations by targeting progression into intermediate and advanced forms of training with specialization for those who targeted muscle growth, strength, power, and endurance enhancement for essentially all healthy adults including the general health and fitness, athletic, and older adult populations. These guidelines were extended in the form of an evidence-based document in 2009. Thus, RT has come a long way to where it is now a scientifically proven and overwhelmingly recommended form of exercise for healthy adults.

Today S&C has grown tremendously. Nearly all athletes follow an S&C program off-season, preseason, and in-season. Because of the overwhelming evidence demonstrating the importance of S&C for optimal performance, the S&C coach position has increased greatly among all levels of competition from middle and high school to the professional levels. Although not all schools or programs have a true S&C coach on staff, most will at least have an assistant coach in charge of supervising S&C sessions. The increased popularity of S&C has given students an exceptional opportunity to major in an S&C-related field in college and enter a promising career where they have the opportunity to work with athletes of varying background.

WHY DO INDIVIDUALS RESISTANCE TRAIN?

The goals and benefits of RT are numerous, and individuals train for different reasons (2,13). The Sidebar (Goals Associated with Resistance Training) and Table 1.1 outline basic goals and benefits of RT. Many engage in RT for recreational purposes where the goals are to increase size, endurance, and strength somewhat but not to a great extent. Others engage in RT to enhance their muscular strength, power, endurance, or size. Some engage in RT for rehabilitation. **Rehabilitation** implies an injury or disease occurred which posed some physical limitation and now the individual trains to strengthen the weakened area. Many individuals engage in RT for **prehabilitation**, where the primary goal is injury prevention. Competitive strength, power, and endurance athletes engage in RT to enhance athletic performance, and some compete in lifting sports. In season, athletes engage in maintenance training. The goal of **maintenance training**

TABLE 1.1 BENEFITS OF RESISTANCE TRAINING

HEALTH BENEFITS	PERFORMANCE BENEFITS
↓ risk factors for disease	↑ muscle power
↓ percent body fat	↑ balance and coordination
↑ dynamic, isometric, and isokinetic muscle strength	↑ speed
↑ muscle hypertrophy	↑ capacity to perform activities of daily living
↑ muscular endurance	↑ vertical jump ability
↑ basal metabolic rate	↑ throwing velocity
↓ blood pressure	↑ kicking performance
↓ blood lipids, LDL cholesterol	↑ running economy
↓ resting heart rate	↑ baseball bat swinging velocity
↓ cardiovascular demand to exercise	↑ tennis serve velocity
↑ bone mineral density	↑ wrestling performance
↑ glucose tolerance and insulin sensitivity	↑ cycling power and performance
↓ age-related muscle atrophy (*Sarcopenia*)	
↓ risk of colon cancer and osteoporosis	
↑ Vo_{2max}	
↑ flexibility	
↓ risk/symptoms of low back pain	

is to maintain off-season training gains and adaptations as best as possible in season as the emphasis shifts to sport-specific conditioning, practice, and competitions/ games. This phase is temporary until the season is completed. However, nonathletes may engage in maintenance training as well depending on their circumstances. Many engage in RT to elicit positive health adaptations to the body, *e.g.*, connective tissue, muscle, nerve, respiratory, and cardiovascular systems. Lastly, one does not need to train specifically for one goal; rather, many resistance train with multiple goals in mind. This is referred to as **integrative training** where multiple goals are sought for training purposes.

SIDEBAR   **GOALS ASSOCIATED WITH RESISTANCE TRAINING**

- **General fitness and recreation**
- **Strength training**
- **Power training**
- **Muscular endurance training**
- **Muscle hypertrophy**
- **Rehabilitation and prehabilitation**
- **Competitive lifting sports (bodybuilding, strength athletics, powerlifting, weightlifting)**
- **Athletics**
- **Maintenance training**
- **Physiological adaptations**
- **Integration training**

BENEFITS OF RESISTANCE TRAINING

Health and performance benefits of RT are shown in Table 1.1 (13). Several studies have shown RT to improve multiple facets of health and performance. Collectively, these studies have been conducted in athletes, general fitness, clinical, or special populations, and children and have shown RT is safe and effective for most individuals. These ramifications are critical to optimal athletic performance, and to any individual striving to enhance performance of activities of daily living.

FITNESS COMPONENTS

HEALTH-RELATED FITNESS COMPONENTS

Strength and conditioning programs target multiple levels of fitness. Thus, fitness components may be classified in two ways: health-related and skill-related fitness components (6). **Health-related fitness components** are those that are designated as improving health, wellness, and one's quality of life. Improvements in these components can enhance physical performance. Health-related components include muscular strength, muscular endurance, cardiovascular endurance, flexibility, and body composition.

Muscular Strength

Muscular strength may be defined as the maximal amount of force one can generate during a specific movement pattern at a specified velocity of contraction (11). For a dynamic muscle action, it may be assessed in the weight room via a 1 RM lift for a given exercise; that is, the maximal amount of weight lifted in one all-out effort. In other cases, it may be estimated from submaximal strength performance. This ultimate magnitude of force development may be defined as *absolute muscular strength* as it represents the limit of physical capacity of an individual for a specific exercise. When maximal strength is expressed relative to body mass or lean body mass (the mass of nonfat tissue, *e.g.*, muscle, bone, water, etc.), it is defined as *relative muscular strength*. Relative muscular strength is

Myths & Misconceptions

Resistance Training is Important for Athletes but has Little Benefit for Nonathletes

Although RT is critical in the training of athletes, nonathletes can benefit greatly as well. Table 1.1 shows many health-enhancing adaptations including reduced blood pressure and blood lipids, increased glucose tolerance and insulin sensitivity, and reduced heart rate to name a few. These adaptations take place in addition to improved health- and skill-related components of fitness. Health improvements benefit all individuals and provide the basis for the ACSM's recommendation of inclusion of RT into a comprehensive exercise program for essentially all adults. Improvements in skill-related fitness components allow the individual to perform activities of daily living more efficiently. The balance and coordination improvements reduce risks of falling, which becomes a concern as one gets older. Thus, everyone benefits from RT and not just athletes.

critical for many athletes who compete in weight classes because the higher the ratio, the more advantageous it is for that athlete.

A high **strength-to-mass ratio** enables high levels of force production without the addition of substantial mass gains. Relative strength measures have been used to compare lifting performances among athletes of different sizes. For example, when weight classes are not used or when the best lifter in a competition among all weight classes is determined, the weight lifted may be divided by the individual's body mass (or lean body mass) to yield a ratio which can be used comparatively (known as *body mass scaling*). However, simply performing this calculation as is tends to strongly favor athletes of smaller mass. For example, a 165-lb lifter who bench pressed 285 lb would generate a factor value of ~1.73 (285/165). Another lifter weighing 245 lb would have to bench press at least 425 lb in order to beat the 165-lb lifter in direct competition. Attempts have been made to correct for this, *e.g.*, by raising the mass to the two-thirds power using *allometric scaling* or by using height as a scaling factor, but still certain somatotypes may gain advantage. Allometric scaling is theoretically based on the two-thirds law where geometric similarity is sought (19). Geometric similarity suggests that strength measures (two-dimensional) and mass (three-dimensional) conform to the relationship: strength $\times$ (mass$^{2/3}$)$^{-1}$ (19). Although allometric scaling may be more practical than body mass scaling, it still has deficiencies favoring middle-sized athletes (19).

In lifting competitions, the Wilks and Sinclair formulas have been used. The *Wilks formula* (developed by Robert Wilks) used mostly in powerlifting is complex, but typically a conversion table (for men and women) is used based on body mass to obtain a conversion factor that is multiplied by the weight lifted to correct for size differences. For example, an athlete with a body mass of 80.5 kg would generate a factor of 0.68 and an athlete with a body mass of 124 kg would generate a factor of 0.57. If the first athlete lifted 200 kg (0.68 × 200 kg = 136 kg) in competition and the second athlete lifted

230 kg (0.57 × 230 kg = 131 kg), the first athlete would place higher. The *Sinclair formula* (18) is a polynomial equation where the coefficients are updated every 4 years (to account for world record totals in each weight class) and primarily used in international weightlifting competitions. The following coefficients will be used through 2012. If the athlete's body mass is greater than 173.96 kg (men) or 125.44 kg (women) than the Sinclair coefficient = 1. For all other athletes the Sinclair coefficient is calculated via the following equation: Sinclair coefficient = 10^{AX2} where $X = \log_{10}(x \cdot b^{-1})$ as x = athlete's body mass and b = 173.96 kg (men) or 125.44 kg (women), A = 0.784780654 (men) or 1.056683941 (women). The coefficient is then multiplied by the athlete's weightlifting total to calculate the Sinclair total. For example, a male athlete with a body mass of 62 kg would generate a Sinclair coefficient of ~1.44. If his total was 280 kg, then his Sinclair total = 403.2 kg (280 kg × 1.44).

Muscular strength is certainly multidimensional and depends on several factors discussed later in this book, *e.g.*, muscle action (concentric, eccentric, isometric), contraction velocity, muscle group and length, joint angle, and other physiological and biomechanical factors concerning the muscular, nervous, metabolic, endocrine, and skeletal systems. The ability to develop muscular strength is critical to health and performance especially as one grows older.

Case Study 1.2

A high strength-to-mass ratio is beneficial for athletes.

Questions for Consideration: **What types of athletes benefit the most from having a high strength-to-mass ratio? Why might this be the case?**

Muscular Endurance

Muscular endurance is the ability to sustain performance and resist fatigue. The intensity of muscle contraction plays a role. *Submaximal muscular endurance* is characterized by the ability to sustain low-intensity muscular contractions for an extended period of time. *High-intensity (or strength) endurance* is the ability to maintain high-intensity muscular contractions over time. For example, it entails the ability to run repeated sprints with similar times or perform a specific number of repetitions for a resistance exercise over a number of sets despite a rest interval in between sets. Another common term used is *local muscular endurance*. Local muscular endurance is still defined by the ability to sustain exercise; however, the term *local* now specifically refers to the muscle groups involved in that exercise. Overall, having good muscular endurance is important for good posture, health, and injury prevention and aids in optimizing sports performance.

Cardiovascular Endurance

Cardiovascular endurance is the ability to perform prolonged aerobic exercise at moderate to high exercise intensities. Cardiovascular endurance is highly related to functioning of the lungs, heart, and circulatory system and the capacity of skeletal muscle to extract oxygen and thereby sustain performance. The key measure of cardiovascular endurance or aerobic capacity is maximal oxygen uptake or Vo_{2max}. A moderately high to high Vo_{2max} is a critical component for success in endurance athletes, and possessing a good aerobic base (>44 and 37 mL $\cdot$ kg^{-1} $\cdot$ min^{-1} for men and women, respectively, younger than 39 years of age) can enhance recovery from anaerobic exercise as well. Cardiovascular endurance is essential to good health and reducing risk factors for disease, as well as improving self-image, cognitive functioning, and stress management.

Flexibility

Flexibility is the ability of a joint to move freely its ROM. Enhanced joint flexibility can reduce injury risk, improve muscle balance and function, increase performance, improve posture, and reduce the incidence of low back pain. The best ways to increase flexibility is to perform exercises in a full ROM and engage in a proper stretching program, preferably at the end of a workout when the muscles are thoroughly warmed up.

Body Composition

Body composition refers to the proportion of fat and fat-free mass throughout the body. Fat-free mass (or **lean body mass**) is that component consisting of bone, muscle, water, and other nonfat tissues. Healthy body composition involves minimizing the fat component while maintaining or increasing the lean body mass component. An individual with an excessive amount of body fat may be considered obese and is at greater risk for disease and other debilitating conditions. The

most effective way to enhance body composition is to eat properly (low saturated fat intake, low simple sugar consumption, moderate protein intake, and appropriate kilocalorie intake) and exercise regularly. Strength training, as well as other forms of anaerobic training, is effective for enhancing body composition as it increases lean body mass (muscle and bone components) while reducing fat. A common term used to describe tissue growth is **hypertrophy**, especially with respect to muscle growth where the term *muscle hypertrophy* is commonly used. Aerobic training plays a large role in reducing fat mass and plays a lesser role in enhancing lean tissue mass. Body composition plays a key role in those sports where weight classes are used (wrestling, weightlifting), where athletes have to overcome their own body mass for success (high jump, gymnastics, endurance sports), or where athletic competition is based on physique development (bodybuilding).

SKILL-RELATED COMPONENTS OF FITNESS

Skill-related components of fitness include power, speed, agility, balance and coordination, and reaction time. These components are essential to athletic performance and the ability to perform activities of daily living. Skill-related components may be developed in a variety of ways including RT, sprint/interval training, agility training and plyometrics, and through sport-specific practice.

Power

Power is the rate of performing work. Because power is the product of force and velocity, there is a strength component to power development (strength at low-to-high velocities of contraction). The optimal expression of muscle power is reliant upon correct exercise technique. Although at times the terms *power* and *strength* are used interchangeably, this is not correct. Power has a time component; thus, if two athletes have similar maximal strength, the one who expresses strength at a higher rate (higher velocity or shorter period of time) will have a distinct advantage during performance of anaerobic sports. In addition, power has been described in terms of strength. For example, terms such as *speed strength* and *acceleration strength* have been used to define force development across a spectrum of velocities. *Starting strength* is a term used to describe power production during the initial segment of movement. **Rate of force development** (a term used primarily in scientific publications) describes power output during an explosive exercise task, *e.g.*, assessed by the time needed to reach a threshold level of force or the amount of force produced per second. The velocity component of the power equation indicates that high contraction velocities (or at least the intent to contract at maximal velocities even against a heavy resistance) of muscle contraction are imperative. Therefore, power development is multidimensional, involving enhancement of both force and velocity components. Muscle power may be enhanced via RT, speed, agility, and plyometric training, and through sport-specific practice/conditioning.

Speed

Speed is the capacity of an individual to perform a motor skill as rapidly as possible. Speed is an integral component of sport. For example, linear running speed may be defined by its three distinct phases: (a) acceleration, (b) maximum speed, and (c) deceleration. The *acceleration* phase is characterized by an increase in speed, and is reliant upon strength, power, and reaction time. The *maximum speed* phase is characterized by the individual's attainment of his or her fastest speed and how long he or she can maintain it, *e.g.*, speed endurance. The *deceleration* phase is a result of fatigue and is characterized by the individual involuntarily decreasing speed after maximum speed has been attained. Speed may be enhanced by a combination of methods including nonassisted and assisted sprint training, strength and power training, plyometrics, technique training, and sport-specific practice.

Agility

Agility is the ability of an individual to change direction rapidly without a significant loss of speed, balance, or bodily control. Being agile requires a great deal of power, strength, balance, coordination, quickness, speed, anticipation, and neuromuscular control. Agility is a critical component to any sport that requires rapid changes of direction, decelerations, and accelerations. Agility training is comprised of predetermined drills (*closed drills*) and drills that force the athlete to anticipate, adjust, and react explosively (*open drills*). Likewise, agility can be enhanced by plyometrics, multidirectional agility and reactive drills, strength and power training, balance training, and sport-specific practice.

Balance and Coordination

Balance is the ability of an individual to maintain equilibrium. It requires control over the athlete's center of gravity and allows him or her to maintain proper body position during complex motor skill performance. Balance can be enhanced by strength and power training, plyometrics, sprint and agility training, specific balance training (with unstable equipment), and through sport-specific practice.

Gross motor coordination refers to the ability of an individual to perform a motor skill with good technique, rhythm, and accuracy. Critical elements to coordination include balance, spatial awareness, timing, and motor learning. Likewise, coordination can be improved by similar training methods. Sport-specific practice is very important as repetitive exposure to different motor patterns is essential to improving motor coordination.

Reaction Time

Reaction time is the ability to respond rapidly to a stimulus. Reaction time is critical to sports performance. The quicker an athlete reacts to a stimulus, the more likely success will be obtained. Some athletic skills require less than half-second response times, *i.e.*, hitting a 90+-mph fastball in baseball. The ability to react quickly is paramount and can be used to separate athletes of different caliber. Reaction time may be improved by explosive exercise (power, sprint, agility, quickness training) and sport-specific practice.

KEYS TO SUCCESS: THE RESISTANCE TRAINING PROGRAM

The key ingredient to RT responses and subsequent training adaptations is the program (2). A RT program is a composite of several variables that may be manipulated in different ways to achieve a desired effect. Although specific recommendations and guidelines for program design will be discussed in subsequent chapters, it is important to define these variables with other terminology. These variables include

- **Muscle Action:** refers to the type of muscular contraction. An *eccentric* (ECC) muscle action involves muscle lengthening, and is sometimes described as a negative component of each repetition. ECC muscle actions produce higher levels of force, are very conducive to muscle growth, and make an athlete more susceptible to muscle damage and soreness. A *concentric* (CON) muscle action involves muscle shortening and is sometimes described as a positive component of each repetition. An *isometric* (ISOM) muscle action involves force development with no noticeable change in joint angle or muscle length. In comparison, greatest muscle force is produced during ECC muscle actions, followed by ISOM and CON. CON and ECC muscle actions are considered to be *dynamic* muscle actions because force production throughout the ROM is variable. However, some authors prefer to use the term *isotonic*. Isotonic implies that equal tension is produced throughout the ROM. Although the weight lifted is constant throughout the ROM, the amount of force (or torque) developed is not. Therefore, *dynamic muscle action* (sometimes called **dynamic constant external resistance**) is a more appropriate and accurate term. The term **isoinertial** has been used because it assumes the mass lifted is constant.
- **Repetition:** a complete movement cycle including an ECC and CON muscle action, *e.g.*, lifting the weight up and down. May also refer to a single ISOM contraction.

- **Set:** a specified group or number of repetitions, *i.e.*, three sets of 10 repetitions.
- **Volume:** the total amount of work performed during a workout. Represented by the total number of sets, resistance, and repetitions performed.
- **Intensity:** describes the magnitude of loading (or weight lifted) during resistance exercise, *e.g.*, 90% of 1RM is high intensity. Some have defined intensity as representing the magnitude of difficulty associated with training. The latter is more representative of *perceived exertion*, and thus the most widely accepted definition of intensity relates to loading.
- **Frequency:** a term used to describe the number of training sessions per week or day. It also has been used to describe the number of times per week a muscle, muscle group, or specific exercise is performed.
- **Exercise Selection:** the exercises selected or chosen to be performed during a workout or throughout a training program.
- **Exercise Order:** the sequence in which exercises are performed.
- **Rest Periods or Intervals:** the amount of rest taken between sets and exercises. This term may also be used to define the amount of rest taken in between reps within a set.
- **Repetition Velocity:** the velocity at which reps are performed.

COMPETITIVE FORMS OF RESISTANCE TRAINING

Many individuals engage in RT for competitive purposes. RT competitions have been popular since the late 1800s. Currently, there are numerous local, state, national, and international competitions, as well as federations, in which an athlete can participate. The competitive RT sports include bodybuilding, weightlifting, powerlifting, and strength competitions. As one might expect, the level of dedication, motivation, and training is much higher as one embarks on a competitive career.

BODYBUILDING

Bodybuilding is a competitive sport in which athletes compete on stage in a physique contest where they are judged subjectively by a panel of judges who assign points based on their aesthetic appearance. Although weights are not lifted during a bodybuilding competition, RT is an essential component of training for bodybuilding competition. Following a precompetition training period accompanied by strict dieting, bodybuilders will attempt to maximize muscle size and minimize body fat and dehydrate to maximize their appearance. Critical to bodybuilding is the presentation of the physique. Following a period of performing compulsory poses (most muscular, front double biceps, lat spread, etc.), or prejudging, bodybuilders

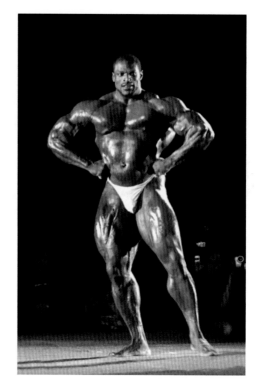

■ **FIGURE 1.9.** A bodybuilder.

pose on stage to music in a choreographed posing routine. They are judged on presentation as well as their physiques. Bodybuilding training is aimed at maximizing muscular hypertrophy, symmetry, shape, and definition while maintaining low levels of body fat. Muscular strength may be a goal but is secondary to hypertrophy. Several bodybuilders (Fig. 1.9) use RT to enhance muscle size; thus, strength gains may be considered a by-product and not the primary goal. However, some bodybuilders include strength training to enhance their muscle growth. This has been helpful for those bodybuilders in attaining large amounts of muscle hypertrophy due to heavier loading required for strength training. Bodybuilding workouts typically consist of multiple exercises per muscle group for moderate to heavy loads for rep ranges from few to many with little rest between sets. These workouts are aimed at maximizing muscular development in all facets, hence a wide spectrum of intensity, volume, exercises, and techniques are used. Off-season training focuses on improving size and strength whereas precompetition is devoted to size maintenance while reducing body fat, weight, and water. Several individuals include bodybuilding training for competition purposes; however, others use it to enhance appearance, performance, and health in a noncompetitive manner.

WEIGHTLIFTING

Weightlifting (Fig. 1.10) was actually the first true competitive lifting sport to develop historically (3). It is

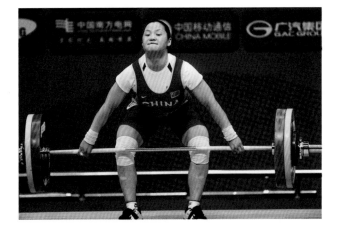

■ **FIGURE 1.10.** A weightlifter.

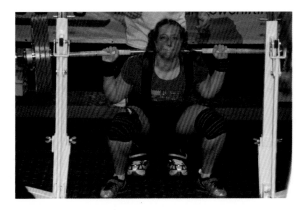

■ **FIGURE 1.11.** A powerlifter.

the only lifting sport that is included in the Olympics. Unlike bodybuilding, weightlifting is a performance sport where athletes place based on how much weight they lift relative to their weight class (there are seven weight classes for women and eight for men). The sport of weightlifting involves two competitive lifts, the *snatch* and *clean and jerk* (although others have been used throughout its >115-year history). The snatch, clean and jerk, and their variations (referred to as the *Olympic lifts*) are the most technically demanding and complex resistance exercises in existence. Thus, good coaching is mandatory. Weightlifters normally begin competitive training at an early age. Hence, the initial phases of training are dedicated to learning proper form and technique whereas subsequent years are dedicated to improving lift performance, strength, and power. Performance of these competition lifts requires total body coordination, power, and speed. Therefore, weightlifters are extremely well-conditioned athletes. Records for the snatch and clean and jerk are ~476 and 586 lb, respectively. Because the Olympic lifts require high degree of balance, coordination, strength, power, and speed, these exercises form the foundation of RT for anaerobic strength and power athletes. Much of the training programs of weightlifters will be developed around these two lifts, and will include variations of these (hang clean, drop snatch), basic strength exercises (squat, deadlift), and assistance exercises (lunge, Romanian deadlift). Weightlifting programs normally consist of high load, low reps with long rest periods between sets. The quality of each repetition is critical as explosive lifting speeds are used. As with strength/power programs, periodized training cycles to peak performance for each competition are used. USA Weightlifting, a very prominent weightlifting organization and governing body of Olympic weightlifting in the United States, offers various coaching certifications including the club, regional, sports performance, and senior coach certifications, as well as the publication *Weightlifting USA.*

POWERLIFTING

Powerlifting (Fig. 1.11) is a competitive lifting sport involving maximal performance of three competition lifts: *squat, bench press,* and *deadlift.* In addition, other types of competitions have evolved based on inclusion of only a few of these lifts (bench press competitions), or in some cases other exercises have been included (strict barbell curl). Placing is based on maximum lifting performance over three trials for each exercise. Judges play a critical role to standardize a technique, *e.g.,* assure parallel position attained in squat, sufficient pause length used in the bench press, rhythmic ascent of the bar during the deadlift (no "hitching"), and will either allow or discard the trial. Like weightlifters, powerlifters compete in weight classes; thus, a high strength-to-mass ratio is desirable, especially for light to middle weights. Records for the bench press and deadlift now exceed 1,000 lb and the squat 1,200 lb. Powerlifting performance has been greatly enhanced by the use of specialized equipment such as bench press shirts, squat suits, erector shirts, and wraps; thus, lifting records in supportive apparel may exceed "raw" records (those without specialized apparel) by more than 200–300 lb. Multiple federations exist and each has slightly different rules regarding gear. The major publication that covers an array of subjects from competitions to training and nutrition advice is *Powerlifting USA* (since 1977). Powerlifting training encompasses focusing on the structural lifts plus additional assistance exercises for low to moderate repetition number with gradual periodized increase in intensity as the competition approaches.

STRENGTH COMPETITIONS

Modern-day strength competitions consist of six to eight events in which an athlete will score a specific amount of points based on how the athlete performs (or what place the athlete attains) (22). After all events have been completed, the leading scorer will win the competition. The events epitomize maximal dynamic and ISOM strength,

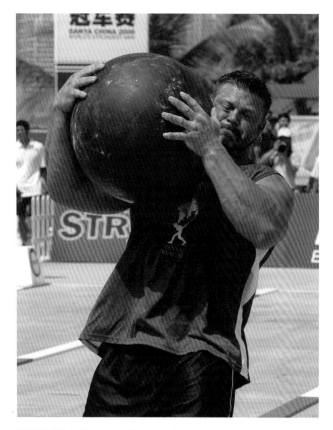

■ **FIGURE 1.12.** A strength competitor.

grip strength and endurance, power, strength endurance, and perhaps a high degree of pain tolerance and determination (Fig. 1.12). Some events commonly contested include the farmer's walk (180–375 lb per arm), tire flipping (450–900 lb), various loading (220–360 lb objects) medleys, barrel loading, various deadlifts (*e.g.*, silver dollar, car), car walk (~800 lb), duck walk (400 lb), log press (185–305 lb) or other overhead lifting, crucifix (isometric holding), Hercules hold, stone circle or Conan's wheel, keg toss, truck/plane pulling, stone lifting (Atlas/McGlashen stones, 220–365 lb or more) and carries (*e.g.*, Husafell stone ~385 lb), incline press for reps, various squatting or backlifts, yoke walk (~904 lb), caber toss, carry and drag (anchor, weights), Fingal's fingers, bar bending, power stairs (with 400–600 lb objects), Thomas Inch dumbbell lift, refrigerator carry, and tug-of-war. Training for strength competitions is very rigorous and multidimensional as multiple components of fitness need to be maximized to perform well across all of the events. Various federations have been formed over the years, with the *World's Strongest Man or Woman* still the epitome of international strength athletics competition.

COMPETITIVE LIFTING MODES AND PERFORMANCE

When comparing the different competitive lifting modes, a high degree of training specificity is observed. For example, best power clean and snatch performances (and their subsequent variations) are observed in Olympic weightlifters by far. Weightlifters produce very high power outputs during Olympic lifting (8). This is a major reason why weightlifting exercises are included in training programs of strength/power athletes. Upon examination of maximal strength during the multiple-joint competitive lifts of the squat, bench press, and deadlift, powerlifters hold the majority of competitive records. However, Olympic weightlifters score very well on the squat and deadlift as they train maximally for these to some extent. In one study, McBride et al. (14) showed similar maximal squat performance among Olympic weightlifters and powerlifters of similar size. However, weightlifters produced more force, velocity, power, and greater heights during the vertical jump and jump squat assessments, thereby showing superiority of weightlifting training for enhancing jumping performance. Powerlifting performance is enhanced to a substantial degree by training accessories (suits, belts, wraps) many Olympic weightlifters do not use. Thus, raw performance of these lifts may be similar when athletes are matched for size. Many times weightlifters do not emphasize the bench press for fear it may limit shoulder ROM for the snatch and power clean. Thus, powerlifters and some bodybuilders may score better on this exercise. Some bodybuilders who also prioritize strength training ("power bodybuilders") score well on these three lifts, better than those bodybuilders who view strength gains as merely a by-product of bodybuilding training. Interestingly, an early study from Sale and MacDougall (16) showed that powerlifters and bodybuilders possessed similar maximal isokinetic strength for most single-joint exercises tested. Bodybuilders may score well on other single-joint exercises as some powerlifters either do not routinely perform them or do not emphasize them. Because of their training principles, bodybuilders tend to score very well on strength-endurance type of events or display a much lower fatigue rate than powerlifters during various lifting tasks with short rest intervals (12).

THE STRENGTH AND CONDITIONING PROFESSION

The S&C professional position has evolved to be one of the most critical coaching positions. The fundamental responsibility of the S&C professional is to design, implement, and supervise sports conditioning programs. Strength and conditioning professionals may work in various settings including middle or high schools, colleges or universities, professional sports teams, health and fitness facilities, and sports complexes, and can run or assist with S&C camps, workshops, and clinics. In addition, personal trainers have filled a role in the S&C field as many upper-level and elite athletes have hired personal trainers for one-on-one specialized training. The roles and responsibilities of the S&C coach have increased over the years owing to the importance of improving conditioning to optimize performance and reduce the risk of injury. Thus, complete preparation is paramount for a student planning on becoming a competent professional in the S&C field. Critical concepts such as education, proficiencies required for the field, the importance of holding professional memberships and certifications, and knowledge gained through practical experience are discussed next. In addition, the duties and responsibilities of the S&C coach are outlined.

EDUCATION AND PROFICIENCIES

Education in the S&C field is gained via three major ways: (a) scholarly study, (b) personal experience, and (c) professional practice. *Scholarly study* entails content knowledge gained through taking college courses; reading scholarly books, journals, and articles; personal research; self-study; viewing videos; and attending conferences, workshops, and seminars (which are also excellent avenues for networking within the field). The S&C professional should at least have a B.S. or B.A. degree in an exercise-related field, *e.g.*, Exercise Physiology or Science, Kinesiology, Physical Education, Athletic Training, and Health and Human Performance. Some colleges and universities now offer a major in S&C. Students take several courses in Biology, Physiology, Chemistry, Health, Mathematics and Statistics, Nutrition, and Exercise Science and Training/Testing that are vital in acquiring the underlying knowledge needed in the field. Most S&C jobs require at least a B.S. or B.A. degree. Some higher-level jobs may require a master's degree in an exercise-related field. A master's degree offers more in-depth knowledge in human physiology, greater specialization in coursework, *e.g.*, Biomechanics, Exercise Science, and other fields, and introduces students to research (for those students who had limited undergraduate research experiences). Another advantage of graduate training is that the student may serve as a graduate assistant or volunteer in the S&C program. This can lead to full-time employment at that facility or is valuable experience for obtaining a position elsewhere upon graduation. Some S&C positions can be difficult to attain, so serving as an assistant (or intern and volunteer) initially can be an excellent means of gaining entry into the field, especially if the student works with an established S&C coach. A competent S&C professional should have an extensive library of scholarly material, which is constantly updated with new texts and articles to keep abreast of current information. Doctoral training is not usually necessary unless an academic position is sought.

Personal experience is the education gained by playing sports, training, and observations of other athletes and coaches training/instructing. The S&C coach should have an extensive background in exercise (RT, speed and agility, plyometric, flexibility, and aerobic training). One must "practice what they preach" in the S&C field. It is very difficult to instruct athletes on proper technique if one has limited or no experience with the exercise or drill. Thus, competent S&C professionals exercise regularly and should have an extensive background performing all of the modalities they will be instructing.

Professional practice refers to the knowledge gained once the individual attains the position and is working in the S&C field. Education gained in the field is unique and in many instances is not directly learned from taking courses or reading textbooks. For example, this is the knowledge gained through interacting with athletes, staff, coaches, parents, and administrators, hands-on experience in training and testing, and the experiences of supervising or working in a facility (equipment maintenance, accidents, facility issues, staff issues, organization and planning, etc.). Professional practice experience (along with success) is critical and may be viewed by many as the key component to resume development.

Proficiency is defined as advancement in knowledge, skill, or expertise in a particular area of interest. Strength and conditioning professionals must be proficient in several areas. That is, they must have at least a rudimentary

SIDEBAR	STRENGTH AND CONDITIONING PROFESSIONAL PROFICIENCIES
Anatomy and physiology	Weight training
Kinesiology	Plyometric training
Sports endocrinology	Aerobic endurance
Bioenergetics and metabolism	training
Neuromuscular physiology	Speed and agility training
Connective tissue physiology	Balance and functional training
Biomechanics and motor learning	Power and ballistic training
Cardiorespiratory physiology	Strength training
Environmental physiology	Flexibility training and warm-ups
Immune function	Muscle endurance and hypertrophy training
Sport psychology	Implement training
Sports nutrition	Sport-specific demands and conditioning
Supplements and ergogenic aids	Advanced program design
Overtraining and detraining	Exercise technique and spotting
Periodization	Performance assessment
Recovery	Injury prevention

(Continued)

Weight loss/body fat reduction	Facility design and management
CPR administration and first aid	Equipment use and maintenance
Special populations (children, older adults, clinical)	Organization and administration
	Risk management and liability

knowledge base in pertinent areas of S&C. The Sidebar (Strength and Conditioning Professional Proficiencies) depicts several proficiencies desired by a competent S&C professional.

In addition, S&C professionals must possess other skills that transcend directly into successful coaching or training. For example, the S&C professional should have excellent organizational and time management skills to handle the rigors of training a large number of athletes at various times of day, keeping training logs of all athletes, designing workout schedules around athletic competitions and practices, and perhaps supervising a staff of employees, graduate assistants, and interns. He or she should have the ability to motivate athletes to train hard and correctly follow procedures. The S&C coach should have good interpersonal, communication, and teaching skills that are mandatory for quality instruction. In addition, the S&C coach should always be well prepared, cautious, and hands-on when instructing. Because the S&C coach works within a team of professionals catering to athletes, e.g., athletic trainers, physical therapists, nutritionists, doctors, head and assistant coaches, etc., he or she must constantly communicate with staff on the athlete's health and performance status. Leadership is a critical component as the S&C coach must set the example for athletes to follow. Lastly, the S&C coach should be dedicated and willing to work long hours.

MEMBERSHIPS AND CERTIFICATIONS

Holding memberships in professional organizations is an important component of professionalism. Membership has many benefits, including access to educational resources, dissemination of current knowledge, networking, career resources and job advertisements, conferences and seminars, certification information, scholarships and grants, merchandise, and in some cases liability insurance. There are several organizations that serve the S&C profession in numerous ways. Many of these serve the Exercise Science or related fields (Athletic Training, Physical Therapy, Sports Medicine, Nutrition, and Personal Training) in general. However, some of the most popular and influential organizations targeting the S&C profession include the NSCA, ACSM, Collegiate Strength

and Conditioning Coaches Association (CSCCa), USA Weightlifting, and the International Sport Sciences Association (ISSA).

Unlike some other professional occupations, e.g., physical therapy, S&C does not require licensure. However, obtaining credible certifications increases the education and marketability of the S&C professional. Strength and conditioning professionals either obtain a specific S&C certification or become certified in a related field, e.g., personal trainer, health and fitness instructor, and/or exercise specialist. The NSCA offers two major certifications, the Certified Strength and Conditioning Specialist (CSCS) and Certified Personal Trainer (NSCA-CPT). The CSCS certification is most popular and widely regarded as the "gold standard" of S&C certifications. It requires at least an undergraduate degree (or a college senior in good standing) and current CPR certification. The ACSM offers several clinical and specialty certifications. Some common certifications for the S&C professional may be the ACSM Certified Personal Trainer (CPT) and ACSM Certified Health Fitness Specialist (HFS). USA Weightlifting offers the Level 1 Sports Performance Coach Certification, which is excellent for coaching the Olympic lifts and variations. This certification has a large practical component. Other organizations offer certifications as well. Once certified, practitioners must maintain certification by generating continuing education units (CEUs). Each certification and organization is specific regarding the number of CEUs needed in a given time span. CEUs can be attained in various ways, but self-study, attending conferences, publishing articles, awards and achievements, experience, and taking courses are just a few ways to earn CEUs. These ensure that the S&C professional is continuing to educate herself or himself and keep current with up-to-date information. Strength and conditioning professionals should obtain at least one major certification upon entering the field. More information regarding certification can be obtained by visiting the following organization Web sites:

- ACSM: www.acsm.org
- NSCA: www.nsca-lift.org
- USA Weightlifting: http://weightlifting.teamusa.org/
- ISSA: www.issaonline.com

DUTIES, ROLES, AND RESPONSIBILITIES

The S&C professional will have numerous duties and responsibilities depending on if the individual is the S&C director or head strength coach, an assistant S&C coach, or facility staff employee (4). The Sidebar (Potential Duties of a Strength and Conditioning Professional) depicts several potential duties and responsibilities of the S&C professional. As defined by the NSCA, "certified strength and conditioning specialists are professionals who practically apply foundational knowledge to assess, motivate, educate, and train athletes for the primary goal of improving sport performance. They conduct sport-specific testing sessions, design and implement safe and effective S&C programs, and provide guidance for athletes in nutrition and injury prevention" (15).

SIDEBAR	POTENTIAL DUTIES OF A STRENGTH AND CONDITIONING PROFESSIONAL

- Design and implement all S&C training programs: this includes developing yearly training plans— programs designed to increase strength, power, endurance, aerobic capacity, flexibility, balance and coordination, speed, agility, hypertrophy, and reduce body fat
- Supervise athletes during training hours: the coaches' office/desk should be in clear view of the entire facility
- Monitor athlete's technique and correct errors
- Assist in spotting athletes during RT when necessary
- Supervise and schedule all performance testing
- Ensure all safety procedures are being used
- Oversee purchase and maintenance of equipment and possibly design of a facility
- Budget allocation
- Facility uptake (cleaning), inspection, and maintenance
- Data collection: storage and examination of all training logs, evaluations, equipment manuals, and health history documents
- When applicable, travel with sport teams and supervise pregame warm-ups
- Instruct and educate athletes on injury prevention, proper nutrition, recovery practices, and use of supplements and banned substances
- Design and enforce facility rules and regulations and have them posted in plain view of athletes
- Staff training, development, and creation of job listings/criteria for new staff hires
- Delegate duties to other staff including assistant coaches, graduate assistants, interns, and volunteers
- Risk management and minimize potential litigation

- Oversee staff meetings and develop staff working schedules
- Control the training environment including music type and volume
- Design athlete's training schedules: organize different groups of athletes into scheduled time slots
- Motivate athletes to train maximally
- Prepare training sheets and other documents to be used in the facility including sign-in sheets, health history forms, and rules and regulations
- Post or distribute educational information that can benefit athletes and perhaps post a motivational "leader board" depicting athlete's weight room accomplishments
- Communicate with other coaches, athletic trainers, physical therapists, doctors, nutritionists, and staff regarding the status of athletes
- Maintain certification CEUs and keep abreast with the latest research and information
- Develop and post emergency procedures and place them (along with pertinent phone numbers and locations) in plain view
- Ensure staff has CPR and first aid certification
- Attend professional conferences and meetings

Summary Points

✔ Strength training is an essential component to improving health and maximizing performance. Virtually all health- and skill-related components of fitness are enhanced when specifically targeted through proper program design.

✔ Scoring highly on various measures of physical fitness can separate athletes of different caliber.

✔ Examination of the history of S&C is important for the practitioner as it magnifies the accomplishments of many pioneering individuals in the field and perhaps may provide insight into future S&C trends.

✔ The key ingredient to RT responses and subsequent training adaptations is proper design of the training program.

✔ Competitive forms of RT include weightlifting, bodybuilding, powerlifting, and strength competitions.

✔ Education in S&C is gained through scholarly study, personal experience, and professional practice.

Review Questions

1. The maximal amount of force one can generate during a specific movement pattern at a specified velocity of contraction is:
   a. Muscle endurance
   b. Muscle power
   c. Muscle strength
   d. Body composition

2. A competitive sport where lifters place based on the amount of weight they lift in the snatch and clean and jerk is:
   a. Bodybuilding
   b. Weightlifting
   c. Powerlifting
   d. Strength competitions

3. A Greek strongman whose training program was ascribed as being the first known example of using progressive overload was:
   a. Milo of Crotona
   b. Galen
   c. Michel de Montaigne
   d. Dudley Sargent

4. The Dynamic Tension philosophy and training course was developed by which legendary strongman?
   a. Louis Cyr
   b. Thomas Inch
   c. Eugen Sandow
   d. Charles Atlas

5. The individual most responsible for increasing the popularity of bodybuilding in the United States from the 1940s to present day is:
   a. Joe Weider
   b. Bob Hoffman
   c. Bernarr McFadden
   d. Hopton Hadley

6. The ability of an athlete to change direction rapidly without a significant loss of speed, balance, or bodily control is:
   a. Speed
   b. Power
   c. Agility
   d. Balance

7. RT can:
   a. Increase bone mineral density
   b. Increase basal metabolic rate
   c. Decrease percent body fat
   d. All of the above

8. The first lifting sport to develop in the late 1800s was bodybuilding. T F

9. During early times a relationship existed between the medical/scientific communities and fascination with muscular strength and development. T F

10. The "health lift" (partial deadlift) was an exercise first promoted by George Barker Windship. T F

11. The first weight training magazine published was *Iron Man* in the 1930s. T F

12. The *Father of American Weightlifting* was Bob Hoffman. T F

13. Certification is a critical component to becoming a competent strength and conditioning professional. T F

References

1. American College of Sports Medicine. Position Stand: the recommended quantity and quality. of exercise for developing and maintaining cardiorespiratory and muscular fitness, and flexibility in healthy adults. *Med Sci Sports Exerc.* 1998;30: 975–991.

2. American College of Sports Medicine. Progression models in resistance training for healthy adults. *Med Sci Sports Exerc.* 2002;34: 364–380.

3. Drechsler A. *The Weightlifting Encyclopedia: A Guide to World Class Performance.* Whitestone (NY): A is A Communications; 1998. pp. 1–15.

4. Epley B, Taylor J. Developing a policies and procedures manual. In: Baechle TR, Earle RW, editors. *Essentials of Strength Training and Conditioning.* 3rd ed. Champaign (IL): Human Kinetics; 2008. pp. 569–588.

5. Fair JD. *Muscletown USA: Bob Hoffman and the Manly Culture of York Barbell.* University Park (PA): The Pennsylvania State University Press; 1999. p. 804.

6. Fahey TD, Insel PM, Roth WT. *Fit and Well: Core Concepts and Labs in Physical Fitness and Wellness.* 6th ed. Boston (MA): McGraw-Hill; 2005. pp. 28–37.

7. Fleisig GS, Barrentine SW, Zheng N, Escamilla RF, Andrews JR. Kinematic and kinetic comparison of baseball pitching among various levels of development. *J Biomech.* 1999;32:1371–1375.

8. Garhammer J. Power production by Olympic weightlifters. *Med Sci Sports Exerc.* 1980;12:54–60.

9. Garstecki MA, Latin RW, Cuppett MM. Comparison of selected physical fitness and performance variables between NCAA Division I and II football players. *J Strength Cond Res.* 2004;18:292–297.

10. Hoffman J. *Norms for Fitness, Performance, and Health*. Champaign (IL): Human Kinetics; 2006. p. 220.

11. Knuttgen HG, Kraemer WJ. Terminology and measurement in exercise performance. *J Appl Sport Sci Res*. 1987;1:1–10.

12. Kraemer WJ, Noble BJ, Clark MJ, Culver BW. Physiologic responses to heavy-resistance exercise with very short rest periods. *Int J Sports Med*. 1987;8:247–252.

13. Kraemer WJ, Ratamess NA, French DN. Resistance training for health and performance. *Curr Sports Med Rep*. 2002;1:165–171.

14. McBride JM, Triplett-McBride T, Davie A, Newton RU. A comparison of strength and power characteristics between power lifters, Olympic lifters, and sprinters. *J Strength Cond Res*. 1999;13:58–66.

15. National Strength and Conditioning Association. *Strength and Conditioning Professional Standards and Guidelines*. Colorado Springs (CO): NSCA; 2009.

16. Sale DG, MacDougall JD. Isokinetic strength in weight-trainers. *Eur J Appl Physiol Occup Physiol*. 1984;53:128–132.

17. Sierer SP, Battaglini CL, Mihalik JP, Shields EW, Tomasini NT. The National Football League combine: performance differences between drafted and nondrafted players entering the 2004 and 2005 drafts. *J Strength Cond Res*. 2008;22:6–12.

18. Sinclair RG. Normalizing the performances of athletes in Olympic weightlifting. *Can J Appl Sport Sci*. 1985;10:94–98.

19. Stone MH, Sands WA, Pierce KC, Carlock J, Cardinale M, Newton RU. Relationship of maximum strength to weightlifting performance. *Med Sci Sports Exerc*. 2005;37:1037–1043.

20. Stoppani J. *Encyclopedia of Muscle and Strength*. Champaign (IL): Human Kinetics; 2006. pp. 1–7.

21. Todd T. The myth of the muscle-bound lifter. *NSCA Journal*. 1985;7:37–41.

22. Waller M, Piper T, Townsend R. Strongman events and strength and conditioning programs. *Strength Condition J*. 2003;25:44–52.

2

Biomechanics of Force Production

objectives

After completing this chapter, you will be able to:

· Understand the biomechanics of the neuromuscular system in relation to strength and power performance
· Understand how muscle force varies depending on its length and contraction velocity
· Understand how acute changes in a pennate muscle's angle of pennation may limit force production, but how chronic increases resulting from muscle hypertrophy can be advantageous for strength and power increases
· Understand the principles of torque and leverage and how altering moment arm length affects joint force production and speed
· Understand how force/torque varies throughout full joint range of motion and the ramifications this has for weight training performance
· Understand how friction affects force production and sports performance
· Understand the principles of stability and how performance is altered via changes in the body's center of gravity
· Understand how mass, inertia, momentum, and impulse affect performance
· Understand how lifting performance can be enhanced via various accessories

Biomechanics is the science of applying the principles of mechanics to biological systems. Basic knowledge of biomechanics is critical to strength and conditioning coaches, practitioners, and athletes to improve technique, prevent injuries, and understand the underlying factors associated with performance enhancement. Biomechanical concepts apply to all motor skills performed in sports as well as all training modalities. There are several physiological and biomechanical properties of skeletal muscle that affect one's acute level of force/power production and subsequent increases in muscle strength that occur concomitant to training. Several properties are discussed in this chapter and others are discussed in subsequent chapters. In biomechanics, the branch that deals with the forces that cause motion is **kinetics** whereas the description of motion, *e.g.*, displacement, position, velocity, acceleration, is **kinematics**. The kinetics of force production embodies numerous mechanisms and interactions between the nervous, muscular, connective tissue, metabolic, and endocrine systems. In this chapter, several mechanical properties of skeletal muscle are discussed.

MUSCLE ACTIONS

Skeletal muscles produce force in three different ways. Muscle shortening is a *concentric* (CON) muscle action, while muscle lengthening is an *eccentric* (ECC) muscle action. A muscle action characteristic of no noticeable change in muscle length or joint position is an *isometric* (ISOM) muscle action. Greatest muscle force is produced during ECC muscle actions, followed by ISOM and CON actions. ECC muscle actions are particularly important for strength and hypertrophy gains. All three muscle actions are commonly used in training and motor skill performance. However, CON and ECC actions predominate during agonist-prescribed movements whereas ISOM actions play a key role in joint stabilization and maintenance of static bodily positions. CON and ECC muscle action velocities can be controlled by specialized dynamometers. Velocity-controlled CON and ECC muscle actions are **isokinetic**, and isokinetic devices enable strength testing or training at slow, moderate, and/or fast velocities.

THE INFLUENCE OF MUSCLE LENGTH

Skeletal muscle length plays a substantial role in force production. This concept has been termed the muscle *length-tension relationship*. Figures 2.1 and 2.2 depict the muscle length-tension relationship. This parabolic curve indicates that greatest tension is produced in the middle slightly past resting muscle length. This sarcomere (the functional component of a muscle fiber) length indicates optimal interaction of the maximal number of

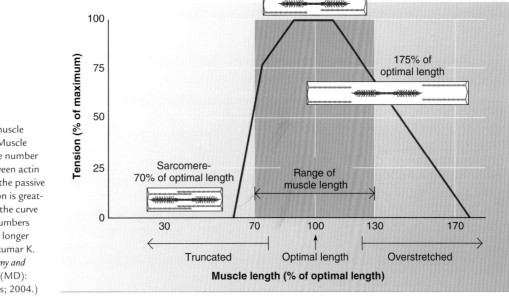

■ FIGURE 2.1. The active muscle length-tension relationship. Muscle tension is proportional to the number of cross-bridges formed between actin and myosin filaments. Here, the passive elements are minimal. Tension is greatest in the middle segment of the curve but lessens as cross-bridge numbers decrease at both shorter and longer muscle lengths. (From Premkumar K. *The Massage Connection: Anatomy and Physiology*. 2nd ed. Baltimore (MD): Lippincott Williams & Wilkins; 2004.)

muscle contractile proteins (actin and myosin). Figure 2.1 depicts the *active* length-tension relationship where passive elements are not considered. When examining total muscle tension, both active and passive elements contribute, with active elements contributing greatly from short to moderate lengths and passive elements contributing greatly at moderate to longer lengths. At shorter muscle lengths, there is overlap of the actin filaments, which reduces actin and myosin interaction. Because muscle tension is proportionate to the number of cross-bridges formed, shorter lengths geometrically pose a problem reducing active muscle tension. Theoretically (as shown in Fig. 2.1), at longer muscle lengths a similar phenomenon may occur where cross-bridge formation is reduced. In this case, myosin filaments cannot reach as many actin filaments. However, the passive neuromuscular elements need to be considered, as shown in Figure 2.2, where at longer lengths they contribute highly to the rebound of muscle tension. Tension developed within the tendon, cross-bridges, and structural proteins (*series elastic component*) and from the muscle fascia (*parallel elastic component*) increases. Although cross-bridge interaction is minimal at long muscle lengths, tension rebounds mostly due to resistance to stretch from tendons and skeletal muscle fascia along with some tension produced within the contractile and structural proteins.

STRETCH-SHORTENING CYCLE

Human movement that begins with a windup or countermovement results in a more powerful action when the movement is reversed. An ECC muscle action that

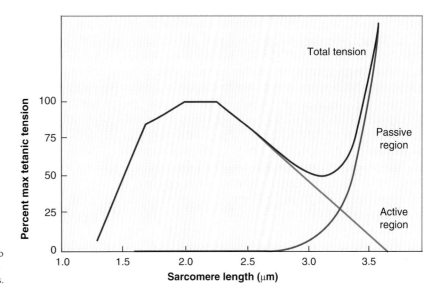

■ FIGURE 2.2. The passive muscle length-tension relationship. This relationship is similar to Figure 2.1 with the exception that the passive elements contribute greatly to longer muscle lengths.

Interpreting Research

Bench Press Performance and the SSC

Wilson GJ, Elliott BC, Wood GA. The effect on performance of imposing a delay during a stretch-shorten cycle movement. *Med Sci Sports Exerc*. 1991;23:364–370.

Wilson et al. (37) examined bench press performance under four conditions: (a) a rebound "touch and go" bench press (RBP), (b) a bench press with a short pause (SPBP) of ~0.6 seconds, a bench press with a long pause (LPBP) of 1.27 seconds, and a purely CON bench press (PCBP) initiated from the bottom starting position. A continuum was found where maximal bench press strength was greatest with RBP (~143.1 kg), followed by SPBP (~137.3 kg), LPBP (~132.9 kg), and PCBP (125.0 kg). Ground reaction force patterns were similar (Fig. 2.3). These data showed that strength performance was maximized with high SSC activity (no pause) and decreased in proportion to pause length. Purely CON actions resulted in the lowest strength values. The take-home message for S&C professionals is that maximal strength performance is observed with no pause, and training, in part, should be centered on maximizing SSC activity. However, some athletes (powerlifters) benefit from including a pause between ECC and CON actions at various points in training because competition necessitates it.

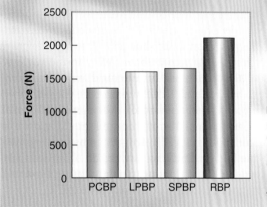

FIGURE 2.3. Bench press performance under various conditions. Bench press ground reaction force was greatest during the rebound bench press (RBP) and was lower in proportion during short-pause bench press (SPBP), long-pause bench press (LPBP), and purely concentric bench press (PCBP). (Adapted with permission from Wilson GJ, Elliott BC, Wood GA. The effect on performance of imposing a delay during a stretch-shorten cycle movement. *Med Sci Sports Exerc*. 1991;23:364–370.)

precedes a CON action results in a more forceful CON action. This phenomenon is known as the stretch-shortening cycle (SSC) and allows the athlete to develop large force and power outputs. The SSC consists of the stretch reflex (see Chapter 3) and the muscle's ability to store elastic energy within its series and parallel elastic components. Of the two primary mechanisms, storage of elastic energy contributes mostly (up to ~70%) to the SSC. The stretch reflex is initiated by a specific sensory receptor, the *muscle spindle*, which responds to both the magnitude and rate of muscle length change. The resultant effect is that the SSC can enhance performance by an average of 15%–20% (33). The SSC is most prominent in **fast-twitch (FT) muscle fibers** (as FT fiber motion is faster resulting in greater elastic energy storage) and is highly trainable via plyometric, sprint, agility, and resistance training (RT).

Critical to SSC performance is that the CON action follows right away. Any pause between the ECC and CON phases (or initiating an action without a countermovement) results in attenuated performance. In skeletal muscle, stored elastic energy can be lost as heat energy. Although elastic energy enhances performance, heat energy provides very little to no ergogenic effects. Subsequently, force and power can be reduced in proportion to the length of the pause between muscle actions. This has been shown to occur during resistance exercise (37). Maximizing SSC activity entails performing ballistic muscle actions with minimal time lapse between ECC and CON muscle actions. Lastly, SSC activity is reduced following periods of high-intensity static stretching (34). Muscle stiffness enhances SSC function; therefore, static stretching that reduces stiffness can lessen force and power production.

THE ROLE OF VELOCITY ON MUSCLE FORCE PRODUCTION

The velocity of muscle contraction plays a critical role in the magnitude of force produced. This *force-velocity relationship* is shown in Figure 2.4. Skeletal muscle fibers

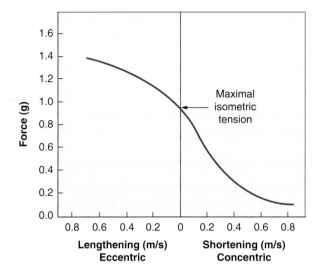

FIGURE 2.4. The force-velocity relationship.

produce force to match external loading, *i.e.*, increasing velocity of shortening during light loading and decreasing velocity of shortening with greater loading. For CON muscle actions, greatest force is produced at slower velocities of contraction whereas less force is produced at fast velocities of contraction. Thus, force increases as velocity slows and decreases as velocity increases. For example, a one-repetition maximum (1RM) bench press is performed

at a slow velocity. Although the individual provides as much force as possible, the overall net velocity is slow due to the high external load. Peak ISOM force occurs at 0 m/s⁻¹ (no movement) that is larger than peak CON force. The force disparity appears related to the number of muscle cross-bridges formed once again. Actin filaments slide rapidly at fast velocities, thereby making it more difficult for myosin to form cross-bridges with actin. As cross-bridge cycling rate increases, less cross-bridges remain intact at any given time. However, cross-bridge formation is enhanced at slow velocities and during ISOM actions where the cross-bridge cycling rate is low. The result is greater force production. On the contrary, muscle force increases as velocity increases during ECC actions. Loading greater than the peak ISOM force level causes muscle fibers to lengthen. Additional loading increases the lengthening velocity. Thus, muscle force increases as lengthening velocity increases because the fibers are contracting as they are lengthening and greater force is present during ECC actions.

MUSCLE ARCHITECTURE

Skeletal muscle architecture refers to the size and arrangement of muscle fibers relative to the muscle's line of pull. The muscle's line of pull dictates the direction of

Myths & Misconceptions

Intentionally Slow Lifting Velocities are the Best Way to Train Based on the Force-Velocity Relationship

When examining the velocity of the external load as it is lifted during resistance exercise, some have argued that intentionally lifting a weight slowly is the best way to maximize strength and point to the force-velocity relationship as supporting evidence. However, the missing element in this argument is the effort level given by the individual and how this impacts the external load's velocity of motion. When maximal effort is given by the athlete against a submaximal external load, the net velocity of movement is fast but this is not the case during maximal loading where the net velocity is slow. The force-velocity relationship assumes that muscles are CON contracting maximally at a given velocity when examining the total system (35). This can be seen when isokinetic strength testing or when 1RM strength testing are performed. During submaximal loading, intentionally slow velocities occur when the individual purposely limits contraction velocity. Albeit intentionally slow velocities may pose a stimulus for endurance and hypertrophy training, slow velocities with submaximal loads are not conducive to maximal strength and power training. The underlying factor is that the individual must purposely slow contraction velocity when lifting a submaximal weight and this in turn limits the neuromuscular response (less recruitment and firing rate of activated muscle fibers). Research has shown that the amount of weight lifted (24) or repetitions performed with a given weight, force (25,35), and neural responses (25) are lower when a weight is intentionally lifted at a slower velocity. Motion of the external load is governed by Sir Isaac Newton's Second Law of Motion (*Law of Acceleration*) where *force = mass × acceleration*. When mass is held constant, greater force produces higher acceleration. As Schilling et al. (35) have pointed out, the required force to lift a slowly moving weight is just slightly larger than the weight itself as the velocity is slightly higher than 0 m/s⁻¹. Greater force is needed to accelerate the weight to a higher velocity. The justification of using intentionally slow reps (for strength improvements) with nonmaximal weights is not supported by the force-velocity relationship.

motion of the joint that ensues as muscle fibers shorten. Architectural features of skeletal muscle include the length of fascicles, fibers, and the arrangement of muscle fibers.

MUSCLE FIBER ARRANGEMENT

The arrangement of skeletal muscle fibers plays an important role in their ability to produce force, power, and speed. Two general fiber arrangements are shown, pennate and nonpennate muscles (Fig. 2.5). **Nonpennate** muscles have their fibers run parallel to the muscle's line of pull. Various types of nonpennate muscles exist. *Longitudinal (strap)* muscles, *e.g.*, sartorius and rectus abdominis, are long in length. *Quadrate (quadrilateral)* muscles, *e.g.*, rhomboids, are flat, four-sided nonpennate muscles. *Fan-shaped (radiate, triangular)* muscles, *e.g.*, pectoralis major, gluteus medius, have fibers that radiate from a narrow point of attachment at one end to a broader point of attachment at the opposite end. *Fusiform* muscles, *e.g.*, biceps brachii and brachioradialis, are rounded, spindle-shaped muscles that taper at both ends. Nonpennate muscles have longer fiber lengths and are typically fewer in number. Thus, nonpennate muscle fiber arrangement is more advantageous for range of motion (ROM) and speed of contraction. Although nonpennate muscles' force-producing capacity can increase with muscle growth, *e.g.*, an increase in its *anatomical cross-sectional area*, they are designed more efficiently for optimizing muscle fiber ROM and contraction velocity.

Pennate muscle fibers (from the Latin "penna" meaning "feather") are arranged obliquely to the central tendon, or line of pull. A *unipennate* muscle, *e.g.*, tibialis posterior, has one column of fibers that are arranged at an angle to the line of pull. A *bipennate* muscle, *e.g.*, rectus

femoris, has a long central tendon with fibers extending diagonally in pairs from either side in two columns. A *multipennate* muscle, *e.g.*, deltoid, has more than two columns of fibers converging on a tendon to form one muscle. The pennate muscle arrangement, *e.g.*, shorter fibers oriented at an angle, is advantageous for strength and power production but not as much for velocity of contraction and ROM.

The Angle of Pennation in Pennate Muscles

In pennate muscles, the *angle of pennation* refers to the angle between the fibers and the central tendon. This angle in the resting state may be low (≤5°) or high (>30°) depending on the muscle and the athlete's level of muscle mass (1,19). The angle of pennation has great functional significance. The larger the angle of pennation, the smaller amount of force transmitted to the tendon. Geometrically, a pennate muscle enables greater fiber number per cross-sectional area. Shorter fiber length coupled with greater fiber packing density yields greater force and power production compared to nonpennate muscles of similar volume. This oblique fiber orientation can be advantageous over time when an athlete trains because a chronic increase in the angle of pennation at rest creates space for muscle hypertrophy. Because there is a positive relationship between a muscle's *physiologic cross-sectional area* (sum total of all fiber cross-sections in a plane perpendicular to fiber orientation) and its force potential, an increase in a muscle's angle of pennation accommodates growth thereby increasing strength and power potential. Several longitudinal (1,21,36) and cross-sectional studies (19) have shown that RT (resulting in muscle growth) increases a muscle's angle of pennation in the resting state over time. However, during acute exercise, the muscle's angle of pennation may increase largely to account for contraction. As a muscle shortens during contraction, fibers must shorten to accommodate the change in muscle belly shape. As a result, muscle fibers rotate and become more oblique (changing contraction leverage) as the fiber shortens (5) thereby increasing the angle of pennation further. This changes the direction of force relative to the muscle's line of action and limits force production. Thus, acute increases in angle of pennation could limit force production but chronic increases in the angle of pennation (resulting from hypertrophy) are advantageous for strength and power development.

Muscle Fascicle Length

Muscle fibers are arranged in parallel within a larger structure known as a *fascicle* (Chapter 4). Fascicle length is another muscle architectural component of interest. Similar to pennation angle, fascicle length tends to decrease with muscle shortening. Chronic changes

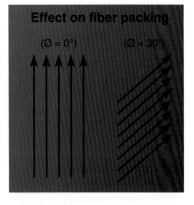

■ **FIGURE 2.5.** Muscle architecture. Pennate and nonpennate muscle arrangements are shown. Shown below is the effect of pennation angle on fiber packing density. More fibers can be located in a given volume when their arrangement is oblique. Geometrically, this has a positive effect on strength and power production. A nonpennate muscle has a pennation angle of 0°. (Oatis CA. *Kinesiology: The Mechanics and Pathomechanics of Human Movement.* Baltimore (MD): Lippincott Williams & Wilkins; 2004. Fiber packing from MKK 7e.)

in fascicle length may be an additional muscular adaptation to training. Although currently unclear as to the role changes in fascicle length plays with training, some research has yielded interesting findings. Some studies have shown greater fascicle lengths in athletes with large levels of muscle hypertrophy (23), perhaps suggesting that increasing fascicle length may be a mechanism contributing to hypertrophy. However, some studies have shown increases in fascicle length early during RT (4,8,36) whereas some studies have reported no changes in fascicle length with smaller levels of muscle hypertrophy (7,20). Sprint/plyometric training has been shown to increase fascicle length during short-term training periods (6). Among comparisons in athletes, soccer players have shorter fascicle lengths in the vastus lateralis and gastrocnemius muscles than swimmers (22), and sprinters have larger fascicle lengths than distance runners in the same muscles (2). It is thought that greater fascicle lengths favor high contraction velocity (greater running speed). In support, fascicle length correlates highly with maximal sprint performance (28).

TORQUE AND LEVERAGE

A force can be defined as a push or pull that has the ability to accelerate, decelerate, stop, or change the direction of an object. Forces are described by their magnitude, direction, and point of application. Linear motion is produced by force application. **Linear motion** occurs when all points on a body or object move the same distance, at the same time, and in the same direction, thereby yielding a straight (*rectilinear motion*) or curved (*curvilinear motion*) pathway. However, angular motion is the counterpart to linear motion. **Angular motion** occurs when all points on a body or object move in circular patterns around the same axis. Angular motion of bodily segments can produce linear and angular motion of the entire body. Angular kinetic and kinematic parameters have analogs to linear motion, and the angular analog to force is torque. Analysis of torque and leverage is critical to studying athletic performance.

Torque (also known as moment) is the rotation caused by a force about a specific axis and is the product of force and moment arm length. The force may be directed through the object's center of gravity (COG) (*centric force*), away from the COG (*eccentric force*), or multiple forces may be equal in size but opposite in direction (*force couple*). Centric and eccentric forces can produce linear motion, and eccentric forces and force couples can produce angular motion. A **moment arm** (or lever arm) is the perpendicular distance between the force's line of action and the fulcrum, but it may also be the perpendicular distance between the resistance and fulcrum. Two types of moment arms exist in human motion. A moment arm is formed between the point of muscle attachment and the joint (*moment arm of force*), and a moment arm is

formed between the joint and where the loading is concentrated (*moment arm of resistance*). Because it is an angular kinetic variable, torque is dependent upon not only the force applied but also the leverage involved. Figure 2.6 depicts an example where an individual pulls at two different angles with the same net force. The torque generated differed because the moment arm length changed. A RT example is the *side lateral raise*. If the athlete selects 20-lb dumbbells to perform this exercise, one can see that the exercise is more difficult or easy by repositioning the arms. With the elbows extended, the exercise is more difficult than if the athlete flexes the elbows. If we assume muscle force to be similar in both cases, less torque is generated to lift the dumbbells with the elbows flexed because the resistance arm is smaller. The athlete can perform more repetitions with the elbows flexed. It is not uncommon to see individuals instinctively bend their arms when this exercise becomes more difficult. The moment arm of resistance can be manipulated many ways to alter exercise performance.

The human body acts as a system of levers (Fig. 2.7). A *lever* is used to overcome a large resistance and is used to enhance speed and ROM. A lever is made up of a *fulcrum* (pivot point), *resistance*, and *force*. The distance from the fulcrum to the concentration of the resistance is the *resistance arm* whereas as the distance from the fulcrum to the concentration of the force is the force or *effort arm*. The relative location of each determines what type of lever is present. A *first-class lever* (the elbow during extension) has its fulcrum lie between the force and resistance. Speed and ROM are maximized with this type of lever and force is secondary. A *second-class lever* (standing plantar flexion onto the toes) has its resistance lie between

$$\text{Torque}_1 = F_1 d_\perp = 30\ N\ (1.0\ m) = 30\ Nm\ \text{of torque}$$
$$\text{Torque}_2 = F_2 d_\perp = 30\ N\ (.5\ m) = 15\ Nm\ \text{of torque}$$

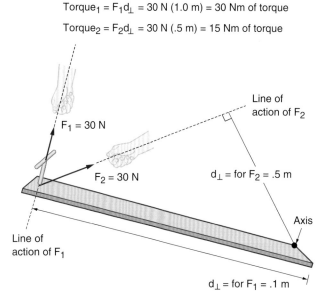

■ **FIGURE 2.6.** Torque generation at two angles of force application.

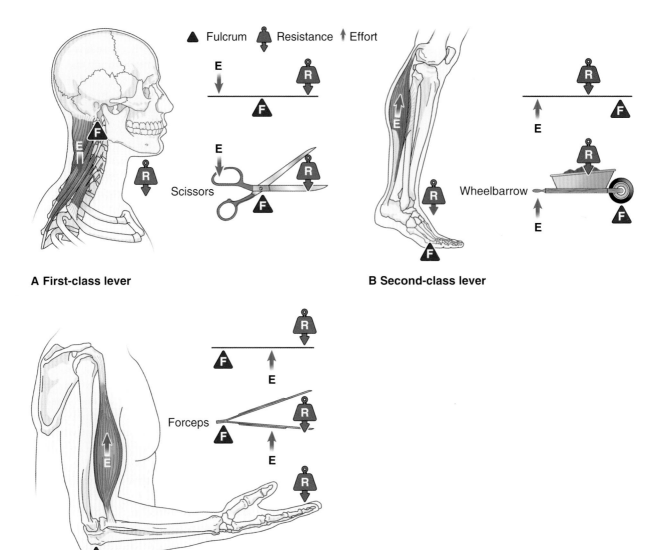

■ **FIGURE 2.7.** Three classes of levers. (Reprinted with permission from Cohen BJ, Taylor JJ. *Memmler's The Human Body in Health and Disease.* 11th ed. Baltimore (MD): Wolters Kluwer Health; 2009.)

the fulcrum and force. An advantage with this type of lever is force. A *third-class lever* (elbow during flexion) has its force lie between the fulcrum and resistance. Similar to a first-class lever, a third-class lever is more advantageous for speed and ROM and not as much for force. Most single-joint movements in the human body operate via third-class levers.

As a leverage system, bones act as levers, joints act as fulcrums, and contracting skeletal muscles act as the force. Weight (or the concentration of the weight) of each segment plus external loading both act as the resistance. A term used to describe a lever's potential for force production is *mechanical advantage*. **Mechanical advantage** is the ratio of the moment arm of muscle force (effort arm) to the moment arm of resistance (resistance arm). A value of 1 indicates balance between the effort

and resistance arms. A value >1 indicates a mechanical advantage where the torque created by the effort force is magnified whereas a value <1 indicates a mechanical disadvantage (although it would be an advantage for speed and ROM) where a larger effort force is needed to overcome the resistance (15). First-class levers in the human body operate mostly at values similar to or less than 1 indicating a mechanical disadvantage under certain conditions during motion (15). Third-class levers pose mechanical disadvantages (<1) and are more suitable for greater joint angular velocities as the resistance arm is larger than the effort arm. However, a second-class lever provides a mechanical advantage (>1) as the effort arm is larger than the resistance arm. Most skeletal muscles produce single-joint movements that operate at a mechanical disadvantage thereby requiring muscles to produce additional force in order to overcome a resistance. Based on lever systems, it appears that the human body was designed to produce motion at higher speeds at the expense of the large force applications.

MOMENT ARMS AND TENDON INSERTION

The location of a muscle's tendon insertion into bone is another factor contributing to maximal strength expression. The distance from the joint center to the point of tendon insertion represents the moment arm of muscle force, or the effort arm. A tendon inserted slightly further away from the joint poses a mechanical advantage for force production whereas insertion closer to the joint is more advantageous for speed. An athlete with a longer force arm has the ability to lift more weight but at the expense of speed. For a given amount of muscle shortening, a muscle that has a tendon inserted closer to the joint will experience a greater change in ROM than a muscle with its tendon inserted farther from the joint. Greater ROM covered in the same period of time reflects greater joint angular velocity. Consequently, a baseball or tennis player might benefit more from a smaller moment arm of force whereas a powerlifter would benefit more from a larger moment arm of force. Tendon insertion is a genetic factor contributing to strength that does not change with training.

Case Study 2.1

Michael is a S&C coach who is strength testing athletes from various sports. Michael is using the 1 RM bench press assessment to test upper-body maximal strength. One athlete, a basketball player, who is 6'8" and weighs 220 lb, maxes out at 225 lb. Another athlete, a wrestler, who is 6'0" and weighs 220 lb, also maxes out at 225 lb.

Question for Consideration: **What mechanically can be deduced from the performance data of both athletes?**

MOMENT ARMS AND BODILY PROPORTIONS

An athlete's stature plays an important role in performance. Longer limbs create a longer resistance arm that can reduce mechanical advantage. However, a longer resistance arm yields greater velocity. This is advantageous for sports such as basketball, volleyball, and pitching in baseball. Longer limb lengths contribute to greater stride length in running and stroke length and frequency in swimming (31). Limb length is a genetic attribute that is not coached but increases the likelihood of success in some sports. However, in lifting sports a longer moment arm of resistance makes it difficult to lift a great deal of weight for many exercises.

Proportions contribute, in part, to the success an individual will have in athletics. As previously discussed, limb lengths affect moment arm sizes and leverage can be gained or lost depending on bodily proportions. Although bodily proportions are stable in adulthood, an athlete can modify technique and/or train specifically to accommodate or compensate for genetic structural attributes. Relative proportion is an area of interest to coaches as certain anthropometric variables have been linked to sporting success. Some commonly used variables include: (a) *crural index* ([ratio of leg length/thigh length] × 100); (b) *brachial index* ([ratio of forearm length/arm length] × 100); (c) *trunk to extremity index*; (d) *lower limb to trunk ratio*; and (e) *seated height to stature index*. As Ackland and de Ridder (3) have pointed out:

- Tennis players with long limbs have an advantage with high-velocity shots whereas players with shorter limbs need to play with more agility to compensate.
- Elite swimmers tend to have a larger stature depending on the event. Sprinters have displayed a higher brachial index, arm span, and lower leg and foot length compared to middle-distance and distance swimmers. Freestyle and backstroke swimmers tend to have longer limbs, and butterfly swimmers tend to have longer trunks.
- Gymnasts tend to have shorter statures with a low crural index and lower limb/trunk ratio.
- Weightlifters and powerlifters tend to have long trunks, low crural index, low lower limb/trunk ratio, low brachial index, and high sitting height/stature ratio.
- Sprinters tend to have a low lower limb/trunk ratio with an average-to-high crural index compared to middle-distance runners.
- High and triple jumpers tend to have a high lower limb/trunk ratio and a high crural index.
- Discus and javelin throwers tend to have longer arms with normal trunk lengths.
- Cyclists tend to have a high crural index that increases mechanical advantage during pedaling.
- Sports such as baseball and football are more variable based on the diversity of different positions.
- Basketball and volleyball players tend to be tall and have long upper and lower limbs, and a high crural index.
- Wrestlers and judo athletes tend to have a low lower limb/trunk ratio and a low crural index to assist in maintaining a low COG.

HUMAN STRENGTH CURVES

An athlete's level of muscular strength varies on the position within the ROM, *e.g.*, peak torque and force varies depending on joint position. This concept can be illustrated by examining any weight training exercise. There are areas that feel easier and there is a point where the

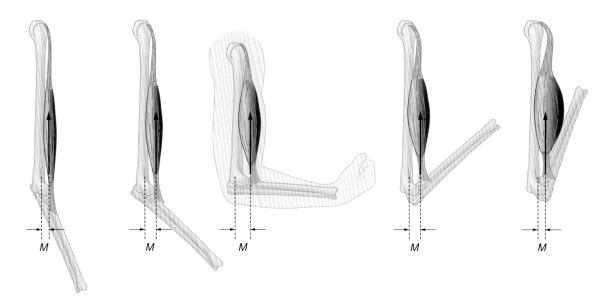

■ **FIGURE 2.8.** Effort arm changes during elbow flexion.

exercise is most difficult. The area of greatest difficulty where the velocity of the weight slows down is known as the **sticking region**. Sticking regions may not be seen during low-intensity repetitions; however, they do become apparent during high-intensity lifts or when fatigue is substantial (12). At this point it is very tempting for the athlete to break form and cheat the weight to its full repetition completion. However, proper technique must be emphasized and weight selection should consider this weak link for a given exercise.

There are several physiological and biomechanical factors that contribute to human strength curves. Some factors are addressed in this and subsequent chapters including neural activation, muscle cross-sectional area, muscle length, and architecture. Perhaps the most significant of these factors is the changes in length of the moment arm of muscle force that takes place throughout full joint ROM. Figure 2.8 depicts moment arm of muscle force changes of the biceps brachii that take places during elbow flexion. The moment arm of force is largest in the middle of the ROM near an elbow angle of 90°. The force arm decreases in length as the arm is flexed or extended towards the limits of the ROM. Graphically, this kinetic pattern yields a parabolic-shaped joint angle-torque curve known as an *ascending-descending torque curve* (Fig. 2.9). Starting from full elbow extension, muscle torque is low but gradually increases to a peak at or near 90° (the ascending segment). Beyond this point, muscle torque gradually decreases until full joint flexion (the descending segment). Although peak ISOM torque may vary slightly amongst different joint actions, single-joint movements are depicted as ascending-descending torque curves (27).

The strength, or force, curves for multiple-joint actions differ. They tend to be more linear (as linear motion is

produced), and either ascend or descend on a joint angle-force curve. An *ascending strength curve* is one where overall net force is lowest initially but gradually increases as the exercise progresses (Fig. 2.10). Many pushing exercises such as the squat, bench press, and shoulder press exemplify an ascending strength curve. In the barbell squat, the exercise is most difficult at the parallel bottom position (or

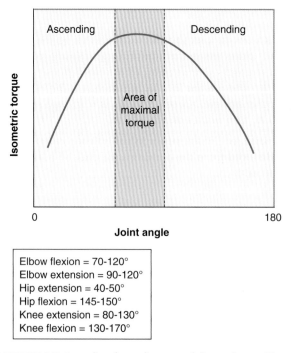

Elbow flexion = 70-120°
Elbow extension = 90-120°
Hip extension = 40-50°
Hip flexion = 145-150°
Knee extension = 80-130°
Knee flexion = 130-170°

■ **FIGURE 2.9.** Ascending-descending strength (torque) curve. The values depict areas of maximal strength determined by several studies. (Redrawn from Kraemer WJ, Fry AC, Ratamess NA, French DN. Strength testing: development and evaluation of methodology. In: Maud PJ, Foster C, eds. *Physiological Assessments of Human Performance.* 2nd ed. Champaign (IL): Human Kinetics; 2006:119–150.)

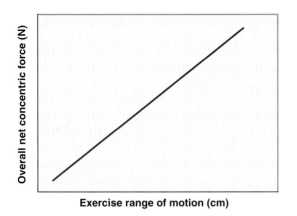

FIGURE 2.10. Ascending strength (force) curve.

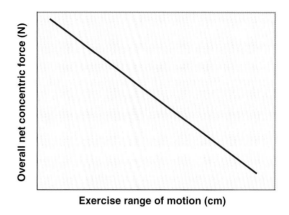

FIGURE 2.11. Descending strength (force) curve.

lower) but easiest at the very top near full knee and hip extension. The difference in the amount of weight lifted between a parallel and a quarter squat is of great significance as this value can be in excess of 200 lb or more in some athletes. This is why it is common to see athletes not descend to the parallel position when the squat exercise becomes more difficult with fatigue or heavy loading.

A *descending strength curve* is one where the overall net force is greatest initially but gradually decreases as the exercise progresses to its final position within the ROM (Fig. 2.11). Many pulling exercises such as the barbell row, pull-up, and lat pull-down exemplify a descending strength curve. In the lat pull-down exercise, the exercise is easiest at the top position (full shoulder flexion and elbow extension) but becomes more difficult as the bar is pulled to below chin level. Hence, a common mistake seen is the use of the lower back and hips to generate momentum to lower the bar near the bottom position of the exercise.

ACTION/REACTION FORCES AND FRICTION

An *action force* is the force (a push or pull) applied by an individual to an object with the intent to accelerate, decelerate, stop, maintain, or change the direction of the object. Muscular contraction, in addition to the effects of gravity, produces action forces in sports and exercise. However, a *reaction force* is produced in response to the action. In his Third Law of Motion, Sir Isaac Newton has stated "for every action there is an equal and opposite reaction." That is, the reactive force is equal and opposite of the action force. The ground supplies an equal and opposite force in response (**ground reaction force**) to a force applied to the ground by the athlete during locomotion. The ground reaction force enables the athlete to run. Figure 2.12 depicts a typical ground reaction force observed during running. Reaction forces are seen in other conditions as well. During weight training, a

reactive force is seen by the barbell in response to the action force provided by the lifter. Critical to our discussion is that the response may differ even though the forces are equal and opposite. When the lifter applies the force to the barbell, the reactive force is equal; however, the barbell does move. Thus, similar forces can lead to dissimilar results in that the object with less mass, stability, and/or leverage may move despite similar kinetics.

Action forces applied to an object or another body will be higher if stable contact is made between the two objects. These action/reaction forces are considered perpendicular but there needs to be a sufficient parallel force present to create stability between the two surfaces in contact. This parallel force is known as **friction**. Friction acts to oppose relative motion of these two surfaces. That is, friction causes stability at the point of contact

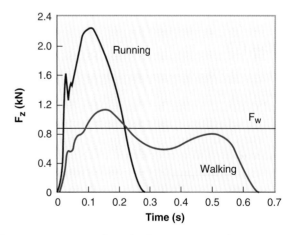

FIGURE 2.12. Ground-reaction force curves. Data demonstrate increased ground reaction forces with increasing speeds of running and walking. Ground-reaction force curve shows two distinct segments (the curves are more visible during running). The first rise in force (or peak) is known as the *peak impact force,* which depicts force produced upon the foot landing on the ground. The second rise (or peak) is known as the *peak propulsion force,* which is the peak force produced during acceleration as the individual's center of gravity moves forward during push-off. Fw indicates the force of body weight.

and prevents one object from sliding past the other. The maximum frictional force is the product of the reactive force and a quantity known as the *coefficient of friction*, which is a numerical representation of the two contact surfaces. Two types of friction, static and dynamic, are relevant to sports and exercise. *Static friction* acts between two objects not moving relative to each other where there is sufficient stability between the contact surfaces. *Dynamic (sliding) friction* acts between two surfaces moving relative to each other, resulting in sliding.

Numerous examples of friction can be seen in athletics and its importance is great. Static friction is critical for nearly all RT exercises. For the bench press, static friction between the lifter's back and bench, feet and floor, and hands and bar are important for stability and lifting performance. For the dead lift, static friction between the lifter's feet and floor and hands and bar are important for lifting performance. Greater friction equals better performance or weight lifted. This is why powerlifters and weightlifters use chalk on their hands and on their backs (powerlifters) as chalk increases the coefficient of static friction. In addition, knurling on a bar enhances friction. Static friction plays critical roles in sports as well. Static friction between a player's feet and the ground is essential and has been a major consideration when examining shoe design. Greater force and power can only be produced when the individual is in the most stable position. Static friction is important when gripping an object whether it is a baseball, basketball, tennis racquet, or football. Some exercise devices (weighted sled) rely on frictional forces to some extent to provide resistance to the trainee. However, some sports strive for low dynamic friction. Skaters and skiers perform much better and achieve better times when the coefficient of sliding friction is ultralow between the skis/skates and the ground/ice.

STABILITY

Stability is the ability of an object or individual to resist changes in equilibrium. Maintaining a stable position is critical to the expression of maximal strength and power. Stability is reliant to a great extent on manipulation of the COG. The COG is the point at which the weight is concentrated. The COG is multiplanar, meaning it has longitudinal, side-to-side, and front-to-back orientations. Thus, the COG can move side to side when limbs are abducted or the trunk is laterally flexed, can be lowered by flexing the trunk, hips, or knees, can be raised by lifting the arms, and can shift from front to back or vice versa during sagittal plane movements. Motion changes the COG in one or more planes, and manipulation of the COG is crucial to maintaining and optimizing stability. Relevant to the COG is an imaginary line that connects the COG to the ground known as the *line of gravity*. As the COG changes, so potentially can the line of gravity, and manipulating the line of gravity affects an object's stability.

Of significance to stability is the object's weight, level of friction, and size of the base support. The *base support* is an area within the lines connecting the outer perimeter of the parts of the body in contact with the ground. For example, a sprinter in 4-point stance would have a larger base support than an individual standing in an upright position with a shoulder-width stance (2-point stance). The size of the base support can be manipulated to increase stability. Increasing the size of the base support leads to greater stability. For example, postural stability is greater when an individual performs the squat with a wide stance versus a narrow stance. Thus, stability is governed by general principles:

- *Greater stability is seen when the COG is lower*, as is the case with a football player or wrestler who maintains a low position to increase the likelihood of success.
- *Greater stability is present when the line of gravity is aligned equidistantly within the base support*, when weight is not shifted from side to side or front to back; stability is greater when the line of gravity is centralized.
- *Greater stability is observed when the base support is wide*, increasing the width of the stance or the number of contact points with ground enhances stability.
- *Greater stability is observed in objects with larger mass*; objects larger in mass possess greater stability.
- *Greater stability is observed when the level of friction is greater*; when the coefficient of friction increases, greater stability is present.
- *Stability decreases when external loading is applied to the upper body*; external loading to the upper extremities raises the COG and reduces stability.

MASS AND INERTIA

Mass is the amount of matter an object takes up whereas *inertia* is the resistance of an object to changing its motion. In linear motion, objects with larger mass and inertia have more stability. Mass is a critical element to many sports especially those that have weight classes. For some sports, increasing mass can be advantageous especially in the form of muscle mass increases, *e.g.*, football. However, sports with weight classes or sports where the athlete must overcome mass for success (high jumper, pole-vaulter, and gymnast) limit the amount of mass an athlete may be willing to gain. For these sports a high strength-to-mass ratio is important. A high strength-to-mass ratio indicates that the athlete produces a high level of force (or power for the *power-to-mass ratio*) with less or similar body mass. A 10% increase in strength with only a 2% increase in body mass could be advantageous for many athletes. Thus, an athlete who competes in weight classes or against gravity could theoretically perform better with strength increases while maintaining a similar mass. Additional mass could be problematic for athletes such as gymnasts or jumpers as the individual has to overcome more inertia to accelerate, potentially resulting in less distance or height jumped. Small mass increases could be beneficial if performance is enhanced. However, some athletes have to weigh the advantages and disadvantages of mass gains via trial and error to possibly increase mass slightly but not too much to limit performance. Training can be designed to enhance strength and power while minimizing mass gains.

In angular motion, mass is still critical. However, the distribution of mass is a major factor of consideration. The angular kinetic analog to mass or inertia is the **moment of inertia**. The moment of inertia is the property of an object to resist changes in angular motion and is the product of the object's mass and a measure of mass distribution about an axis of rotation known as the *radius of gyration*, e.g., moment of inertia (I_a) = mass (m) × radius of gyration (r)^2. The radius of gyration is the distance from the axis of rotation to where the object's mass is concentrated. Because the radius of gyration is a squared term, a small change yields a large change in the moment of inertia. Changing an object's center of mass changes the moment of inertia. Some examples of decreasing the moment of inertia in sports are "choking up" in baseball or softball to increase bat velocity; flexing the hips, knees, and trunk in diving or gymnastics to facilitate aerial rotations; and flexing the knee during the swing phase in sprinting to enhance leg angular velocity by decreasing the moments of inertia about the hip joint. For RT, increasing the moment of inertia places greater tension on the muscles (performing a torso rotation with the arms straight rather than bent) as it becomes more difficult to start and stop the movement and requires greater muscle activation.

MOMENTUM AND IMPULSE

In linear terms, Newton's Law of Acceleration ($F = ma$) could be rewritten to yield two additional biomechanical variables. If we substitute the equation for acceleration (Δvelocity/time) and multiply both sides by time to remove the denominator, we end up with an equation $F \times T = m \times \Delta v$. The left side of the equation ($F \times T$) is the linear *impulse* whereas the right side of the equation ($m \times \Delta v$) is linear *momentum*. Impulse represents the level of force applied over time (N seconds) and causes and is equal to changes in momentum. Increasing force and/or time in which it is applied increases impulse. Momentum can be increased by increasing either the mass or the velocity. Increasing linear momentum can be advantageous especially with *collisions*. A football player who increases mass (via an off-season S&C program) and maintains or increases velocity can generate more linear momentum at the point of contact with an opponent. There are many examples in sports where decreasing momentum is positive. For example, catching a ball decreases ball momentum, blocking or tackling decreases

an opponent's momentum and protective equipment reduces momentum and lessens the peak force absorbed by an athlete. For weight training, momentum can be increased or decreased by manipulating the repetition velocity for a given submaximal weight. Changes in momentum are proportional to the force applied. A large force application can increase impulse throughout the remainder of the exercise. Some argue that the generation of too much momentum can reduce muscle development as lower momentum generated requires a longer period of force application. The choice is based on training goals as increasing momentum may play a greater role in strength and power development with submaximal lifting intensities.

Angular motion analogs are seen for momentum and impulse as well. Angular impulse is equivalent to torque × time and angular momentum is the product of the joint angular velocity and the moment of inertia. Similar to linear momentum, maximizing angular momentum necessitates the optimal combination of angular velocity and the moment of inertia. Baseball and softball can be used to illustrate this point. Choking up on a bat reduces the moment of inertia to increase velocity. However, choking up on the bat is not a formula for success in power hitting. Less angular momentum is generated upon contact with the ball yielding less velocity of the ball after it is struck. When a player "extends the arms," the ball generally travels farther and faster. The moment of inertia is increased at minimal expense to angular velocity thereby increasing angular momentum. Thus, an athlete with the power to swing a heavier (or more concentrated) bat at a fast velocity presents a greater power hitting threat at the plate. A similar scenario is presented in golf where the driver (longest club resulting in a longer radius of gyration) yields farther ball distances upon contact. Some sports depend on increasing and decreasing angular momentum during performance. For example, a discus thrower will spin fast initially to use a larger moment of inertia to maximize the time of torque application. After this phase, the moment of inertia is reduced to maximize angular velocity before release.

BODY SIZE

An athlete's body size is an influential factor for maximal force production. In general, the larger the body size the larger the force potential. However, this only applies relative to muscle mass as a positive relationship exists between muscle mass and absolute force production. Several coaches and practitioners have used relative strength measures to compare athletes of different sizes in lifting events (see Chapter 1). Body mass scaling clearly favors smaller individuals. As body size increases, body mass increases to a greater extent than muscle strength. Larger athletes have a higher absolute segment of their body mass in the form of bone mass or nonmuscle mass that does not contribute directly to greater muscle force production. In addition, potential reductions in leverage (larger moment arms of resistance in taller athletes) could limit the maximal amount of weight lifted. Other scaling methods, *e.g.*, allometric scaling, tend to favor middle-weight individuals. Perhaps the best solution is to use weight classes and compare absolute performances when possible.

OTHER KINETIC FACTORS IN STRENGTH AND CONDITIONING

INTRA-ABDOMINAL AND INTRATHORACIC PRESSURES

Intra-abdominal pressure (IAP) is the pressure developed within the abdominal cavity during contraction of deep trunk muscles and the diaphragm. The abdominal cavity contains a large fluid element that provides great stability (Fig. 2.13). This element has been described as a fluid ball that assists in stabilizing the vertebral column and reducing compressive forces on spinal disks. This fluid component is structurally greater than the support seen in gaseous environments such as the thoracic cavity, *e.g.*, *intrathoracic pressure* (ITP) (16). IAP pushes against the spine and helps keep the torso upright, which is important for preventing lower-back injuries especially during exercises involving high-intensity trunk flexion, extension, and jumping (9) and during fatiguing back extension exercises (14). Both IAP and ITP have been shown to increase with heavier loads lifted (16). A study has shown that increasing IAP by up to 60% increased spinal stiffness up to 31% (18). Thus,

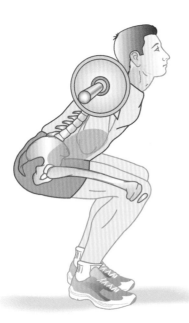

■ **FIGURE 2.13.** Intra-abdominal pressure. (Reprinted with permission from Harman E. Biomechanics of resistance exercise. In: *Essentials of Strength Training and Conditioning.* 3rd ed. Champaign (IL): Human Kinetics, 2008, pp. 85.)

methods used to increase IAP play a role in increasing postural stability and reducing risks of injury.

Ways to Increase Intra-Abdominal Pressure

Because higher IAP provides a protective effect against lumbar spinal injuries, increasing IAP has important training ramifications. There are three ways to increase IAP during training: (a) abdominal contraction and subsequent trunk muscle training, (b) breath holding, and (c) lifting belts. Contraction of abdominal (transversus abdominis, rectus abdominis, and external and internal obliques) and lumbar (erector spinae) muscles contribute greatly to the development of IAP (10). Consistent core training allows athletes to develop greater IAP and increase the rate of IAP development (11). Breath holding, *e.g.*, a *Valsalva maneuver*, also results in an increased IAP. Air cannot escape the lungs and the glottis is closed, thereby creating torso rigidity. Although negative side effects are associated with the Valsalva maneuver (see Chapter 9), breath holding has been shown to result in high levels of IAP (16,32). This is why many experienced lifters temporarily hold their breath during the most difficult area (sticking region) of a heavy exercise. Lastly, weight lifting belts increase IAP (29). However, caution must be used as overuse of lifting belts can actually weaken muscles and make it more difficult for core musculature to generate IAP over time.

LIFTING ACCESSORIES

Lifting accessories have been developed to reduce the risk of injury and increase the efficiency of RT. Although these accessories provide substantial joint support and reduce injury risk, most strength athletes use them for their ergogenic potential. For example, many athletes use straps and gym chalk to enhance grip during performance of heavy pulling exercises. Other training accessories are commonly used and are discussed in this section.

Lifting Belts

Many different types of lifting belts are sold on the market. Athletes use belts for support and for the assumed lower risk of back injuries. Lifting belts augment IAP during lifting by 13%–40% and reduce compressive forces on the back by ~6% (29). During performance of a near-maximal squat, belts were shown to increase the magnitude of IAP, peak rate of IAP, and IAP over time compared to performing the same exercise with no belt (17). Belts allow athletes to use more weight, perform more reps, and perform faster reps during exercises such as the squat and deadlift (30). The magnitude depends on the type and tightness of the belt as tighter belts are more supportive. Quadriceps muscle activity increases during the back squat when belts are used. In contrast, core muscle activation is lower with belt use as muscle activity was greater by 8%–24% in the rectus abdominis, 13%–44% in the external obliques, and 12%–23% in the erector spinae without a belt during the squat (29). It is important to recognize that belts should not be overused as they limit potential core strength development. It is recommended that lifting belts be used only during performance of exercises that involve trunk flexion/extension (squats, dead lift, bent-over row) with maximal or near-maximal weights. Powerlifters and strength athletes commonly use belts but very few weightlifters use belts during performance of the Olympic lifts. Intense core training allows the musculature to increase strength and IAP-generating capacity, thus reducing the need to use a belt. Lastly, belts should only be used during a set and should be loosened or removed between sets as they reduce blood flow back to the heart and increase blood pressure (32).

Wraps

Some athletes use various types of wraps on their knees, elbows, or wrists. Knee wraps can enhance performance of exercises involving knee extension by providing support that resists knee flexion. The magnitude is dependent upon the type of wraps used, wrapping technique, and the angle of knee flexion during wrapping, and tightness of the wraps. Thick, heavy wraps long in length with sufficient elasticity provide the most support. Some athletes anecdotally claim increased squat lifts of 50 lb or more. Elbow wraps are effective for reducing elbow pressure and enhancing performance of extension exercises (bench press, shoulder press). Wrist wraps reduce pressure on the wrist by limiting joint flexion and extension, and allow for greater stability during exercises using heavy weights. Likewise, wraps should not be overused in order to maximize muscular involvement in the exercise.

Bench Press Shirts

A bench press shirt is very tight, supportive gear that several powerlifters use during competition and during the final stages of precompetition training. Bench press shirts can enhance 1 RM strength greatly. Although research is lacking, gains of at least 25–50 lb are expected, with some elite lifters suggesting increases of >100 lb. The amount of increase is dependent on the type (polyester, denim, canvas; single or double layer) and tightness of shirt used, biomechanics of the lifter, and prior experience of bench press shirt use. These shirts tend to provide the greatest support near full descent where the bar is close to the chest and favors lifters who use wide grips. Bench press shirts are tight enough to potentially cause bruising and require assistance from one or two experienced individuals to put on in a systematic manner. Powerlifters tend to start with a basic single-layer polyester shirt and progress with training. The tighter the shirt, the greater the support gained by the lifter. Athletes need to train with and accustom themselves to bench press shirts in order to maximize bench press performance. It is recommended that powerlifters use the shirt several times during the precompetition preparation phase.

Lifting Suits

Lifting suits include super suits, briefs, and erector shirts. *Super suits* and briefs are tight compression garments used primarily by powerlifters to enhance stability and performance of the squat and deadlift. The super suits extend from the upper quadriceps area to the upper abdomen with straps that are placed over the shoulders. Greater support is gained as the lifter descends and it assists the lifter in the "up" phase through the sticking region. Some lifters estimate at least a 50- to 60-lb increase in the squat, whereas some experienced lifters estimate >150 lb. The magnitude is dependent upon quadriceps and lumbar extension strength during the top of the ROM where the suit is less supportive. Escamilla (13) stated individuals with knee wraps and suits lifted an average of ~13% more weight than without. The mean total time needed to complete a repetition was almost half a second less when suits and wraps were used (2.82 seconds with gear; 3.29 seconds without gear). Erector shirts are the opposite of the bench press shirt in that the majority of the support is in the core. Lifters use erector shirts to maintain an erect posture during the squat and deadlift.

▐ Summary Points

✔ Skeletal muscles produce greater force during ECC actions, followed by ISOM and CON actions.
✔ A relationship between muscle length and force exists where muscles are strongest near resting sarcomere lengths (where the optimal number of myofilament cross-bridges are formed) but weaken as the muscle shortens. At longer lengths, passive elements become more engaged and enhance muscle force production.
✔ When maximal intensity contractions are used, greatest muscle force is produced at slow velocities whereas less force is produced at fast velocities.
✔ Muscle architectural changes, *e.g.*, in a pennate muscle's angle of pennation and/or fascicle length, take place during training that enhances muscular strength.
✔ Strength and speed performance is based, in part, upon stature, leverage, and mechanical advantage, *e.g.*, the ratio of the moment arm of force to the moment arm of resistance.
✔ Torque production changes throughout joint ROM. An ascending-descending curve is seen with single-joint movements, an ascending curve is seen with pushing movements, and descending curves are seen with pulling movements.
✔ Friction is a critical component to force production and stability.
✔ The development of intra-abdominal pressure is important for relieving spinal stress during lifting.
✔ Various lifting accessories have been developed that can reduce the risk of injury but also can significantly enhance lifting performance.

Review Questions

1. A muscle action characteristic of muscle shortening is a(n) _____ muscle action
   a. Eccentric
   b. Concentric
   c. Isokinetic
   d. Isometric

2. The biceps brachii is an example of a(n) _____ muscle
   a. Pennate
   b. Fusiform
   c. Quadrilateral
   d. Triangular

3. The shoulder press exercise displays a(n)
   a. Ascending-descending strength curve
   b. Ascending strength curve
   c. Descending strength curve
   d. Isometric strength curve

4. During isokinetic maximal strength testing, which of the following velocities would result in the greatest muscle torque produced?
   a. $30°·s^{-1}$
   b. $90°·s^{-1}$
   c. $150°·s^{-1}$
   d. $300°·s^{-1}$

5. Muscle tension is reduced at short muscle lengths primarily because
   a. The stretch-shortening cycle is maximally engaged
   b. Actin filaments are extended excessively thereby making it difficult to reach a large number of myosin heads
   c. Actin filaments slide past each other thereby reducing the number of active sites available to bind with myosin heads
   d. No actin-myosin cross-bridges can be formed

6. The perpendicular distance between the force's line of action to the fulcrum is known as a(n)
   a. Torque
   b. Mechanical advantage
   c. Inertia
   d. Moment arm

7. Which of the following scenarios would decrease an individual's stability?
   a. Increasing the level of friction between the feet and the ground
   b. Lowering the size of the base support
   c. Lowering the center of gravity
   d. Increasing the mass of the individual

8. The branch of biomechanics that deals with the forces that cause motion is kinetics.   T F

9. Stretch-shortening cycle activity is highest in slow-twitch muscle fibers.   T F

10. Muscle hypertrophy can increase the angle of pennation at rest in a pennate muscle.   T F

11. Increasing the length of the resistance arm increases mechanical advantage.   T F

12. Choking up on a baseball bat increases the moment of inertia.   T F

References

1. Aagaard P, Andersen JL, Dyhre-Poulsen P, Letters AM, et al. A mechanism for increased contractile strength of human pennate muscle in response to strength training: changes in muscle architecture. *J Physiol*. 2001;534:613–623.
2. Abe T, Kumagai K, Brechue WF. Fascicle length of leg muscles is greater in sprinters than distance runners. *Med Sci Sports Exerc*. 2000;32:1125–1129.
3. Ackland TR, de Ridder JH. Proportionality. In: Ackland TR, Elliott BC, Bloomfield J, editors. *Applied Anatomy and Biomechanics in Sport*. 2nd ed. Champaign (IL): Human Kinetics; 2009. pp. 87–101.
4. Alegre LM, Jimenez F, Gonzalo-Orden JM, Martin-Acero R, Aguado X. Effects of dynamic resistance training on fascicle length and isometric strength. *J Sports Sci*. 2006;24:501–508.
5. Azizi E, Brainerd EL, Roberts TJ. Variable gearing in pennate muscles. *PNAS*. 2008;105:1745–1750.
6. Blazevich AJ, Gill ND, Bronks R, Newton RU. Training-specific muscle architecture adaptation after 5-wk training in athletes. *Med Sci Sports Exerc*. 2003;35:2013–2022.
7. Blazevich AJ, Gill ND, Deans N, Zhou S. Lack of human muscle architectural adaptation after short-term strength training. *Muscle Nerve*. 2007;35:78–86.
8. Blazevich AJ, Cannavan D, Coleman DR, Horne S. Influence of concentric and eccentric resistance training on architectural adaptation in human quadriceps muscles. *J Appl Physiol*. 2007;103: 1565–1575.
9. Cholewicki J, Juluru K, McGill SM. Intra-abdominal pressure mechanism for stabilizing the lumbar spine. *J Biomech*. 1999;32:13–17.
10. Cresswell AG, Grundstrom H, Thorstensson A. Observations on intra-abdominal pressure and patterns of abdominal intramuscular activity in man. *Acta Physiol Scand*. 1992;144:409–418.

11. Cresswell AG, Blake PL, Thorstensson A. The effect of an abdominal muscle training program on intra-abdominal pressure. *Scand J Rehabil Med*. 1994;26:79–86.

12. Elliott BC, Wilson GJ, Kerr GK. A biomechanical analysis of the sticking region in the bench press. *Med Sci Sports Exerc*. 1989;21:450–462.

13. Escamilla R. The use of powerlifting aids in the squat. *Powerlifting USA*. 1988;12:14–15.

14. Essendrop M, Schibye B, Hye-Knudsen C. Intra-abdominal pressure increases during exhausting back extension in humans. *Eur J Appl Physiol*. 2002;87:167–173.

15. Hamill J, Knutzen KM. *Biomechanical Basis of Human Movement*. 3rd ed. Philadelphia (PA): Wolters Kluwer Lippincott Williams & Wilkins; 2009. pp. 411–461.

16. Harman EA, Frykman PN, Clagett ER, Kraemer WJ. Intra-abdominal and intra-thoracic pressures during lifting and jumping. *Med Sci Sports Exerc*. 1988;20:195–201.

17. Harman EA, Rosenstein RM, Frykman PN, Nigro GA. Effects of a belt on intra-abdominal pressure during weight lifting. *Med Sci Sports Exerc*. 1989;21:186–190.

18. Hodges PW, Eriksson AE, Shirley D, Gandevia SC. Intra-abdominal pressure increases stiffness of the lumbar spine. *J Biomech*. 2005;38:1873–1880.

19. Kawakami Y, Abe T, Fukunaga T. Muscle-fiber pennation angles are greater in hypertrophied than in normal muscles. *J Appl Physiol*. 1993;74:2740–2744.

20. Kawakami Y, Abe T, Kuno SY, Fukunaga T. Training-induced changes in muscle architecture and specific tension. *Eur J Appl Physiol Occup Physiol*. 1995;72:37–43.

21. Kanehisa H, Nagareda H, Kawakami Y, Akima H, Masani K, Kouzaki M, et al. Effects of equivolume isometric training programs comprising medium or high resistance on muscle size and strength. *Eur J Appl Physiol*. 2002;87:112–119.

22. Kanehisa H, Muraoka Y, Kawakami Y, Fukunaga T. Fascicle arrangements of vastus lateralis and gastrocnemius muscles in highly trained soccer players and swimmers of both genders. *Int J Sports Med*. 2003;24:90–95.

23. Kearns CF, Abe T, Brechue WF. Muscle enlargement in sumo wrestlers includes increased muscle fascicle length. *Eur J Appl Physiol*. 2000;83:289–296.

24. Keeler LK, Finkelstein LH, Miller W, Fernhall B. Early-phase adaptations of traditional-speed vs. superslow resistance training on strength and aerobic capacity in sedentary individuals. *J Strength Cond Res*. 2001;15:309–314.

25. Keogh JWL, Wilson GJ, Weatherby RP. A cross-sectional comparison of different resistance training techniques in the bench press. *J Strength Cond Res*. 1999;13:247–258.

26. Kraemer WJ, Fry AC, Ratamess NA, French DN. Strength testing: development and evaluation of methodology. In: Maud PJ, Foster C, editors. *Physiological Assessments of Human Performance*. 2nd ed. Champaign (IL): Human Kinetics; 2006. pp. 119–150.

27. Kulig K, Andrews JG, Hay JG. Human strength curves. *Exerc Sports Sci Rev*. 1984;12:417–466.

28. Kumagai K, Abe T, Brechue WF, Ryushi T, Takano S, Mizuno M. Sprint performance is related to muscle fascicle length in male 100-m sprinters. *J Appl Physiol*. 2000;88:811–816.

29. Lander JE, Simonton RL, Giacobbe JKF. The effectiveness of weight-belts during the squat exercise. *Med Sci Sports Exerc*. 1990;22:117–126.

30. Lander JE, Hundley JR, Simonton RL. The effectiveness of weight-belts during multiple repetitions of the squat exercise. *Med Sci Sports Exerc*. 1992;24:603–609.

31. McArdle WD, Katch FI, Katch VL. *Exercise Physiology: Energy, Nutrition, and Human Performance*. 6th ed. Philadelphia (PA): Lippincott Williams & Wilkins; 2007.

32. McGill SM, Norman RW, Sharratt MT. The effect of an abdominal belt on trunk muscle activity and intra-abdominal pressure during squat lifts. *Ergonomics*. 1990;33:147–160.

33. Newton RU. Biomechanics of Conditioning Exercises. In: Chandler TJ, Brown LE, editors. *Conditioning for Strength and Performance*. Philadelphia, PA: Lippincott Williams & Wilkins; 2008. pp. 77–93.

34. Power K, Behm D, Cahill F, Carroll M, Young W. An acute bout of static stretching: effects on force and jumping performance. *Med Sci Sports Exerc*. 2004;36:1389–1396.

35. Schilling BK, Falvo MJ, Chiu LZF. Force-velocity, impulse-momentum relationships: Implications for efficacy of purposely slow resistance training. *J Sports Sci Med*. 2008;7:299–304.

36. Seynnes OR, de Boer M, Narici MV. Early skeletal muscle hypertrophy and architectural changes in response to high-intensity resistance training. *J Appl Physiol*. 2007;102:368–373.

37. Wilson GJ, Elliott BC, Wood GA. The effect on performance of imposing a delay during a stretch-shorten cycle movement. *Med Sci Sports Exerc*. 1991;23:364–370.

Part Two

Physiological Responses and Adaptations

Neural Adaptations to Training

After completing this chapter, you will be able to:

· Describe the central and peripheral nervous systems
· Describe the anatomy and functions of neurons
· Describe the major sites of adaptation within the brain and spinal cord
· Define a motor unit and discuss how changes in recruitment, firing rate, and firing patterns affect muscular strength and power
· Describe changes that take place at the neuromuscular junction in response to training
· Describe the roles of sensory receptors, especially Golgi tendon organs and muscle spindles
· Describe how training variables can affect the neural responses and training adaptations
· Discuss the role of the autonomic nervous system during exercise

The nervous system is extremely important for modulating acute exercise performance and the subsequent training adaptations. Nerves provide the major lines of communication between the brain and bodily tissues including skeletal muscles. They ensure the message or signal travels to the appropriate location. From a training perspective, the magnitude (or strength) of the signal is critical in determining the final output, which could be the expression of muscular strength and power. This quantity is termed *neural drive* and an increase in neural drive is critical to the individual striving to maximize performance. The increase in neural drive is thought to occur via increases in *agonist* (i.e., those major muscles involved in a specific movement or exercise) muscle recruitment, firing rate, and the timing/pattern of discharge during high-intensity muscular contractions. A reduction in inhibitory mechanisms is thought to occur. Although it is not exactly clear how these mechanisms coexist, it is clear that neural adaptations are complex and may precede changes in skeletal muscle.

FUNCTIONAL ORGANIZATION OF THE NERVOUS SYSTEM

The nervous system is one major control system contained within the human body (the other being the endocrine system). It has the ability to receive sensory information (pain, pressure, hot/cold temperatures, joint position, muscle length), integrate this information in appropriate places, and control the output or response (voluntary and involuntary) from every tissue, gland, and organ. It also controls our emotions, personality, and other cerebral functions.

The nervous system is composed of two major divisions, the central and peripheral nervous systems (Fig. 3.1). The *central nervous system* (CNS) consists of the brain and spinal cord. The *peripheral nervous system* consists of two major divisions: the sensory and motor divisions. Thirty-one pairs of spinal nerves exist and exit on the posterior (sensory) and anterior (motor) roots of the spinal cord. The *sensory nervous system* detects various stimuli and conveys this information afferently to the CNS. The *motor nervous system* consists of two major divisions: the somatic and autonomic nervous systems (ANS). The *somatic nervous system* conveys information from the CNS efferently (*e.g.*, away from CNS) to skeletal muscle ultimately leading to muscle contraction (and fatigue). The ANS consists of nerves conveying efferent information to smooth muscle, cardiac muscle, and other glands, tissues, and organs. The ANS consists of the *sympathetic* and *parasympathetic* nervous systems, both of which are essential for preparing the body for the stress of exercise and returning the body back to normal resting conditions. Training may elicit adaptations along the neuromuscular chain initiating in the higher brain centers and continuing down to the level of individual muscle fibers. Aerobic training imposes specific neural demands although the pattern of neural activation appears less complex than anaerobic, high-intensity training where high levels of muscle strength, power, and speed are required.

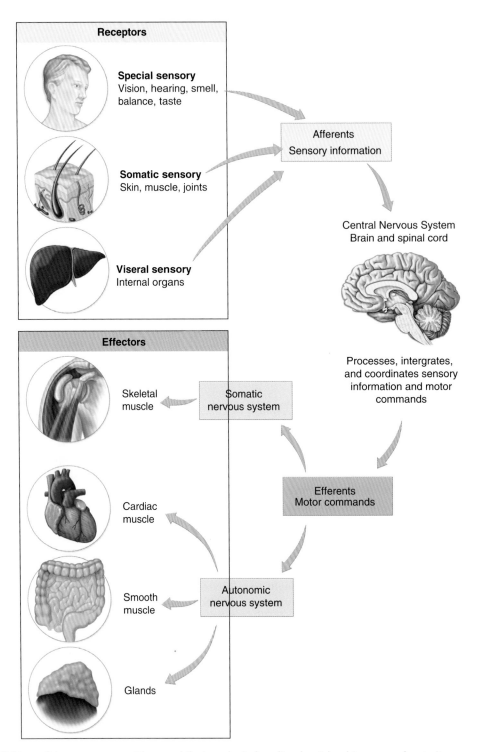

■ **FIGURE 3.1.** Divisions of the nervous system. The central (brain and spinal cord) and peripheral (sensory and motor) nervous systems are shown. (From Premkumar K. *The Massage Connection: Anatomy and Physiology*. Baltimore (MD): Lippincott Williams & Wilkins; 2004.)

NERVE CELLS

Nervous tissue comes in two forms: (a) *supporting cells* and (b) *neurons*. Supporting cells play key stability roles throughout the CNS. Neurons are the actual nerve cells with the ability to communicate with other tissues and nerves. Sensory neurons tend to be unipolar whereas

motor neurons are multipolar (Fig. 3.2). Neurons possess several key features. *Dendrites* receive input from other nerve cells. The *cell body* contains the organelles responsible for protein synthesis, transport, energy metabolism, and packaging and plays the critical role in integrating stimuli from other neurons from within the CNS to determine if and how much stimuli will make its

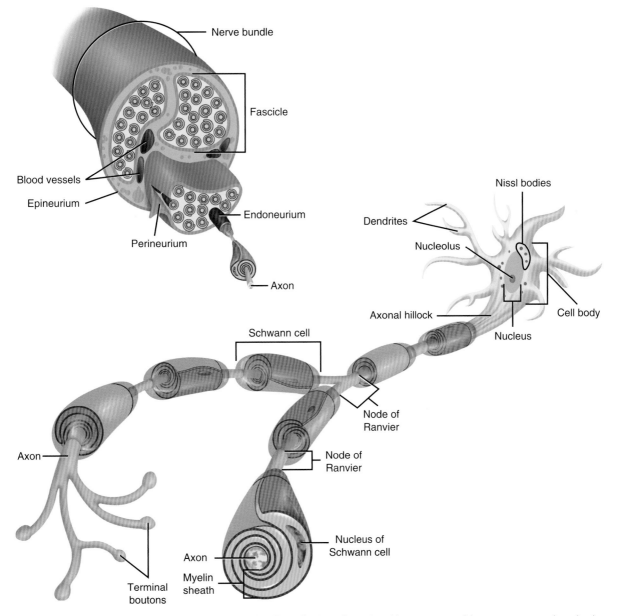

■ FIGURE 3.2. Motoneuron anatomy. The peripheral nerve bundle (collection of axons) and key structures of the motoneuron such as the dendrites, cell body, axon, axon hillock, myelin sheath, and nodes of Ranvier are shown. (From Eroschenko VP. *di Fiore's Atlas of Histology, with Functional Correlations.* 9th ed. Baltimore (MD): Lippincott Williams & Wilkins; 2000.)

way to skeletal muscle. *Axons* are long processes that are responsible for communicating with target tissues. The *axon hillock* is the area where the action potential is initiated once the critical threshold is reached. *Myelin sheath* (fatty tissue) is wrapped around the axons, which greatly increases the speed of transmission. The end of the axon branches and is known as the *presynaptic terminal*.

NEURAL COMMUNICATION

Nerves communicate with other nerves and tissue via generation of an electrical current (signal) called the *action potential*. The action potential (Fig. 3.3) consists of three major events: (a) integration, (b) propagation, and (c) neurotransmitter release. Integration occurs within the cell body (within the CNS) and determines whether or not the action potential will be sent to the target tissue. The cell body integrates charges from other neurons (excitatory, inhibitory) known as miniature end plate potentials. If the threshold voltage is reached, the action potential will travel in all-or-none fashion to the end of the nerve terminal. Propagation is brought about by ion movement (sodium and potassium) down the axon at the nodes of Ranvier via a process called *saltatory conduction*. This drives the electrical current rapidly down the axon to the terminal. The presence of myelin sheath

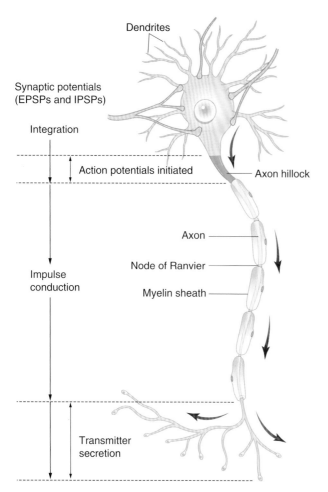

FIGURE 3.3. The action potential. The dendrites receive information from other neurons in the spinal cord. The resultant messages (excitatory post-synaptic potential [EPSP] and inhibitory post-synaptic potential [IPSP]) are integrated in the cell body and an action potential is produced if the threshold voltage is reached. The action potential is propagated down the axon to the terminal where neurotransmitters are released to allow communication with target tissues, *i.e.*, skeletal muscle. (Cohen BJ. *Medical Terminology*. 4th ed. Philadelphia (PA): Lippincott Williams & Wilkins; 2003.)

greatly accelerates this process. At the nerve terminal, neurotransmitters (chemical signaling molecules) are released, thereby allowing communication to take place with the target tissue. This entire process occurs at a very fast speed, which enables several action potentials to be conducted in a second.

HIGHER BRAIN CENTERS

The brain contains billions of neurons each with the ability to communicate with nearly 10,000 others (Fig. 3.4). Ultimately, the brain controls nearly all aspects of human bodily function from psychological/emotional factors to motor performance. Although complete discussion of the brain is beyond the scope of this text, some critical areas need to be mentioned because they serve as potential sites of adaptations to training. The *brainstem* (consisting of

the medulla oblongata, midbrain, pons, and reticular formation) contains neuronal centers that control cardiac heart rate and force of contraction, blood pressure, blood vessel diameter, breathing, hearing, vision, sleep, and consciousness. The *diencephalon* (consisting of the thalamus, hypothalamus, and pineal body or epithalamus) is the major relay area of the brain (thalamus) and control center for sleep (pineal body). The *hypothalamus* is the major link between the nervous and endocrine systems because it is an endocrine gland under neural control. It releases several hormones that either cause or inhibit the release of hormones from the anterior pituitary, ultimately controlling *homeostasis*, autonomic control, body temperature, emotions, and essentially most functions within the body. The *cerebrum* is the largest part of the brain, with 75% of the neurons within the nervous system located in the outermost region of the cerebrum known as the *cerebral cortex*. Although many areas of the cerebral cortex have important functions, critical areas include the *primary sensory area* (where sensory information is integrated), the *premotor cortex* (where a voluntary muscle contraction begins and also a memory bank for skilled motor activities), and the *primary motor cortex* (where voluntary muscle contraction is controlled). The *cerebellum* integrates sensory information and coordinates skeletal muscle activity, *e.g.*, it provides a blueprint of how the motor skill should be performed. Lastly, the *basal ganglia* is involved with planning and control of muscle function, posture, and controlling unwanted movements.

The ability to increase neural output begins in the higher brain centers, *i.e.*, motor cortex, with the volitional intent to produce high levels of force and power. Studies have shown that neural activity increases in the primary motor cortex as force increases (13). Motor learning results in functional organization of the cerebral cortex. In fact, visualization training (*i.e.*, performing mental contractions or visualizing lifting weights without actually lifting them) has been shown to result in significant strength increases in untrained individuals (46,63). These studies suggest that adaptations in higher brain centers may result in strength gain. Cerebral adaptations are paramount for enhanced coordination, motor learning, skill acquisition, strength, power, and speed.

DESCENDING CORTICOSPINAL TRACTS

The descending corticospinal (or *pyramidal*) tracts are a large collection of axons linking the cerebral cortex to the spinal cord. The motor pathway is characterized by neurons in the brain (primarily in the motor areas) forming synapses with other nerves that eventually make their way down the spinal cord to the exact anterior root of exit for innervation of skeletal muscle. A substantial proportion of potential neural changes take place in the spinal cord along the descending corticospinal tracts. Untrained individuals display limited ability to maximally recruit

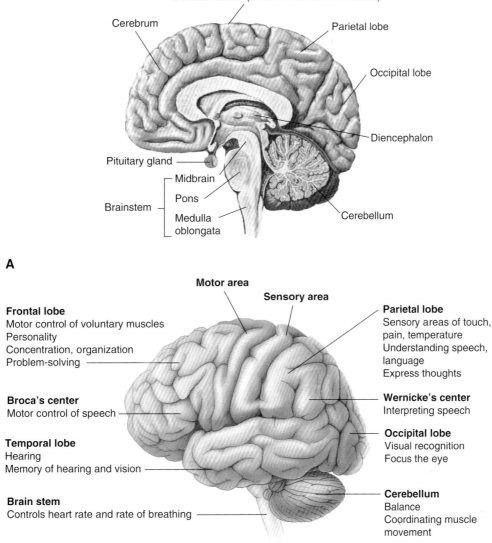

■ **FIGURE 3.4.** The brain. **A** shows the anatomy of the brain. Key areas of the brain such as the medulla oblongata, cerebrum, cerebellum, cerebral cortex, diencephalon, primary motor area, and sensory area are identified. (From Bickley LS, Szilagyi P. *Bates' Guide to Physical Examination and History Taking*. 8th ed. Philadelphia (PA): Lippincott Williams & Wilkins; 2003.) **B** shows the various areas of the brain and their control over body systems and function.

all of their muscle fibers. A study by Adams et al. (4) showed that only 71% of muscle mass was activated during maximal effort in untrained individuals. It is believed that a limitation in this central drive reduces strength and power and much of the inhibition originates from these descending corticospinal tracts (7). However, training can greatly reduce this deficit (9,42,45), thereby showing a greater potential to recruit a larger percent of one's muscle mass with training.

MOTOR UNITS

The functional unit of the nervous system is the *motor unit*. A motor unit consists of a single alpha motor nerve

and all of the muscle fibers it innervates (Fig. 3.5). Cell bodies and dendrites are located within the spinal cord (to receive excitatory and inhibitory signals from other neurons), whereas axons extend beyond the spinal cord and innervate skeletal muscles in the periphery. Motor neurons may innervate only a few muscle fibers for small muscles (for greater coordination and control) and >1,000 for large trunk and limb muscles (for greater force and power). Greater force is produced when excitatory signals increase, inhibitory signals decrease, or a combination of both. When maximal force and power is desired from a muscle, all available motor units must be activated. This generally results from an increase in recruitment, rate of firing, synchronization of firing, or a combination of these factors.

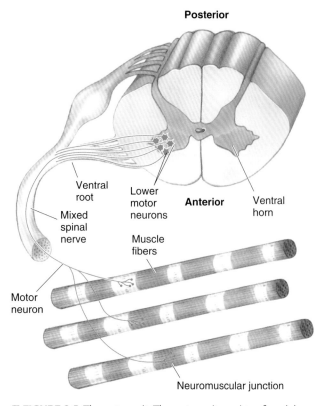

Posterior

Ventral root
Lower motor neurons
Anterior
Ventral horn
Mixed spinal nerve
Muscle fibers
Motor neuron
Neuromuscular junction

■ **FIGURE 3.5.** The motor unit. The motor unit consists of an alpha motoneuron and all of the muscle fibers it innervates. (From Bear M, Conner B, Paradiso M. *Neuroscience, Exploring the Brain*. 2nd ed. Baltimore (MD): Lippincott Williams and Wilkins; 2000.)

RECRUITMENT

Recruitment refers to the voluntary activation of motor units during effort. Motor units are recruited and decruited in an orderly progression based on the *size principle* (Fig. 3.6), which states that motor units are recruited in succession from smaller (slow-twitch [ST] or type I) to larger (fast-twitch [FT] or type II) units based on each activation threshold and firing rate (28). Small units are recruited first for more intricate control and larger units are recruited later to supply substantial force for high-intensity contractions. The activation threshold is the most critical determinant of motor unit recruitment especially among units of similar size. Force and power production may vary greatly because most muscles contain a range of type I and II motor units. Thus, type II motor units are not recruited unless there is a high force, power, or speed requirement. Interestingly, the ability for type II motor units for recruitment is based on previous activation history. Once a motor unit is recruited, less activation is needed for it to be rerecruited (17). This has important ramifications for acute strength and power performance as type II motor units are more readily recruited. Likewise, motor units are decruited (inactivated) in the reverse order where type II motor units relax first.

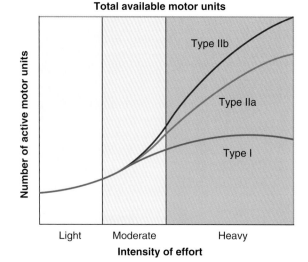

Total available motor units

Type IIb
Type IIa
Type I

Number of active motor units

Light   Moderate   Heavy
Intensity of effort

■ **FIGURE 3.6.** The size principle. Motor units are recruited under most conditions based on their size where smaller (ST) units are recruited first and larger (FT) units may be recruited later if a substantial amount of force or power is required. (From McArdle WD, Katch FI, Katch VL. *Exercise Physiology: Nutrition, Energy, and Human Performance.* 7th ed. Baltimore (MD): Lippincott Williams & Wilkins; 2010.)

Selective Recruitment

Under normal conditions, 84%–90% of motor units are recruited in accordance with the size principle (57). However, variations in recruitment order exist. *Selective recruitment*, or the preferential recruitment of type II motor units, can occur during change in direction of exerted forces (59) and explosive muscle actions (40). These variations in recruitment order may benefit high-velocity power training where activation of type II motor units can provide the needed explosive bursts of power. Inhibition of type I motor units during explosive exercise can be beneficial because it allows the individual to preferentially recruit type II units.

Muscle Mass Activation

The amount of muscle mass activated to lift a specific amount of weight depends on the magnitude of muscle hypertrophy. A training adaptation that takes place is that the level of muscle mass activation may decrease when muscle size increases. A larger muscle does not require as much neural activation to lift a standard weight as it did before the growth took place (because the muscle fibers themselves are larger and stronger and therefore require less stimuli to produce a certain level of force). A landmark study by Ploutz et al. (44) showed that less quadriceps muscle tissue was activated to lift a standard pretraining load after 9 weeks of resistance training (RT) (3–6 sets × 12 reps) that resulted in a 5% increase in muscle size. Thus, progressive overload during training is mandatory in order to continually activate an optimal amount of muscle mass.

Myths & Misconceptions

Lifting Light Weights Optimally Stimulates Muscle Fiber Activation

Some have postulated that lifting light weights can maximally recruit all available motor units during an exercise. However, research has shown that motor unit recruitment is intensity dependent. Greater numbers of muscle fibers are recruited only when needed and the need is high during the lifting of heavy weights. Thus, heavy RT is required to maximally recruit type II motor units.

Postactivation Potentiation

Activated motor units stay facilitated for a period of time following use. Maximal or near-maximal muscle contractions elicit a *postactivation potentiation* (PAP) for subsequent muscle contractions occurring within several seconds to a few minutes (25,27). That is, when an individual performs a moderately high to high-intensity contraction, there is a window of time following where it is easier to recruit type II motor units. During this time, lifting a certain amount of weight may feel lighter or jumping a certain height may seem easier. Ultimately, acute strength and power may be enhanced (16). PAP is more prominent in explosive power athletes (8), although endurance athletes demonstrate PAP (26). Some examples of how PAP can be used to enhance athletic performance include

1. swinging a weighted bat prior to stepping in the batter's box for a baseball of softball player;
2. performing a few sets of squats prior to testing for max vertical jump performance (29);
3. using a weighted vest as part of a warm-up prior to speed or agility events (14); and
4. including a few sets of weight training as a warm-up prior to sports performance.

PAP also serves as a mechanism of training to be targeted for advanced techniques such as complex training (discussed later in this book).

Case Study 3.1

Steve is an athlete who is preparing to maximally test his vertical jump. He was told he might enhance his vertical jump height by utilizing a loaded warm-up. In this case, the loaded warm-up refers to a scenario where PAP can be used to augment performance. Steve approaches you for advice on how he can design a prejump warm-up to perform better.

Question for Consideration: **What would you advise him to do?**

FIRING RATE

Firing rate refers to the number of times per second a motor unit discharges. Firing rate is affected by the nerve's conduction velocity as conduction velocities are higher in type II motor units. Conduction velocity tends to be higher in power athletes compared with endurance athletes (31) possibly due to a larger contingent of type II motor units in power athletes. At rest, motor units have low firing rates; however, a positive relationship exists between the amount of force produced and firing rate (37,45). The role of increasing firing rate (vs. recruitment) depends on muscle size as some, especially smaller muscles, rely more on increasing rate to enhance force and power production, whereas larger muscles rely more on recruitment (10) and may depend upon the muscle action, *i.e.*, dynamic versus isometric (45). Anaerobic training enhances the firing rates of recruited motor units (1,2,61). High firing rates at the onset of ballistic muscle contraction are especially critical to increasing the rate of force development (1).

MOTOR UNIT SYNCHRONIZATION

Synchronization occurs when two or more motor units fire at fixed time intervals. Although motor units typically fire asynchronously, it is thought motor synchronization may be advantageous for bursts of strength or power needed in a short period of time. Greater motor unit synchronization has been shown following RT (15,36,54). Although it is unclear as to the exact role synchronization plays during training, the bursts of grouped motor unit discharges may be advantageous for the timing of force production and may not be advantageous for the overall level of force produced.

ANTAGONIST MUSCLE ACTIVATION

The cocontraction of *antagonist* muscles during movement increases joint stability, movement coordination, and reduces the risk of injury. However, there are occasions when cocontraction can be counterproductive because it may counteract the effects of agonist muscles. Muscle group, velocity and type of muscle action, intensity, joint position, and injury status affect the magnitude of antagonist cocontraction (49). Neural adaptations of antagonist musculature may take place with training that benefit performance enhancement. For sprint or plyometric training, the timing of coactivation may change, *i.e.*, it is higher during the precontact phase with the ground but less during propulsion or acceleration phases (32). During RT, studies have shown no change in antagonist cocontractions (2,53) and reductions (6,24,42). Thus, cocontraction of antagonist musculature appears to be a mechanism in place when there is a lack of familiarity with the exercise and the magnitude of decrease may be minor compared with the improvements in strength.

COMMUNICATION WITH SKELETAL MUSCLE: THE NEUROMUSCULAR JUNCTION

The nerve and muscle are not continuous, meaning there is a gap between the two (Fig. 3.7). A chemical messenger must be released in order for the action potential

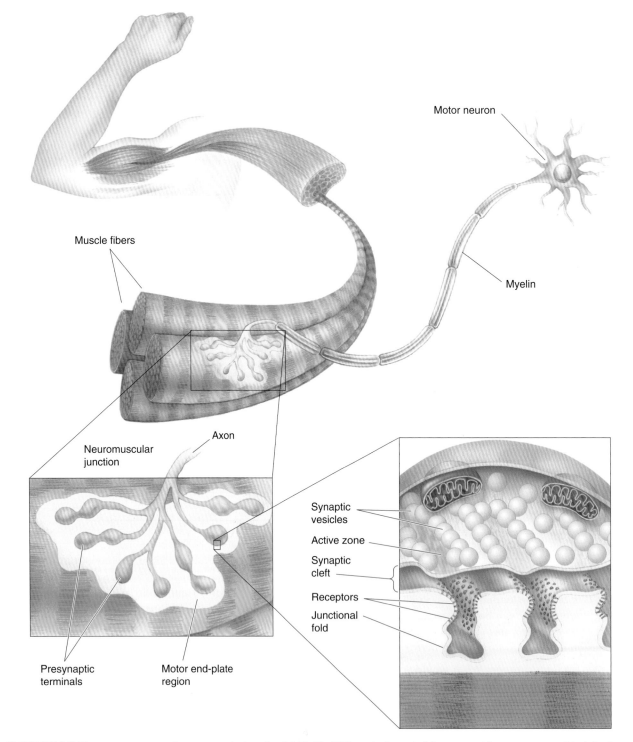

■ FIGURE 3.7. The motor neuron and neuromuscular junction (NMJ). The NMJ marks the end of the axon and forms a synapse with skeletal muscle. Synaptic vesicles migrate to the terminal membrane and release neurotransmitters into the synaptic cleft via exocytosis where they bind to receptors on the surface of the sarcolemma membrane (From Bear MF, Connors BW, Paradiso MA. *Neuroscience, Exploring the Brain*. 2nd ed. Baltimore (MD): Lippincott Williams & Wilkins; 2001.)

to reach the muscle. The chemical messenger is called a *neurotransmitter*, and there are several excitatory and inhibitory neurotransmitters found at synapses between neurons and other neurons, tissues, and organs. The key neurotransmitter released between a motor nerve and skeletal muscle is *acetylcholine*. When the action potential reaches the terminal, neurotransmitters are ultimately released into the space (*cleft*) where they bind to specific receptors on muscle and spread the action potential to muscle. The neuromuscular junction (NMJ) refers to the nerve terminal, space, and muscle fiber membrane.

Critical to training adaptations is the nerve terminal (also called *presynaptic terminal*). The NMJ in type I motor units tends to be less complex than type II (56), which is not surprising since type II units are advantageous for strength and power. Aerobic training results in greater presynaptic nerve terminal area, increased number of nerve terminal branches, increased perimeter of nerve terminal, and increased average length of individual nerve terminals (11). However, NMJ changes are much more pronounced during high-intensity training because the terminal branches become more dispersed, longer, asymmetrical, and irregularly shaped (11). RT may result in greater terminal area and greater dispersion of acetylcholine receptors (12). These changes in the NMJ are conducive to enhanced neural transmission to skeletal muscle, which increases force and power production.

SENSORY NERVOUS SYSTEM

The sensory nervous system contains receptors that send information to the CNS via afferent pathways. Sensory receptors pick up various stimuli such as pain, hot/cold temperatures, and pressure. Proprioceptors are important because they pick up information concerning muscle length, joint position, movement, and tension. Although several types of sensory receptors function within the human body, two proprioceptors critical to exercise and sports performance are the Golgi tendon organs (GTOs) and muscle spindles.

GOLGI TENDON ORGANS

GTOs are proprioceptors located at the muscle-tendon junction (Fig. 3.8). Because of their location, their primary role is to convey information regarding muscle tension to the CNS. As muscle tension increases, so does the amount of stretch to the GTOs. Once a threshold level of tension is attained, GTO activity increases greatly and its response is to cause agonist muscle relaxation (or fatigue) and antagonist muscle excitation. GTOs may be considered to be a defense mechanism to protect the body from excessive damage. This may help explain why untrained individuals are only able to voluntarily recruit a smaller portion of their muscle mass in large muscle groups. However, their role inhibits performance to some

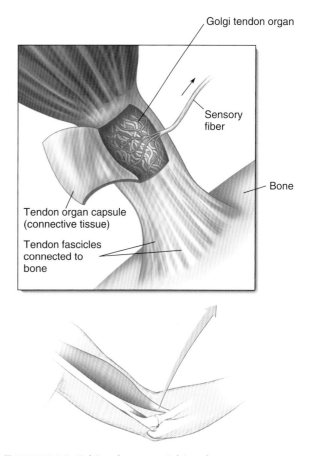

FIGURE 3.8. Golgi tendon organ. Golgi tendon organs are located in the muscle-tendon junction and respond to tension. (From Premkumar K. *The Massage Connection: Anatomy and Physiology.* Baltimore (MD): Lippincott Williams & Wilkins; 2004.)

extent. Although not sufficiently studied, many experts believe that gradual training reduces GTO sensitivity, which enables many neural adaptations to take place, *e.g.*, recruitment, rate, synchronization, and less antagonist cocontraction.

MUSCLE SPINDLES

Muscle spindles are proprioceptors (Fig. 3.9) located within muscle fibers (*i.e.*, intrafusal fibers). They consist of two components called nuclear chain and nuclear bag fibers. Muscle spindles respond to the magnitude of change in muscle length, the rate of change of length, and convey information to the CNS regarding static changes in muscle length or joint angle. Unlike GTOs, muscle spindles enhance human performance. Muscle spindles are critical because they initiate the stretch reflex. The *stretch reflex* is a monosynaptic reflex (a sensory nerve directly synapses with motor nerve in spinal cord) where muscle force production is enhanced when the muscle is previously stretched. A reflex itself is an involuntary response and reflects a time component because more force is produced in a short period of time. When a muscle is stretched, information is sent from the muscle

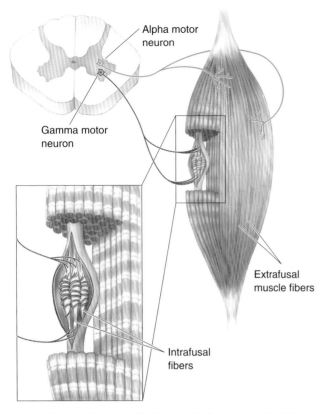

■ FIGURE 3.9. Muscle spindle. Muscle spindles are located within muscle fibers and respond to changes in length. (From Bear MF, Connors BW, Paradiso MA. *Neuroscience, Exploring the Brain.* 2nd ed. Baltimore (MD): Lippincott Williams & Wilkins; 2001.)

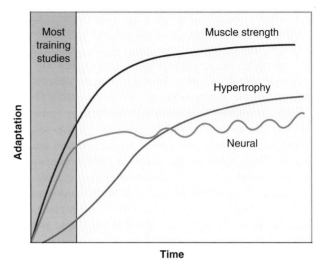

■ FIGURE 3.10. Contributions of neural and hypertrophic adaptations to resistance training. Neural adaptations predominate as the major mechanism for strength increases early in training. Muscle hypertrophy takes places after the first few weeks of training and becomes the major mechanism for further strength increases as training advances. The shaded area denotes a time frame examined by most studies. Thus, the remaining segment is theoretical and based partly on some cross-sectional data. It appears that there is interplay between neural and hypertrophic factors during advanced RT. That is, muscle hypertrophy lessens the need for optimal neural activation unless progressive overload is applied. Progressive overload in the form of high intensity loading and/or fast lifting velocities are needed to optimally stimulate the nervous system with advanced training. (Adapted with permission from Sale DG. Neural adaptations to strength training. In: Komi PV, editor. *Strength and Power in Sport,* 2nd ed. Malden (MA): Blackwell Science; 2003. pp. 281–314.)

spindles to the spinal cord where a potent muscular response ensues. The stretch reflex enhances muscular performance, efficiency, and is trainable.

Reflex Potentiation

Training can enhance reflex potentiation or the efficacy of the stretch reflex. RT can increase reflex potentiation by 15%–55% (3,30,50,52). Strength-trained athletes (weightlifters, bodybuilders) have greater reflex potentiation in the soleus muscle compared to untrained individuals (51). Enhanced reflex potentiation is associated with increases in rate of force development and power (30).

TRAINING STUDIES

Most studies examining changes in neural function with training have used *electromyography* (EMG). EMG quantifies the level of electrical activity to a skeletal muscle. An increase in EMG reflects greater neural activation; however, the precise mechanism(s) (increased recruitment, rate, synchronization, Golgi tendon inhibition) cannot be determined using surface EMG. Most studies have shown increases in EMG with some showing no

change following RT despite increases in muscle strength of >70% in some studies (47). Training status is critical. Training is initially characterized by neural adaptations, *e.g.*, increased motor learning and coordination (41,48). When muscle hypertrophy takes place, declines in EMG are seen (38) because muscle fibers are capable of providing more tension. Beyond this point, it has been suggested that training exhibits an interplay between neural and hypertrophic mechanisms (Fig. 3.10) for strength and power improvements (49). That is, lifters must specifically stress the nervous system in training when hypertrophy occurs, *i.e.*, by lifting heavier weights or fast lifting velocities. Advanced weightlifters show limited potential for further neural adaptations over the course of 1 year (20).

Case Study 3.2

William is a 20-year-old, healthy man who has no previous weight training experience. He begins a progressive weight training program and he realizes his strength has improved over the course of his first six workouts. For example, his bench press weight increased 10 lb and he is now performing

12 reps on the bent-over row with a weight he initially was only able to lift for 8 reps. William is amazed yet surprised he got stronger without any noticeable changes in muscle size.

Questions for Consideration: What mechanisms may have accounted for William's strength increases in the absence of noticeable muscle growth?

The training program dictates the pattern of adaptation. EMG, or neural activation, has been shown

- To be higher for high-intensity muscular effort versus low-intensity muscular effort (18).
- To be higher during ballistic or explosive resistance exercise compared to slower velocities (18,19,33).
- To be higher for concentric (CON) versus eccentric (ECC) muscle actions when matched for intensity (34).

Myths & Misconceptions

Performing Repetitions with Light to Moderate Loading at an Intentionally Slow Velocity Yields Similar Neuromuscular Responses to Heavier Loading at Moderate to Fast Velocities

Some have stated that performing an intentionally slow lifting velocity (longer than 3–5-s CON and ECC phases) produces similar neuromuscular responses to either heavier loading with a moderate velocity (1–2-s CON and ECC phases) or lighter loading with explosive velocity (<1-s CON and ECC phases). However, this is not the case. Intentionally slowing the repetition velocity limits motor unit recruitment and results in less muscular force and power. This was shown in a study by Keogh et al. (33). They compared several aspects of bench press performance. Three comparisons were made between standard heavy weight training (HWT; 6 reps performed with a 6 RM load or 80%–85% of 1 RM), super-slow (SS) training (5-s CON phase, 5-s ECC phase with 55% of 1 RM for 5–6 reps), and ballistic bench press (BBP) training (6 explosive reps where the bar was released at the end of each repetition with 30% of 1 RM). It is important to note that in order to perform the SS reps in 10 seconds, a significant weight reduction was needed. They measured force and power characteristics as well as EMG activity of the pectoralis major and triceps brachii muscles. Figure 3.11 shows the EMG results during the CON muscle actions from this study. For the pectoralis major muscle, HWT produced much higher EMG activity than SS and BBP. For the triceps brachii muscle, HWT and BBP produced much higher EMG than SS. These results showed that for each muscle, HWT produced much greater neural activation than SS and for the triceps brachii, ballistic reps with less weight produced higher neural activation than SS. Therefore, faster lifting velocities produce a greater neural response to resistance exercise than intentionally slow velocities.

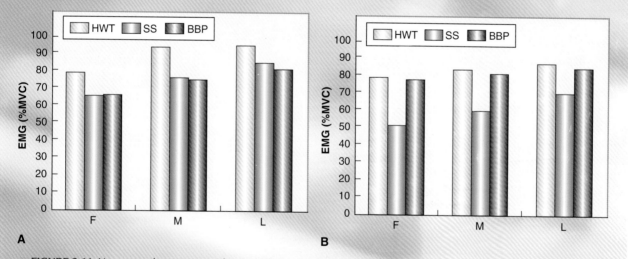

FIGURE 3.11. Neuromuscular responses to heavy weight training (HWT), super slow training (SS), and ballistic bench press training (BBP). **A:** Pectoralis major EMG data (expressed as a percent of maximal voluntary effort). **B:** Triceps brachii EMG data (expressed as a percent of maximal voluntary effort). *F,* first repetition; *M,* middle repetition; *L,* last repetition. (Adapted with permission from Keogh JWL, Wilson GJ, Weatherby RP. A cross-sectional comparison of different resistance training techniques in the bench press. *J Strength Cond Res.* 1999;13:247–258.)

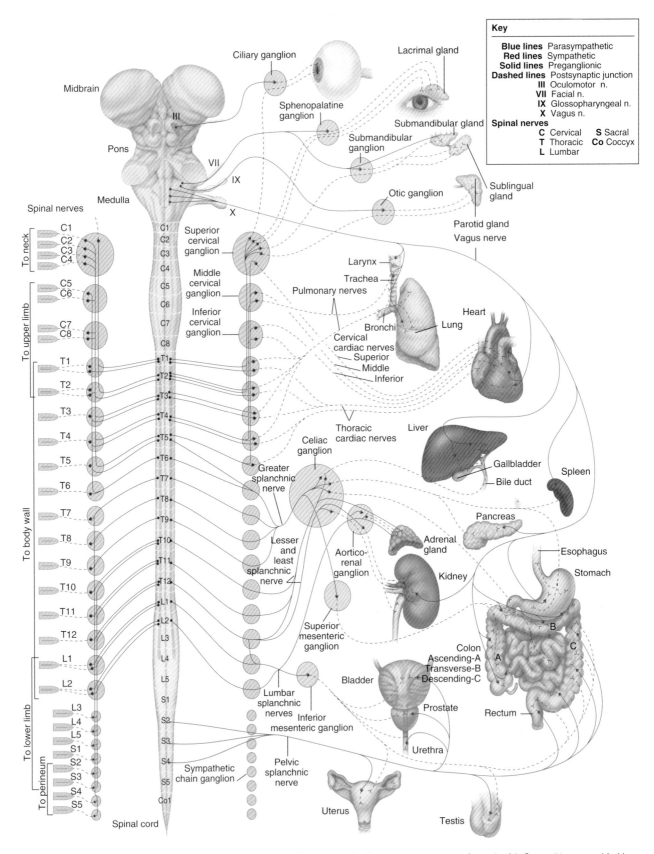

FIGURE 3.12. Autonomic nervous system. The sympathetic and parasympathetic nervous systems are shown in this figure. (Asset provided by Anatomical Chart Co.)

- To increase as fatigue ensues in CON and ECC muscle actions during a submaximal resistance exercise set (33,43,60).
- To be reduced following a workout compared to preworkout, *e.g.*, a fatigue-induced state from training (5).
- To be lower for high-volume, high-intensity training (*i.e.*, overreaching) but return to baseline during "tapering" (*i.e.*, reduced training volume) (21,22).
- To be reduced during periods of detraining (18).

Collectively, these studies show that EMG increases or is higher when the intensity is high, the lifting velocity is fast, and CON muscle actions are used. Training programs targeting the nervous system are ones that emphasize heavy weight lifting and explosive movements such as plyometrics, ballistic RT, speed, and agility training. Fatigue is another factor affecting neural responses and adaptations to training. With submaximal exercise (*e.g.*, performing a 10-repetition set), EMG increases as the set progresses. This is thought to reflect greater motor unit recruitment to replace fatigued units as the set duration increases. However, the fatigue associated with a complete workout is high and results in a lower EMG response if assessed immediately after the workout ends. Fatigue limits motor unit activation to some extent; subsequently, EMG responses are lower. Therefore, recovery after a workout is critical before the next training session to restore maximal neural function.

UNILATERAL VERSUS BILATERAL TRAINING

Training with one or two limbs simultaneously affects neural adaptations to training. *Cross education* refers to strength and endurance gained in the nontrained limb during unilateral training. Several studies have shown an average strength increase of up to 22% with a mean increase of nearly 8% compared to pretraining in the untrained limb (39). The strength increase is accompanied by greater EMG activity in the trained and nontrained limbs (41,55,62); endurance may increase in the untrained limb as well (64). The practical ramification is that training only one limb at a time induces a novel stimulus to the nervous system. Adaptations are carried over to the opposite limb. Unilateral training may be useful in improving functional performance and very useful for injured individuals because a partial training effect may be gained by the injured (nontrained) limb during a time of immobilization or greatly reduced activity.

In reference to unilateral and bilateral training, a bilateral deficit has been shown. The *bilateral deficit*

refers to the maximal force produced by both limbs contracting bilaterally (together) is smaller than the sum of the limbs contracting unilaterally. Unilateral training increases unilateral strength to a greater extent and bilateral training increases bilateral strength to a greater extent with a corresponding greater specific EMG response (23,35,58). The bilateral deficit is seen especially in lesser-trained individuals because it is reduced with bilateral training. Practically, it is important to include unilateral and bilateral exercises in a training program.

AUTONOMIC NERVOUS SYSTEM

The ANS is a branch of the peripheral nervous system highly involved in bodily control (Fig. 3.12). Target tissues of autonomic nerves include cardiac muscle, smooth muscle, and other glands, organs, and tissues. The ANS controls such functions such as heart rate and force of contraction, respiration rate, digestion, blood pressure and flow, and fuel mobilization, to name a few. The sympathetic branch (also called the "fight or flight" system) prepares the body for stress or exercise by increasing heart rate and force of contraction, increasing breathing rate, increasing blood glucose and muscle glycogen breakdown, fat mobilization, increasing blood pressure, redirecting blood flow toward skeletal muscle, and pupil dilation for enhanced performance. The parasympathetic branch has the opposite effect by returning the body back to normal (or *homeostasis*). Several facets of the ANS are enhanced through aerobic and anaerobic training, as well as the target tissues and organs (several of which are discussed in other chapters). Ultimately, these changes enhance acute exercise performance and increase recovery post exercise.

■ Summary Points

✔ Exercise training may elicit adaptations along the neuromuscular chain initiating in the higher brain centers and continuing down to the level of individual muscle fibers.

✔ Cerebral adaptations are important for technique enhancement, coordination, and strength and power increases.

✔ Greater motor unit recruitment, firing rates, synchronization, reflex potentiation, and decreased Golgi tendon organ sensitivity enhance muscular strength, power, speed, and performance.

✔ Neural activation is highest during high-intensity and ballistic muscular efforts and is lower during times of overreaching and detraining.

Review Questions

1. An athlete is performing a 1 RM bench press to evaluate the off-season conditioning program. His previous best was 280 lb. After a warm-up, he attempts 315 lb and is unable to lift the weight. Which of the following mechanisms was most responsible for this failure?
   a. Increase in muscle spindle activity
   b. Increase in Golgi tendon organ activity
   c. Decrease in Golgi tendon organ activity
   d. Decrease in antagonist muscle cocontraction

2. The preferential activation of FT motor units during explosive exercise is known as
   a. Action potential
   b. Motor unit synchronization
   c. Postactivation potentiation
   d. Selective recruitment

3. The part of the neuron that receives information from other neurons is a
   a. Cell body
   b. Dendrite
   c. Axon
   d. Myelin sheath

4. After 10 weeks of RT, an athlete comes into the lab and performs an EMG assessment during a strength test. His strength increases and subsequently his EMG increases as well. The increase in EMG may have resulted from
   a. Greater motor unit recruitment
   b. Higher firing rates
   c. Motor unit synchronization
   d. All of the above

5. Unilateral training that results in a strength increase in the nontrained limb is known as
   a. Motor unit
   b. Bilateral deficit
   c. Cross education
   d. Size principle

6. Which of the following is true regarding EMG changes/responses to training?
   a. EMG is higher during low- versus high-intensity contractions
   b. EMG does not change over the course of a resistance exercise set
   c. EMG is higher during fast versus intentionally slow velocity contractions (using a standard load)
   d. EMG is higher during ECC versus CON muscle actions (using a standard load)

7. The CNS consists of the brain and spinal cord.   T F

8. Based on the size principle, FT motor units are recruited before ST motor units.   T F

9. The parasympathetic nervous system helps prepare the body for the stress of exercise by increasing heart rate, blood pressure, and skeletal muscle force of contraction.   T F

10. The bilateral deficit refers to the maximal force produced by both limbs contracting together is smaller than the sum of the limbs contracting individually.   T F

11. Muscle hypertrophy increases the need to recruit additional motor units in order to lift a standard amount of weight.   T F

12. Cocontraction of antagonist skeletal muscles is an important mechanism to increase joint stability and reduce the risk of injury.   T F

References

1. Aagaard P. Training-induced changes in neural function. *Exerc Sports Sci Rev.* 2003;31:61–67.
2. Aagaard P, Simonsen EB, Andersen JL, Magnusson P, Dyhre-Poulsen P. Increased rate of force development and neural drive of human skeletal muscle following resistance training. *J Appl Physiol.* 2002;93:1318–1326.
3. Aagaard P, Simonsen EB, Andersen JL, Magnusson P, Dyhre-Poulsen P. Neural adaptation to resistance training: changes in evoked V-wave and H-reflex responses. *J Appl Physiol.* 2002; 92:2309–2318.
4. Adams GR, Harris RT, Woodard D, Dudley G. Mapping of electrical muscle stimulation using MRI. *J Appl Physiol.* 1993;74:532–537.
5. Benson C, Docherty D, Brandenburg J. Acute neuromuscular responses to resistance training performed at different loads. *J Sci Med Sport.* 2006;9:135–142.
6. Carolan B, Cafarelli E. Adaptations in coactivation after isometric resistance training. *J Appl Physiol.* 1992;73:911–917.
7. Carroll TJ, Riek S, Carson RG. The sites of neural adaptation induced by resistance training in humans. *J Physiol.* 2002;544: 641–652.

8. Chiu LZ, Fry AC, Weiss LW, Schilling BK, Brown LE, Smith SL. Postactivation potentiation response in athletic and recreationally trained individuals. *J Strength Cond Res.* 2003;17:671–677.

9. Del Olmo MF, Reimunde P, Viana O, Acero RM, Cudeiro J. Chronic neural adaptation induced by long-term resistance training in humans. *Eur J Appl Physiol.* 2006;96:722–728.

10. DeLuca CJ, LeFever RS, McCue MP, Xenakis AP. Behaviour of human motor units in different muscles during linearly varying contractions. *J Physiol.* 1982;329:113–128.

11. Deschenes MR, Maresh CM, Crivello JF, Armstrong LE, Kraemer WJ, Covault J. The effects of exercise training of different intensities on neuromuscular junction morphology. *J Neurocytol.* 1993; 22:603–615.

12. Deschenes MR, Judelson DA, Kraemer WJ, et al. Effects of resistance training on neuromuscular junction morphology. *Muscle Nerve.* 2000;23:1576–1581.

13. Dettmers C, Ridding MC, Stephan KM, et al. Comparison of regional cerebral blood flow with transcranial magnetic stimulation at different forces. *J Appl Physiol.* 1996;81:596–603.

14. Faigenbaum AD, McFarland JE, Schwerdtman JA, Ratamess NA, Kang J, Hoffman JR. Dynamic warm-up protocols, with and without a weighted vest, and fitness performance in high school female athletes. *J Athl Train.* 2006;41:357–363.

15. Felici F, Rosponi A, Sbriccoli P, Filligoi C, Fattorini L, Marchetti M. Linear and non-linear analysis of surface electromyograms in weightlifters. *Eur J Appl Physiol.* 2001;84:337–342.

16. French DN, Kraemer WJ, Cooke CB. Changes in dynamic exercise performance following a sequence of preconditioning isometric muscle actions. *J Strength Cond Res.* 2003;17:678–685.

17. Gorassini M, Yang JF, Siu M, Bennett DJ. Intrinsic activation of human motor units: reduction of motor unit recruitment thresholds by repeated contractions. *J Neurophysiol.* 2002;87: 1859–1866.

18. Häkkinen K, Alen M, Komi PV. Changes in isometric force-and relaxation-time, electromyographic and muscle fibre characteristics of human skeletal muscle during strength training and detraining. *Acta Physiol Scand.* 1985;125:573–585.

19. Häkkinen K, Komi PV, Alen M. Effect of explosive type strength training on isometric force- and relaxation-time, electromyographic and muscle fibre characteristics of leg extensor muscles. *Acta Physiol Scand.* 1985;125:587–600.

20. Häkkinen K, Komi PV, Alen M, Kauhanen H. EMG, muscle fibre and force production characteristics during a 1 year training period in elite weight-lifters. *Eur J Appl Physiol.* 1987;56:419–427.

21. Häkkinen K, Kauhanen H. Daily changes in neural activation, force-time and relaxation-time characteristics in athletes during very intense training for one week. *Electromyogr Clin Neurophysiol.* 1989;29:243–249.

22. Häkkinen K, Kallinen M, Komi PV, Kauhanen H. Neuromuscular adaptations during short-term "normal" and reduced training periods in strength athletes. *Electromyogr Clin Neurophysiol.* 1991; 31:35–42.

23. Häkkinen K, Kallinen M, Linnamo V, Pastinen UM, Newton RU, Kraemer WJ. Neuromuscular adaptations during bilateral versus unilateral strength training in middle-aged and elderly men and women. *Acta Physiol Scand.* 1996;158:77–88.

24. Häkkinen K, Kallinen M, Izquierdo M, et al. Changes in agonist-antagonist EMG, muscle CSA, and force during strength training in middle-aged and older people. *J Appl Physiol.* 1998;84: 1341–1349.

25. Hamada T, Sale DG, MacDougall JD, Tarnopolsky MA. Postactivation potentiation, fiber type, and twitch contraction time in human knee extensor muscles. *J Appl Physiol.* 2000;88: 2131–2137.

26. Hamada T, Sale DG, MacDougall JD. Postactivation potentiation in endurance-trained male athletes. *Med Sci Sports Exerc.* 2000; 32:403–411.

27. Hamada T, Sale DG, MacDougall JD, Tarnopolsky MA. Interaction of fibre type, potentiation and fatigue in human knee extensor muscles. *Acta Physiol Scand.* 2003;178:165–173.

28. Henneman E, Somjen G, Carpenter DO. Excitability and inhabitability of motoneurons of different sizes. *J Neurophysiol.* 1965; 28:599–620.

29. Hoffman JR, Ratamess NA, Faigenbaum AD, Mangine GT, Kang J. Effects of maximal squat exercise testing on vertical jump performance in American college football players. *J Sports Sci Med.* 2007; 6:149–150.

30. Holtermann A, Roeleveld K, Engstrøm M, Sand T. Enhanced H-reflex with resistance training is related to increased rate of force development. *Eur J Appl Physiol.* 2007;101:301–331.

31. Kamen G, Kroll W, Zignon ST. Exercise effects upon reflex time components in weight lifters and distance runners. *Med Sci Sports Exerc.* 1981;13:198–204.

32. Kellis E, Arabatzi F, Papadopoulos C. Muscle co-activation around the knee in drop jumping using the co-contraction index. *J Electromyogr Kines.* 2003;13:229–238.

33. Keogh JWL, Wilson GJ, Weatherby RP. A cross-sectional comparison of different resistance training techniques in the bench press. *J Strength Cond Res.* 1999;13:247–258.

34. Komi PV, Kaneko M, Aura O. EMG activity of leg extensor muscles with special reference to mechanical efficiency in concentric and eccentric exercise. *Int J Sports Med.* 1987;8(suppl):22–29.

35. Kuruganti U, Parker P, Rickards J, Tingley M, Sexsmith J. Bilateral isokinetic training reduces the bilateral leg strength deficit for both old and young adults. *Eur J Appl Physiol.* 2005;94: 175–179.

36. Milner-Brown HS, Stein RB, Lee RG. Synchronization of human motor units: possible roles of exercise and supraspinal reflexes. *EEG Clin Neurophysiol.* 1975;38:245–254.

37. Monster AW, Chan H. Isometric force production by motor units of extensor digitorum communis muscles in man. *J Neurophysiol.* 1977;40:1432–1443.

38. Moritani T, deVries HA. Neural factors versus hypertrophy in the time course of muscle strength gain. *Am J Phys Med.* 1979;58:115–130.

39. Munn J, Herbert RD, Gandevia SC. Contralateral effects of unilateral resistance training: a meta-analysis. *J Appl Physiol.* 2004;96:1861–1866.

40. Nardone A, Romano C, Schieppati M. Selective recruitment of high-threshold human motor units during voluntary isotonic lengthening of active muscles. *J Physiol.* 1989;409:451–471.

41. Narici MV, Roi GS, Landoni L, Minetti AE, Cerretelli E. Changes in force, cross-sectional area and neural activation during strength training and detraining of the human quadriceps. *Eur J Appl Physiol.* 1989;59:310–319.

42. Pensini M, Martin A, Maffiuletti MA. Central versus peripheral adaptations following eccentric resistance training. *Int J Sports Med.* 2002;23:567–574.

43. Pincivero DM, Gandhi V, Timmons MK, Coelho AJ. Quadriceps femoris electromyogram during concentric, isometric, and eccentric phases of fatiguing dynamic knee extensions. *J Biomech.* 2006; 39:246–254.

44. Ploutz LL, Tesch PA, Biro RL, Dudley GA. Effect of resistance training on muscle use during exercise. *J Appl Physiol.* 1994;76:1675–1681.

45. Pucci AR, Griffin L, Cafarelli E. Maximal motor unit firing rates during isometric resistance training in man. *Exp Physiol.* 2006; 91:171–178.

46. Ranganathan VK, Siemionow V, Liu JZ, Sahgal V, Yue GH. From mental power to muscle power – gaining strength by using the mind. *Neuropsychol.* 2004;42:944–956.

47. Ratamess NA, Izquierdo M. Neuromuscular adaptations to training. In: Schwellnus, M, ed. *The Olympic Textbook of Medicine in Sport.* Hoboken, NJ: Wiley-Blackwell, 2008.

48. Rutherford OM, Jones DA. The role of learning and coordination in strength training. *Eur J Appl Physiol.* 1986;55:100–105.

49. Sale DG. Neural adaptations to strength training. In: Komi PV, editor. *Strength and Power in Sport*. 2nd ed. Malden (MA): Blackwell Science; 2003. pp. 281–314.

50. Sale DG, McComas AJ, MacDougall JD, Upton, ARM. Neuromuscular adaptation in human thenar muscles following strength training and immobilization. *J Appl Physiol*. 1982;53:419–424.

51. Sale DG, Upton ARM, McComas AJ, MacDougall JD. Neuromuscular functions in weight-trainers. *Exp Neurol*. 1883;82:521–531.

52. Sale DG, MacDougall JD, Upton ARM, McComas AJ. Effect of strength training upon motoneuron excitability in man. *Med Sci Sports Exerc*. 1983;15:57–62.

53. Seger JY, Thorstensson A. Effects of eccentric versus concentric training on thigh muscle strength and EMG. *Int J Sports Med*. 2005;26:45–52.

54. Semmler JG, Sale MV, Meyer FG, Nordstrom MA. Motor-unit coherence and its relation with synchrony are influenced by training. *J Neurophysiol*. 2004;92:3320–3331.

55. Shima SN, Ishida K, Katayama K, Morotome Y, Sato Y, Miyamura M. Cross education of muscular strength during unilateral resistance training and detraining. *Eur J Appl Physiol*. 2002;86:287–294.

56. Sieck GC, Prakash YS. Morphological adaptations of neuromuscular junctions depend on fiber type. *Can J Appl Physiol*. 1997;22:197–230.

57. Somjen G, Carpenter DO, Henneman E. Responses of motoneurons of different sizes to graded stimulation of supraspinal centers of the brain. *J Neurophysiol*. 1965;28:958–965.

58. Taniguchi Y. Lateral specificity in resistance training: the effect of bilateral and unilateral training. *Eur J Appl Physiol*. 1997;75:144–150.

59. Ter Haar Romeny BM, Dernier Van Der Goen JJ, Gielen CCAM. Changes in recruitment order of motor units in the human biceps muscle. *Exp Neurol*. 1982;78:360–368.

60. Tesch PA, Dudley GA, Duvoisin MR, Hather BM, Harris RT. Force and EMG signal patterns during repeated bouts of concentric or eccentric muscle actions. *Acta Physiol Scand*. 1990;138:263–271.

61. Van Custem M, Duchateau J, Hainut K. Changes in single motor unit behaviour contribute to the increase in contraction speed after dynamic training in humans. *J Physiol*. 1998;513:295–305.

62. Weir JP, Housh TJ, Weir LL. Electromyographic evaluation of joint angle specificity and cross-training after isometric training. *J Appl Physiol*. 1994;77:197–201.

63. Yue G, Cole KJ. Strength increases from the motor program: comparison of training with maximal voluntary and imagined muscle contractions. *J Neurophysiol*. 1992;67:1114–1123.

64. Yuza N, Ishida K, Miyamura M. Cross transfer effects of muscular endurance during training and detraining. *J Sports Med Phys Fit*. 2000;40:110–117.

4

Muscular Adaptations to Training

After completing this chapter, you will be able to:
- Discuss the differences between cardiac, smooth, and skeletal muscles
- Describe the various roles skeletal muscles play within the human body
- Describe the gross anatomy of skeletal muscle
- Diagram the organization of a myofibril
- Describe the processes involved in skeletal muscle contraction
- Distinguish between different fiber types and discuss the importance of fiber types on performance
- Discuss factors that influence muscle hypertrophy
- Describe structural changes to skeletal muscle and discuss how they enhance muscular performance

Muscles perform a multitude of functions in the human body. There are three types of muscles: cardiac, smooth, and skeletal. **Cardiac muscle** is found in the heart. It contracts involuntarily with strong force and is responsible for creating a rhythmic pressure head and moving blood throughout the body. **Smooth muscle** is found in the walls of hollow organs and blood vessels. It contracts involuntarily resulting in a squeezing-type phenomenon where constriction takes place. **Skeletal muscle** is larger, constitutes nearly 40% of body mass, contracts voluntarily, contracts and relaxes rapidly, and contains multiple *nuclei* (which is critical to the exercise adaptation process). Skeletal muscle performs several important functions. Skeletal muscle contraction enables movement to occur. Contraction of skeletal muscle helps produce body heat, maintain posture, and assists with communication. Lastly, rhythmic skeletal muscle contraction enables ventilation to occur.

ROLES OF SKELETAL MUSCLES

Contraction of skeletal muscles produces tension and acts on bones to produce movement. The human body contains more than 660 skeletal muscles. Muscles are attached to bones in two general locations. The *proximal* attachment, or attachment closest to the midline, is known as the **origin**. The *distal* attachment, or attachment farther from the midline, is known as the **insertion**. Some muscles may have multiple points of origin or insertion. A muscle (tendon) must cross a joint in order for movement to occur. Several muscles' points of origin and

insertion may span one joint (*e.g.*, vastus lateralis). These muscles are *uniarticular* because they produce movement at one joint. Some muscles' origins and insertions span two joints. These muscles are *multiarticular* because they produce movement about two joints (*e.g.*, hamstrings). A muscle will shorten when it contracts, thereby pulling on its ends at the origin and insertion. However, movement will take place at only one end. One end will be held fixed or stable by muscle contraction and/or by the mass of the skeletal attachment point. Many times movement will take place at the point of insertion; however, movement may take place at the origin as well. One example is the *psoas* muscle group of the hip. When an individual is standing, contraction of the psoas muscle will flex the hip by raising the thigh (movement at the insertion). However, when lying supine with the lower body, stable, contraction of this muscle will produce hip flexion by lifting up on the trunk (*e.g.*, a sit-up), thereby causing movement at the point of origin.

When a muscle contracts to perform a specific movement, it is known as an **agonist**. In contrast, a muscle that opposes agonist movement is known as an **antagonist**. For example, during elbow flexion, the biceps brachii is an agonist muscle whereas the triceps brachii is an antagonist muscle. However, upon lowering the weight, the biceps brachii becomes the antagonist and the triceps brachii is the agonist. Antagonist muscles must relax to some degree to allow agonist movement to take place. Antagonist muscle contraction plays a key role in stabilizing the joint, decelerating agonist movement, and reducing the risk of joint injury. When a muscle contracts to stabilize either the point of origin or insertion for a corresponding muscle, it is known as a **stabilizer** or **fixator**. When a muscle contracts to eliminate one movement of a multiarticular muscle, it is known as a **neutralizer**. For example, the hamstrings muscle group is a knee flexor and hip extensor. When only hip extension takes place, the quadriceps muscles will contract to eliminate knee flexion. Muscles can function under any of these roles depending on the situation.

SKELETAL MUSCLE GROSS ANATOMY

The structure of skeletal muscle is shown in Figure 4.1. Skeletal muscle is designed to generate high levels of force efficiently and to have these forces effectively transmitted to bone. Muscular structures are stacked in parallel. That is, smaller units are arranged in parallel to form larger units, and these units are stacked in parallel to form still larger units, etc. The most basic structural units of skeletal muscle are the myofilaments. Myofilaments are composed primarily of the contractile proteins *actin* and *myosin*. The myofilaments form the basic functional unit of muscle, the **sarcomere**. Sarcomeres are stacked in series to form a **myofibril**. Myofibrils are stacked in parallel to form **muscle fibers** (the muscle cells). A muscle fiber may have a diameter of 10–100 μm on average while the length may range up to 30 cm. Groups of muscle fibers form **fascicles** that are separated by fascia known as *endomysium*. Groups of fascicles form the muscle belly that is separated by fascia known as *perimysium*. The muscle belly is surrounded by fascia known as the *epimysium*. At the polar regions of muscle, tendons are located. The tendon connects muscle to bone. Fascia (endomysium, perimysium, and epimysium) located throughout the muscle assists in transferring forces produced by the shortening sarcomeres to the tendons and then ultimately to bone. Fascia (especially the endomysium) also assists in stabilizing blood vessels and nerves surrounding muscle fibers. Thus, a continuum of tissues involved in muscle contraction exists and force transmission from basic proteins to fascia to strong tendons.

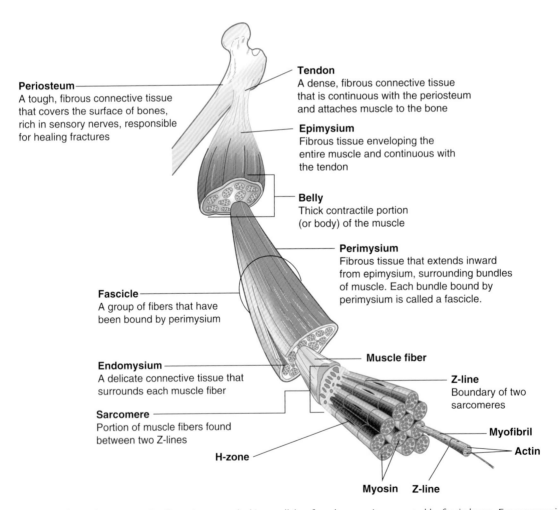

Periosteum
A tough, fibrous connective tissue that covers the surface of bones, rich in sensory nerves, responsible for healing fractures

Tendon
A dense, fibrous connective tissue that is continuous with the periosteum and attaches muscle to the bone

Epimysium
Fibrous tissue enveloping the entire muscle and continuous with the tendon

Belly
Thick contractile portion (or body) of the muscle

Perimysium
Fibrous tissue that extends inward from epimysium, surrounding bundles of muscle. Each bundle bound by perimysium is called a fascicle.

Fascicle
A group of fibers that have been bound by perimysium

Endomysium
A delicate connective tissue that surrounds each muscle fiber

Sarcomere
Portion of muscle fibers found between two Z-lines

Muscle fiber

Z-line
Boundary of two sarcomeres

Myofibril

Actin

H-zone

Myosin **Z-line**

■ **FIGURE 4.1.** Skeletal muscle anatomy. Smaller units are stacked in parallel to form larger units separated by fascia layers. Force transmission is efficient from shortening of the sarcomeres and cross-bridge cycling of the myofilaments to the endomysium, perimysium, epimysium, tendons, and ultimately to bone. (Asset provided by Anatomical Chart Co.)

MUSCLE FIBER ORGANIZATION

The organization of a skeletal muscle fiber is shown in Figure 4.2. Surrounding the muscle fiber (beneath the endomysium) is the cell membrane, also known as the **sarcolemma**. The sarcolemma encloses the fiber and regulates what enters and exits. It is important for propagating the action potential along the periphery of the fiber. The sarcolemma contains an outer plasma membrane and an inner basement membrane that is associated with structures of the basal lamina. Extending from openings in the sarcolemma to the interior of the fiber are transverse tubules (**T tubules**). The T tubules propagate the action potential deeper into the muscle fiber. Surrounding the myofibrils is the liquid cytoplasm (**sarcoplasm**) of the muscle fiber. The sarcoplasm contains enzymes, fat, glycogen, **mitochondrion** (site of aerobic energy production), multiple nuclei, and other organelles. The sarcoplasmic reticulum is a latticework of conductile tissue that penetrates deep into the muscle fiber allowing propagation of the action potential. It surrounds the myofilaments and carves them into myofibrils. On either side of the T tubules lies an extension of the sarcoplasmic reticulum known as the **terminal cisternae** or lateral sacs that are storage houses for calcium. The two terminal cisternae and the associated T tubule are collectively known as a *triad*. The **nucleus** contains the muscle fiber's genetic material and is especially important for initiating processes involved in protein synthesis. The muscle fiber has many peripherally located nuclei.

FUNCTIONAL UNIT OF A MUSCLE FIBER: THE SARCOMERE

The sarcomere spans from one *Z line* to the next adjacent Z line and is the functional unit of the muscle fiber.

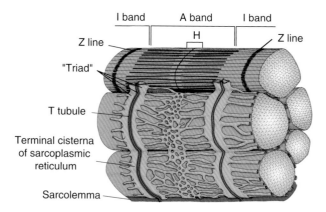

FIGURE 4.2. Muscle fiber organization. Key structures such as the sarcolemma, T tubules, and sarcoplasmic reticulum are shown. The conductile structures shown are important for propagating the action potential throughout the muscle fiber and mobilizing calcium from its intracellular storage site. (From Rubin R, Strayer DS. *Rubin's Pathology: Clinicopathologic Foundations of Medicine.* 5th ed. Philadelphia (PA): Lippincott Williams & Wilkins; 2008.)

A sarcomere on average is ~2.5 μm and is arranged in series with other sarcomeres within a myofibril. Figure 4.3 depicts the sarcomere and its constituents. Anchored to each Z line are the **actin** filaments. Several structural proteins anchor and structurally stabilize actin including the protein *nebulin*. Actin and its associated proteins make up the thin filament. The M line represents the central region of the sarcomere. The thick filaments consist of **myosin** and its associated proteins. Myosin is anchored (to the M line) and stabilized by structural proteins including the protein *titin*. Cross-section of a myofibril shows that a myosin filament has the opportunity to interact with any of six actin filaments surrounding it. Both actin and myosin are key proteins involved in muscle contraction. However, muscle contraction would be highly limited without the structural and cytoskeletal proteins maintaining stability of the sarcomere and proper orientation of the myofilaments. Under a microscope, areas of the sarcomere housed predominantly by actin stain very light (*isotropic*) and are referred to as the **I band**. Areas of the sarcomere housed predominantly by myosin stain dark (anisotropic) and are referred to as the **A band**. Alternating light and dark bands from sequential sarcomeres give the muscle fiber a striated, or striped appearance. The area surrounding the M line is devoid of actin filaments and is known as the *H zone*. This area may be thought of as a spacer as it will disappear during full sarcomere shortening.

THE MYOFILAMENTS

The myofilaments (shown in Fig. 4.4) are actin and myosin that account for nearly 85% of the protein content of the myofilaments. Actin is structured in a helical chain. Each strand of actin (known as fibrous or *F actin*) comprises a chain of smaller monomers (known as globular or *G actin*). A segment on G actin has a very high binding affinity to myosin. This region is known as an *active site* on actin. At rest, this area is not exposed but rather is covered by a barrier protein known as *tropomyosin*. Tropomyosin is a long protein that is associated with another critical protein, *troponin*. Troponin (Tn) consists of three major subunits: TnI, TnC, and TnT. TnI is the subunit that binds to actin. TnC is the subunit with high affinity for the mineral calcium. TnT is the subunit that binds to tropomyosin. We will discuss the roles of these proteins in a moment during our discussion of muscle contraction. Myosin is a large protein known as a "molecular motor" due to its involvement in muscle contraction. It is composed of two heavy chains that form a helix. Each heavy chain binds two light chains, an *essential* and a *regulatory* light chain. The chain (part of the heavy chain and the light chains) complexes form two globular regions shaped like golf clubs known as *myosin heads*. One light chain is important for regulating the activity of a key metabolic enzyme **myosin ATPase** in the myosin head.

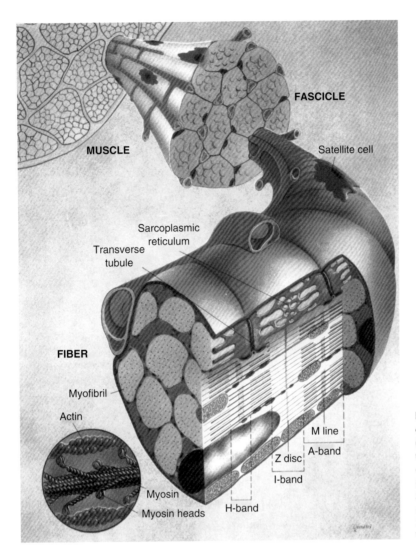

FIGURE 4.3. Structure of the sarcomere. The sarcomere spans from a Z line (disc) to an adjacent Z line (disc). The A band represents area comprised of the thick filaments. The I band represents area comprised of the thin filaments. The centrally located H zone (band) disappears during full muscle shortening. Sarcomeres are arranged in series spanning the length of the myofibril. (From Rubin E, Farber JL. *Pathology*. 3rd ed. Philadelphia (PA): Lippincott Williams & Wilkins; 1999.)

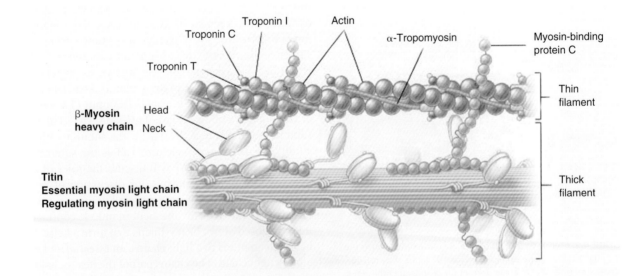

FIGURE 4.4. The myofibrillar proteins. The key contractile proteins actin and myosin and barrier proteins troponin (I [actin], C [calcium], and T [tropomyosin] subunits) and tropomyosin are shown. Myosin binding proteins Myosin-Binding Protein C and Titin are also shown. (Reprinted with permission from Nabel EG. Cardiovascular disease. *N Engl J Med*. 2003;349:60–72, Fig. 3.)

The tail of myosin forms the thick filament backbone whereas the two heads (head region) form **cross-bridges** with actin during muscle contraction. The *hinge region* (at the neck) allows for mobility of the myosin heads.

MUSCLE CONTRACTION: THE SLIDING FILAMENT THEORY

The *Sliding Filament* theory or model of muscle contraction was proposed by Hugh Huxley and Andrew Huxley in the early 1950s. It was so named because the underlying principle was that the thick and thin filaments slide past each other without changing length (although the sarcomere shortens). Ultimately, sarcomere shortening in series leads to shortening of the muscle fibers and muscle belly leading to movement and force generation. Muscle contraction occurs in stages: (a) excitation-contraction coupling, (b) cross-bridge cycling, and (c) relaxation.

Excitation-Contraction Coupling

The electrical signal propagated along the motor nerve must be propagated throughout the muscle fibers. Skeletal muscle contains conductile tissue able to propagate the action potential throughout at a high speed. The action potential first propagates along the sarcolemma. Neurotransmitters (acetylcholine) released from the motor nerve bind to receptors and open adjacent sodium channels, initiating the spread of depolarization throughout the sarcolemma. From the sarcolemma the action potential spreads through the T tubules and sarcoplasmic reticulum where calcium is stored in the terminal cisternae. The goal of the electrical discharge, or *excitation*, is to mobilize calcium. Calcium concentrations are low in the sarcoplasm at rest. An increase in calcium initiates subsequent events of muscle contraction. Depolarization causes a conformational change in channel proteins thereby opening and allowing calcium from the SR to diffuse into the sarcoplasm. Once in the sarcoplasm, calcium rapidly binds to troponin (TnC) that triggers a conformational change in the protein configuration. That is, binding of calcium to TnC pushes the tropomyosin off of the actin active site (via TnT). The active site of actin is now exposed and will immediately bind to a myosin head forming a cross-bridge (also called an *actomyosin* complex). Troponin-tropomyosin complex can be viewed as a barrier protein complex that inhibits muscle contraction. However, once it is removed, cross-bridges can form and muscle contraction can take place. Therefore, one can view *excitation-contraction coupling* as a mechanism where electrical discharge at the muscle level leads to chemical events stimulating muscle contraction.

Cross-Bridge Cycling

Figure 4.5 depicts the events involved in cross-bridge cycling. Formation of the cross-bridge is only an initial step. For muscle contraction to proceed, numerous cross-bridges need to form until the sarcomere shortens. The term for multiple cross-bridge formation is *cross-bridge cycling*. Cross-bridge cycling can most simply be described by events analogous to a "tug-of-war" where the competitors are analogous to myosin (or the thick filament), their arms analogous to myosin heads, and the rope analogous to the thin filament. The goal of cross-bridge cycling is for the centrally stabilized myosin filaments to pull the structurally stabilized thin filaments inward to shorten the sarcomere. When a cross-bridge is formed, immediately movement of the myosin head pulls actin slightly. This movement is referred to as the *power stroke* and is analogous to a tug-of-war participant pulling the rope inward. The power stroke involves a pivot of the myosin head. However, this motion of the myosin head is not complete. Rather, the myosin head must disengage and bind to another active site on actin further upstream. This is referred to as *cross-bridge cycling* as myosin heads form multiple cross-bridges with actin until sarcomere shortening ceases. This process occurs asynchronously. That is, there are always cross-bridges formed (keeping tension on the thin filaments) while other myosin heads and actin monomers are disengaged. In our tug-of-war example, there is no part of the competition where all participants on a team will let go of the rope at the same time to switch hand position. That would result in losing all tension on the rope and the competition. The same applies here. Myosin heads rotate asynchronously as cross-bridges form and detach. Detachment is a process that requires energy. The power stroke releases ADP + P already in the myosin head and binds a new ATP. Myosin ATPase (in the head of myosin) splits ATP for energy enabling the head of myosin to detach and subsequently bind to another exposed active site on actin further upstream. Cross-bridge formation and cycling continue (while calcium concentrations are elevated in the sarcoplasm) until relaxation takes place. Subsequently, cross-bridge cycling pulls the thin filaments in sliding past the thick filaments, thereby causing muscle contraction. All muscle fibers within a motor unit will be activated accordingly, and motor unit recruitment, rate, and firing patterns will depend upon the amount of force and power needed.

Relaxation

Relaxation begins with a reduction in neural stimuli. As force production requirements decrease, action potentials along the motor nerve will decrease. This will reduce action potentials through the muscle fiber and remove the stimulus for calcium mobilization. In the sarcoplasm, calcium is restored by the actions of energy-requiring protein "pumps" located in the SR (*calcium ATPase* pumps). The barrier proteins return to their

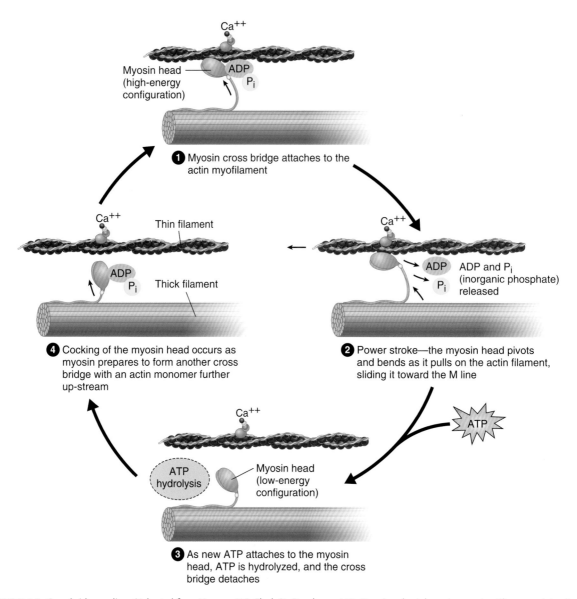

Ca⁺⁺

Myosin head — (high-energy configuration)

ADP
Pᵢ

❶ Myosin cross bridge attaches to the actin myofilament

Ca⁺⁺

Thin filament

ADP
Pᵢ

Thick filament

❹ Cocking of the myosin head occurs as myosin prepares to form another cross bridge with an actin monomer further up-stream

Ca⁺⁺

ADP
Pᵢ

ADP and Pᵢ (inorganic phosphate) released

❷ Power stroke—the myosin head pivots and bends as it pulls on the actin filament, sliding it toward the M line

ATP

Ca⁺⁺

ATP hydrolysis

Myosin head (low-energy configuration)

❸ As new ATP attaches to the myosin head, ATP is hydrolyzed, and the cross bridge detaches

■ **FIGURE 4.5.** Crossbridge cycling. (Adapted from Kraemer WJ, Fleck SJ, Deschenes MR. Exercise physiology: Integrating Theory and Application. Battimore: Wolterskluwer Health; 2012.)

resting configuration blocking the actin active sites, and the myofilaments return to their resting state.

SKELETAL MUSCLE'S GRADED RESPONSES

The contraction of muscle in response to a stimulus is known as a **twitch**. Multiple twitches are needed as tension requirements increase. The effect of multiple twitches is known as **summation**. When multiple motor units are activated thereby contributing to force development, it is known as *spatial summation*. When a motor unit increases its frequency of discharge to increase force, it is known as *temporal summation*. Both types of summation increase force and power production dramatically. **Tetanus** refers to maximal force production (graphically depicted as a plateau or flat line) when summation is peaked.

SKELETAL MUSCLE CHARACTERISTICS AND ADAPTATIONS

Skeletal muscle adapts to exercise in various and specific ways. Training up-regulates the activity of numerous genes that enhance muscle function. Skeletal muscle can enlarge (hypertrophy) when subjected to stress demanding greater force production. Fiber-type and architectural transitions can occur, increasing one's force, power, and endurance. Changes in skeletal muscle enzyme activity, substrate content, receptor content, capillary and mitochondrial density, and protein content also enhance athletic performance. Several of these changes are discussed in the next section while a few are discussed in subsequent chapters in relation to other physiological systems.

TABLE 4.1 MUSCLE FIBER-TYPE CHARACTERISTICS

CHARACTERISTIC	SLOW-TWITCH	FAST-TWITCH
Motor nerve size	Smaller	Larger
Nerve conduction velocity	Slower	Faster
Nerve recruitment threshold	Lower	Higher
Size	Smaller	Larger
Contraction speed	Slower	Faster
Type of myosin	Slower	Faster
Myosin ATPase activity	Lower	Higher
Sarcoplasmic reticulum development	Poor	Great
Troponin affinity for calcium	Poor	Great
Force	Lower	Higher
Muscle efficiency	Great	Poor
Fatigability	Lower	Higher
Anaerobic energy stores	Lower	Higher
Relaxation time	Slower	Faster
Glycolytic enzyme activity	Lower	Higher
Glycogen stores	Moderate	Higher
Endurance	Higher	Lower
Triglyceride stores	Higher	Lower
Myoglobin	Higher	Lower
Aerobic enzyme activity	Higher	Lower
Capillary density	Higher	Lower
Mitochondrial density	Higher	Lower

MUSCLE FIBER FORMATION

The formation of new muscle fibers is critical to normal muscle function. Although muscle fiber number remains constant for the most part, new muscle fibers must be formed to replace old or damaged muscle fibers as part of tissue *remodeling*. The process of muscle fiber formation is known as **myogenesis**. Satellite cells (stem cells) are released from the basal lamina and migrate to the area of fiber formation. Satellite cells proliferate (increase in number) and differentiate into a more functional cell called a *myoblast*. Myoblasts fuse to form a multinucleated *myotube*. Myotubes form the scaffold of the new fiber, and further maturation results in a new muscle fiber. The process of myogenesis is enhanced by several intermediates including *MyoD*, *Myf5*, and *myogenin* but is inhibited by a protein called **myostatin**. Stimulators of myogenesis increase muscle growth whereas inhibitors limit muscle growth. Myostatin has been of great interest to scientists since the late 1990s when it was discovered that animals not expressing the gene that produces myostatin were shown to have extremely large muscles. Since then, markers of myogenesis have been studied during training.

Most, but not all (3), studies have shown that an acute resistance exercise workout up-regulates myogenesis markers (myogenin, MyoD) within a few hours (up to 24–48 hours) postexercise (4,8,14,22,42). Interestingly, the acute response to a workout may be enhanced by chronic resistance training (RT) (22). Endurance exercise has shown a modest effect on these responses (7). Longer-term studies (*e.g.*, 12–16 weeks) have shown RT up-regulates myogenic marker expression over time

(22,23,63). On the other hand, myostatin expression has been shown to be lower following training in most studies (22,49) even when very low training intensities were used (8). These changes play a role in muscle growth and fiber changes taking place with chronic training.

MUSCLE FIBER TYPES

Muscle fibers reflect the type of stimulation they receive from the nervous system. Two general fiber-type classifications exist based on muscle's contractile and metabolic properties: *slow-twitch* (ST) and *fast-twitch* (FT). ST (type I) fibers are predominantly endurance fibers whereas FT (type II) fibers are strength/power fibers. Each fiber type has distinct characteristics leading to its force/endurance profile (Table 4.1). Within these major classifications, muscle fibers exist on a continuum. That is, intermediate fibers exist such that there are six fiber-type subclassifications. Figure 4.6 depicts the fiber-type intermediates. Because fiber types operate on a continuum,

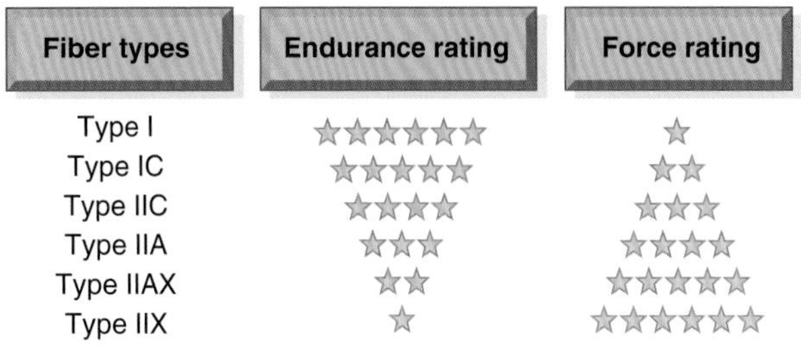

Fiber types	Endurance rating	Force rating
Type I	★★★★★★	★
Type IC	★★★★★	★★
Type IIC	★★★★	★★★
Type IIA	★★★	★★★★
Type IIAX	★★	★★★★★
Type IIX	★	★★★★★★

■ **FIGURE 4.6.** Fiber-type continuum with force and endurance ratings. (Adapted with permission from Staron RS. The classification of human skeletal muscle fiber types. *J Strength Cond Res.* 1997;11:67.)

the type I fibers possess the least generated-force capacity but are highest in endurance whereas the type II fiber has the least endurance but the greatest strength. Other fibers lie somewhere in between on a continuum. The continuum (I, IC, IIC, IIAC, IIA, IIAB [or IIAX], and IIB [or IIX]) exists concomitant to myosin heavy chain expression, *i.e.*, MHCI, IIA, and IIB or IIX (54).

Fiber Types in Athletes

Skeletal muscle is composed of both ST and FT fibers. The ratio of the two assists in determining the muscle's functional capacity. Each muscle will have a distinct ratio and may favor one type or the other; the gastrocnemius muscle is predominantly FT in most individuals whereas the soleus muscle is predominantly ST. Endurance athletes (*e.g.*, long- and middle-distance runners, cyclists) display larger percentages of type I fibers whereas strength/power athletes (*e.g.*, sprinters, throwers, weightlifters, jumpers) display larger percentages of type II fibers. For example, Häkkinen et al. (15) showed that the percentage of FT fibers in the vastus lateralis muscles of powerlifters, bodybuilders, and wrestlers were 60%, 59%, and 42%, respectively. Other reviews have shown endurance athletes to have 18%–25% of type II fibers in the same muscle (35). In a review of studies, Tesch and Alkner (57) compared fiber-type composition of various lifters. For the vastus lateralis muscle, powerlifters possessed ~55%–56% FT fibers, bodybuilders had ~45%–48% FT fibers, and weightlifters had ~54%–62% FT fibers. Bodybuilders possess a relatively higher percentage of ST fibers than weightlifters, powerlifters, and other power athletes. Muscle fiber-type composition is genetically determined and is one attribute that may lead athletes toward participation in certain sports.

Fiber-Type Transitions

Although the proportions of type I and II fibers are mostly genetically determined, transitions have been shown to occur within each subpopulation. Changes in myosin heavy chain (MHC) content (IIX to IIA) can occur within the first few workouts (10,18) that precede changes in fiber types. With RT, transitions take place from IIX to IIA (10,24,53) (Fig. 4.7). type IIX fibers have been considered reservoir fibers that transform into a more oxidative form upon training (*i.e.*, to an intermediate fiber type IIAX to IIA) (5). The advantage of this transition is that more force can be produced over time. Although type IIX fibers are stronger, their fatigability renders them less useful when performing many strength/power tasks. The transition appears to be more beneficial for performance enhancement. It is important to note that type IIX fibers are not readily recruited (based on the size principle; see Chapter 3). The intensity of exercise needs to be high to activate this fiber type. Once activated consistently through training, however, recruitment of these fibers leads to transitions to type IIAX and

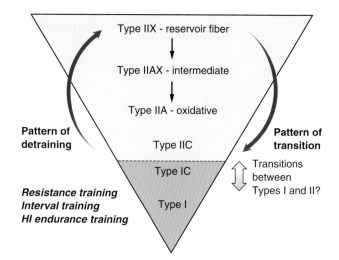

■ FIGURE 4.7. Fiber-type transitions with training and detraining. Resistance training, interval training, and high-intensity endurance training have been shown to reduce type IIX population with a concomitant increase in type IIA fiber percent. Type IIAX fiber changes may reflect fibers in transition (to type IIA). Detraining produces the opposite direction of transition. The line reflects a lack of sufficient evidence to indicate transitions between type I and II fibers.

IIA fibers. Interestingly, detraining results in an increase in type IIX fibers and reduction in type IIA fibers, with a possible overshoot (*i.e.*, a larger percentage seen after detraining than what was seen before training) of type IIX fibers (2). Moderate-to-high-intensity aerobic training has produced similar fiber-type transitions (38,51). In a review, McComas (35) reported reduced type IIX percentages and slight increases in type IIA and I populations in nearly all studies examined. The magnitude of type IIX fiber percent reduction is greater following strength than endurance training (24). Simultaneous aerobic and RT result in a reduction in MHCIIX (43).

Of interest to exercise scientists has been the capacity to transform between muscle fiber types, *e.g.*, transformations from a type I to type II or vice versa. It is believed currently that muscle fibers will only transform within each population (*e.g.*, from a type IIX to IIA) and not between fiber types. However, there have been a few studies that have shown a significant change in type I and type II muscle fiber populations as a result of training (35). Some methods have been criticized in these studies making it difficult to conclusively state for sure if these changes occurred. Cross-sectional comparisons of different athletes have shown substantial differences in type I and II populations for a given muscle especially when strength/power athletes are compared to endurance athletes. However, one cannot determine the effects of genetics when viewing cross-sectional studies. For example, were these athletes genetically gifted with this fiber-type variation, did training affect these percentages, or both? But these data pose an interesting question; can training lead to increases in type I or II populations? Based on the fact that fiber types function on a continuum, it

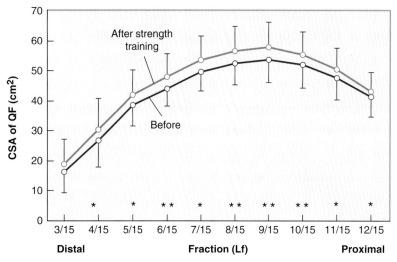

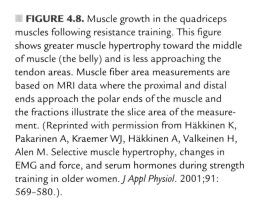

FIGURE 4.8. Muscle growth in the quadriceps muscles following resistance training. This figure shows greater muscle hypertrophy toward the middle of muscle (the belly) and is less approaching the tendon areas. Muscle fiber area measurements are based on MRI data where the proximal and distal ends approach the polar ends of the muscle and the fractions illustrate the slice area of the measurement. (Reprinted with permission from Häkkinen K, Pakarinen A, Kraemer WJ, Häkkinen A, Valkeinen H, Alen M. Selective muscle hypertrophy, changes in EMG and force, and serum hormones during strength training in older women. *J Appl Physiol.* 2001;91: 569–580.).

seems plausible that the possibility may exist under certain circumstances. The identification of type IC and IIC fibers have supported this contention to some degree. For example, what if a cross-country runner stopped endurance training and began a lifting program? Or, what if a powerlifter ceased lifting weights and began a distance running program? These are two extreme examples but certainly situations where one might expect at least some small fiber-type transitions to occur. However, further research is needed to analyze this concept.

MUSCLE HYPERTROPHY

An increase in muscle size is a common adaptation to anaerobic training, especially RT. There is a positive relationship between a muscle's size and its force potential; thus, a larger muscle is a stronger muscle. Muscle hypertrophy can result from an increase in *protein synthesis*, a decrease in protein breakdown, or a combination of both. Protein synthesis increases following a workout and may be elevated up to 48 hours after an acute bout of exercise (41). Protein breakdown is common while one is lifting but protein synthesis (and muscle growth) occurs during the recovery period. The repeated pattern of protein

breakdown and synthesis eventually leads to a supercompensation resulting in muscle growth. Enhanced postworkout protein synthesis depends on several factors including amino acid availability from nutrient intake, the timing of nutrient intake (before, during, or immediately after a workout), the intensity and volume of the workout (mechanical stress), and the hormonal and growth factor response (26). Muscle growth results in a proportional greater size and number of actin/myosin filaments and the addition of peripheral sarcomeres, which is highly important for strength and power development. Although neural adaptations predominate early in training, hypertrophy becomes increasingly important as RT continues. Changes in muscle proteins take place within a couple of workouts (53). However, a longer period of time (>8 workouts) is needed to demonstrate significant muscle growth and this is only provided the workout stimulus surpasses one's own threshold of conditioning. Both men and women experience increases in muscle size during training. However, in absolute terms, men experience more hypertrophy than women predominantly due to the higher concentrations of the hormone *testosterone*. Lastly, muscle growth typically occurs in higher magnitude along the muscle belly in a nonuniform manner (Fig. 4.8) (17).

Myths & Misconceptions

Muscles Grow While the Individual is in the Gym Lifting Weights

Some have postulated that muscles grow mostly while the athlete is working out. Although the stimulus for muscle growth is the workout, muscles actually grow during the recovery period postexercise. Part of the misconception is due to the fact the muscle blood flow increases during resistance exercise leading to a "muscle pump." The pump temporarily increases the size of the muscles during acute exercise. Rather, protein breakdown is high during and immediately following the workout but muscle protein synthesis is elevated for up to 24–48 hours following the workout. Consistent training over time where there is a pattern of breakdown and synthesis leads to greater net protein deposition. Greater protein accretion leads to muscle hypertrophy and an increase in muscle CSA. Thus, muscles grow during recovery and not during the act of lifting weights.

Interpreting Research

Fiber Hypertrophy and Resistance Training

McCall GE, Byrnes WC, Dickinson A, Pattany PM, Fleck SJ. Muscle fiber hypertrophy, hyperplasia, and capillary density in college men after resistance training. *J Appl Physiol*. 1996;81:2004–2012.

McCall et al. (34) had individuals resistance train 3 days per week for 12 weeks. The program consisted of performing eight exercises for 3 sets of 10 reps (with 10RM [repetition maximum] loading). Muscle biopsies from the biceps brachii showed that muscle fiber area increased 17% for type II fibers and 10% for type I fibers. Because type I fibers were much smaller to begin with, the percent improvement may be somewhat hyperinflated as shown in Figure 4.9. This was one of several studies to show differential hypertrophy patterns between ST and FT fibers.

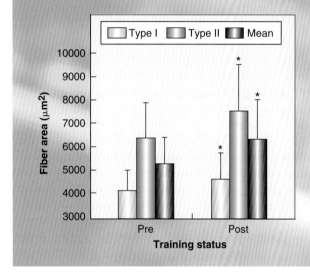

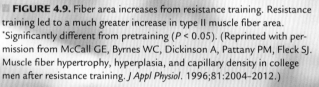

FIGURE 4.9. Fiber area increases from resistance training. Resistance training led to a much greater increase in type II muscle fiber area. *Significantly different from pretraining (*P* < 0.05). (Reprinted with permission from McCall GE, Byrnes WC, Dickinson A, Pattany PM, Fleck SJ. Muscle fiber hypertrophy, hyperplasia, and capillary density in college men after resistance training. *J Appl Physiol*. 1996;81:2004–2012.)

Muscle Hypertrophy and Fiber Types

Muscle growth occurs in both ST and FT muscle fibers. However, growth potential is higher in FT fibers. As FT fibers are known for their strength and power, it is not surprising that they increase in size to a greater extent. For example, Tesch et al. (59) showed that the size of vastus lateralis FT fibers in athletes was 118%–144% larger than untrained individuals whereas ST fiber size was only 55%–78% greater. MacDougall et al. (28) showed that FT fiber area increased 33% whereas ST fiber area increased 27% after 6 months of RT. Hortobagyi et al. (20) found no increase in ST fiber area but a large increase in FT fiber area following 12 weeks of training. ST fibers increase in size to a certain extent but, because of their vital role in muscular endurance, too much hypertrophy may be counterproductive. In fact, aerobic training has been shown to reduce muscle fiber size in some lower-body muscles (25). Lower ST fiber area may improve oxygen kinetics within the muscle thereby improving endurance.

Factors Influencing Muscle Hypertrophy

Several factors influence the magnitude of muscle growth resulting from training. *Mechanical factors* focus on the tension/force produced by muscle fibers. These include the type of muscle actions trained, the intensity and volume of training, and perhaps muscle damage to some extent. *Circulatory factors* focus on blood flow (and/or restriction of blood flow) and muscle metabolism during training. Both mechanical and circulatory factors elicited by a training session done for hypertrophy may influence muscle gene expression, protein synthesis, growth factor expression, and hormonal responses. Lastly, *nutritional factors* play a significant role. This includes diet, supplement use, and perhaps anabolic drug use. Important factors influencing muscle growth include:

- Greater gains in muscle size are seen when ECC muscle actions are used or emphasized in training (9). A study by Vikne et al. (60) compared 12 weeks of CON-only training to ECC-only training in resistance-trained men and showed that types I and II fiber area changed by –2% and 5%, respectively, following CON-only training but increased by 25% and 40%, respectively, following ECC-only training. Similar findings were obtained from Hortobagyi et al. (20) who trained subjects for 12 weeks and found

You Need to Damage Muscles to Make Them Grow!

For some time it was thought that muscle damage was a necessary precursor to growth (one use of the phrase "no pain no gain"). Although damage to skeletal muscle is a stimulus that increases protein synthesis and muscle growth, repeated exposure to a similar training program lessens the amount of muscle damage. Yet, muscle growth still occurs despite minimal to no damage. Mair et al. (33) subjected participants to an intense ECC RT protocol, and then repeated the protocol 4 and 13 days after the initial day. After the first day, muscle soreness was high, *creatine kinase* (an indirect marker of muscle damage) was high, and performance was reduced. However, when this protocol was performed on day 13, subjects did not experience soreness, performance was not reduced, and creatine kinase concentrations did not change. There appears to be a protective effect on skeletal muscle to reduce damage with consistent training. This was shown by Chen (6) who found that performing an ECC protocol 3 days after the first day it was performed (which produced significant damage) did not exacerbate the damage any further or impede recovery. This repeated exercise protective effect has been shown by others as well (21,36). However, the effect lessens as the time between workouts increases greatly (37). It appears that muscle damage is a product of high levels of muscle tension, and that muscle tension is a key factor influencing muscle growth. These studies show the rapidity by which skeletal muscle adapts to exercise and demonstrates the need for progressive overload, specificity, and variation to enhance the stimuli to produce further gains.

ECC-only trained increased type II fiber area 10 times more than CON-only training. The importance of ECC muscle actions, or muscle lengthening, has been noted for several years especially in animal studies where muscles exposed to chronic stretch hypertrophied or maintained mass during immobilization. Mechanical stretch on muscle fibers increases protein synthesis and the number of sarcomeres in series, and with the added tension (and potential for muscle damage) from loaded ECC actions, presents a potent stimulus for muscle growth.

- Tension produced by muscle is another key factor. Tension, as a function of the intensity and volume of training, increases muscle growth in many ways. Resistance training may alter the activity of nearly 70 genes (48). Muscle tension disrupts muscle fiber membranes increasing the production of several muscle growth factors (*e.g.*, *mechanogrowth factor*, *calcineurin*), which ultimately increase gene transcription and protein synthesis. Muscle tension increases myogenic pathway activity leading to muscle growth. Muscle tension is a stimulus for an anabolic hormonal response and up-regulation of anabolic hormone receptors. Muscle tension on a muscle fiber increases a multitude of intracellular pathway signaling mechanisms that enhance muscle hypertrophy.

- Circulatory factors related to blood flow or a lack of blood flow play a role in muscle growth. Studies that have restricted blood flow during lifting weights and used light loading of 10%–50% of 1 RM (to purposely increase metabolite production such as lactic acid making the workout more anaerobic) have shown prominent increases in muscle growth comparable to heavier lifting (46,50,52,56). These studies suggest a possible role (either direct or indirect) of metabolic stress in muscle growth. It has been shown that **occlusive resistance exercise** (where blood flow is mechanically reduced) elicits a more pronounced lactate and growth hormone response (55) than low-intensity training with no occlusion. This may, in part, give one explanation as to the efficacy of bodybuilding programs that use moderate loading and high volumes with short rest intervals for increasing muscle hypertrophy. It is important to note that the use of occlusion during training can reduce acute muscular endurance (*i.e.*, the number of repetitions performed with occlusion vs. the number of repetitions performed without occlusion) presumably due to the acidic environment (62).

- The water content of skeletal muscle plays a role in muscle hypertrophy. Studies show that increased cellular hydration decreases protein breakdown and increases protein synthesis (61). This is especially seen when individuals supplement with *creatine*. Creatine supplementation increases cellular hydration, leads to initial weight gain, and ultimately increases muscle growth during training.

- Nutritional factors influence muscle growth. Carbohydrate and protein intake significantly affect protein synthesis. Carbohydrates increase the synthesis and secretion of the potent anabolic hormone *insulin*. Insulin plays an important role in regulating muscle mass in addition to the many metabolic roles it plays. It has been recommended that an athlete

Interpreting Research

Use of Occlusion During Resistance Training

Madarame H, Neya M, Ochi E, Nakazato K, Sato Y, Ishii N. Cross-transfer effects of resistance training with blood flow restriction. *Med Sci Sports Exerc*. 2008;40:258-263.

In order to study the effects of restricted blood flow on RT adaptations, tourniquets and cuffs at various pressures have been used. Madarame et al. (31) trained individuals two times per week for 10 weeks. The participants trained with 30%–50% of their 1RM for the knee extension and biceps curl exercises. In one condition participants performed 3 sets of 10 reps with 50% of 1RM for the arms and 3 sets of 15–30 reps with 30% of 1RM for the legs. The other condition had participants perform the same protocol with occlusion. Occlusion was brought about by the use of elastic belts with >160 mm Hg of pressure. For the legs, knee extensor and flexor muscle CSA did not change with normal training but did increase by 4%–6% in the occlusive training condition. Muscle strength increased by 9%–16% (depending on the assessment) in the occluded group whereas muscle strength increased by 2%–10% in the normal group. For the arms, elbow muscle CSA only increased in the occluded condition by >11%. No further augmentation in growth hormone or testosterone was shown following a workout (although the occluded group had higher mean values of both hormones), but the occluded group had a larger *catecholamine* (adrenaline) response. These data, as well as data from other studies, show that increasing the anaerobic nature of the exercise workout via occlusion does present a potent stimulus for muscle growth.

consume ~55%–65% of calories from carbohydrates at levels approaching 6 g CHO · kg^{-1} body mass per day. Protein is a macronutrient made up of *amino acids*. Out of the 20 identified amino acids, 9 are essential and 11 are nonessential. *Nonessential* amino acids can be produced within the body whereas *essential* amino acids must be obtained through the diet. Muscle growth and recovery necessitate the amount of protein synthesized be greater than the amount broken down. Protein intake (amino acid availability) should be high when training to increase muscle size. Studies have shown that athletes require higher protein intake (in a range of 1.7–2.2 g kg^{-1} of body mass of protein per day) depending on the intensity, volume, and frequency of training (44,45). Protein supplementation is recommended if the athlete does not consume an adequate amount from the diet (44,45). Protein supplements contain various amounts of protein (from various sources as well) per serving. Protein and/or amino acid intake before, during, or immediately after a workout very important for increasing protein synthesis and enhancing recovery prior to the next workout. Lastly, a few supplements and anabolic drugs increase muscle growth. Creatine supplementation can increase muscle mass. Other supplements that enhance the training stimulus have the potential to increase muscle growth over time. Anabolic drugs (*e.g.*, anabolic steroids, testosterone esters, growth hormone, testosterone enhancers) have potent muscle-building effects and are very effective for increasing muscle hypertrophy (19,45). However, these are banned for use for athletic purposes and are not ethical to consume.

Case Study 4.1

Michael is a college track and field athlete who has just completed his first full year of serious and consistent RT. Over the course of the year, Michael's body weight increased from 165 to 178 lb. In addition, his body fat decreased from 12.1% to 11.2%. Based on these assessments, Michael's coach calculates that he gained 13.1 lb of lean tissue mass. Much of this gain in lean tissue mass was attributed to muscular hypertrophy.

Questions for Consideration: **Based on our previous discussions of skeletal muscle, what mechanisms may have contributed to Michael's muscle growth? What types of fiber composition changes may have been expected?**

Muscle Hypertrophy and Other Training Modalities

Sprint and power training can increase muscle size to a lesser extent (47). Linossier et al. (27) found type II fiber hypertrophy after 9 weeks of high-intensity cycle ergometry training. Häkkinen et al. (16) found greater muscle fiber area after 24 weeks of plyometric training compared to before training. Sprint, agility, and plyometric training require high levels of force and power; thus, muscle fiber recruitment is high (especially FT fibers). Fiber transitions and subsequent muscle growth occur. However, the magnitude of muscle growth is less than what is gained through weight training. When combined with weight training, gains in muscle size are more substantial from sprint, agility, and plyometric training (40). Aerobic training results in no change (43) or a reduction in muscle size (24,25). Reductions in muscle size occur mostly in type I and IIC fiber populations (24). Simultaneous strength and aerobic training results in substantial increases in CSA of type IIA muscle fibers (24,43).

HYPERPLASIA

Hyperplasia is thought to involve longitudinal splitting of existing muscle fibers (new fiber development), subsequently resulting in an increased number of muscle cells. In addition, hyperplasia has been suggested to occur via increased satellite cell proliferation following muscle damage (35). Hyperplasia was first shown in laboratory animals (11). However, it has been controversial in humans. Bodybuilders and powerlifters have shown greater number of muscle fibers than untrained individuals (29,58). However, it was not known if this was a result of training or genetics as other research has shown similar muscle fiber number between strength athletes and untrained controls (30). Although some data indicate the potential for hyperplasia in humans (34), it is still not known conclusively if it is a viable mechanism leading to muscle fiber growth. If hyperplasia does occur, it may represent an adaptation to RT when certain muscle fibers reach a theoretical upper limit in cell size. For example, large increases in muscle size over years of training or perhaps use of anabolic drugs where one's level of muscle mass may surpass the drug-free genetic potential pose interesting scenarios testing the viability of hyperplasia as a mechanism of adaptation. In these cases, hyperplasia may seem possible due to large increases in muscle size where the human body may be viewed as possessing secondary mechanisms to take muscle growth to higher levels. However, if hyperplasia does occur, it is thought to account for only a minor portion of the increase in muscle size.

STRUCTURAL CHANGES TO MUSCLE

Structural changes to skeletal muscle occur leading to enhanced performance. We have previously discussed several components of skeletal muscle with regards to muscle contraction. The structures discussed, proteins, and enzymes all have the ability to adapt to training enabling muscle to increase its strength, power, size, and endurance. Resistance training increases the number of myofibrils, the density of the sarcoplasm, sarcoplasm reticulum, and T tubules, and sodium-potassium ATPase pump activity (1,12,28,29). As protein synthesis increases, proteins appear to be synthesized relative to their distribution within muscle fibers to maintain optimal proportions. Actin-to-myosin ratio remains constant, structural proteins increase in proportion, and sarcomere length remains constant although sarcomere number increases. In addition to these changes,

sprint training improves calcium kinetics which assists in speed development (39). Endurance training has been shown to decrease calcium kinetics and increase sodium-potassium ATPase pump activity (12,13,32).

OTHER CHANGES TO SKELETAL MUSCLE

Other changes may take place within skeletal muscle that improves performance. These changes are discussed in subsequent chapters more specifically (because different physiological systems interact within skeletal muscle) but need to be mentioned here as well. Sprint and RT increase anaerobic substrate content, alter enzyme activity, and increase a muscle's buffer capacity. Aerobic training increases the activity of aerobic enzymes. Resistance training up-regulates anabolic hormone receptors. Aerobic training increases mitochondrial and capillary density; however, RT decreases these variables. Connective tissue within skeletal muscle increases in capacity, which helps support strength development and hypertrophy. Lastly, the length of fascicles and muscle fiber orientation may change in response to sprint and resistance training, which favor force production and power.

▓ Summary Points

✔ Skeletal muscles play several important roles upon contraction, including agonist, antagonist, stabilizer, and neutralizer functions.

✔ Skeletal muscle is designed such that structures are stacked in parallel, *i.e.*, smaller units are arranged in parallel to form larger units and so on, to increase force production and transmission to tendons and bones.

✔ The functional unit of muscle fibers is the sarcomeres. Sarcomeres contain actin and myosin, as well as other structural proteins, critical to muscle contraction.

✔ Muscle contraction consists of a series of events beginning with spreading the action potential throughout each muscle fiber, mobilization of calcium, cross-bridge formation and cycling (theoretically similar to a "tug-of-war"), and culminating in relaxation.

✔ Myogenesis is the process by which new muscle fibers are formed (as part of remodeling and regeneration after injury).

✔ Muscle fibers are either slow-twitch (ST) or fast-twitch (FT). ST fibers are high in endurance whereas FT fibers are strength/power fibers. The relative distribution of each type within each muscle is a genetic attribute that points athletes toward competing and succeeding in certain sports.

✔ Fiber-type transitions occur during resistance, sprint, and endurance training. type IIX (reservoir fibers) percents decrease with a concomitant increase in the percent of type IIA and/or type IIAX fibers. type II to I fiber transitions and vice versa have not been consistently shown and appear debatable at this point in time.

✔ Muscle hypertrophy increases in response to anaerobic training and appears related to the training intensity and volume, muscle actions used (especially ECC muscle actions), fiber type, nutritional intake, metabolite formation, and the water content of muscle.

✔ Hyperplasia has been shown to occur in animals but its influence on muscle growth in humans is debatable at the current time.

✔ Structural changes in skeletal muscle occur in response to training. These include increases in the number of myofibrils, the density of the sarcoplasm, sarcoplasm reticulum, and T tubules, and sodium-potassium ATPase pump activity.

✔ Other adaptations in skeletal muscle include increased buffer capacity, anaerobic substrate content, altered enzyme activity, increased connective tissue strength, anabolic hormone receptor up-regulation, increased fascicle length and fiber orientation, and, in some cases (aerobic training) increased mitochondrial and capillary density.

Review Questions

1. A muscle that opposes agonist movement is known as a(n)
   a. Fixator
   b. Antagonist
   c. Stabilizer
   d. Origin

2. A structural barrier protein that needs to be displaced in order for muscle contraction to occur is
   a. Titin
   b. Myosin
   c. Tropomyosin
   d. Actin

3. An untrained individual begins a 10-week resistance training program. Which of the following fiber-type transitions would be expected in this individual after 10 weeks of training?
   a. Type IC to type I
   b. Type IIA to type IIX
   c. Type IIX to type IIA
   d. Type IIX to type I

4. The longitudinal splitting of muscle fibers resulting in an increase in muscle fiber number is
   a. Myogenesis
   b. Hyperplasia
   c. Hypertrophy
   d. Myoblast

5. Which of the following statements is true concerning muscle hypertrophy and training?
   a. Metabolites may play a direct or indirect role in muscle growth
   b. Concentric muscle actions are most critical to muscle growth
   c. Type I fibers hypertrophy to the greatest extent
   d. Tension plays a minimal role in muscle growth

6. Which of the following proteins has an inhibiting effect on muscle growth?
   a. Myostatin
   b. Myosin
   c. Actin
   d. Myogenin

7. Fast-twitch muscle fibers have _____ compared to slow-twitch fibers
   a. Slower myosin
   b. Lower cross-sectional area
   c. Greater capillary density
   d. Greater glycogen stores

8. Myofibrils stacked in parallel form muscle fascicles.   T F

9. The process of muscle fiber generation is known as myogenesis.   T F

10. Endurance training leads to substantial muscle hypertrophy.   T F

11. Occlusive resistance exercise using light to moderate loading has been shown to produce increases in muscle hypertrophy.   T F

12. Consistent progressive resistance training leads to a greater net amount of protein content within skeletal muscle.   T F

References

1. Alway SE, MacDougall JD, Sale DG. Contractile adaptations in the human triceps surae after isometric exercise. *J Appl Physiol*. 1989; 66:2725–2732.

2. Andersen JL, Aagaard P. Myosin heavy chain IIX overshoot in human skeletal muscle. *Muscle Nerve*. 2000;23:1095–1104.

3. Bamman MM, Ragan RC, Kim JS, Cross JM, Hill VJ, Tuggle SC, et al. Myogenic protein expression before and after resistance loading in 26- and 64-yr-old men and women. *J Appl Physiol*. 2004; 97:1329–1337.

4. Bickel CS, Slade J, Mahoney E, Haddad F, Dudley GA, Adams GR. Time course of molecular responses of human skeletal muscle to acute bouts of resistance exercise. *J Appl Physiol*. 2005;98: 482–488.

5. Campos GE, Luecke TJ, Wendeln HK, et al. Muscular adaptations in response to three different resistance-training regimens: specificity of repetition maximum training zones. *Eur J Appl Physiol*. 2002; 88:50–60.

6. Chen TC. Effects of a second bout of maximal eccentric exercise on muscle damage and electromyographic activity. *Eur J Appl Physiol*. 2003;89:115–121.

7. Coffey VG, Shield A, Canny BJ, Carey KA, Cameron-Smith D, Hawley JA. Interaction of contractile activity and training history on mRNA abundance in skeletal muscle from trained athletes. *Am J Physiol Endocrinol Metab*. 2006;290:E849–E855.

8. Drummond MJ, Fujita S, Takashi A, Dreyer HC, Volpi E, Rasmussen BB. Human muscle gene expression following resistance exercise and blood flow restriction. *Med Sci Sports Exerc*. 2008;40:691–698.

9. Dudley GA, Tesch PA, Miller BJ, Buchanan MD. Importance of eccentric actions in performance adaptations to resistance training. *Aviat Space Environ Med*. 1991;62:543–550.

10. Fry AC, Allemeier CA, Staron RS. Correlation between percentage fiber type area and myosin heavy chain content in human skeletal muscle. *Eur J Appl Physiol*. 1994;68:246–251.

11. Gonyea W, Ericson GC, Bonde-Peterson F. Skeletal muscle fiber splitting induced by weight lifting exercise in cats. *Acta Physiol Scand*. 1977;99:105–109.

12. Green HJ, Ballantyne CS, MacDougall JD, Tarnopolsky MA, Schertzer JD. Adaptations in human muscle sarcoplasmic reticulum to prolonged submaximal training. *J Appl Physiol*. 2003; 94:2034–2042.

13. Green HJ, Barr DJ, Fowles JR, Sandiford SD, Ouyang J. Malleability of human skeletal muscle Na⁺-K⁺-ATPase pump with short-term training. *J Appl Physiol*. 2004;97:143–148.

14. Haddad F, Adams GR. Selected contribution: acute cellular and molecular responses to resistance exercise. *J Appl Physiol*. 2002; 93:394–403.

15. Häkkinen K, Alen M, Komi PV. Neuromuscular, anaerobic, and aerobic performance characteristics of elite power athletes. *Eur J Appl Physiol Occup Physiol*. 1984;53:97–105.

16. Häkkinen K, Alen M, Komi PV. Changes in isometric force-and relaxation-time, electromyographic and muscle fibre characteristics of human skeletal muscle during strength training and detraining. *Acta Physiol Scand*. 1985;125:573–585.

17. Häkkinen K, Pakarinen A, Kraemer WJ, Häkkinen A, Valkeinen H, Alen M. Selective muscle hypertrophy, changes in EMG and force, and serum hormones during strength training in older women. *J Appl Physiol*. 2001;91:569–580.

18. Harber MP, Fry AC, Rubin MR, Smith JC, Weiss LW. Skeletal muscle and hormonal adaptations to circuit weight training in untrained men. *Scand J Med Sci Sports*. 2004;14:176–185.

19. Hoffman JR, Ratamess NA. Medical issues of anabolic steroids: are they over-exaggerated? *J Sports Sci Med*. 2006;5:182–193.

20. Hortobagyi T, Hill JP, Houmard JA, Fraser DD, Lambert NJ, Israel RG. Adaptive responses to muscle lengthening and shortening in humans. *J Appl Physiol*. 1996;80:765–772.

21. Howatson G, Van Someren K, Hortobagyi T. Repeated bout effect after maximal eccentric exercise. *Int J Sports Med*. 2007;28: 557–563.

22. Hulmi JJ, Ahtiainen JT, Kaasalainen T, et al. Postexercise myostatin and activin IIb mRNA levels: effects of strength training. *Med Sci Sports Exerc*. 2007;39:289–297.

23. Kosek DJ, Kim JS, Petrella JK, Cross JM, Bamman MM. Efficacy of 3 days/wk resistance training on myofiber hypertrophy and myogenic mechanisms in young vs. older adults. *J Appl Physiol*. 2006;101:531–544.

24. Kraemer WJ, Patton JF, Gordon SE, et al. Compatibility of high-intensity strength and endurance training on hormonal and skeletal muscle adaptations. *J Appl Physiol*. 1995;78:976–989.

25. Kraemer WJ, Nindl BC, Ratamess NA, et al. Changes in muscle hypertrophy in women with periodized resistance training. *Med Sci Sports Exerc*. 2004;36:697–708.

26. Kraemer WJ, Ratamess NA. Fundamentals of resistance training: progression and exercise prescription. *Med Sci Sport Exerc*. 2004; 36:674–678.

27. Linossier MT, Dormois D, Geyssant A, Denis C. Performance and fibre characteristics of human skeletal muscle during short sprint training and detraining on a cycle ergometer. *Eur J Appl Physiol*. 1997; 75:491–498.

28. MacDougall JD, Sale DG, Moroz JR, Elder GC, Sutton JR, Howald H. Mitochondrial volume density in human skeletal muscle following heavy resistance training. *Med Sci Sports*. 1979;11: 164–166.

29. MacDougall JD, Sale DG, Elder GC, Sutton JR. Muscle ultrastructural characteristics of elite powerlifters and bodybuilders. *Eur J Appl Physiol*. 1982;48:117–126.

30. MacDougall JD, Sale DG, Alway SE, Sutton JR. Muscle fiber number in biceps brachii in body builders and control subjects. *J Appl Physiol*. 1984;57:1399–1403.

31. Madarame H, Neya M, Ochi E, Nakazato K, Sato Y, Ishii N. Cross-transfer effects of resistance training with blood flow restriction. *Med Sci Sports Exerc*. 2008;40:258–263.

32. Madsen K, Franch J, Clausen T. Effects of intensified endurance training on the concentration of Na,K-ATPase and Ca-ATPase in human skeletal muscle. *Acta Physiol Scand*. 1994;150:251–258.

33. Mair J, Mayr M, Muller E, et al. Rapid adaptation to eccentric exercise-induced muscle damage. *Int J Sports Med*. 1995;16:352–356.

34. McCall GE, Byrnes WC, Dickinson A, Pattany PM, Fleck SJ. Muscle fiber hypertrophy, hyperplasia, and capillary density in college men after resistance training. *J Appl Physiol*. 1996;81: 2004–2012.

35. McComas AJ. *Skeletal Muscle: Form and Function*. Champaign (IL): Human Kinetics; 1996.

36. Nosaka K, Sakamoto K, Newton M, Sacco P. The repeated bout effect of reduced-load eccentric exercise on elbow flexor muscle damage. *Eur J Appl Physiol*. 2001;85:34–40.

37. Nosaka K, Newton MJ, Sacco P. Attenuation of protective effect against eccentric exercise-induced muscle damage. *Can J Appl Physiol*. 2005;30:529–542.

38. O'Neill DS, Zheng D, Anderson WK, Dohm GL, Houmard JA. Effect of endurance exercise on myosin heavy chain gene regulation in human skeletal muscle. *Am J Physiol*. 1999;276:R414–R419.

39. Ortenblad N, Lunde PK, Levin K, Andersen JL, Pedersen PK. Enhanced sarcoplasmic reticulum Ca(2+) release following intermittent sprint training. *Am J Physiol*. 2000;279:R152–R160.

40. Perez-Gomez J, Olmedillas H, Delgado-Guerra S, et al. Effects of weight lifting training combined with plyometric exercises on physical fitness, body composition, and knee extension velocity during kicking in football. *Appl Physiol Nutr Metab*. 2008;33: 501–510.

41. Phillips S, Tipton K, Aarsland A, Wolf S, Wolfe R. Mixed muscle protein synthesis and breakdown after resistance exercise in humans. *Am J Physiol.* 1997;273:E99–E107.

42. Psilander N, Damsgaard R, Pilegaard H. Resistance exercise alters MRF and IGF-I mRNA content in human skeletal muscle. *J Appl Physiol.* 2003;95:1038–1044.

43. Putnam CT, Xu X, Gillies E, MacLean IM, Bell GJ. Effects of strength, endurance and combined training on myosin heavy chain content and fibre-type distribution in humans. *Eur J Appl Physiol.* 2004;92:376–384.

44. Ratamess NA. Amino acid supplementation: what can it really do for you? *Pure Power* 2004;4:38–42.

45. Ratamess NA. *Coaches Guide to Performance-Enhancing Supplements.* Monterey (CA): Coaches Choice Books; 2006.

46. Rooney KJ, Herbert RD, Balwave RJ. Fatigue contributes to the strength training stimulus. *Med Sci Sports Exerc.* 1994;26:1160–1164.

47. Ross A, Leveritt M. Long-term metabolic and skeletal muscle adaptations to short-sprint training: implications for sprint training and tapering. *Sports Med.* 2001;31:1063–1082.

48. Roth SM, Ferrell RE, Peters DG, et al. Influence of age, sex, and strength training on human muscle gene expression determined by microarray. *Physiol Genomics.* 2002;10:181–190.

49. Roth SM, Martel GF, Ferrell RE, Metter EJ, Hurley BF, Rogers MA. Myostatin gene expression is reduced in humans with heavy-resistance strength training: a brief communication. *Exp Biol Med.* 2003;228:706–709.

50. Shinohara M, Kouzaki M, Yoshihisa T, Fukunaga T. Efficacy of tourniquet ischemia for strength training with low resistance. *Eur J Appl Physiol.* 1998;77:189–191.

51. Short KR, Vittone JL, Bigelow ML, et al. Changes in myosin heavy chain mRNA and protein expression in human skeletal muscle with age and endurance exercise training. *J Appl Physiol.* 2005;99:95–102.

52. Smith RC, Rutherford OM. The role of metabolites in strength training. I. A comparison of eccentric and concentric contractions. *Eur J Appl Physiol.* 1995;71:332–336.

53. Staron RS, Karapondo DL, Kraemer WJ, et al. Skeletal muscle adaptations during early phase of heavy-resistance training in men and women. *J Appl Physiol.* 1994;76:1247–1255.

54. Staron RS. The classification of human skeletal muscle fiber types. *J Strength Cond Res.* 1997;11:67.

55. Takarada Y, Nakamura Y, Aruga S, Onda T, Miyazaki S, Ishii N. Rapid increase in plasma growth hormone after low-intensity resistance exercise with vascular occlusion. *J Appl Physiol.* 2000; 88:61–65.

56. Takarada Y, Tsuruta T, Ishii N. Cooperative effects of exercise and occlusive stimuli on muscular function in low-intensity resistance exercise with moderate vascular occlusion. *Jpn J Physiol.* 2004; 54:585–592.

57. Tesch PA, Alkner BA. Acute and chronic muscle metabolic adaptations to strength training. In: Komi PV, editor. *Strength and Power in Sport.* 2nd ed. Boston (MA): Blackwell Science; 2002. pp. 265–280.

58. Tesch PA, Larsson L. Muscle hypertrophy in bodybuilders. *Eur J Appl Physiol.* 1982;49:301–306.

59. Tesch PA, Thorsson A, Essen-Gustavsson B. Enzyme activities of FT and ST muscle fibers in heavy-resistance trained athletes. *J Appl Physiol.* 1989;67:83–87.

60. Vikne H, Refsnes PE, Ekmark M, Medbo JI, Gundersen V, Gundersen K. Muscular performance after concentric and eccentric exercise in trained men. *Med Sci Sports Exerc.* 2006;38:1770–1781.

61. Waldegger S, Busch GL, Kaba NK, et al. Effect of cellular hydration on protein metabolism. *Miner Electrolyte Metab.* 1997;23: 201–205.

62. Wernbom M, Augustsson J, Thomee R. Effects of vascular occlusion on muscular endurance in dynamic knee extension exercise at different submaximal loads. *J Strength Cond Res.* 2006;20: 372–377.

63. Willoughby DS, Rosene JM. Effects of oral creatine and resistance training on myogenic regulatory factor expression. *Med Sci Sports Exerc.* 2003;35:923–929.

5 Connective Tissue Adaptations to Training

After completing this chapter, you will be able to:

- Identify the types of stresses and subsequent strain that lead to connective tissue adaptations
- Understand the internal and external features of a bone
- Understand how bones hypertrophy in response to loading
- Discuss ways to alter training programs to target increased bone strength and size
- Describe the components of connective tissue structures and understand adaptations to exercise training
- Discuss the functions of cartilage and subsequent adaptations to exercise

Increases in muscle size, strength, endurance, and power can only be maximized when the supporting structures adapt proportionally. That is, increases in connective tissue (CT) size, strength, and endurance need to take place in order to accommodate changes in skeletal muscle performance. CT structures include bones, tendons, ligaments, fascia, and cartilage. Adaptations in CT resulting from training are critical for how muscle force is transmitted to bone, joint stability, and injury prevention. This chapter discusses various types of CT structures and concurrent adaptations to training.

STIMULI FOR CONNECTIVE TISSUE ADAPTATIONS

Before discussing CT, it is important to overview terminology associated with loading, which initiates the adaptation process. CT can only adapt when it is progressively overloaded by increasing stress. **Mechanical stress** is defined by the internal force observed divided by the cross-sectional area of the CT structure. By definition, less mechanical stress is placed on CT when the cross-sectional area (denominator in the equation) increases per level of force encountered. Thus, CT increases tolerance for loading by increasing size and/or by altering structural properties. These have important ramifications for injury prevention in sports and force transmission from muscle to bone. CT adaptations must take place to accommodate changes in muscle performance. However, CT adaptations take place at a slower rate compared to skeletal muscle.

TYPES OF STRESS

Stress relates to the force applied to CT. The three most common types of stress associated with CT are tension, compression, and shear stresses. *Tension* stresses result in pulling forces on the tissue. Stretching or elongation occurs as is the case with tendons during muscle contraction. *Compression* stresses result in pushing the structure inward, or compressing its longitudinal length. Some examples include the spine when performing the squat exercise or the humerus (upper arm bone) when performing a push-up. *Shear* stresses result in skewing where force is encountered obliquely. Examples include scissors during cutting and the knee during a knee extension exercise. Shear stresses tend to be more injurious when encountered athletically. In some cases a twisting effect, or *torsion*, is seen. The result of stress is deformation to CT. Deformation leads to adaptation and is proportional to the level of stress encountered.

Stress-Strain Relationship

As stress is the level of force encountered by a tissue, **strain** is the magnitude of deformation that takes place in proportion to the amount of stress applied. Two types of strain are shown in CT, linear and shear. *Linear strain* results from compressive and tensile stresses where the tissue (tendons, ligaments) changes length, and the quantification of linear strain is expressed as a percentage relative to resting length. *Shear strain* results in bending of the tissue (bone) and is quantified by the angle of deformation. For circular-type tissues (cartilage), another

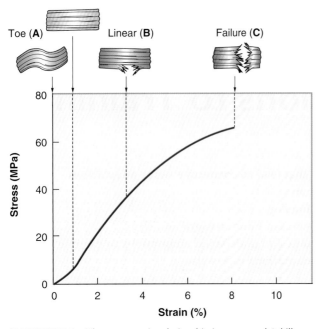

■ FIGURE 5.1. The stress-strain relationship in a ruptured Achilles tendon. The three distinct regions are (**A**) toe region, (**B**) linear region, and (**C**) failure region.

type of strain can be seen. When a tissue is compressed, its longitudinal height decreases but it laterally expands. The ratio of strain in the longitudinal direction to strain in the lateral direction is known as **Poisson's ratio**. This is a useful measure to examine compression in articular cartilage and intervertebral disks (where too great of a strain can lead to a rupture).

The stress-strain relationship for a tendon is shown in Figure 5.1. Stress is shown on the Y axis whereas strain (%) is shown on the X axis. At complete rest, there is a small degree of slack in the tendon. Upon low level of muscle contraction, the tendon elongates to its normal length and is denoted as the *toe region* on the graph. With greater stress, there is a proportional increase in strain depicted as the *linear region* on the graph. If the level of stress is too high, injury can result as denoted as the *failure region* on the graph. Upon elongation as a result of stress, the tendon can return to its normal length when the stress is removed. The property of CT to return to its original length after being stretched is **elasticity**. However, chronic stretching to a tissue can cause transient or permanent deformation where the tissue remains at least partially elongated and does not return entirely to its original length. This property is known as **plasticity**. There are times where plasticity is good (tendons in response to chronic flexibility training) or bad (ligaments in response to damage over time).

SKELETAL SYSTEM

The skeletal system consists of 206 bones, 177 of which are involved in human voluntary movement (Fig. 5.2).

The skeletal system is divided into two major subdivisions: axial and appendicular. The *axial skeleton* consists of 80 bones of the skull and trunk (vertebral column, ribs, sternum, sacrum, and coccyx) whereas the *appendicular skeleton* consists of 126 bones of the limbs, shoulder, and pelvic girdle. The skeletal system plays several important roles in human function. It provides support, area for muscular attachment, and protection to several organs. Bones produce movement upon skeletal muscle contraction. Bones provide a storage site for minerals in times where dietary intake may be low. Lastly, bones produce red blood cells which are essential for transporting oxygen.

BONE ANATOMY

Bones exist in five forms. *Long bones* (femur, humerus) contribute greatly to human height and limb lengths. *Short bones* (carpals and tarsals of hands and feet) are typically found in areas where mobility is critical. *Flat bones* (ribs, scapula, bones of the skull, sternum) are especially important for protection. *Irregular bones* (vertebrae) are uniquely shaped because they perform a multitude of functions. *Sesamoid bones* (patella) help create a more favorable line of pull for muscles that span their surface area.

To understand how bones adapt to exercise, it is important to examine the anatomy of a bone. Figure 5.3 depicts the anatomy of a long bone. The polar ends of the bone are known as the *epiphyses*. Growth plates (epiphyseal plates) are located here and are the sites of longitudinal bone growth during the developmental years. The long region of the bone is known as the shaft, or *diaphysis*. Long bones consist of two types of bone: compact and spongy. *Compact bone* is located on the perimeter and is much stronger than *spongy (trabecular) bone* which is located within and helps give bone its pliability. The ratio of each within a bone dictates the degree of strength and pliability of the bone. The outermost layer of the bone is the *periosteum*. The periosteum consists of two layers of importance. The outermost layer provides a firm base for CT attachment. The innermost layer secretes cells involved in bone remodeling. The *endosteum* is the innermost layer that surrounds the medullary cavity which also secretes cells involved in bone remodeling. The medullary cavity houses bone marrow.

The internal anatomy of a long bone is shown in Figure 5.4. The layer of compact bone is highly organized. Compact bone is comprised of osteons. The *osteon* resembles a concentric layer with a central canal that provides a conduit for nerves and blood vessels. A cellular look shows the mature bone cells, the *osteocytes*, as well as the surrounding bone matrix comprise osteons. Below, it is shown that the osteocyte is housed within the *lacunae* (space) and is surrounded by canaliculi. The *canaliculi* act similar to a capillary bed in that nutrients are dispersed

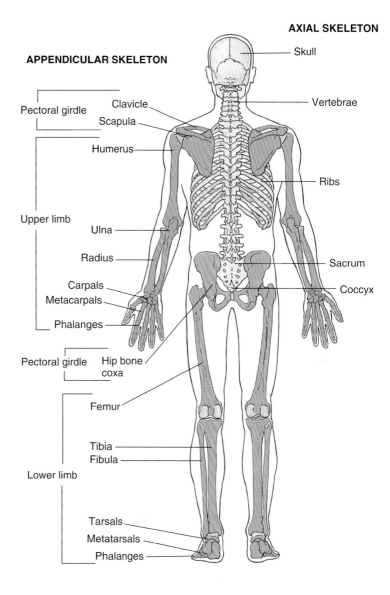

APPENDICULAR SKELETON

AXIAL SKELETON

Skull

Pectoral girdle

Clavicle

Scapula

Vertebrae

Humerus

Ribs

Upper limb

Ulna

Radius

Sacrum

Coccyx

Carpals

Metacarpals

Phalanges

Pectoral girdle

Hip bone
coxa

Femur

Lower limb

Tibia

Fibula

Tarsals

Metatarsals

Phalanges

■ **FIGURE 5.2.** The axial and appendicular skeletons. (From Moore KL, Agur AMR. *Essential Clinical Anatomy*. 2nd Ed. Baltimore (MD): Lippincott Williams & Wilkins; 2004.)

throughout thereby supplying the osteocyte. Canaliculi play a major role in how bones adapt to loading as they deform during fluid movement which stimulates the osteocytes. The area surrounding the osteocyte is known as the *bone matrix*. The bone matrix consists of an organic (~35%) and inorganic (~65%) region. The organic region consists primarily of protein, most of which is in the form of **collagen** which helps give bone strength and pliability. The inorganic region consists of minerals and specialized cells that help ossify bone known as *hydroxyapatites*. The inorganic region is important for giving bone its stiffness and compression strength. Overall, bone consists of approximately 25%–30% of its content in water.

BONE REMODELING

Remodeling is a process that affects bone. Bone is constantly broken down and built up again. In order for remodeling to occur, functional cells must be activated to alter bone metabolism. Bone formation is brought

about by specialized activated cells known as *osteoblasts*. Osteoblasts are cells that secrete a collagen-rich ground substance (to help form the bone matrix) that aids in bone formation. They are secreted by the periosteum and endosteum and secrete a substance called *osteocalcin*, which serves as a blood marker for bone metabolism. Osteoblasts secrete an enzyme known as *bone alkaline phosphatase* (involved in bone mineralization), which has been used as a blood marker of bone metabolism. *Osteoclasts* are cells involved in bone resorption, or breakdown. They digest the mineralized bone matrix via acids and lysosomal enzymes thereby breaking down bone. Both osteoblasts and osteoclasts develop from stem cells and are activated from parent molecules under the control of hormones, growth factors, immune cells, nutrients, and physical activity. Because it takes 3–4 months for one complete bone remodeling cycle consisting of bone resorption, formation, and mineralization to occur, measurable changes in bone mass take at least 6–8 months (1).

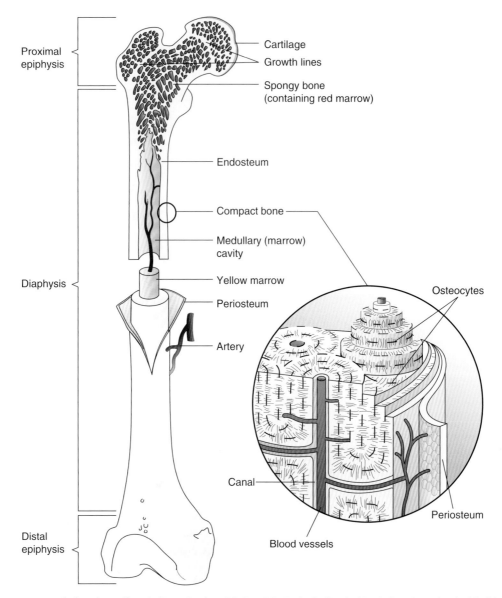

■ **FIGURE 5.3.** Anatomy of a long bone (femur). (From Smeltzer SC, Bare BG. *Textbook of Medical-Surgical Nursing*. 9th Ed. Philadelphia (PA): Lippincott Williams & Wilkins; 2000.)

Bone Growth

Bones grow in both length and width. Longitudinal bone growth occurs during our developmental years and occurs primarily in two ways. Bone growth resulting from CT membranes is known as *intramembranous ossification* whereas growth from cartilage is known as *endochondral ossification*. After the first few years of life, bones continue to develop mostly by endochondral ossification. Longitudinal bone growth takes place at the **growth plate**. The epiphyses enlarge by growth of cartilage and bone replacement as the diaphysis extends. Each bone has its own rate of metabolism; therefore, some bones fully reach their final length by age 18 and some may take as long as 25 years of age. Changes in longitudinal length are supported by changes in bone width, or *appositional growth*.

Of interest to discussion of adaptations to exercise is the process by which skeletal loading increases bone width. An increase in bone cross-sectional area (CSA) allows bone to tolerate greater loading (Fig. 5.5). Muscle strength and size gains increase the force exerted on the bones. Stronger forces of contraction increase the mechanical stress (and strain) on bone, and bone must increase its size to accommodate larger muscles. Bone responds to loading intracellularly by a general process known as **mechanotransduction**, or the transduction of a mechanical force into a local cellular signal. In this model, mechanical loading applied to bone causes deformation, or bending of the bone. Bending is proportional to the magnitude and rate of loading applied, thereby demonstrating the importance of exercise intensity. Bending may occur as a result of direct compressive loading to the

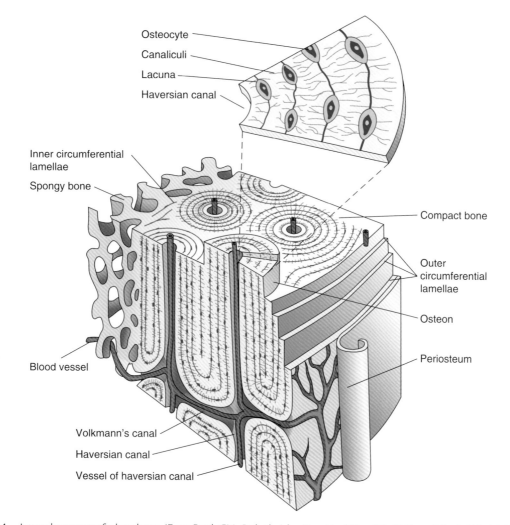

FIGURE 5.4. Internal anatomy of a long bone. (From Porth CM. *Pathophysiology Concepts of Altered Health States.* 7th ed. Philadelphia (PA): Lippincott Williams & Wilkins; 2005.)

skeletal system or by forces associated with tendons pulling during muscular contraction. Deformation to bone causes fluids to move within the bone (bones are approximately 25%–30% water). In order for this model to be effective, a sensor is needed to perceive this stimulus. The sensor in bone is the mature bone cell, the osteocyte. The osteocyte is activated in a few ways, either by stretching the membrane (via fluid movement) or by electrical charges resulting from ion movement within the fluids. Both stimuli open ion channels (calcium, sodium) on the osteocyte, and calcium influx is critical to mediating a slew of reactions within the osteocyte. The main result is to increase gene transcription and translation of proteins ultimately leading to bone deposition and structural changes. Collagen fibers form a scaffold, minerals and hydroxyapatites (adhesive cells) migrate, and osteoblasts reach the targeted area resulting in bone ossification. Although these processes are engaged quickly, measurable bone growth is very slow and may take several months.

BONE ADAPTATIONS TO EXERCISE

Exercise poses a potent stress to the skeletal system. However, the stress must reach a certain level in order for bones to adapt. The term **minimal essential strain** has been defined as the minimal threshold stimulus (volume and intensity) that is needed for new bone formation (25). If the exercise stimulus does not reach this threshold, then there is no need for bones to adapt favorably. In fact, some studies that have shown no effect of training on bone mass used low training intensities (1). The minimal essential strain depends upon an athlete's training status and age. Exercise needs to be of sufficient intensity and volume to elicit increases in **bone mineral density (BMD)**. Bone mineral density is commonly used to study bone adaptations. However, bone strength can increase independently of changes in BMD (1). Bones can become stronger at a much larger rate and magnitude (via architectural changes) than the potential increases seen

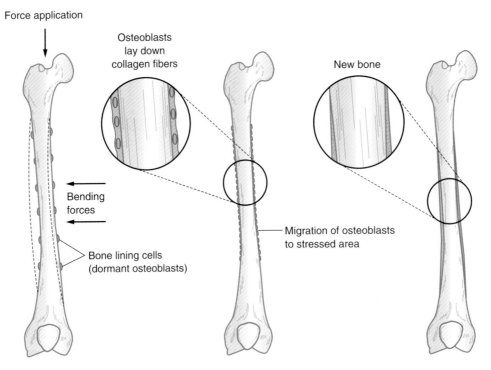

FIGURE 5.5.   Model for bone adaptation to loading.

in BMD. It has been suggested that the minimal essential strain is approximately one-tenth of the force required to fracture bone. Certain exercises are better than others for increasing BMD. Dynamic, high-intensity loading to the skeletal system is paramount. Weight-bearing exercise is more effective than non-weight-bearing exercise for increasing BMD as loading magnitude and rate is higher when an individual has to bear his or her body weight. Lifting and contact sports, and sports/activities requiring explosive running/jumping (plyometrics, sprint, and agility) are excellent means to increase BMD whereas swimming is less effective because of the buoyancy of water decreasing stress on the skeletal system. In 2004, the American College of Sports Medicine (ACSM)

(1) published a position stand recommending the following training guidelines for increasing bone mass:

- Weight-bearing endurance exercises, activities that involve jumping, and resistance training (RT)
- Moderate to high exercise intensities
- Endurance exercise frequency of 3–5 days per week, RT frequency of 2–3 days per week
- Exercise for 30–60 minutes per day involving multiple training modalities (RT, endurance training)

Research shows a positive relationship between BMD and muscle mass and strength (31). Stronger individuals tend to have higher BMD values than less-fit populations. Athletes tend to have greater BMD than age-matched,

Interpreting Research

Bone Mineral Density Changes Following 1 Year of Training

Cussler EC, Lohman TG, Going SB, et al. Weight lifted in strength training predicts bone change in post-menopausal women. *Med Sci Sports Exerc.* 2003;35:10–17.

Although it has long been speculated that heavier weights yield greater increases in BMD, very little long-term research has been conducted to explore this phenomenon. Cussler et al. (8) studied postmenopausal women over the course of 1 year of RT, *i.e.,* eight exercises, 2 sets of 6–8 reps (70%–80% of 1 RM), and 3 days per week. They measured BMD before and after 1 year of RT. They found a linear relationship between changes in BMD in site-specific regions and the amount of weight lifted during training. The weights lifted in the squat exercise showed the highest relationship to BMD increases in the femur. This study demonstrated the importance of lifting progressively heavier loads when training to increase BMD.

untrained populations (1). Resistance-trained athletes have higher BMD than age-matched sedentary individuals (6,28). However, bones have a much longer adaptational period. A short-term training program may not increase BMD. BMD changes are typically seen after 6 months of training (5) and only if an individual trains beyond their current threshold level of adaptation, or minimal essential strain. The quantitative deposition of bone is a long process. Interestingly, the initial bone growth processes begin after the first few workouts. Osteogenic bone markers in the blood can be measured to investigate potential increases in activation of bone anabolic processes despite no changes in bone size taking place at that time. Two markers of bone growth include *bone alkaline phosphatase* and *osteocalcin*. High-intensity anaerobic exercise can elevate osteocalcin concentrations (7,32). Weightlifters have higher osteocalcin concentrations (by 35%) than age-matched control subjects (14). Resistance training elevates osteocalcin (and bone alkaline phosphatase) (13,23) and the magnitude is affected by protein intake (2,26). The mechanisms of bone growth are engaged within the first few workouts but take several months before measurable changes are seen.

TRAINING TO INCREASE BONE SIZE AND STRENGTH

Training programs designed to stimulate bone growth need to incorporate specificity of loading, speed and direction of loading, volume, proper exercise selection, progressive overload, and variation (1,25). Although the scientific study of program differentiation on bone growth is limited, the following general recommendations may be helpful:

- Multijoint exercises (squats, power cleans, dead lifts, bench press) are preferred because they enable the individual to lift greater loads.
- Loading should be high with moderate to low volume (10 reps and less).
- Fast velocities of contraction are preferred as force is proportional to acceleration, and increasing the force requirement on skeletal muscles produces greater stress on bone.
- Rest intervals should be moderate to long in length (at least 2–3 min) to accommodate greater loading during each set.
- Variation in the training stress is important for altering the stimuli to bone.

Case Study 5.1

Brenda is a 35-year-old woman who has been weight training for 5 years. A primary goal she wanted to attain was to increase her bone mass to prevent osteoporosis as she ages. At a recent checkup, her physician ordered a bone scan to assess her BMD. It was reported that her BMD did not change in the past 5 years (since the last time she had the test performed). Brenda is confused because she had joined a health club and was working out consistently over the past 5 years. Thus, she anticipated increasing her BMD to some extent. Upon examination of her program, Brenda exercised aerobically 1 day per week and worked out with weights 2 days per week during this time period. Her cardiovascular exercise consisted of stationary cycling for 20 minutes and her weight training consisted of predominantly machine-based exercises for 3 sets of 10–15 reps with loads corresponding to ~30%–45% of her maximal potential. She has performed this same training routine for the majority of the 5 years with little change to the intensity, volume, and exercise selection.

Question for Consideration: What advice would you give to Brenda regarding how she could change her program to more effectively target bone growth?

COMPONENTS OF DENSE CONNECTIVE TISSUE

Tendons and ligaments are dense fibrous CT structures composed of predominantly water (60%–70% of content), *fibroblasts* (collagen-producing cells) and *fibrocytes* (mature cells), elastin, collagen, and ground substances. Ground substances help provide structural stability to CT. *Elastin* is a protein that gives CT its elastic quality whereas collagen is the strongest, most abundant (20%–25% of total protein) protein in the human body. Collagen provides great tensile strength which is why it is found in tissues requiring support and strength. There are many types of collagen. Type I is found in skin, bones, tendons, and ligaments whereas type II is found in cartilage. Figure 5.6 shows a collagen fiber. Collagen provides strength primarily for two reasons. It is stacked in parallel to form larger components. Collagen molecules are self-assembled or stacked in parallel to form microfibrils, microfibrils are stacked in parallel to form fibrils, fibrils are stacked in parallel to form fibers, and fibers form a collagen bundle that forms the structure of tendons, for example. The fibril is the load-bearing unit. The second major reason is its structure. Collagen is activated from its parent molecule, *procollagen*, and consists of three chains of >1,400 amino acids in each. Collagen consists mostly of three amino acids, proline (~25%), hydroxyproline (~25%), and glycine (~33%). These amino acids are essential because they help form very tight hydrogen bonds in between the three chains. These bonds are called **cross-links** and provide great strength to the collagen fibers similar to what may be seen in

Myths & Misconceptions

Resistance Training will Stunt Bone Growth in Children and Adolescents

One common myth and misconception is RT will stunt a child's growth. However, this is not the case. Of primary concern for a child or adolescent is that the epiphyseal (growth) plates have not fully ossified. Depending on the bone in question, growth plates completely ossify between the ages of 18 and 25 years but occur a few years earlier in females compared to males (11). A concern exists that a growth plate injury can occur to a child via trauma or overuse. In general, most injuries (fractures) occurring to growth plates will have full recovery provided that blood flow is adequate during healing. Although growth can be temporarily stunted during the injury period, bone metabolism will increase higher than normal following this period resulting in bone growth reaching its normal level (a phenomenon known as **catch-up growth**). Although some growth plate injuries are very serious and pose potential growth problems, full recovery is seen in most cases. Resistance training is a very safe form of exercise for children and adolescents provided that it is supervised and proper recommendations are followed. Although some injuries to children and adolescents have occurred during RT, these were mostly the result of lack of supervision leading to very poor technique, loading, or accidents (11). Research has shown that RT in children and adolescents is very safe when properly supervised, and has concluded that RT does not negatively impact growth and maturation (9–12,22). In fact, position stands developed by the National Strength and Conditioning Association and Canadian Society for Exercise Physiology (endorsed by the ACSM) recommend RT as a suitable exercise modality in children and adolescents (3,9). Although there is no minimal age requirement (children should be mature enough to be able to listen and follow directions), children as young as 6 years of age have participated safely in RT programs. Some recommendations (3,9–11) include

- Low to moderate intensities for 6–15 reps with gradual increase in intensity
- 1–3 sets per exercise
- 2–3 nonconsecutive days per week
- Single- and multijoint exercises

a rope. Collagen turnover (the net change in collagen content from synthesis and degradation) is important for determining CT strength and is highly related to stretch and loading (15).

Tendons have a higher proportion of collagen whereas ligaments possess a higher proportion of elastin. In fact, the collagen content in tendons and ligaments are both higher than bone and much larger than skeletal muscle (15). Tendons provide great strength and passive energy absorption whereas ligaments tend to be more pliable. This is critical as tendons connect muscles to bones whereas ligaments connect bones to other bones. Tendon metabolism is slower because of poor circulation. CTs that surround and separate different organizational levels within skeletal muscle are referred to as *fascia*. Fascia contains bundles of collagen fibers arranged in different planes to provide resistance to forces from different directions. Fascia within skeletal muscle converges to form a tendon through which the force of muscle contraction is transmitted to bone.

TENDON, LIGAMENT, AND FASCIAL ADAPTATIONS TO TRAINING

The major stimulus for growth of tendons, ligaments, and fascia is mechanical loading which leads to a cascade of events leading to hypertrophy. These processes may be analogous to the mechanotransduction of bone previously discussed. Stretching of the cytoskeleton in response to loading appears to be the stimulus leading to greater net collagen synthesis and CT growth (15,16). The degree of adaptation is proportional to the intensity of exercise. The sites where CT can increase strength are (a) at the junctions between the tendon/ligament and bone surface, (b) within the body of the tendon/ligament, and (c) in the network of fascia within skeletal muscle. Within CT, an increase in collagen fibril number, density, and diameter, and greater number of cross-links may occur, thereby increasing its strength. Muscle hypertrophy necessitates structural and/or CSA changes to tendons to accommodate the larger force output.

Exercise initiates the processes of tendon adaptations. Acute exercise (aerobic and anaerobic) initially results in collagen degradation; however, subsequent days following collagen synthesis rate increases significantly (15). Type I collagen synthesis may be elevated during chronic training (15,16). It has been suggested that training initially results in increased type I collagen turnover to allow for organizational restructuring of the tissue, and prolonged training results in an increase in tendon CSA (15,16). Tendons hypertrophy following as little

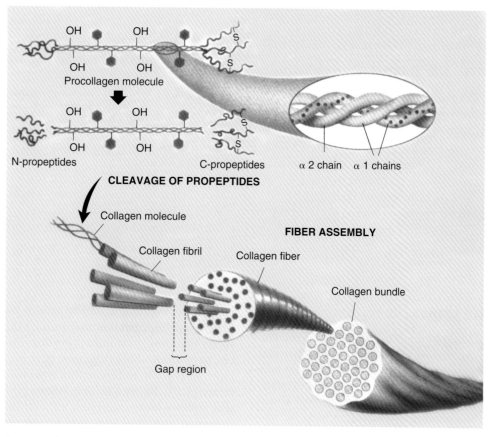

■ FIGURE 5.6. Structure of collagen.

as 12 weeks of RT (17), and runners have shown larger Achilles tendon CSA than untrained, age-matched sedentary individuals (15). **Tendon stiffness** (force transmitted per unit of strain) increases as a result of RT (16,20), and may comprise collagen organizational restructuring changes leading to increased tendon strength initially in the absence of hypertrophy. Kubo et al. (18) showed a 15%–19% increase in Achilles tendon stiffness following 8 weeks of RT. Of great importance is the intensity as heavy loads (80% of 1 RM) increase tendon stiffness but light loads (20% of 1 RM) may not (18). Interestingly, the response to training may be more prominent in men than women (30). Lastly, collagen synthesis in skeletal muscle has been shown during training indicating adaptations taking place within fascia to accommodate skeletal muscle growth (16).

Myths & Misconceptions

Connective Tissue Adapts at a Similar Rate to Skeletal Muscle

Some athletes and trainees have assumed that skeletal muscle and CT adapt at similar rates to training. Although changes in CT structure and strength are needed to accommodate enhanced muscle function, CT adaptations lag behind muscular adaptations. Skeletal muscles begin adapting after the first few workouts. Muscle strength may increase after the first workout. However, tendons, ligaments, and bone have a longer adaptation period. Bone adapts the slowest, taking several months for new deposition to occur. This can become a concern for the athlete who rapidly increases strength and power in a short period of time. The added strength and power (and subsequent increased training loads) can result in overuse injuries if CT structures do not have sufficient time to catch up. This is one reason why anabolic steroid use can lead to higher risks of injuries.

Interpreting Research

Tendon Growth and Resistance Training Loading

Kongsgaard M, Reitelseder S, Pedersen TG, et al. Region specific patellar tendon hypertrophy in humans following resistance training. *Acta Physiol.* 2007;191:111–121.

Kongsgaard et al. (17) examined patellar tendon CSA before and following a RT program. Subjects trained for 12 weeks using unilateral knee extensions. One group trained with heavy weights whereas another group trained with light weights. After RT, maximal strength increased by 15% in the heavy weight group but did not significantly increase in the light weight group (~6%). Quadriceps muscle CSA increased (by 6%) in the heavy weight group. Light weight training increased proximal patellar tendon CSA and heavy weight training increased proximal and distal tendon CSA. Patellar tendon stiffness increased only after heavy weight training. The results showed RT increased tendon CSA and that the changes were more comprehensive following heavy weight training.

CARTILAGE ADAPTATIONS TO TRAINING

Cartilage is composed of fluid (60%–80%), type II collagen, electrolytes, and other ground substances. *Articular (hyaline) cartilage* is the type that covers the ends of long bones at joints and is found within the growth plate. *Fibrous cartilage* is found within intervertebral disks, menisci, and at the point of insertion into bone for tendons and ligaments. *Elastic cartilage* is flexible and found in the ear. Articular and fibrous cartilages are the types central to adaptations resulting from exercise as collectively they provide a smooth surface for joint motion, act as a shock absorber, and assist in providing strength to tendon and ligament attachments to bone. Unique to cartilage is that it lacks its own blood supply and must receive its nutrients from *synovial fluid*. Thus, cartilage injuries have very long recovery periods and oftentimes require surgery. The process by which cartilage is perfused with synovial fluid highly depends upon physical activity. Compression and decompression of cartilage creates a pressure gradient by which synovial fluid may be absorbed into cartilage. Animal studies have shown aerobic exercise can increase articular cartilage thickness (27). However, less is known in humans although it is thought that moderate amounts of exercise can maintain cartilage thickness.

A major concern regarding articular cartilage is the potential for joint degeneration. Degeneration of articular cartilage can result in a pathological condition known as **osteoarthritis**. In animal studies, running can result in no change or an increase in articular cartilage thickness (4). In humans, moderate exercise appears to reduce cartilage degradation. For example, long-time runners have shown no greater prevalence for osteoarthritis compared to sedentary, age-matched controls (21,24). However, joint injuries and highly repetitive intense exercise upon injured or improperly healed joints pose a scenario where joint degeneration may ensue (4). Athletes from sports requiring great impact loading, *e.g.*, football, soccer, baseball, ice hockey, tennis, have been shown to be more susceptible to osteoarthritis primarily due to past injury (4,29). Buckwalter and Martin (4) have suggested that athletes most susceptible to joint degeneration are those with abnormal joint anatomy, previous joint injury and/or surgery, joint instability, heavy body weight, inadequate muscle strength, or altered muscle innervation.

Summary Points

✔ Stress is the level of force placed upon CT and strain quantifies the magnitude of deformation resulting from stress. Strain is a potent stimulus for CT adaptations to training.

✔ Bone remodeling is a cycle of catabolic and anabolic activities. Chronic training above the minimal essential strain results in remodeling favoring bone anabolism, or growth, via mechanotransduction.

✔ Bone mineral density increases during training are typically greater during weight-bearing exercise, explosive exercise, and high-intensity contact sports.

✔ Recommendations for increasing BMD during RT include multiple-joint (especially free weight) exercises of high-intensity for 10 reps or less performed with high levels of force and/or velocity.

✔ Tendons, ligaments, and fascia adapt to training favorably by increasing stiffness or CSA in order to accommodate greater muscle size and force production.

✔ Cartilage adaptations to training are less clear and appear related to the duration, intensity, and volume of training, as well as an individual's injury history. The most critical concern may be the effect of training on prevention of cartilage degeneration.

Review Questions

1. According to the ACSM, which of the following is recommended for enhancing bone mineral density in adults?
   a. Non-weight-bearing activities, low to moderate intensity, 15–30 min day^{-1}
   b. Non-weight-bearing activities, high intensity, 30–60 min day^{-1}
   c. Weight-bearing activities, low to moderate intensity, 15–30 min day^{-1}
   d. Weight-bearing activities, high intensity, 30–60 min day^{-1}

2. An untrained individual begins a weight training program. What would be the expected increase in BMD during the first 4 months?
   a. <1%–2%
   b. 5%–10%
   c. 15%–20%
   d. 25%–30%

3. The protein which gives CT an abundance of strength is
   a. Elastin
   b. Collagen
   c. Osteon
   d. Endosteum

4. A joint pathology characterized by degeneration of articular cartilage is
   a. Osteoporosis
   b. Osteogenesis
   c. Osteoarthritis
   d. Osteoblast

5. Which of the following statements is true concerning CT adaptations to exercise?
   a. Connective tissue structures rapidly adapt to training at a pace quicker than skeletal muscle
   b. Connective tissue growth will only take place if the individual trains consistently beyond his or her minimal threshold level of strain
   c. Activities that are non-weight-bearing and low in intensity are most effective for eliciting CT growth
   d. None of the above

6. Loading on the spine from placing a loaded barbell on the shoulders in preparation for performing the squat exercise is an example of a(n) _____ stress
   a. Shear
   b. Tensile
   c. Compressive
   d. Torsion

7. The property of CT to return to its original length after being stretched is elasticity.   T F

8. Bone cells that help build up bone are osteoclasts.   T F

9. The mature bone cell is known as an osteocyte.   T F

10. The magnitude of changes in BMD are due, in part, to the level of strain encountered during exercise.   T F

11. Injuries to articular cartilage heal relatively quickly because of the cartilage's great blood supply.   T F

12. An elevation in a blood biomarker such as osteocalcin indicates bone anabolism may be taking place despite no noticeable changes in BMD.   T F

References

1. American College of Sports Medicine. Position stand: Physical activity and bone health. *Med Sci Sports Exerc.* 2004;36:1985–1996.
2. Ballard TLP, Clapper JA, Specker BL, Binkley TL, Vukovich MD. Effect of protein supplementation during a 6-mo strength and conditioning program on insulin-like growth factor 1 and markers of bone turnover in young adults. *Am J Clin Nutr.* 2005;81:1442–1448.
3. Behm DG, Faigenbaum AD, Falk B, Klentrou P. Canadian Society for Exercise Physiology position paper: resistance training in children and adolescents. *Appl Physiol Nutr Metab.* 2008;33:547–561.
4. Buckwalter JA, Martin JA. Sports and osteoarthritis. *Curr Opin Rheumatol.* 2004;16:634–639.
5. Chilibeck PD, Calder A, Sale DG, Webber CE. Twenty weeks of weight training increases lean tissue mass but not bone mineral mass or density in healthy, active young women. *Can J Physiol Pharmacol.* 1996;74:1180–1185.
6. Conroy BP, Kraemer WJ, Maresh CM, et al. Bone mineral density in elite junior Olympic weightlifters. *Med Sci Sports Exerc.* 1993;25:1103–1109.
7. Creighton DL, Morgan AL, Boardley D, Brolinson PG. Weight-bearing exercise and markers of bone turnover in female athletes. *J Appl Physiol.* 2001;90:565–570.
8. Cussler EC, Lohman TG, Going SB, et al. Weight lifted in strength training predicts bone change in postmenopausal women. *Med Sci Sports Exerc.* 2003;35:10–17.
9. Faigenbaum AD, Kraemer WJ, Cahill B, et al. Youth resistance training: position statement paper and literature review: position statement. *Strength Cond.* 1996;18:62–76.
10. Faigenbaum AD. Strength training for children and adolescents. *Clin Sports Med.* 2000;19:593–619.

11. Faigenbaum AD. Age- and sex-related differences and their implications for resistance exercise. In: Baechle TR, Earle RW, editors. *Essentials of Strength Training and Conditioning.* 3rd ed. Champaign (IL): Human Kinetics; 2008. pp. 141–158.

12. Falk B, Eliakim A. Resistance training, skeletal muscle and growth. *Pediatr Endocrinol Rev.* 2003;1:120–127.

13. Fujimura R, Ashizawa N, Watanabe M, et al. Effect of resistance exercise training on bone formation and resorption in young male subjects assessed by biomarkers of bone metabolism. *J Bone Miner Res.* 1997;12:656–662.

14. Karlsson MK, Vergnaud P, Delmas PD, Obrant KJ. Indicators of bone formation in weight lifters. *Calcif Tissue Int.* 1995;56:177–180.

15. Kjaer M, Langberg H, Miller BF, et al. Metabolic activity and collagen turnover in human tendon in response to physical activity. *J Musculoskelet Neuronal Interact.* 2005;5:41–52.

16. Kjaer M, Magnusson P, Krogsgaard M, et al. Extracellular matrix adaptation of tendon and skeletal muscle to exercise. *J Anat.* 2006;208:445–450.

17. Kongsgaard M, Reitelseder S, Pedersen TG, Holm L, Aagaard PL, Kjaer M, et al. Region specific patellar tendon hypertrophy in humans following resistance training. *Acta Physiol.* 2007;191: 111–121.

18. Kubo K, Kanehisa H, Fukunaga T. Effects of resistance and stretching training programmes on the viscoelastic properties of human tendon structures in vivo. *J Physiol.* 2002;538:219–226.

19. Kubo K, Komuro T, Ishiguro N, et al. Effects of low-load resistance training with vascular occlusion on the mechanical properties of muscle and tendon. *J Appl Biomech.* 2006;22:112–119.

20. Kubo K, Yata H, Kanehisa H, Fukunaga T. Effects of isometric squat training on the tendon stiffness and jump performance. *Eur J Appl Physiol.* 2006;96:305–314.

21. Lane NE, Michel B, Bjorkengren A, et al. The risk of osteoarthritis with running and aging: a five year longitudinal study. *J Rheumatol.* 1993;20:461–468.

22. Malina RM. Weight training in youth — growth, maturation, and safety: an evidence-based review. *Clin J Sport Med.* 2006;16:478–487.

23. Menkes A, Mazel S, Redmond RA, et al. Strength training increases regional bone mineral density and bone remodeling in middle-aged and older women. *J Appl Physiol.* 1993;74:2478–2484.

24. Puranen J, Ala-Ketola L, Peltokallio P, Saarela J. Running and primary osteoarthritis of the hip. *Br Med J.* 1975;2:424–425.

25. Ratamess NA. Adaptations to anaerobic training programs. In: Baechle TR, Earle RW, editors. *Essentials of Strength Training and Conditioning.* 3rd ed. Champaign (IL): Human Kinetics; 2008; pp. 93–119.

26. Ratamess NA, Hoffman JR, Faigenbaum AD, Mangine G, Falvo MJ, Kang J. The combined effects of protein intake and resistance training on serum osteocalcin concentrations in strength and power athletes. *J Strength Cond Res.* 2007;21:1197–1203.

27. Saaf RB. Effect of exercise on adult cartilage. *Acta Orthop Scand Suppl.* 1950;7:1–83.

28. Sabo D, Bernd L, Pfeil J, Reiter A. Bone quality in the lumbar spine in high-performance athletes. *Eur Spine J.* 1996;5:258–263.

29. Thelin N, Holmberg S, Thelin A. Knee injuries account for the sports-related increased risk of knee osteoarthritis. *Scand J Med Sci Sports.* 2006;16:329–333.

30. Westh E, Kongsgaard M, Bojsen-Moller J, et al. Effect of habitual exercise on the structural and mechanical properties of human tendon, in vivo, in men and women. *Scand J Med Sci Sports.* 2008;18:23–30.

31. Wittich A, Mautalen CA, Oliveri MB, Bagur A, Somoza F, Rotemberg E. Professional football (soccer) players have a markedly greater skeletal mineral content, density, and size than age- and BMI-matched controls. *Calcif Tiss Int.* 1998;63:112–117.

32. Woitge HW, Friedmann B, Suttner S, Farahmand I, Muller M, Schmidt-Gayk H, et al. Changes in bone turnover induced by aerobic and anaerobic exercise in young males. *J Bone Miner Res.* 1998;13:1797–1804.

Endocrine System Responses and Adaptations

objectives

After completing this chapter, you will be able to:
- Define a hormone and explain autocrine, paracrine, and endocrine hormonal actions
- Identify and explain the types of hormones that play key roles in exercise performance
- Discuss general functions of various hormones and relate these to their importance for acute exercise performance and chronic training adaptations
- Discuss how hormones are released, travel through circulation, bind to specific receptors, and their cellular signaling properties
- Discuss how acute hormonal responses and changes in resting concentrations during training contribute to performance enhancement and physiologic adaptations

The endocrine system is one of two major systems of control in the human body; the nervous system is the other. It helps the body maintain normal function, prepares the body for exercise, mediates several adaptations, and is involved to some extent in every system. The actions help facilitate exercise performance and mediate chronic adaptations to training. The endocrine system operates by releasing a chemical messenger, transporting the chemical to specific target tissues, and eliciting a chain of events leading to the desired function. The chemical messenger is a **hormone**. Hormones come in various types and perform a multitude of functions. Most hormones are released from *endocrine glands* although some are released from nerve, muscle, cardiac, fat cells, and other tissues. Figure 6.1 depicts major endocrine glands.

HORMONE ACTIONS

When released, hormones act as signal molecules and may regulate the cells that released them, adjacent cells, or enter circulation and travel throughout the body. When a hormone is produced by cells and acts upon the same cells that produced it, this is known as an **autocrine** action. Some hormones are produced by cells, released by these cells, and then regulate activity of adjacent cells. This action is known as a **paracrine** action. When released, most hormones enter general circulation where they travel systemically to specific target tissues, *e.g.*, an **endocrine** action.

ROLE OF RELEASING HORMONES

Some hormones cause the release of other hormones and are referred to as **releasing hormones**. For example, the *hypothalamus* is a segment of the brain that acts as an endocrine gland. It provides a link between the nervous and endocrine systems. The hypothalamus synthesizes and releases neurohormones that are transported to the pituitary gland (anterior segment). The hypothalamus releases the hormones *corticotrophin-releasing hormone* (CRH), *gonadotropin-releasing hormone* (GnRH), *growth hormone-releasing hormone*, *growth hormone-inhibiting hormone* (somatostatin), *thyrotropin-releasing hormone* (TRH), and *prolactin-inhibiting hormone* (PIH) that control the release of other hormones including growth hormone (GH), follicle-stimulating hormone (FSH), luteinizing hormone (LH), adrenocorticotropic hormone (ACTH), thyroid-stimulating hormone (TSH), prolactin, and beta-endorphins. The posterior pituitary releases two hormones in response to stimuli, *antidiuretic hormone* (ADH or vasopressin [AVP]) and *oxytocin*. Unlike the anterior pituitary, the posterior pituitary does not require releasing hormones to secrete these hormones. Hormones released from the pituitary travel to all tissues to elicit specific physiologic actions. Some of these hormones (FSH, LH, GnRH, TSH, GH, and ACTH) cause the release of other hormones from endocrine glands.

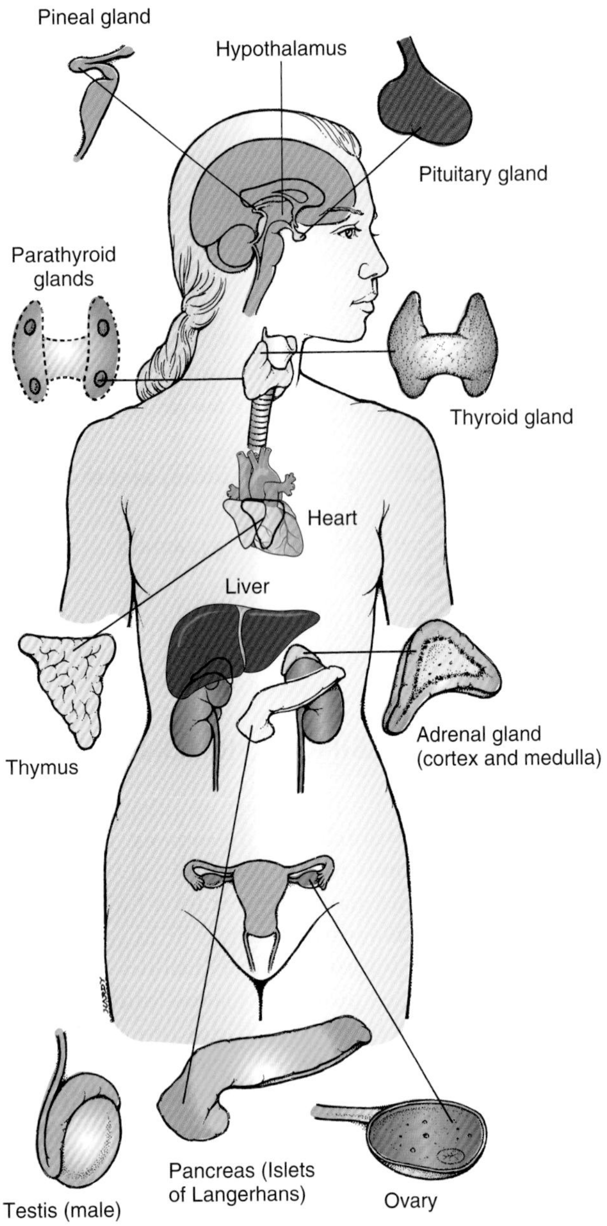

■ FIGURE 6.1. Major endocrine glands in the human body. (From *Stedman's Medical Dictionary*. 27th ed. Baltimore (MD): Lippincott Williams & Wilkins; 2000.)

TYPES OF HORMONES

Hormones come in three forms. **Steroid hormones** are made of three 6-carbon rings and one 5-carbon ring. All steroids are synthesized from *cholesterol* via synthetic pathways consisting of many intermediates, some of which are biologically active. Steroids are released into circulation; arrive at the target tissue, diffuse through the cell membrane, and bind to a specific cytoplasmic- or nuclear-bound receptor within the cell. Common steroids include androgens (testosterone [TE]), estrogens, mineralocorticoids (aldosterone), glucocorticoids (cortisone), progesterone, and prostaglandins. **Anabolic**

steroids, a common type of steroids used/abused by athletes, are just one type, as steroids have other applications, including anti-inflammation, fluid balance, and gender characteristics.

Peptide hormones are proteins of various sizes. Small chains (<20 amino acids) are *peptides*, and large chains are *polypeptides*. Peptide hormones are the direct product of mRNA translation, cleavage from larger parent molecules, and/or other postsynthesis modifications. The quantity and sequence of amino acids determine the function of each hormone although some partial sequences of amino acids (*secratogues*) may have biologic significance. Several hormones are proteins, including insulin, insulin-like growth factor-1 (IGF-1) and the superfamily of GH molecules. Peptides are prone to degradation, so pharmaceuticals (insulin and GH) are not consumed orally and need direct routes into circulation (injection). Peptides circulate and bind to specific receptors on the cell membranes of target tissues. They are lipophobic and cannot pass through cell membranes so receptors need to be external for binding.

A third type is an **amine hormone**. These have an amine (NH_2) group at the end of the molecule. Because they are derived from amino acids, amines may be classified as protein hormones. Amines include epinephrine, norepinephrine, and dopamine (collectively known as *catecholamines*). Catecholamines are synthesized from the amino acid tyrosine, sometimes phenylalanine (via conversion to tyrosine), and tryptophan. Similar to peptides, amines must bind to a surface-bound receptor on the target tissue. Catecholamines can act as neurotransmitters in the autonomic nervous system.

ENDOCRINE GLANDS AND HORMONAL FUNCTIONS

Several glands release hormones into circulation. Figure 6.1 depicts some major endocrine glands including the hypothalamus, pituitary, thyroid, parathyroid, heart, liver, adrenals, pancreas, kidneys, testes, and ovaries. There are a multitude of hormones functioning within the human body. Table 6.1 presents some of the major hormones and their basic functions. Several hormones released can alter the concentrations and potency of other hormones. The endocrine system is quite complex where there are multiple levels of control and interaction between numerous tissues, cells, and other hormones.

HORMONE ACTIVITY: PRODUCTION, RELEASE, AND TRANSPORTATION

The production, release, and transportation of hormones to target tissues is critical for mediating the desired effects. Production depends upon the type of hormone. For example, peptides and amines are synthesized in advance and stored within vesicles until they are needed. Amines

TABLE 6.1 HORMONES AND RELATED FUNCTIONS

GLAND	HORMONE	FUNCTIONS
Anterior pituitary	Growth hormone	Tissue growth, protein synthesis, fat mobilization, release of IGF-1, decreased glucose utilization, increased collagen synthesis and cartilage growth
	ACTH	Stimulate secretion of glucocorticoids
	Beta-endorphins	Analgesia
	LH	Produces testosterone (males), ovulation and secretion of sex hormones (females)
	FSH	Spermatogenesis in males, maturation of Graafian follicles of ovaries in females
	TSH	Secretion of thyroxine (T4) and triiodothyronine (T3)
	Prolactin	Stimulates milk production in mammary glands, secretion of progesterone
	Melanocyte-stimulating hormone (MSH)	Stimulates melanocytes, skin pigmentation
Posterior pituitary	ADH	Increased reabsorption of water in kidneys
	Oxytocin	Stimulates uterine contractions and milk release from mammary glands
Thyroid	T3, T4	Increased BMR and sensitivity to catecholamines, protein synthesis
	Calcitonin	Decrease blood calcium levels, increased calcium uptake into bone
Parathyroid	Parathyroid hormone (PTH)	Increased osteoclast activity in bone, increased blood calcium, decreased blood phosphates
Pancreas	Insulin	Glucose/amino acid transport into cells, protein synthesis
	Glucagon	Increase blood glucose
Adrenal cortex	Cortisol	Gluconeogenesis, spares glucose, fat breakdown, inhibit amino acid incorporation into proteins
	Aldosterone	Sodium and water reabsorption
Adrenal medulla	Catecholamines	"Fight or flight" response, preparation for stress and exercise
	Peptide F	Analgesia, immune function
Liver	Insulin-like growth factors (IGFs)	Increased protein synthesis, growth, development
	Angiotensin	Vasoconstriction, release of aldosterone
Ovaries	Estrogens	Female sex characteristics, growth, bone formation, increase HDLs
	Progesterone	Female sex characteristics, pregnancy maintenance
Testes	Testosterone (androgens)	Growth, male sex characteristics, protein synthesis, neural stimulation, blood volume
Heart	Atrial peptide	Regulates sodium, potassium, fluid volume
Kidney	Renin	Kidney function
	Erythropoietin	Increased red blood cells
Adipose tissue	Leptin	Increased energy expenditure, decreased appetite
Stomach	Ghrelin	Stimulate appetite, GH
	Neuropeptide Y	Increased food intake, decreased activity

are produced from precursor molecules and stored in vesicles until release. Tyrosine is converted to dopamine, norepinephrine, and epinephrine in the adrenal medulla. Dopamine and norepinephrine also act as neurotransmitters. Thyroid hormones are produced in follicular cells of the thyroid gland (with incorporation of iodine) and stored in vesicles until released. Steroids are synthesized from cholesterol (see Fig. 6.2) via several enzymatic reactions as they are released upon completion (they are not stored) via diffusion through the cell membrane. Steroids are synthesized in adrenal glands, ovaries, testes (Leydig cells), and to a lesser extent in other peripheral tissues. Hormonal synthesis/release is modified at several levels for greater control.

Hormones must be transported to target tissues. The time a hormone remains active in circulation affects transportation. Some hormones have a short **half-life** (the time it takes for half of the hormone secreted to be degraded) of a few minutes, *e.g.*, catecholamines, thereby limiting interaction with target tissues. However, some hormones have long half-lives of several minutes (peptides, steroids) to hours that increase the likelihood of receptor interaction (assuming the hormone arrives before it is metabolized). Thyroid hormones have half-lives of 1–7 days. Preservation of a hormone is critical. Many hormones are transported via **transport (binding) proteins** that protect the hormone from metabolism and help deliver the hormone to its receptor. Thyroid hormones (by thyroid hormone-binding globulin), GH molecules (by GH-binding protein), IGF-1 (by IGF-binding proteins), and steroid hormones (by sex hormone-binding globulin [SHBG] for TE mostly, corticosteroid-binding globulin for cortisol and progesterone) are chaperoned by transport proteins whereas some hormones such as catecholamines and some peptides circulate unbound and partially dissolved in plasma. The hormone-binding protein complex travels in circulation but must dissociate prior to receptor binding. The free hormone binds to

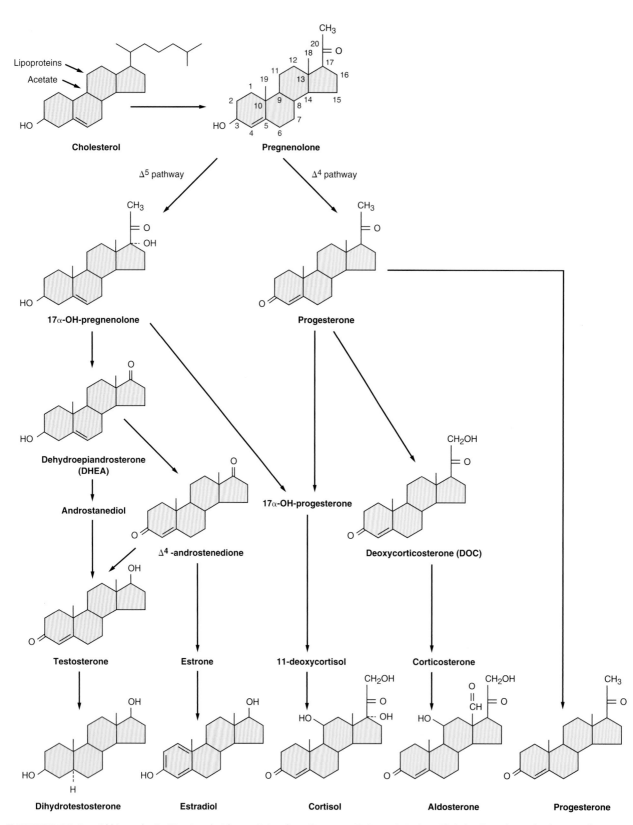

FIGURE 6.2. Steroid biosynthesis. (Reprinted with permission from Greenspan F, Baxter J. *Basic & Clinical Endocrinology*. 4th ed. Norwalk (CT): Appleton and Lange; 1994.)

its receptor although some new research is investigating potential roles of cellular uptake of the complex (hormone and binding protein) among steroids.

WHAT DETERMINES HORMONAL CONCENTRATIONS IN THE BLOOD?

Several factors affect hormonal concentrations in the blood (Fig. 6.3; Table 6.2). Hormonal concentrations are transient and depend upon several factors including the amount of hormone released, the pattern of release (*pulsatility*), rate of metabolism, quantity of transport proteins, the time of day, and plasma volume shifts (74). Genetics, gender, age, diet, and various stimuli (in addition to regulation from other hormones) affect hormone synthesis and secretion rates. For example, men have higher concentrations of TE whereas women have higher concentrations of estrogens, and the hormonal responses tend to decrease with age. The insulin response is highly dependent upon blood sugar levels whereas hormones such as TE, cortisol, and

the GH superfamily are responsive to the stress of exercise. Most hormones are released in periodic pulsatile bursts where the concentration will vary between peaks. The frequency and amplitude of the pulses dictate hormone concentrations and depends on circadian patterns and cellular stimulation. This is true for GH that is released in a series of pulses overnight, *i.e.*, ~50% of GH secretion may occur during the third and fourth rapid eye movement (REM) stages of sleep. The quantum of hormone released in a pulse provides enough quantity to maintain physiologic function until the next pulse is released.

Hormonal concentrations vary in circadian patterns depending on the time of day. For example, TE concentrations in men are highest in the morning but are gradually reduced throughout the day (69,106). As a result, some strength and conditioning professionals have recommended afternoon/early evening workouts to stimulate TE concentrations, *e.g.*, the workout can provide a stimulus to low TE concentrations. Afternoon resistance exercise-induced elevations in TE may be greater than

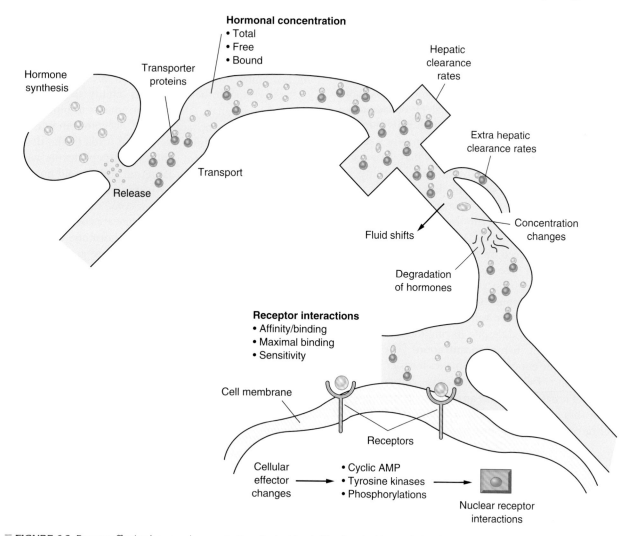

FIGURE 6.3. Factors affecting hormonal concentrations in the blood. (Reprinted with permission from Kraemer WJ, Ratamess NA. Endocrine responses and adaptations to strength and power training. In: Komi PV, editor. *Strength and Power in Sport*. 2nd ed. Malden (MA): Blackwell Scientific Publications; 2003. pp. 361–386.)

TABLE 6.2 ADULT RESTING HORMONAL VALUES

HORMONE	RANGE
Testosterone	
Men	10–35 nmol L^{-1}, 3–10 ng mL^{-1}
Women	<3.5 nmol L^{-1}, <0.1 ng mL^{-1}
Cortisol	50–410 nmol L^{-1}, 2–15 µg dL^{-1}
Growth hormone	
Men	0–5 µg L^{-1}
Women	0–10 µg L^{-1}
IGF-1	
Men	0.45–2.2 U mL^{-1}
Women	0.34–1.9 U mL^{-1}
Insulin (fasting)	5–20 µU mL^{-1}
Triiodothyronine	1.2–3.4 nmol L^{-1}
Thyroxine	42–51 nmol L^{-1}

Modified from Fry AC, Hoffman JR. Training responses and adaptations of the endocrine system. In: Chandler TJ, Brown LE, editors. *Conditioning for Strength and Human Performance*. Philadelphia (PA): Lippincott Williams & Wilkins; 2008. pp. 94–122.

that observed in the morning (36) but the long-term training ramifications are unknown. Morning or afternoon workouts do not alter diurnal TE concentrations (106). Cortisol concentrations are highest in the early morning (4–7 a.m.) and lower throughout the day (106). When measuring hormones in the blood, it is important to standardize the times of measurements as two different times will yield two different values. Circadian patterns are consistent under most circumstances. Resistance exercise has limited effects on normal TE circadian patterns (69,106) as normal circadian rhythm (within 1 h) is quickly reestablished upon completion of a workout. However, nocturnal circadian patterns may be affected (86). Nindl et al. (94) showed that GH pulsatility was higher during the second phase of sleep on a day where high-volume resistance exercise was performed.

Plasma volume shifts occur during exercise. Plasma is the liquid portion of blood. During exercise, fluid lost intracellularly is replaced by extracellular fluid (plasma). Coupled with fluid loss to thermoregulation, plasma volume is reduced during exercise. Hormone measurements express the amount of hormone per volume of blood. A higher hormone value will be obtained when fluid volume is reduced despite having the same amount of hormone present (**hemoconcentration**). The resultant elevated hormone concentration makes it easier for receptor interaction (71–74). During exercise, hormone elevations do not necessarily reflect an increase in synthesis and secretion, but rather reflect plasma volume reductions and slower rates of tissue clearance and degradation (72,74).

NEGATIVE FEEDBACK CONTROL

Hormonal concentrations are controlled by **negative feedback** systems. A negative feedback system will elevate a hormone when it is low or reduce a hormone when it is elevated. Negative feedback system can be seen with TE. A male athlete who uses anabolic steroids will experience reductions in his own TE production. As a result,

testicular shrinkage can occur due to negative feedback inhibition of *endogenous* (produced within one's body) TE production. Negative feedback systems predominate and provide multiple levels of control.

RECEPTOR INTERACTION

As hormones are messengers, their message would be useless without other molecules' ability to receive the signal. The ultimate fate of a hormone is to bind to specific receptors on the target tissue. Receptor binding leads to a cascade of cellular events that leads to the desired function. Receptors for amines and peptides lie within the cell membrane whereas steroid and thyroid hormone receptors are located either in the nucleus (thyroid) or cytoplasm (steroids). Receptors come in different forms but are specific to the hormone they are coupled with via a lock-and-key principle. Only one hormone will unlock or activate the receptor. However, there are exceptions. Some molecules that are similar to the hormone may act as a barrier for hormonal interaction whereas some bind to the receptor leading to activation. This **cross-reactivity** allows more than one hormone or molecule to activate a receptor. This can be of great value in the pharmaceutical industry where drug analogues are produced. Upon binding to a receptor, second messenger systems or the nucleus will be activated.

SECOND MESSENGER SYSTEMS

Because some hormones (amines, peptides) bind to a membrane-bound receptor on the surface of the cell, other molecules must mediate this signal intracellularly. Thus, several second messengers are activated and initiate a cascade of events leading to the desired cellular response. Many second messenger systems are mediated by guanylyl (G) proteins that can stimulate or inhibit further cellular activity. Figure 6.4 depicts the adenylate cyclase-cyclic AMP second messenger system.

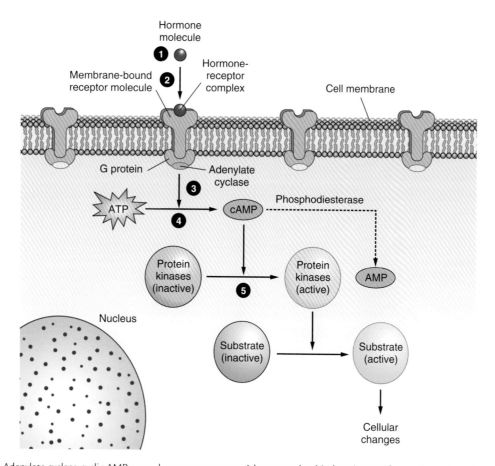

FIGURE 6.4. Adenylate cyclase-cyclic AMP second messenger system. A hormone that binds to its specific membrane-bound receptor can stimulate or inhibit this system. A stimulatory hormone binds to its receptor and activates a stimulating G protein that activates the enzyme adenylate cyclase to produce cyclic AMP from ATP. Cyclic AMP activates protein kinases (*i.e.*, protein kinase A). Protein kinase A phosphorylates several proteins/substrates yielding numerous cellular effects. An inhibitory hormone activates an inhibiting G protein to limit these reactions. Cyclic AMP has a short half-life and is rapidly degraded by the enzyme *phosphodiesterase*, which itself is inhibited by caffeine.

STEROID AND THYROID HORMONES

Because steroids are lipophilic, they diffuse through target cell membranes and bind to receptors in the cytoplasm or nucleus (Fig. 6.5). Many steroids bind to receptors in the cytoplasm. Receptors are bound to heat-shock proteins in the cytoplasm prior to hormone binding. Heat-shock proteins dissociate and the hormone-receptor complex moves to the nucleus where it binds to response elements on DNA (leading to protein synthesis). Thyroid hormones (T3, T4) enter the cell membrane via transporter proteins, travel to the nucleus, and bind with receptors (mostly T3) to stimulate or inhibit gene transcription.

HORMONES AND EXERCISE

Exercise presents a potent stimulus for hormonal adaptations. For resistance training (RT), the manipulation of the acute program variables (intensity, volume, rest intervals, exercise selection and sequence, repetition velocity, frequency) ensures an optimal endocrine response.

Intensity, volume and duration, modality, work:rest ratio, and frequency are critical variables for aerobic training and other anaerobic modalities including plyometric, sprint, and agility training. The training program as well as genetic predisposition, gender, fitness level, nutritional intake, and the potential for adaptation all play roles in the hormonal responses. Hormonal responses and adaptations entail four classifications: (a) acute responses during exercise; (b) chronic changes in resting concentrations; (c) chronic changes in the acute response to exercise; and (d) receptor changes.

TESTOSTERONE

More than 95% of TE in men is secreted from the Leydig cells of the testes, with the remainder produced by the adrenals. In women, ovarian/adrenal production of TE is the major source. Skeletal muscle contains the necessary enzymes and may have the potential to produce small amounts of androgens as well (116). Most (~98%) of TE travels bound to SHBG (60%) and a protein *albumin* (38%); however, it is the unbound free TE that diffuses

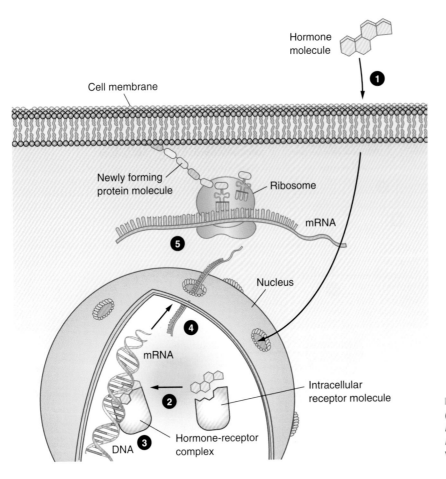

FIGURE 6.5. Steroid hormone action. (From Golan DE, Tashjian AH, Armstrong EJ. *Principles of Pharmacology: The Pathophysiologic Basis of Drug Therapy.* 2nd ed. Baltimore (MD): Wolters Kluwer Health; 2008.)

into cells and interacts with receptors. Testosterone is a potent hormone. However, some TE is converted to a more potent (about six times that of TE) analyte dihydrotestosterone (DHT) in peripheral tissues via the 5α reductase enzyme. This enzyme is limited in skeletal muscle. It is TE that is the major androgen mediating anabolic processes in men. Testosterone has many ergogenic effects on performance (see the Sidebar appearing next). Some TE is aromatized to estrogens, and final metabolism of TE occurs in the liver and kidneys where inactivated metabolites are excreted in urine.

- Increases red blood cell formation, hemoglobin, hematocrit, and endurance
- Increases osteoblast activity and BMD
- Increases glycogen storage
- Increases lipolysis (fat breakdown) and low-density lipoproteins and decreases high-density lipoproteins
- Increases neural transmission, neurotransmitter release, and regrowth of damaged peripheral nerves
- Increases aggression

SIDEBAR ERGOGENIC EFFECTS OF TESTOSTERONE

- Increases LBM and muscle CSA
- Increases cardiac tissue mass
- Decreases body fat percentage
- Increases ISOM and dynamic muscle strength and power
- Enhances recovery ability between workouts
- Increases protein synthesis
- Increases satellite cell proliferation and differentiation

Acute Responses to Exercise

Testosterone concentrations are elevated during and immediately following exercise (88). Resistance exercise is a potent modality of exercise that elevates total and free TE concentrations in men (1,38,49,66–68,99) and women (93) if a threshold volume, muscle mass, and intensity are reached/activated. The acute TE response in women appears limited compared to men (38,63). Rather, it appears that other anabolic hormones such as the GH superfamily may be more influential for increasing muscle size and strength in women. The response may be greater in resistance-trained men than endurance-trained men (115), and may be enhanced with training experience (62,68), although some research has shown training status may not affect the acute TE response (2). These elevations are attributed to plasma volume reductions, sympathetic nervous system stimulation, lactate-stimulated secretion, and possible adaptations in TE synthesis and secretion capacity (74). Acute elevations in TE during a workout may enhance neural function and augment the effects of other hormones (GH) leading to greater strength and power. However, some recent studies have shown moderate strength and size gains during RT despite a lack of acute TE elevations (120–122). It is difficult to parcel out the effects of an acute TE elevation versus the chronic influence TE may have on tissue growth. Thus, the impact of acute TE elevations during exercise is unknown although it is thought to, in part, mediate some training adaptations. Several other factors affect the acute TE response. These include

- Exercise selection and muscle mass involvement: the acute TE response is greater with large muscle mass exercises (41,117).
- Intensity and volume: the acute TE response is greater with high- versus low-intensity resistance exercise and the response is greater with moderate- to high-volume programs compared to low-volume workouts (29,60,61,96,97,103). The interaction between intensity and volume is critical as those programs with a high glycolytic component (*e.g.*, moderate to high intensity, high volume, and short rest intervals like bodybuilding programs) yield substantial acute TE elevations, even greater so than strength training programs with longer rest intervals between sets (16,60,61,79,85). Short rest intervals

(1 min) elicit a more substantial response than longer rest intervals (2.5 min) at least early in training but this effect may subside as training progresses (9). Low-intensity workouts may not elicit an acute TE response (79). McCaulley et al. (85) compared three programs of similar volume: (a) hypertrophy: 4 sets of 10 squats at 75% of 1 RM (90-s rest intervals; (b) strength: 11 sets 3 squats at 90% of 1 RM (5-min rest intervals); and (c) power: 8 sets of 6 jump squats with no weight (3-min rest intervals) and showed that the hypertrophy workout produced a 32% TE elevation whereas the strength and power workouts produced nonsignificant 19.6% and 10.7% elevations, respectively. Similar results were shown by Crewther et al. (16).

- Training frequency: the acute TE response may be more substantial when training volume is divided into two sessions instead of one (33).
- Nutritional intake: the acute TE response is limited with carbohydrate/protein intake before, during, or immediately after a workout (48,49,66,105), possibly due to antagonism with insulin elevations. Caffeine intake prior to resistance exercise may augment the acute TE response in a dose-dependent manner (6).
- Overtraining and dehydration: The TE response may be less when athletes are overtrained (32) and dehydrated prior to resistance exercise (54).

Chronic Changes in Resting Testosterone Concentrations

Changes in resting TE concentrations during RT have been inconsistent (4). Although some studies have shown elevations (2,34,44,68,83,111), no changes (31,32,84), and reductions (76) in resting TE concentrations after RT, it

Interpreting Research

Exercise Sequencing, Testosterone Response, and Changes in Strength

Hansen S, Kvorning T, Kjaer M, Szogaard G. The effect of short-term strength training on human skeletal muscle: the importance of physiologically elevated hormone levels. *Scand J Med Sci Sport*. 2001;11:347–354.

Some have theorized that performing large and small muscle mass exercises poses an advantage for the smaller mass exercises due to an augmented hormonal environment. Exercises such as the squat, deadlift, and power clean performed early in the workout may produce substantial TE elevations that could expose smaller muscles to a greater response. Hansen et al. (41) measured elbow flexor strength changes after 9 weeks of unilateral RT. One group performed elbow flexion exercises only and a second group performed lower body exercises following elbow flexion exercises. Isometric strength increased by 37% in the combination group but only 9% in the arm-only group. No difference was seen between groups in other strength measures. Performing elbow flexion exercises only did not acutely elevate TE concentrations. However, TE was elevated when lower-body exercises were performed after the arm exercises. This study provided partial support for performing large muscle mass, multijoint exercises in a workout to stimulate smaller mass exercises when strength training.

Myths & Misconceptions

Resistance Training will Increase Resting Testosterone Concentrations

One misconception is that consistent RT will increase TE in men at rest over time. Although some elevations in resting TE may take place, these tend to be transient and return to a normal baseline level upon accommodation to training. Resting TE values reflect a diurnal pattern and change throughout the day. Basal TE levels decrease as one ages independent of training status. Thus, an expectation of large resting TE elevations is not warranted. Although elevations in TE at rest may be advantageous to some extent, long-term elevations could be counterproductive when one views potential negative health risk factors (elevated low-density lipoprotein (LDL) cholesterol, prostate ailments) and receptor desensitization (down-regulation). *Receptor down-regulation*, or *tolerance*, is a term used to describe a reduction in receptors from chronic exposure to high levels of hormones or drugs. It takes a larger hormonal output to generate a given response once tolerance develops. Many anabolic steroid users cycle drugs to prevent tolerance and keep receptors primed for adaptation. Thus, it seems beneficial to an athlete to have acute bursts of TE output rather than chronic elevations. TE could potentially have negative side effects (some seen in anabolic steroid users) at chronically high levels and it appears that the body safeguards against this.

seems that resting concentrations reflect the current state of muscle such that elevations or reductions may occur at various stages depending on the volume and intensity of training. A study examining elite Olympic weightlifters showed no differences in 1 year of training (32); however, elevations were shown following a second year of training (34). Changes in volume and intensity can produce transient changes in resting TE (2,76) but it appears that values return to a homeostatic level upon adaptation to the change in program design. These data have prompted suggestions that chronic hormonal changes may not be paramount to mediating strength and size changes (74). Lastly, short-term (7–10 d) detraining in strength/power athletes may result in elevated TE concentrations (47); however, long-term detraining (>8 weeks) may result in TE reductions (4,31).

Luteinizing Hormone

LH is a protein hormone secreted from basophilic cells of the anterior pituitary (under the control of GnRH),

which is the primary regulator of TE secretion from the testes. LH stimulation of TE requires sufficient time (at least 15 min) (23) so TE elevations during a workout appear to be the result of other mechanisms (reduced clearance, plasma volume shifts), at least during the first part of the workout. A workout may not induce LH secretion (35) although a delayed response may occur later during recovery (115). Some studies have shown no change (31) or an elevation (36) in LH at rest, again reflecting the transient nature of resting hormonal concentrations. Resistance-trained men have shown a more pronounced response than endurance-trained men during exercise (115).

Sex Hormone-Binding Globulin

Circulating TE is mostly bound to SHBG. A change in SHBG concentrations may influence the binding capacity of TE and the availability of free TE. During RT, differential responses (elevations, reductions, and no change) have been reported (74,122).

Myths & Misconceptions

Testosterone is Long-Lasting and Does Not Produce Rapid Effects

Although TE has long-term actions, studies have shown that TE may exert rapid (within seconds to minutes) nongenomic effects in target tissues that can be beneficial for exercise. Androgen receptors (ARs) (located in cell membranes) may mediate these effects. In addition to normal steroid-receptor genomic activity (which takes at least 30 min), nongenomic activities of TE involve the induction of a second messenger signal transduction cascade (89). Research has identified SHBG receptors on cell membranes, thereby reflecting a possible receptor-mediated role of SHBG in mediating androgen actions (55). Elevated TE concentrations during exercise may augment performance as well as mediate critical adaptations in skeletal muscle to training.

Testosterone Precursors (Prohormones)

The synthesis of TE contains many steps involving precursors such as dehydroepiandrosterone (DHEA), androstendione, and androstenediol. In comparison to TE, these precursors are less potent as evidenced by a lack of ergogenic effects seen with prohormone supplementation (74). Androgens such as DHEA may play a greater role in women because of their lower levels of TE. Women can convert a larger percentage of DHEA to androstenedione and TE and have higher baseline concentrations of androstenedione than men (119). Elevations in circulating androstenedione and DHEA sulfate in men and women have been shown during resistance exercise (115,119). During RT, elevations, reductions, and no changes have been shown in androstenedione, DHEA, and DHEA sulfate, reflecting the lack of consistency in hormonal changes at rest (3,4,39).

The Androgen Receptor

The AR consists of ~919 amino acids and is found in nearly all tissues in the human body (except the spleen and adrenal medulla). A truncated version has been identified. The presence of ARs correlates highly with the functions of androgens. The AR consists of four functional domains: a C-terminal hormone-binding domain, a DNA-binding domain, a hinge region, and an N-terminal transcription activation domain. The goal of AR-DNA interaction is to induce transcription and translation of proteins necessary to fulfill specific functions. AR function is enhanced by coactivators that form a bridge between the DNA-bound AR and the transcriptional machinery and by facilitating hormonal binding.

The concentration of ARs in skeletal muscle depends on the muscle fiber type (high in FT fibers), training status, and androgen concentrations. Modifications of AR content are critical to strength and hypertrophy enhancement. Animals with AR deficiency have low levels of muscle mass (80) and may experience up to 70% less muscle growth (51). Significant correlations between AR content and 1 RM squat have been shown (98). Resistance exercise and sequential workouts up-regulate AR content 48 hours postexercise (5,49,125). However, the initial response may be down-regulation within 1 hour when no nutrients are consumed (98) but is prevented with protein/carbohydrate consumption before and after the workout (75).

Interpreting Research

Testosterone Elevations and the Androgen Receptor Response to Resistance Exercise

Spiering BA, Kraemer WJ, Vingren JL, et al. Elevated endogenous testosterone concentrations potentiate muscle androgen receptor responses to resistance exercise. *J Steroid Biochem Mol Biol.* 2009;114:195–199.

Kvorning T, Andersen M, Brixen K, Schjerling P, Suetta C, Madesn K. Suppression of testosterone does not blunt mRNA expression of myoD, myogenin, IGF, myostatin or androgen receptor post strength training in humans. *J Physiol.* 2007;578:579–593.

TE administration up-regulates AR content in a dose-dependent manner. However, less is known concerning the importance of increasing one's own concentrations (endogenous) of TE acutely during resistance exercise. Spiering et al. (110) examined two protocols: (a) 5 sets of 5 RM knee extensions with 90%–95% of 1 RM with 3-minute rest intervals; and (b) upper-body protocol consisting of the bench press, bench row, and seated press for 4 sets of 10 RM (80% of 1 RM) with 2-minute rest intervals with the same lower-body protocol performed after the upper-body protocol. Protocol 2 elicited a 16% TE elevation whereas protocol 1 had no effect. AR content slightly decreased following protocol 1 but remained constant following protocol 2. AR content was higher 180 minutes following the second protocol compared to the first. Kvorning et al. (78) examined acute responses to resistance exercise (4 sets of body weight squats for 20 reps with 1-min rest intervals) and 8 weeks of RT (seven exercises, 3–4 sets of 6–10 RM with 2–3-min rest intervals, 3 days per week) under two conditions: a placebo or a drug administered to inhibit TE secretion. Throughout the study, TE concentrations were low in the drug group (<2 nmol L^{-1} compared to 22–24 nmol L^{-1} in the placebo group). During a workout, TE was elevated by 15% in the placebo group versus a decrease in the drug group. After RT, both groups increased muscle growth factors (myogenin, IGF-1) and decreased myostatin. These changes were seen within 24 hours after the initial protocol. AR mRNA did not change in either group. Interestingly, only the placebo group increased maximal ISOM strength, and the increase in leg muscle mass seen in the placebo group was greater than the drug group. The authors concluded that blocking TE did not reduce growth factor up-regulation but the suppression of TE limited changes in muscle strength and growth.

Selective Androgen Receptor Modulators

Since 1998 it has been shown that other nonsteroidal molecules can activate the AR. These molecules have been termed **selective androgen receptor modulators** (SARMs) because they bind to the AR and have shown anabolic properties in bone and skeletal muscle. However, unlike other androgens, SARMs produce minimal effects on prostate and secondary sexual organs (91). They have the potential to separate androgenic and anabolic effects. There may be great clinical potential for these molecules but potential for abuse by athletes may exist.

GROWTH HORMONE SUPERFAMILY

The anterior pituitary secretes molecules that make up the GH family. The most commonly studied GH isoform, the 22 kD molecule, consists of 191 amino acids. GH is released in a pulsatile manner (especially during sleep) under the control of GHRH and is inhibited by somatostatin; both are hypothalamic hormones. Other biologically active GH fragments are released and this superfamily of GH molecules operates in a complex manner in mediating GH-related effects (77). Many anabolic effects of GH are mediated through IGF-1. Upon release, GH circulates, attaches to a binding protein (GH-binding protein), and has a half-life of 20–50 minutes.

Acute Responses to Exercises

Exercise is a potent stimulus for GH secretion. Although most studies have examined changes in the 22 kD GH molecule, resistance and aerobic exercises produce acute elevations in other GH variants (50,72,73). The GH variant response is affected by muscular strength in women (73). Resistance exercise elevates 22 kD GH through 30-minute postexercise similarly in men (79,99) and women (79) although resting concentrations of GH are often higher in women (63), and the response is limited when amino acids and carbohydrates are consumed (48,99). The GH response depends on exercise selection and amount of muscle mass recruited, muscle actions used (greater response during CON than ECC muscle actions), intensity, volume, rest intervals between sets, and training status (greater elevations based on strength and the magnitude of work performed) (74). Higher-volume multiple-set workouts elicit larger GH elevations than single-set workouts (15,29,90). Bodybuilding workouts produce larger responses than strength training workouts (60,61,79). These workouts produce substantial blood lactate responses and high correlations between lactate and GH have been shown (37). Zafeiridis et al. (127) compared a strength (4 sets of 5 reps, 88% of 1 RM, 3-min rest intervals), hypertrophy (4 sets of 10 reps, 75% of 1 RM, 2-min rest intervals), and an endurance protocol (4 sets of 15 reps, 60% of 1 RM, 1-min rest intervals) and showed the GH response matched total work where the largest

response was seen in the endurance protocol. Häkkinen and Pakarinen (37) showed that 20 sets of 1 RM squats only produced a slight elevation in GH whereas a substantial increase in GH was shown following 10 sets of 10 reps with 70% of 1 RM. Bottaro et al. (8) showed the GH response was greatest with 30-second rest intervals compared to 60 and 120 seconds. The addition of a single set of high repetitions with 50% of 1 RM to the end of a strength protocol can augment the GH response (28). A lower-body strength training program produces less of a GH elevation than the same program performed after an upper-body hypertrophy workout (109). Exertion is a major stimulus as research has shown an augmented GH response in experienced subjects when workload is greater (14,45).

Chronic Changes in Resting Growth Hormone Concentrations

Consistent exercise does not appear to alter resting GH concentrations. One reason may be that GH needs to be measured over a long period of time because of its pulsatile nature. Several studies examining single GH measures have shown no changes in resting GH concentrations during RT in men and women (44,68,83). Elite strength and power athletes have similar resting GH concentrations to lesser-trained individuals (2,34). The acute GH response to exercise appears to be more critical to adaptations although the anabolic role GH plays in skeletal muscle is unclear. The exercise-induced elevation correlates with type I and type II muscle fiber hypertrophy (84). Interestingly, GH pulsatility during sleep may be altered following resistance exercise where lower GH pulses may be seen early in sleep but greater pulses may be seen later in sleep (91).

Growth Hormone-Binding Protein

About 50% of GH binds to GH-specific binding proteins (GHBPs) that extend its half-life and enhance its effects. The GHBP arises from cleavage of the GH receptor in the liver or wherever the GH receptor exists. Little is known about GHBP and exercise. An elevation in GHBP was shown at rest after 2 weeks of endurance training (100). Aerobic exercise (60 min at 75% of Vo_{2max}) produces elevations in GH and GHBP (18). Resistance exercise (6 sets of squats, 80%–85% of 1 RM, 10 reps, 2-min rest intervals) produces elevations of GHBP; however, no differences between resistance-trained and untrained individuals are seen, suggesting RT may not alter GHBP or change GH receptor expression (101).

INSULIN-LIKE GROWTH FACTORS

IGFs are structurally related to insulin and mediate many actions of GH. IGFs are small polypeptide hormones (70 and 67 amino acids for IGF-1 and IGF-2, respectively) secreted by the liver in response to GH stimulation. IGFs increase proliferation and differentiation of satellite cells, protein synthesis, and enhance muscle hypertrophy. Of the two, IGF-1 has been extensively studied. IGFs are affected by other hormones including TE and thyroid hormones. Once released, IGFs bind to IGF binding proteins (approximately seven different binding proteins exist) and circulate to the target tissues.

Acute Responses to Exercise

The IGF-1 response to exercise is unclear. Some studies showed acute elevations during aerobic and high-intensity, interval exercise (13,19). Studies have shown no change (66) and elevations (60,61,101) in IGF-1 during or immediately following resistance exercise. Elevations are expected when plasma volume is reduced. However, the lack of change may be attributed to delayed secretion of IGF-1, i.e., 3–9 hours, following GH stimulation, as peak values may not be reached until 16–28 hours after exercise.

Chronic Changes in IGF-1 Concentrations

There is not a consistent pattern of change in IGF-1 concentrations during exercise. Because IGF-1 secretion depends upon GH stimulation, resting concentrations are variable due, in part, to the delay in signaling. Reductions in IGF-1 were shown after 11–12 weeks of RT and endurance training (52,102). No changes in resting IGF-1 were shown during short-term RT (68,84,95) and overreaching (76), unless concurrent with carbohydrate/protein supplementation (66). Elevations in IGF-1 may occur during periods of single- and multiple-set RT (7), RT tapering (53), and RT plus protein/amino acid supplementation (126). Resistance-trained men have higher resting IGF-1 concentrations than untrained men (101). A few studies in women have shown elevated resting IGF-1 during long-term RT (57,83). Similar to GH, the measurement of IGF-1 over wider time windows may be more informative.

Muscle IGF-1 Adaptations to Training

IGF-1 has autocrine/paracrine functions within muscle cells. Three isoforms have been identified, each functioning independently. Two isoforms are similar to circulating IGF-1 (IGF-1Ea and IGF-1Eb), and the third muscle-specific isoform (IGF-1Ec) is known as *mechano growth factor* (MGF) (27). MGF acts independently, is expressed earlier than other IGF-1 isoforms in response to exercise, and may have greater anabolic potency (27). Overloaded muscle and mechanical damage from RT are potent stimuli (26). Resistance exercise increases IGF-1, IGF-1Ea, and MGF mRNA (5,40), and the effect is greater with protein supplementation (126). High-intensity workouts produce great mechanical loading (and a substantial ECC component) and hypertrophy, in part, via up-regulation of muscle IGF-1 and MGF.

Insulin-Like Growth Factor Binding Proteins

Nearly all circulating IGFs are bound to IGF-binding proteins (IGFBPs, mostly IGFBP-3). These regulate IGF availability and prolong IGF circulation. Aerobic, sprint, and resistance exercise elevate IGFBP-3 (13,88,94). Less is known about chronic circulating IGFBP-3 and IGFBP-1. Reductions have been shown (7) and some have suggested IGFBP-3 (a reduction) may serve as marker of overtraining (21). Other research has shown no changes in IGFBP-3 or IGFBP-1 after 16 weeks of RT (95).

Case Study 6.1

Troy is a college football player who has begun his off-season strength and conditioning program. Troy's coach would like him to increase his muscle mass as well as his strength and power. Troy's first phase of his training cycle is designated as a *hypertrophy phase* where the goal is to increase muscle mass and prepare the body for subsequent high-intensity training phases. One attribute for Troy is to maximize his acute TE and GH response to each workout.

Questions for Consideration: **If you were coaching Troy, what training advice would you give him? What types of exercises would you suggest, and what order would you sequence them? What types of training volume, intensity, and rest intervals would you incorporate into the program design?**

INSULIN

Insulin is secreted from the Islets of Langerhans (B cells) in the pancreas after modification from its parent molecules, preproinsulin and proinsulin. Proinsulin (86 amino acids) is converted into insulin (51 amino acids) and *C peptide* (31 amino acids). Insulin is secreted in response to glucose intake and has a half-life of 3–5 minutes. Insulin increases muscle protein synthesis when adequate amino acid concentrations are available. Insulin concentrations parallel changes in blood glucose, and the response is enhanced when protein/carbohydrates are ingested prior to, during, or following exercise (66,105). Insulin concentrations decrease during prolonged aerobic exercise (23) and resistance exercise (97). Insulin elevations are mostly affected by blood glucose and/or dietary intake rather than exercise levels. Consumption of carbohydrates, amino acids, or combinations of both prior to, during, and/or immediately after exercise is recommended for maximizing insulin's effects on tissue growth.

Aerobic and anaerobic training improves **insulin sensitivity** and reduces **insulin resistance**. Insulin resistance is a condition (prominent in obese individuals, elderly, and diabetics) where normal amounts of insulin are inadequate to produce a response. Insulin sensitivity is the opposite. Muscle contraction and hypoxia produce similar muscular effects as insulin performs when it binds to its membrane-bound receptor. Muscle contraction activates glucose transport proteins (known as GLUT proteins, mostly GLUT4) similar to insulin although the intracellular pathways differ (46). Glucose transport into muscles occurs during exercise independent of insulin and exercise has a sparing effect on insulin production.

GLUCAGON

Glucagon is a protein hormone consisting of 29 amino acids synthesized (from *proglucagon*) in A cells in the Islets of Langerhans of the pancreas. The half-life of glucagon is 3–6 minutes until it is removed by the liver and kidneys. Glucagon secretion is inhibited by glucose levels and when secreted, glucagon stimulates the breakdown of glycogen and increases energy availability. Glucagon elevation occurs during exercise as energy demands increase (23).

CORTISOL

Cortisol is a catabolic glucocorticoid released from the adrenal cortex in response to stress under the control of CRH and ACTH. Cortisol accounts for ~95% of all glucocorticoid activity. About 10% of circulating cortisol is free, whereas ~15% is bound to albumin and 75% is bound to corticosteroid-binding globulin. Cortisol stimulates lipolysis in adipose cells, and increases protein degradation and decreases protein synthesis in muscle cells, with greater effects in type II muscle fibers. Glucocorticoid administration can up-regulate myostatin expression and limit muscle growth. Because of its role in tissue remodeling, acute and chronic changes in cortisol during exercise is often studied.

Acute Cortisol Responses to Exercise

Exercise is a potent stimulus for cortisol elevations. Aerobic exercise elevates cortisol with the response more prominent as intensity increases (43). Anaerobic exercise produces similar responses and the response is augmented by dehydration (54). Resistance exercise elevates cortisol and ACTH (33,67,68) with similar responses in men and women (63). Cortisol elevations occur despite corrections for plasma volume changes (84). Interestingly, workouts that elicit the greatest cortisol response also elicit the greatest GH and lactate responses. Workouts that are high in volume and moderate to high in intensity and use short rest periods elicit the greatest lactate and cortisol responses with little change during conventional strength/power training sessions (16,37,59,63,85). High-volume programs (4–6 sets vs. 2 sets; 6 sets vs. 1 set) produce greater cortisol responses (98,108). Greater cortisol responses occur during workouts using short (1 min) rest intervals compared to long rest intervals (3 min) (59,65) but are blunted to some extent when carbohydrate supplementation is consumed

(66,112) and augmented with a large consumption of caffeine (6). Although a catabolic hormone and one that is often intended to be minimized, cortisol elevations are necessary for tissue remodeling and recovery.

Chronic Changes in Resting Cortisol Concentrations

Resting cortisol concentrations reflect a long-term training stress and are transient. No change, reductions, and elevations occur during normal strength and power training in men and women (74). Overtraining, resulting from a large increase in volume, elevates cortisol and reduces resting total and free TE concentrations (22), and reduces the testosterone/cortisol (T/C) ratio. The T/C ratio has been used as an indicator of the anabolic/catabolic status of skeletal muscle. Some studies have shown increases during RT whereas some have not (74).

The Glucocorticoid Receptor

The catabolic effects of cortisol are mediated through glucocorticoid receptors. Cortisol and possibly androgen concentrations may determine the level of up- or down-regulation of glucocorticoid receptors. ECC resistance exercise up-regulates glucocorticoid receptor content and protein breakdown (123). However, up-regulation is reduced following the second workout, thereby indicating a protective effect with exposure to ECC exercise. Glucocorticoid receptor up-regulation occurs following 6 and 12 weeks of RT (125) so its role requires further research.

CATECHOLAMINES

The adrenal medulla secretes catecholamines (also known as *adrenaline*) that are synthesized from the amino acid *tyrosine*. Epinephrine (~80%) is predominantly secreted with norepinephrine (15%–20%) and dopamine is also secreted. Norepinephrine and dopamine also serve as neurotransmitters in the autonomic nervous system. Catecholamines are secreted in response to stress (physical, heat, hypoxia, hypoglycemia), reflect the demands of exercise, and are important for increasing force production, muscle contraction rate, energy availability, as well as performing other functions including the augmentation of hormones such as TE. Catecholamine actions are terminated quickly as they bind with low affinity to their receptors and are dissociated rapidly. Catecholamine concentrations are increased during aerobic and anaerobic exercise with the magnitude dependent on the muscle mass involved, posture (upright position yields a higher response), intensity, and duration (56,128). At a standard submaximal workload, endurance-trained athletes may exhibit a smaller catecholamine response (56). However, some studies have shown that endurance athletes produce a more substantial catecholamine response to exercise (at a similar relative workload) than untrained individuals (56,128), termed a

sports adrenal medulla. Similar findings were shown with anaerobic (sprint) training where some studies indicate a greater potential to secrete catecholamines during exercise in trained individuals (128).

Resistance exercise increases plasma concentrations of epinephrine (67), norepinephrine (67), and dopamine (59,67). The magnitude is dependent upon the force of muscle contraction, amount of muscle stimulated, intensity and volume, rest intervals utilized, and level of dehydration (54,74). Trained lifters may experience an anticipatory rise in catecholamines to help prepare the body to perform maximally (61,67). Chronic adaptations are less clear although it has been suggested that training reduces the catecholamine response (30).

β-ENDORPHINS

β-endorphin is a 31-amino acid peptide cleaved in the anterior pituitary from a parent molecule (*proopiomelanocortin*). It also acts as a neurotransmitter in the nervous system. β-endorphins act as analgesics, increase relaxation, and enhance immune function. Exercise is a potent stimulus for β-endorphin secretion with the response dependent on the intensity and duration (104). Anaerobic exercise elevates β-endorphins in proportion to blood lactate and ACTH increases (104,113). Aerobic exercise increases β-endorphins with a rise in intensity (82). A threshold intensity and volume may be necessary for elevations (at least 70% of Vo_{2max}) (25). β-endorphin elevations occur during resistance exercise in men and women in most (20,118) but not all studies (58). Workouts (bodybuilding-type workouts high in volume, moderate to high in intensity, and with short rest intervals) that produce high levels of blood lactate and cortisol also stimulate a rise in β-endorphins. The elevation has been attributed to the magnitude of muscle mass used, rest interval length, intensity, and volume (74). The rise in β-endorphins may help offset the acidosis by improving mood state and pain tolerance (104).

THYROID HORMONES

The thyroid hormones thyroxine (T4) and triiodothyronine (T3) are released into circulation where they travel mostly bound to transport proteins (thyroxine-binding globulin, prealbumin, and albumin). Mostly T4 (~20 times more) circulates as it has a longer half-life than T3. In target tissues T4 is mostly converted to the more potent T3. The thyroid hormones increase basal metabolic rate, protein synthesis, and augment the actions of catecholamines. The response of thyroid hormones to exercise and training is not clear. Aerobic exercise elevates T3 and T4 in an intensity-dependent manner (10). However, some studies showed no acute elevations (96). Inconsistent changes have been shown over long-term training periods (87). The role of thyroid hormones during RT is unclear but may be permissive in its interaction (augmentation) with other hormones, *e.g.*, ARs. Some studies have shown no changes or reductions in resting T4, free T4, T3, and TSH during RT (72,74). Due to the tight control of thyroid hormones, elevations during RT may not be expected.

FLUID-REGULATORY HORMONES

Fluid homeostasis is critical to exercise performance. Elevations in fluid regulatory hormones such as AVP, atrial peptide, renin, aldosterone, and angiotensin II are seen during exercise, with the magnitude dependent on intensity, duration, fitness level, and hydration status (12,81). Resistance exercise elevates atrial peptide, renin, angiotensin II, and plasma osmolality as early as after the first set (67). Fluid shifts elicit a hormonal response to restore fluid balance. Arginine vasopressin is released from the posterior pituitary where it acts on the kidneys and blood vessels to increase fluid reabsorption, sodium, potassium, and chloride reabsorption, and vasoconstriction. Atrial peptide is a 28-amino-acid hormone released from the heart in response to increases in blood pressure to induce *natriuresis* (sodium excretion in urine and decrease in blood fluid volume). Renin is a renal enzyme released in response to low blood pressure and reduced renal blood flow that stimulates production of angiotensin I (from angiotensinogen). Angiotensin I is converted to angiotensin II via the enzyme angiotensin converting enzyme (ACE) which stimulates the release of aldosterone from the adrenal cortex (Fig. 6.6). Aldosterone secretion is controlled by changes in fluid volume, sodium and potassium content in the blood, stress, and changes in blood pressure. The resultant effect of aldosterone is to increase sodium retention and fluid volume to increase blood pressure.

LEPTIN

Leptin, a product of the *ob* gene in adipose tissue, is a hormone that relays satiety signal to the hypothalamus to regulate energy balance and appetite, but is involved in a milieu of bodily responses. Blood leptin concentrations reflect the amount of energy stored in adipose tissue. Obese humans have approximately four times more leptin than lean individuals, and women show higher concentrations than men. Leptin is released and circulates to the brain where it crosses the blood-brain barrier to act with receptors to affect appetite, energy intake and expenditure, thermogenesis, and a number of other actions. Leptin concentrations may be influenced by insulin, glucocorticoids, catecholamines, thyroid hormones, TE, GH, and stimulants. Exercise may not affect leptin concentrations independent of percent body fat (24,101,127). Leptin is a critical mediator of several endocrine pathways pertinent to RT. Leptin directly reduces steroidogenesis (114) resulting in lower TE concentrations in obese men. Body fat can play an indirect role via leptin concentrations (from **leptin resistance**) in adaptations to exercise.

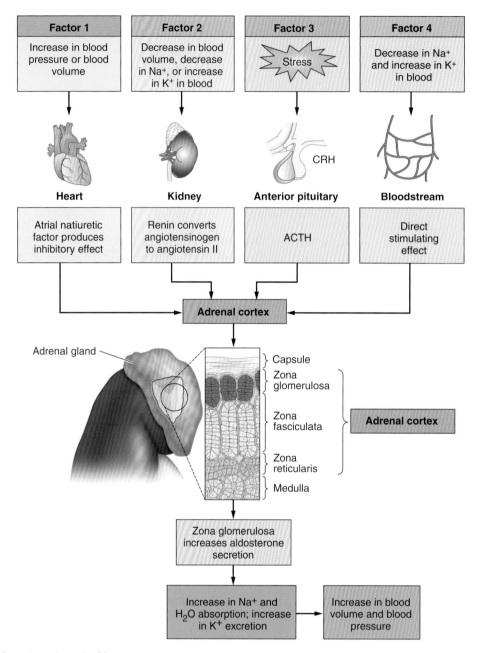

■ **FIGURE 6.6.** The renin-angiotensin-aldosterone system.

ESTROGENS

Estrogens (estradiol, estriol, and estrone) are steroids with long half-lives synthesized and secreted primarily by the ovaries (and adrenals to a lesser extent) in women under the control of LH and FSH, but are produced from conversion of androgens in men. Estrogens circulate bound to SHBG or albumin until they reach the target tissue or become metabolized by the liver. Estrogens perform many functions, including promoting secondary female characteristics, reducing bone resorption (and stimulating growth plate closure), enhancing metabolism, retaining sodium and water, reducing muscle damage, and increasing HDLs (decreasing LDLs). However, estrogens inhibit collagen synthesis (42) that can weaken tendons and

ligaments. Susceptibility to injury is a concern for female athletes or males using anabolic steroids.

Estrogen responses to exercise are less clear. Aerobic exercise may elevate estradiol in women (11). The response to RT is minimal. The phase of the menstrual cycle is critical as estradiol levels are low during the follicular phase (days 1–13), but peak value is attained near ovulation. After a short-term reduction, estradiol levels rise and are higher during the luteal phase (days 15–28). Muscle strength, endurance, power, and Vo_{2max} do not change during various phases of the menstrual cycle (17,74,107). However, prolonged exercise in the heat may be compromised during the mid-luteal phase where body temperature tends to be elevated (17).

▨ Summary Points

✔ The endocrine system is one of two major control systems (along with the nervous system) in the human body.

✔ The human body contains a multitude of hormones that perform numerous functions.

✔ Systemic hormones are released into circulation, many bind to transport proteins, travel to the target tissues, and bind to either membrane-bound or cytoplasmic/nuclear receptors to elicit intracellular signaling mechanisms ultimately leading to the target effect.

✔ Exercise is a potent stimulus eliciting acute hormonal elevations in several key hormones known to enhance exercise performance and subsequent adaptations.

✔ Chronic changes in resting hormonal concentrations are not common, but when they do occur, they usually reflect some substantial changes in the training program, nutritional intake, or recovery activities.

✔ The acute hormonal (TE, GH) response to resistance exercise has been suggested to be important in mediating some of the ensuing changes in muscle size, strength, and power. Some studies have shown modest strength and size increases without significant acute elevations during workouts suggesting that other neuromuscular mechanisms play large roles in the adaptational process. However, the magnitude of strength and size increases appears more substantial when acute hormonal elevations are present during and immediately following a workout.

Review Questions

1. The hormone produced by the liver that is critical to mediating many of the anabolic effects of GH is
   a. Insulin
   b. IGF-1
   c. Cortisol
   d. Glucagon

2. Many side effects associated from excessive TE arise from its conversion into
   a. Estrogens
   b. DHEA
   c. Androstenediol
   d. Cholesterol

3. A major anabolic substance that is produced by muscle cells in response to mechanical stress is
   a. Cortisol
   b. Mechano-growth factor
   c. Insulin
   d. Parathyroid hormone

4. Which of the following hormones plays the most substantial role in fluid volume regulation?
   a. Aldosterone
   b. Leptin
   c. Glucagon
   d. Insulin

5. A hormone known to regulate hunger and energy expenditure is
   a. Leptin
   b. Cortisol
   c. Glucagon
   d. AVP

6. Which of the following hormones does not increase muscle mass?
   a. Insulin
   b. IGF-1
   c. Glucagon
   d. Testosterone

7. LH causes the secretion of cortisol in men.   T F

8. A negative feedback system is one that will reduce secretion of a hormone if it is already high in concentration.   T F

9. Because protein hormones have their receptors on the surface of the cell membrane a second messenger system is needed intracellularly.   T F

10. Plasma volume reductions have no effect on exercise hormonal concentrations.   T F

11. An elevation in TE during a workout is an important factor for androgen receptor up-regulation.   T F

12. Workouts that are low intensity and low volume and use long rest intervals maximize the acute GH response to resistance exercise.   T F

References

1. Ahtiainen JP, Pakarinen A, Kraemer WJ, Häkkinen K. Acute hormonal and neuromuscular responses and recovery to forced vs maximum repetitions multiple resistance exercises. *Int J Sports Med.* 2003;24:410–418.

2. Ahtiainen JP, Pakarinen A, Alen M, et al. Muscle hypertrophy, hormonal adaptations and strength development during strength training in strength-trained and untrained men. *Eur J Appl Physiol.* 2003;89:555–563.

3. Aizawa K, Akimoto T, Inoue H, et al. Resting serum dehydroepiandrosterone sulfate level increases after 8-week resistance training among young females. *Eur J Appl Physiol.* 2003;90:575–580.

4. Alen M, Pakarinen A, Häkkinen K, Komi PV. Responses of serum androgenic-anabolic and catabolic hormones to prolonged strength training. *Int J Sports Med.* 1988;9:229–233.

5. Bamman MM, Shipp JR, Jiang J, et al. Mechanical load increases muscle IGF-1 and androgen receptor mRNA concentrations in humans. *Am J Physiol.* 2001;280:E383–E390.

6. Beaven CM, Hopkins WG, Hansen KT, et al. Dose effect of caffeine on testosterone and cortisol responses to resistance exercise. *Int J Sport Nutr Exerc Metab.* 2008;18:131–141.

7. Borst SE, De Hoyos DV, Garzarella L, et al. Effects of resistance training on insulin-like growth factor-I and IGF binding proteins. *Med Sci Sports Exerc.* 2001;33:648–653.

8. Bottaro M, Martins B, Gentil P, Wagner D. Effects of rest duration between sets of resistance training on acute hormonal responses in trained women. *J Sci Med Sport.* 2009;12:73–78.

9. Buresh R, Berg K, French J. The effect of resistive exercise rest interval on hormonal responses, strength, and hypertrophy with training. *J Strength Cond Res.* 2009;23:62–71.

10. Ciloglu F, Peker I, Pehlivan A, et al. Exercise intensity and its effects on thyroid hormones. *Neuro Endocrinol Lett.* 2005;26: 830–834.

11. Consitt LA, Copeland JL, Tremblay MS. Endogenous anabolic hormone responses to endurance versus resistance exercise and training in women. *Sports Med.* 2002;32:1–22.

12. Convertino VA, Keil LC, Bernauer EM, Greenleaf JE. Plasma volume, osmolality, vasopressin, and renin activity during graded exercise in man. *J Appl Physiol.* 1981;50:123–128.

13. Copeland JL, Heggie L. IGF-I and IGFBP-3 during continuous and interval exercise. *Int J Sports Med.* 2008;29:182–187.

14. Craig BW, Brown R, Everhart J. Effects of progressive resistance training on growth hormone and testosterone levels in young and elderly subjects. *Mech Ageing Dev.* 1989;49:159–169.

15. Craig BW, Kang H. Growth hormone release following single versus multiple sets of back squats: total work versus power. *J Strength Cond Res.* 1994;8:270–275.

16. Crewther B, Cronin J, Keogh J, Cook C. The salivary testosterone and cortisol response to three loading schemes. *J Strength Cond Res.* 2008;22:250–255.

17. De Jonge JAX. Effects of the menstrual cycle on exercise performance. *Sports Med.* 2003;33:833–851.

18. De Palo EF, Gatti R, Cappellin E, Schiraldi C, De Palo CB, Spinella P. Plasma lactate, GH and GH-binding protein levels in exercise following BCAA supplementation in athletes. *Amino Acids.* 2001; 20:1–11.

19. De Palo EF, Antonelli G, Gatti R, Chiappin S, Spinella P, Cappellin E. Effects of two different types of exercise on GH/IGF axis in athletes. Is the free/total IGF-I ratio a new investigative approach? *Clin Chim Acta.* 2008;387:71–74.

20. Eliot DL, Goldberg L, Watts WJ, Orwoll E. Resistance exercise and plasma beta-endorphin/beta-lipotrophin immunoreactivity. *Life Sci.* 1984;34:515–518.

21. Elloumi M, El Elj N, Zaouali M, et al. IGFBP-3, a sensitive marker of physical training and overtraining. *Br J Sports Med.* 2005; 39:604–610.

22. Fry AC, Kraemer WJ. Resistance exercise overtraining and overreaching. Neuroendocrine responses. *Sports Med.* 1997;23: 106–129.

23. Fry AC, Hoffman JR. Training responses and adaptations of the endocrine system. In: Chandler TJ, Brown LE, editors. *Conditioning for Strength and Human Performance.* Philadelphia (PA): Lippincott Williams & Wilkins; 2008. pp. 94–122.

24. Gippini A, Mato A, Peino R, et al. Effect of resistance exercise (body building) training on serum leptin levels in young men. Implications for relationship between body mass index and serum leptin. *J Endocrinol Invest.* 1999;22:824–828.

25. Goldfarb AH, Hatfield BD, Armstrong D, Potts J. Plasma beta-endorphin concentration: response to intensity and duration of exercise. *Med Sci Sports Exerc.* 1990;22:241–244.

26. Goldspink G. Changes in muscle mass and phenotype and the expression of autocrine and systemic growth factors by muscle in response to stretch and overload. *J Anat.* 1999;194:323–334.

27. Goldspink G. Mechanical signals, IGF-1 gene splicing, and muscle adaptation. *Physiology* 2005;20:232–238.

28. Goto K, Sato K, Takamatsu K. A single set of low intensity resistance exercise immediately following high intensity resistance exercise stimulates growth hormone secretion in men. *J Sports Med Phys Fitness.* 2003;43:243–249.

29. Gotshalk LA, Loebel CC, Nindl BC, et al. Hormonal responses to multiset versus single-set heavy-resistance exercise protocols. *Can J Appl Physiol.* 1997;22:244–255.

30. Guezennec Y, Leger L, Lhoste F, et al. Hormone and metabolite response to weight-lifting training sessions. *Int J Sports Med.* 1986; 7:100–105.

31. Häkkinen K, Pakarinen A, Alen M, Komi PV. Serum hormones during prolonged training of neuromuscular performance. *Eur J Appl Physiol.* 1985;53:287–293.

32. Häkkinen K, Pakarinen A, Alen M, et al. Relationships between training volume, physical performance capacity, and serum hormone concentrations during prolonged training in elite weight lifters. *Int J Sports Med.* 1987;8(suppl):61–65.

33. Häkkinen K, Pakarinen A, Alen M, et al. Neuromuscular and hormonal responses in elite athletes to two successive strength training sessions in one day. *Eur J Appl Physiol.* 1988;57:133–139.

34. Häkkinen K, Pakarinen A, Alen M, et al. Neuromuscular and hormonal adaptations in athletes to strength training in two years. *J Appl Physiol.* 1988;65:2406–2412.

35. Häkkinen K, Pakarinen A, Alen M, et al. Daily hormonal and neuromuscular responses to intensive strength training in 1 week. *Int J Sports Med.* 1988;9:422–428.

36. Häkkinen K, Pakarinen A. Serum hormones in male strength athletes during intensive short term strength training. *Eur J Appl Physiol.* 1991;63:191–199.

37. Häkkinen K, Pakarinen A. Acute hormonal responses to two different fatiguing heavy-resistance protocols in male athletes. *J Appl Physiol.* 1993;74:882–887.

38. Häkkinen K, Pakarinen A. Acute hormonal responses to heavy resistance exercise in men and women at different ages. *Int J Sports Med.* 1995;16:507–513.

39. Häkkinen K, Pakarinen A, Kraemer WJ, et al. Basal concentrations and acute responses of serum hormones and strength development during heavy resistance training in middle-aged and elderly men and women. *J Gerontol A Biol Sci Med Sci.* 2000;55:B95–105.

40. Hameed M, Orrel RW, Cobbold G, et al. Expression of IGF-1 splice variants in young and old human skeletal muscle after high resistance exercise. *J Physiol.* 2003;547:247–254.

41. Hansen S, Kvorning T, Kjaer M, Szogaard G. The effect of short-term strength training on human skeletal muscle: the importance of physiologically elevated hormone levels. *Scand J Med Sci Sport.* 2001;11:347–354.

42. Hansen M, Miller BF, Holm L, et al. Effect of administration of oral contraceptives in vivo on collagen synthesis in tendon and muscle connective tissue in young women. *J Appl Physiol*. 2009; 106(4):1435–1443 [2008; ahead of print].

43. Hill EE, Zack E, Battaglini C, Viru M, Viru A, Hackney AC. Exercise and circulating cortisol levels: the intensity threshold effect. *J Endocrinol Invest*. 2008;31:587–591.

44. Hoffman JR, Ratamess NA, Kang J, et al. Effect of creatine and beta-alanine supplementation on performance and endocrine responses in strength/power athletes. *Int J Sport Nutr Exerc Metab*. 2006;16:430–446.

45. Hoffman JR, Ratamess NA, Ross R, et al. Effect of a pre-exercise energy supplement on the acute hormonal response to resistance exercise. *J Strength Cond Res*. 2008;22:874–882.

46. Holloszy JO. Exercise-induced increase in muscle insulin sensitivity. *J Appl Physiol*. 2005;99:338–343.

47. Hortobagyi T, Houmard JA, Stevenson JR, et al. The effects of detraining on power athletes. *Med Sci Sports Exerc*. 1993;25: 929–935.

48. Hulmi JJ, Volek JS, Selanne H, Mero AA. Protein ingestion prior to strength exercise affects blood hormones and metabolism. *Med Sci Sports Exerc*. 2005;37:1990–1997.

49. Hulmi JJ, Ahtiainen JP, Selanne H, et al. Androgen receptors and testosterone in men — effects of protein ingestion, resistance exercise and fiber type. *J Steroid Biochem Mol Biol*. 2008;110:130–137.

50. Hymer WC, Kraemer WJ, Nindl BC, et al. Characteristics of circulating growth hormone in women after acute heavy resistance exercise. *Am J Physiol Endocrinol Metab*. 2001;281:E878–E887.

51. Inoue K, Yamasaki S, Fushiki T, et al. Androgen receptor antagonist suppresses exercise-induced hypertrophy of skeletal muscle. *Eur J Appl Physiol*. 1994;69:88–91.

52. Izquierdo M, Ibanez J, Gonzalez-Badillo JJ, et al. Differential effects of strength training leading to failure versus not to failure on hormonal responses, strength, and muscle power gains. *J Appl Physiol*. 2006;100:1647–1656.

53. Izquierdo M, Ibanez J, Gonzalez-Badillo JJ, et al. Detraining and tapering effects on hormonal responses and strength performance. *J Strength Cond Res*. 2007;21:768–775.

54. Judelson DA, Maresh CM, Yamamoto LM, et al. Effect of hydration state on resistance exercise-induced endocrine markers of anabolism, catabolism, and metabolism. *J Appl Physiol*. 2008;105: 816–824.

55. Kahn SM, Hryb DJ, Nakhla AM, Romas NA, Rosner W. Sex hormone-binding globulin is synthesized in target cells. *J Endocrinol*. 2002;175:113–120.

56. Kjaer M. Adrenal medulla and exercise training. *Eur J Appl Physiol*. 1998;77:195–199.

57. Koziris LP, Hickson RC, Chatterton RT, et al. Serum levels of total and free IGF-1 and IGFBP-3 are increased and maintained in long-term training. *J Appl Physiol*. 1999;86:1436–1442.

58. Kraemer RR, Acevedo EO, Dzewaltowski D, et al. Effects of low-volume resistive exercise on beta-endorphin and cortisol concentrations. *Int J Sports Med*. 1996;17:12–16.

59. Kraemer WJ, Noble BJ, Clark MJ, Culver BW. Physiologic responses to heavy-resistance exercise with very short rest periods. *Int J Sports Med*. 1987;8:247–252.

60. Kraemer WJ, Marchitelli L, Gordon SE, et al. Hormonal and growth factor responses to heavy resistance exercise protocols. *J Appl Physiol*. 1990;69:1442–1450.

61. Kraemer WJ, Gordon SE, Fleck SJ, et al. Endogenous anabolic hormonal and growth factor responses to heavy resistance exercise in males and females. *Int J Sports Med*. 1991;12:228–235.

62. Kraemer WJ, Fry AC, Warren BJ, et al. Acute hormonal responses in elite junior weightlifters. *Int J Sports Med*. 1992;13:103–109.

63. Kraemer WJ, Fleck SJ, Dziados JE, et al. Changes in hormonal concentrations after different heavy-resistance exercise protocols in women. *J Appl Physiol*. 1993;75:594–604.

64. Kraemer WJ, Dziados JE, Marchitelli LJ, et al. Effects of different heavy-resistance exercise protocols on plasma β-endorphin concentrations. *J Appl Physiol*. 1993;74:450–459.

65. Kraemer WJ, Clemson A, Triplett NT, et al. The effects of plasma cortisol elevation on total and differential leukocyte counts in response to heavy-resistance exercise. *Eur J Appl Physiol*. 1996; 73:93–97.

66. Kraemer WJ, Volek JS, Bush JA, et al. Hormonal responses to consecutive days of heavy-resistance exercise with or without nutritional supplementation. *J Appl Physiol*. 1998;85:1544–1555.

67. Kraemer WJ, Fleck SJ, Maresh CM, et al. Acute hormonal responses to a single bout of heavy resistance exercise in trained power lifters and untrained men. *Can J Appl Physiol*. 1999;24:524–537.

68. Kraemer WJ, Häkkinen K, Newton RU, et al. Effects of heavy-resistance training on hormonal response patterns in younger vs. older men. *J Appl Physiol*. 1999;87:982–992.

69. Kraemer WJ, Loebel CC, Volek JS, et al. The effect of heavy resistance exercise on the circadian rhythm of salivary testosterone in men. *Eur J Appl Physiol*. 2001;84:13–18.

70. Kraemer WJ, Dudley GA, Tesch PA, et al. The influence of muscle action on the acute growth hormone response to resistance exercise and short-term detraining. *Growth Horm IGF Res*. 2001;11: 75–83.

71. Kraemer WJ, Mazzetti SA. Hormonal mechanisms related to the expression of muscular strength and power. In: Komi PV, editor. *Strength and Power in Sport*. 2nd ed. Malden (MA): Blackwell Science; 2003. pp. 73–95.

72. Kraemer WJ, Ratamess NA. Endocrine responses and adaptations to strength and power training. In: Komi PV, editor. *Strength and Power in Sport*. 2nd ed. Malden (MA): Blackwell Scientific Publications; 2003. pp. 361–386.

73. Kraemer WJ, Rubin MR, Häkkinen K, et al. Influence of muscle strength and total work on exercise-induced plasma growth hormone isoforms in women. *J Sci Med Sport*. 2003;6:295–306.

74. Kraemer WJ, Ratamess NA. Hormonal responses and adaptations to resistance exercise and training. *Sports Med*. 2005;35:339–361.

75. Kraemer WJ, Spiering BA, Volek JS, et al. Androgenic responses to resistance exercise: effects of feeding and L-carnitine. *Med Sci Sports Exerc*. 2006;38:1288–1296.

76. Kraemer WJ, Ratamess NA, Volek JS, et al. The effects of amino acid supplementation on hormonal responses to resistance training overreaching. *Metabolism*. 2006;55:282–291.

77. Kraemer WJ, Dunn-Lewis C, Comstock BA, Thomas GA, Clark JE, Nindl BC. Growth hormone, exercise, and athletic performance: a continued evolution of complexity. *Curr Sports Med Rep*. 2010; 9:242–252.

78. Kvorning T, Andersen M, Brixen K, Schjerling P, Suetta C, Madesn K. Suppression of testosterone does not blunt mRNA expression of myoD, myogenin, IGF, myostatin or androgen receptor post strength training in humans. *J Physiol*. 2007;578:579–593.

79. Linnamo V, Pakarinen A, Komi PV, Kraemer WJ, Häkkinen K. Acute hormonal responses to submaximal and maximal heavy resistance and explosive exercises in men and women. *J Strength Cond Res*. 2005;19:566–571.

80. MacLean HE, Chiu WS, Notini AJ, et al. Impaired skeletal muscle development and function in male, but not female, genomic androgen receptor knockout mice. *FASEB J*. 2008;22:2676–2689.

81. Mannix ET, Palange P, Aronoff GR, et al. Atrial natriuretic peptide and the renin-aldosterone axis during exercise in man. *Med Sci Sports Exerc*. 1990;22:785–789.

82. Maresh CM, Sokmen B, Kraemer WJ, et al. Pituitary-adrenal responses to arm versus leg exercise in untrained man. *Eur J Appl Physiol*. 2006;97:471–477.

83. Marx JO, Ratamess NA, Nindl BC, et al. Low-volume circuit versus high-volume periodized resistance training in women. *Med Sci Sports Exerc*. 2001;33:635–643.

84. McCall GE, Byrnes WC, Fleck SJ, et al. Acute and chronic hormonal responses to resistance training designed to promote muscle hypertrophy. *Can J Appl Physiol.* 1999;24:96–107.

85. McCaulley GO, McBride JM, Cormie P, et al. Acute hormonal and neuromuscular responses to hypertrophy, strength and power type resistance exercise. *Eur J Appl Physiol.* 2009;105: 695–704.

86. McMurray RG, Eubank TK, Hackney AC. Nocturnal hormonal responses to resistance exercise. *Eur J Appl Physiol.* 1995;72: 121–126.

87. McMurray RG, Hackney AC. Interactions of metabolic hormones, adipose tissue and exercise. *Sports Med.* 2005;35:393–412.

88. Meckel Y, Eliakim A, Seraev M, et al. The effect of a brief sprint interval exercise on growth factors and inflammatory mediators. *J Strength Cond Res.* 2009;23:225–230.

89. Michels G, Hoppe UC. Rapid actions of androgens. *Front Neuroendocrinol.* 2008;29:182–198.

90. Mulligan SE, Fleck SJ, Gordon SE, et al. Influence of resistance exercise volume on serum growth hormone and cortisol concentrations in women. *J Strength Cond Res.* 1996;10: 256–262.

91. Narayanan R, Mohler ML, Bohl CE, Miller DD, Dalton JT. Selective androgen receptor modulators in preclinical and clinical development. *Nucl Recept Signal.* 2008;6:e010.

92. Nindl BC, Hymer WC, Deaver DR, Kraemer WJ. Growth hormone pulsatility profile characteristics following acute heavy resistance exercise. *J Appl Physiol.* 2001;91:163–172.

93. Nindl BC, Kraemer WJ, Gotshalk LA, et al. Testosterone responses after resistance exercise in women: influence of regional fat distribution. *Int J Sport Nutr Exerc Metab.* 2001;11:451–465.

94. Nindl BC, Kraemer WJ, Marx JO, et al. Overnight responses of the circulating IGF-1 system after acute heavy-resistance exercise. *J Appl Physiol.* 2001;90:1319–1326.

95. Petrella JK, Kim J, Mayhew DL, Cross JM, Bamman MM. Potent myofiber hypertrophy during resistance training in humans is associated with satellite cell-mediated myonuclear addition: a cluster analysis. *J Appl Physiol.* 2008;104:1736–1742.

96. Premachandra BN, Winder WW, Hickson R, Lang S, Holloszy JO. Circulating reverse triiodothyronine in humans during exercise. *Eur J Appl Physiol Occup Physiol.* 1981;47:281–288.

97. Raastad T, Bjoro T, Hallen J. Hormonal responses to high- and moderate-intensity strength exercise. *Eur J Appl Physiol.* 2000; 82:121–128.

98. Ratamess NA, Kraemer WJ, Volek JS, et al. Androgen receptor content following heavy resistance exercise in men. *J Steroid Biochem Mol Biol.* 2005;93:35–42.

99. Ratamess NA, Hoffman JR, Ross R, et al. Effects of an amino acid/creatine energy supplement on the acute hormonal response to resistance exercise. *Int J Sport Nutr Exerc Metab.* 2007;17: 608–623.

100. Roelen CA, deVries WR, Koppeschaar HR, Vervoorn C, Thijssen JH, Blankenstein MA. Plasma insulin-like growth factor-I and high affinity growth hormone-binding protein levels increase after two weeks of strenuous physical training. *Int J Sports Med.* 1997;18:238–241.

101. Rubin MR, Kraemer WJ, Maresh CM, et al. Response of high-affinity growth hormone binding protein to acute heavy resistance exercise in resistance-trained and untrained men. *Med Sci Sports Exerc.* 2005; 37: 395–403.

102. Schiffer T, Schulte S, Hollmann W, Bloch W, Struder HK. Effects of strength and endurance training on brain-derived neurotrophic factor and insulin-like growth factor 1 in humans. *Horm Metab Res.* 2009;41(3):250–254 [2008; (ahead of print).]

103. Schwab R, Johnson GO, Housh TJ, et al. Acute effects of different intensities of weight lifting on serum testosterone. *Med Sci Sports Exerc.* 1993;25:1381–1385.

104. Schwartz L, Kindermann W. Changes in beta-endorphin levels in response to aerobic and anaerobic exercise. *Sports Med.* 1992; 13:25–36.

105. Schumm SR, Triplett NT, McBride JM, Dumke CL. Hormonal response to carbohydrate supplementation at rest and after resistance exercise. *Int J Sport Nutr Exerc Metab.* 2008;18: 260–280.

106. Sedliak M, Finni T, Cheng S, Kraemer WJ, Häkkinen K. Effect of time-of-day-specific strength training on serum hormone concentrations and isometric strength in men. *Chronobiol Int.* 2007; 24:1159–1177.

107. Smekal G, von Duvillard SP, Frigo P, et al. Menstrual cycle: no effect on exercise cardiorespiratory variables or blood lactate concentration. *Med Sci Sports Exerc.* 2007;39:1098–1106.

108. Smilios I, Pilianidis T, Karamouzis M, Tokmakidis SP. Hormonal responses after various resistance exercise protocols. *Med Sci Sports Exerc.* 2003;35:644–654.

109. Spiering BA, Kraemer WJ, Anderson JM, et al. Effects of elevated circulating hormones on resistance exercise-induced Akt signaling. *Med Sci Sports Exerc.* 2008;40:1039–1048.

110. Spiering BA, Kraemer WJ, Vingren JL, et al. Elevated endogenous testosterone concentrations potentiate muscle androgen receptor responses to resistance exercise. *J Steroid Biochem Mol Biol.* 2009;114:195–199.

111. Staron RS, Karapondo DL, Kraemer WJ, et al. Skeletal muscle adaptations during early phase of heavy-resistance training in men and women. *J Appl Physiol.* 1994;76:1247–1255.

112. Tarpenning KM, Wiswell RA, Hawkins SA, Marcell TJ. Influence of weight training exercise and modification of hormonal response on skeletal muscle growth. *J Sci Med Sport* 2001; 4:431–446.

113. Taylor DV, Boyajian JG, James N, et al. Acidosis stimulates beta-endorphin release during exercise. *J Appl Physiol.* 1994;77: 1913–1918.

114. Tena-Sempere M, Manna PR, Zhang FP, et al. Molecular mechanisms of leptin action in adult rat testis: potential targets for leptin-induced inhibition of steroidogenesis and pattern of leptin receptor messenger ribonucleic acid expression. *J Endocrinol.* 2001; 170:413–423.

115. Tremblay MS, Copeland JL, Van Helder W. Effect of training status and exercise mode on endogenous steroid hormones in men. *J Appl Physiol.* 2004;96:531–539.

116. Vingren JL, Kraemer WJ, Hatfield DL, et al. Effect of resistance exercise on muscle steroidogenesis. *J Appl Physiol.* 2008; 105:1754–1760.

117. Volek JS, Kraemer WJ, Bush, JA, et al. Testosterone and cortisol in relationship to dietary nutrients and resistance exercise. *J Appl Physiol.* 1997;8:49–54.

118. Walberg-Rankin J, Franke WD, Gwazdauskas FC. Response of beta-endorphin and estradiol to resistance exercise females during energy balance and energy restriction. *Int J Sports Med.* 1992;13:542–547.

119. Weiss LW, Cureton KJ, Thompson FN. Comparison of serum testosterone and androstenedione responses to weight lifting in men and women. *Eur J Appl Physiol.* 1983;50:413–419.

120. West DWD, Kujbida GW, Moore DR, et al. Resistance exercise-induced increases in putative anabolic hormones do not enhance muscle protein synthesis or intracellular signaling in young men. *J Physiol.* 2009;587:5239–5247.

121. West DWD, Burd NA, Tang JE, et al. Elevations in ostensibly anabolic hormones with resistance exercise enhance neither training-induced muscle hypertrophy nor strength of the elbow flexors. *J Appl Physiol.* 2010;108:60–67.

122. Wilkinson SB, Tarnopolsky MA, Grant EJ, Correia CE, Phillips SM. Hypertrophy with unilateral resistance exercise occurs without increases in endogenous anabolic hormone concentration. *Eur J Appl Physiol.* 2006;98:546–555.

123. Willoughby DS, Taylor M, Taylor L. Glucocorticoid receptor and ubiquitin expression after repeated eccentric exercise. *Med Sci Sports Exerc.* 2003;35:2023–2031.

124. Willoughby DS. Effects of heavy resistance training on myostatin mRNA and protein expression. *Med Sci Sports Exerc.* 2004;36:574–582.

125. Willoughby DS, Taylor L. Effects of sequential bouts of resistance exercise on androgen receptor expression. *Med Sci Sports Exerc.* 2004;36:1499–1506.

126. Willoughby DS, Stout JR, Wilborn CD. Effects of resistance training and protein plus amino acid supplementation on muscle anabolism, mass, and strength. *Amino Acids* 2007;32:467–477.

127. Zafeiridis A, Smilios I, Considine RV, Tokmakidis SP. Serum leptin responses after acute resistance exercise protocols. *J Appl Physiol.* 2003;94:591–597.

128. Zouhal H, Jacob C, Delamarche P, Gratas-Delamarche A. Catecholamines and the effects of exercise, training and gender. *Sports Med.* 2008;38:401–423.

7 Metabolic Responses and Adaptations to Training

objectives

After completing this chapter, you will be able to:

· Discuss adenosine triphosphate (ATP) and understand the major metabolic systems in the human body that resynthesize ATP
· Discuss how training results in substrate and enzymatic changes in the ATP-phosphocreatine, glycolytic, and aerobic energy systems
· Discuss the physiologic effects of metabolic acidosis and how the body buffers acids
· Discuss oxygen consumption and energy expenditure during exercise and understand how one can increase basal metabolic rate through diet and exercise
· Discuss how manipulating training programs affects oxygen consumption during exercise
· Discuss strategies to reduce body fat via exercise and diet

Metabolism is the sum of all chemical reactions in the human body to sustain life. **Exergonic** reactions result in energy release whereas **endergonic** reactions result in stored or absorbed energy. **Bioenergetics** refers to the flow of energy change within the human body. It is concerned mostly with the extraction of energy from carbohydrates (CHOs), fats, and proteins. Although CHOs, fats, and in some instances, proteins are sources of dietary energy, biochemical conversion of these large molecules is necessary to extract chemical energy and transfer energy to skeletal muscle contractile proteins. **Energy** is defined as the ability to perform work, and energy will change in proportion to the magnitude of work performed. Although several types of energy are important to human function, chemical energy is needed for several metabolic processes. As the first law of thermodynamics states, energy cannot be created or destroyed but can transform from one form to another. Understanding the body's metabolic systems is critical to developing optimal aerobic and anaerobic training programs.

ADENOSINE TRIPHOSPHATE AND METABOLIC SYSTEMS

The human body requires continuous chemical energy to support life and exercise. Large amounts of potential energy from storage or food sources can be transferred to fuel muscle performance. The high-energy compound is known as **adenosine triphosphate** (ATP).

Figure 7.1 depicts ATP, which is composed of adenine and ribose (adenosine) linked to three phosphates. The bonds that link the outermost two phosphates possess the ability to release chemical energy via **hydrolysis**. Energy is released upon cleavage of the last phosphate bond. Hydrolysis of ATP (via ATPase) reaction yields 7.3 kilocalories (kcal) of free energy in addition to *adenosine diphosphate* (ADP) and *free inorganic phosphate* (P_i) (74).

$$ATP + H_2O \rightarrow ADP + P_i + energy$$

The energy liberated transfers to other molecules and is used to perform physiologic work. Energy is liberated aerobically (with oxygen) and anaerobically (without oxygen). Two major anaerobic energy systems include the ATP-phosphocreatine (ATP-PC) and glycolysis systems and one major aerobic energy system.

ATP AND PHOSPHOCREATINE SYSTEMS

There are three ways chemical energy can be utilized very quickly. One way is to use skeletal muscle ATP stores. The human body has a limited capacity to store ATP, i.e., ~80–100 g of ATP at any given time (74), enough to sustain only a few seconds of exercise. Cells must constantly replenish ATP stores and our metabolic systems are the primary modes. A second way is the **phosphocreatine** (PC) system. PC (or creatine phosphate) is a high-energy phosphate that provides energy for high-intensity activities lasting up to 5–10 seconds. The PC system is

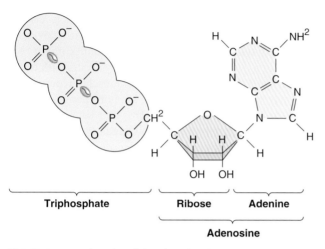

FIGURE 7.1. Adenosine triphosphate (ATP).

engaged initially during low-intensity activities. Its concentration within skeletal muscle is approximately four to five times greater than ATP (59,76), and is more prominent in FT than ST fibers (24) although highly trained endurance athletes may have higher PC content in ST fibers (95). Maximal rates of PC turnover are ~7–9 mmol kg^{-1} s^{-1} dry mass (109), which can be exhausted within 10 seconds. The PC system is the predominant energy source for explosive, anaerobic exercise such as sprinting, jumping, and resistance training (RT), and force declines as PC depletes. Because of limited PC stores, the ATP-PC system cannot provide sufficient energy to sustain exercise beyond 10 seconds. The PC system operates via the following equation:

$$ADP + \text{phosphocreatine} \leftrightarrow ATP + \text{creatine}$$

PC rephosphorylates ADP. Substantial free energy is released when the bond between creatine and phosphate is cleaved. Hydrolysis of PC drives ADP to form ATP. This reaction is catalyzed rapidly by *creatine kinase* (CK) (76). CK, because of its location within skeletal muscle fibers, tends to leak into circulation when muscle damage takes place and serves as an indirect marker of muscle damage. CK has several isoforms that identify the source of damage, *i.e.*, skeletal or cardiac muscle, or the brain.

A third way is to produce ATP from multiple ADP sources. An enzyme *adenylate kinase* (known as *myokinase* in skeletal muscle) catalyzes the following reaction:

$$2\ ADP \leftrightarrow ATP + AMP$$

Two ADPs are hydrolyzed to form ATP and a molecule of adenosine monophosphate (AMP). The adenylate kinase reaction augments the muscle's ability for rapid energy turnover and produces AMP, which is a potent stimulator of glycolysis (24).

Energy systems operate under the *Law of Mass Action*, which states chemical reactions taking place in solutions progress to the right with the addition of reactants or progress to the left with the addition of products (74). With enzyme-mediated reactions the rate of product formation is highly influenced by the amount of reactants. For example, greater amounts of ADP formed during exercise increases the rate of the CK and adenylate kinase reactions. This continues until exercise is terminated or performed at an intensity low enough that other metabolic systems can predominate. Having larger amounts of stored substrates shifts the reactions to generate higher ATP resynthesis during high-intensity exercise. This is the rationale for creatine supplementation (see the Sidebar below) where a larger amount of energy can be liberated from the ATP-PC system. All metabolic systems are engaged at all times. However, one may predominate depending on the exercise intensity, duration, and oxygen availability.

SIDEBAR | **CREATINE SUPPLEMENTATION AND EXERCISE PERFORMANCE**

Creatine is one of the most commonly used supplements by athletes since the early 1990s. The rationale for creatine supplementation derives from two major roles: (a) anaerobic energy metabolism, and (b) its ability to act as an osmotic agent. When muscle creatine stores increase via supplementation, this process attracts water to enter the cells (**osmosis**) causing increased body weight and muscle protein synthesis. Creatine is naturally found in foods but is synthesized in the body from the amino acids arginine, glycine, and methionine. Although creatine is absorbed in other tissues, ~95% of creatine is absorbed in skeletal muscle. A specific creatine transporter protein is located within the muscle's cell membrane that helps creatine enter muscle. Creatine supplementation can increase muscle levels of total creatine substantially by ~11%–22% (90). The majority of muscle creatine elevation occurs within the first few days of supplementation, especially when a loading phase is used. Further supplementation with lower doses can maintain this level. Some individuals are nonresponders whereas some experience large elevations. There are many creatine supplements available on the market with creatine monohydrate in powder form the most popular. Creatine supplementation increases body mass ranging from 0.6 to 5.2 kg (129) and improves muscle strength, endurance, power, vertical jump height, sprint speed, agility, and sport-specific performance (cycling power, swim performance, skating speed) (90). The benefits of creatine supplementation have extended beyond athletes to clinical populations. Creatine is one of a few sports supplements shown to be **ergogenic**.

Phosphagen Repletion

ATP-PC resynthesis is critical to explosive exercise performance. High-intensity exercise may deplete PC by 60%–80% during the first 30 seconds with up to 70% depletion taking place within 12 seconds (76,109). Longer-duration high-intensity exercise (400-m sprint) may reduce PC by 89% (48). The rate of PC depletion may be higher in trained sprinters versus sprinters who cannot run as fast (47). The greater the PC degradation, the longer the time needed to fully recover PC to preexercise values. Resynthesis of PC occurs in a biphasic response where there is a faster followed by a slower component, and the rate of PC resynthesis may be affected by the type of recovery (active vs. passive) (109). The half-life of PC resynthesis ranges from 21 to 57 seconds depending on intensity and volume (76,109). Within 90 seconds of recovery 65% of recovery may be seen, but less than 90% of recovery occurs within 6 minutes (76). Other critical factors affecting PC resynthesis rates are muscle pH, ADP levels, and oxygen availability. The half-life of PC resynthesis is longer when muscle pH decreases (76). It is thought that accumulation of H^+ inhibits PC resynthesis primarily during the slow component of recovery (76). Oxygen availability and ADP levels are critical during the fast component. ATP used to resynthesize PC is derived from oxidative metabolism, and a faster rate of PC resynthesis in ST compared to FT fibers is seen (76). The kinetics of PC resynthesis is important when determining rest intervals for RT and interval training. Less recovery limits PC resynthesis and reduces performance.

Training Adaptations

Anaerobic training induces positive adaptations in the ATP-PC and adenylate kinase metabolic systems. Adaptations take place in three general ways: (a) greater substrate storage at rest, (b) altered enzyme activity, and (c) limited accumulation of fatiguing metabolites. Repeated bouts of high-intensity exercise can increase ATP and PC storage via a supercompensation effect (68). An early study by MacDougall et al. (68) showed a 22% increase in resting PC, 39% increase in muscle creatine, and 18% increase in ATP concentrations following 5 months of RT (3–5 sets of 8–10 reps with 2-min rest intervals). Other studies showed increased resting PC concentrations after 5 weeks of RT (127) and no change (118). Sprint training results in no change or a decrease in resting ATP and PC concentrations (27,101). Trained sprinters may possess a similar resting PC/ATP ratio (despite a higher rate of PC breakdown during exercise) to endurance-trained athletes (55). Resting substrate elevations are most prominent during RT with little changes seen during sprint training.

Enzyme changes occur during training. Two enzymes often studied are CK and adenylate kinase (myokinase). Early studies showed increased activity of CK and myokinase during RT, especially in FT fibers (22,123).

However, the magnitude of muscle growth is critical when examining enzyme changes. Enzyme activity is expressed relative to total muscle protein content. No change or a decrease in enzyme activity occurs with training-induced hypertrophy. During muscle hypertrophy, CK may decrease (62,115,122) or not change whereas increases (117), no change (118), and decreases (115) in myokinase activity have been shown. Powerlifters and Olympic weightlifters have similar myokinase to controls whereas bodybuilders have the highest myokinase activity (116). Myokinase activity may not change or increase up to 20% during sprint and plyometric training of 2–15 weeks (101). Although elite sprinters use PC more rapidly, sprint training does not change CK activity much. A long-term (8-month) combined sprint, plyometric, and RT program showed no change in CK activity as well (18). Metabolic adaptations from sprint training do not appear mediated by greater CK activity.

GLYCOLYSIS

Glycolysis is the breakdown of CHOs to resynthesize ATP in the cytoplasm. It is another anaerobic metabolic system that can provide energy for high-intensity exercise for up to 2 minutes. Its rate of ATP resynthesis is not as rapid as PC; however, the human body has a larger **glycogen** supply, so high energy liberation is sustained for a longer period of time. The free energy released in this series of reactions forms ATP and nicotinamide adenine dinucleotide (NADH). The source of CHOs could be blood glucose or muscle glycogen stores. Glycolysis is a series of 10 reactions breaking down the 6-carbon glucose ($C_6H_{12}O_6$) to a 3-carbon pyruvate ($C_3H_4O_3$). The net result is 2 or 3 ATP formed (3 ATP from muscle glycogen, 2 ATP from a molecule of blood glucose) in the following reaction:

$$\text{glucose} + 2 \text{ NAD}^+ + 2 \text{ ADP} + 2 \text{ P}_i \rightarrow 2 \text{ pyruvate} + 2 \text{ NADH} + 2 \text{ H}^+ + 2 \text{ ATP} + 2 \text{ H}_2\text{O}$$

Figure 7.2 depicts the reactions of glycolysis. The first five steps consume energy (invest) whereas the second half results in net gain of ATP and NADH. The first step is the formation of glucose-6-phosphate. For blood glucose, the enzyme *hexokinase* adds a phosphate to glucose so it cannot leave the cell (and promotes more glucose uptake into muscle). This requires ATP. Remember, glucose must first enter the cell via a glucose transporter (GLUT 4). For muscle glycogen, the enzyme *phosphorylase* breaks a molecule of glucose-1-phosphate from glycogen, which will be converted to glucose-6-phosphate (**glycogenolysis**). This reaction, however, does not require energy. At rest, phosphorylase is inactive (b form) but becomes activated (a form) during exercise in response to greater epinephrine secretion and elevated calcium concentrations (44). Glucose-6-phosphate must then be converted to fructose-6-phosphate (via an *isomerase* enzyme) and to fructose-1,6-biphosphate. The enzyme *phosphofructokinase* (PFK)

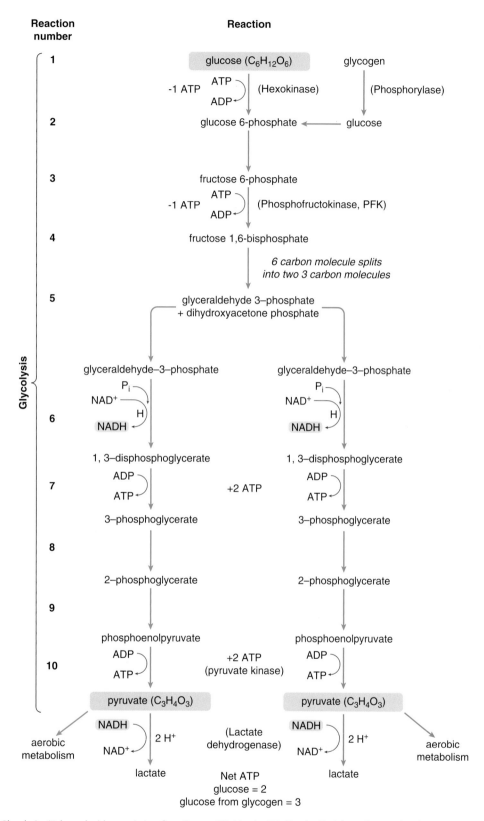

■ **FIGURE 7.2.** Glycolysis. (Adapted with permission from Powers SK, Howley ET. *Exercise Physiology: Theory and Application to Fitness and Performance.* 5th ed. New York (NY): McGraw Hill; 2004.)

phosphorylates fructose-6-phosphate and is considered the rate-limiting reaction of glycolysis. The regulation of PFK is critical to the magnitude of energy liberation derived from glycolysis. This reaction requires energy so up to this point in glycolysis we have used 2 ATPs but have not produced any. These reactions are reversible so glucose could be formed during **gluconeogenesis** (a process by which glucose is reformed in the opposite direction of glycolysis). From this point, our initial 6-carbon molecule is split via an enzyme, *aldolase*, into two 3-carbon molecules, dihydroxyacetone phosphate (DHAP) and glyceraldehyde-3-phosphate. DHAP is rapidly converted to glyceraldehyde-3-phosphate via an isomerase enzyme. Both 3-carbon glyceraldehyde-3-phosphate molecules undergo a series of reactions (where net ATP will be formed) yielding 1,3-bisphosphoglycerate, 3-phosphoglycerate, and 2-phosphoglycerate. Accompanying these reactions is the formation of 2 ATP and 2 NADH. We now have formed a total of 0 ATP for glycolysis to this point (we have used 2 ATP and formed 2 ATP, netting 0 ATP). Phosphoenolpyruvate (PEP) is formed from 2-phosphoglycerate via an enzyme *enolase* and PEP then forms pyruvate via the enzyme *pyruvate kinase*. This reaction produces 2 ATP (one from each PEP molecule) thereby netting 2 ATP formed from glycolysis.

Pyruvate is the end product but can be further modified to meet metabolic demands. If inadequate oxygen is present, pyruvate can be converted into lactate via the enzyme *lactate dehydrogenase* (LDH). This sequence has been called anaerobic or **fast glycolysis**. This reaction leads to some accumulation of H^+ that contributes, in part, to muscle fatigue. Pyruvate can travel to the mitochondria, lose a carbon (forming *acetyl CoA*), and enter the Kreb's cycle (aerobic respiration). This is called aerobic or **slow glycolysis**. The terms *aerobic* and *anaerobic glycolysis* are probably not practical because glycolysis is an anaerobic process.

Control of Glycolysis

Glycolysis can be controlled in several ways. Glycolysis is inhibited by sufficient oxygen levels, *i.e.*, steady-state aerobic exercise or during rest. Glycolysis is stimulated by high concentrations of ADP, P_i, ammonia, and by slight decreases in pH and AMP. Intense exercise results in a marked increase in ATP hydrolysis, thereby yielding higher concentrations of ADP and P_i. Ammonia is a by-product of AMP metabolism, and an increase in ammonia stimulates glycolysis. Glycolysis is inhibited by reductions in pH, increased ATP, PC, citrate, and free fatty acids. High ATP and PC levels signify a recovery (or resynthesis) state, thus a further need for glycolysis is reduced. Energy substrates can regulate glycolysis via negative feedback where high concentrations of ATP will limit production. Acidosis (decreased pH) inhibits glycolysis and is a major component of muscle fatigue. Citrate and free fatty acids are molecules indicative of aerobic metabolism, thereby reflecting adequate oxygen supply/demand.

A substantial portion of glycolysis is regulated through enzyme control. The enzymes hexokinase, PFK, phosphorylase (enzyme that breaks down glycogen), and pyruvate kinase are controlled by other molecules. Enzymes have two major binding areas, a catalytic unit that speeds up reactions and an allosteric unit that binds to regulatory molecules (*i.e.*, hormones, proteins). Negative feedback systems regulate glycolysis via the allosteric unit. For example, hexokinase is inhibited by glucose-6-phosphate. PFK is inhibited by ATP, and H^+ and stimulated by AMP. Pyruvate kinase is inhibited by ATP and acetyl CoA and is stimulated by AMP and fructose-1,6-bisphosphate (24). Phosphorylase is stimulated by hormones (*e.g.*, epinephrine) and is inhibited when another antagonistic enzyme, *glycogen synthase* (enzyme that stores glycogen), is active. This elaborate negative feedback control of glycolysis can stimulate or inhibit key glycolytic enzymes based on the energy needs of the human body.

Glycogen Metabolism

Muscle glycogen supplies a quick source of glucose and greater glycogen availability preexercise enhances endurance performance (44). Glycogen use is most rapid at the beginning of exercise and increases exponentially as intensity increases. On average, humans can store ~500 g (1%–2% of muscle mass) of glycogen in skeletal muscle (depending on body size) and ~80–120 g in the liver. High CHO intake increases muscle glycogen utilization whereas higher dietary fat intake may spare muscle glycogen (44). During exercise, glycogen breakdown takes place at a high rate. Liver glycogen breakdown helps maintain blood glucose and provides glucose for muscle uptake. Phosphorylase breaks down glycogen and glycogen breakdown takes place during exercise, and the magnitude depends on intensity, volume/duration, and rest intervals. Glycogen depletion in some muscle fibers serves as a stimulus for recruitment of other FT fibers. Glycogen is a major source of energy for exercise >50%–60% of Vo_{2max} (44), and glycogen depletion causes muscle fatigue during aerobic exercise or repeated, intermittent high-intensity anaerobic exercise of sufficient duration (1). During aerobic exercise, the pattern of glycogen depletion is related to fiber-type recruitment as substantial depletion occurs in ST fibers with secondary depletion occurring in FT fibers (1). During resistance exercise, glycogen breakdown predominates in FT fibers (85) and the rate is intensity dependent (97). The pattern of glycogen breakdown is similar between trained and untrained individuals (7) and resistance exercise may deplete muscle glycogen by 30%–60% (24,85,114) with some cells completely depleting glycogen stores. Initiating a resistance exercise workout with low muscle glycogen may limit up-regulation of some muscle growth factors (20). Sprint exercise of sufficient distance with short recovery intervals leads to high rates of glycogen depletion (especially in FT fibers) but this glycogen depletion is not thought to contribute highly to fatigue (1).

Muscle and liver glycogen repletion is critical to recovery following exercise. It involves many factors such as hormonal action, glucose uptake into muscle cells, and blood flow, but one critical factor is the amount of CHOs consumed. An enzyme in promoting glycogen storage is *glycogen synthase*, which is very active following exercise. Glycogen repletion is biphasic, with a rapid early phase followed by a slower phase. Most, if not all, muscle glycogen can be replenished within 24 hours provided adequate CHO consumption occurs, although repletion can be slowed by muscle damage (24). Restoration of muscle glycogen can exceed normal levels with consistent training via glycogen supercompensation (44).

SIDEBAR	CARBOHYDRATE INTAKE, MUSCLE GLYCOGEN, AND EXERCISE PERFORMANCE

CHOs (monosaccharides, disaccharides, and oligo-saccharides/polysaccharides) are macromolecules consisting of carbon, hydrogen, and oxygen atoms. CHOs perform many functions including energy liberation, cell structure and integrity, regulation of lipid metabolism, amino acid metabolism, and protein synthesis; enhance immune function; and serve as a structural component of genetic material (90). It is recommended that athletes consume ~55%–65% of their daily caloric intake from CHOs, with the majority complex CHOs with <10% consumed from simple CHOs (3). The American College of Sports Medicine (ACSM) recommends athletes consume 6–10 g CHOs kg body mass^{-1} day^{-1} to perform optimally and recover in between workouts (3). Studies show *CHO loading* or high-CHO diets (500–650 g of CHOs per day; 8–10.5 g of CHO kg of body mass^{-1} consumed for at least 3 days) increase muscle and liver glycogen content for ~3 days after loading and up to 1.8 times that of a normal diet in men and women (4,37,86,94). However, performance may or may not improve depending on the volume and intensity, *i.e.*, performance may increase with long-duration exercise. CHO intake during prolonged exercise helps maintain blood sugar levels, spare muscle and liver glycogen, and promote glycogen synthesis (during rest periods or periods of low-intensity activity). The ACSM recommends that athletes consume ~30–60 g of CHOs h^{-1} during long-term exercise (3) depending on intensity, size, type of CHOs consumed, and conditioning of the individual. For optimal glycogen repletion following long-duration exercise, CHOs (plus some amino acids) should be consumed as soon as possible at ~1.0–1.5 g of CHOs/kg of body mass within 30 minutes (3). This should be repeated every 2 hours for 4–6 hours. For slower repletion, the individual should consume 8–10 g per kg of body mass over a 24-hour period (90).

Training Adaptations

Changes in substrate storage and enzyme activity occur during training. Training that relies on glycolysis provides a potent stimulus for enhanced glycogen storage. Aerobic training (AT) increases muscle glycogen in FT and ST fibers (1). Steady-state AT and high-intensity interval training can increase resting muscle glycogen (65,134). A recent study showed 6 weeks of interval AT (10 × 4-min bouts at 90% of Vo$_{2max}$ with 2-min rest intervals) increased muscle glycogen content by 59% (87). AT results in a glycogen-sparing effect during low-to-moderate-intensity exercise with an increased proportion of energy provided by fat use (51,65). Sprint training may not change or increase glycogen content (101). The magnitude depends on how much sprint training affects the glycolytic metabolic system. Longer sprints with short to moderate rest intervals increases reliance upon glycolysis and may pose a more potent stimulus for glycogen storage than short sprints with long rest intervals. RT increases resting glycogen content by up to 112% (68). Bodybuilders have greater glycogen content than untrained individuals (119). RT with light loads with restricted blood flow can increase muscle glycogen more than RT without occlusion (16).

Glycolytic enzyme activity may decrease, not change, or increase during training. Sprint training may increase (16%–49%) or not change PFK activity, increase LDH (9%–20%), and increase phosphorylase (9%–41%) activity (100,101). AT does not increase anaerobic enzyme activity at rest (119) especially since AT induces changes in substrate utilization, *i.e.*, greater fat use versus CHO. During exercise (80% of Vo$_{2max}$), AT reduces activation of phosphorylase and reduces glycogen breakdown thereby showing a glycogen-sparing effect (19,65). Trained individuals have a higher activity of glycogen synthase. RT may alter enzyme activity depending on the program and magnitude of hypertrophy. RT programs that stress the ATP-PC system (high weight, low repetitions, and long rest intervals) may show reductions in glycolytic enzyme activity with pronounced hypertrophy (70). Phosphorylase activity may increase (22,39), PFK activity may increase (22) or not change (39,115,123), and LDH activity may slightly increase or not change after RT (22,116). Hexokinase may increase after RT (128).

Lactate

Lactate has a negative impact on performance. The production of lactate from pyruvate yields H$^+$, which contributes to muscle fatigue. An accumulation of H$^+$ reduces pH and leads to a rapid onset of fatigue. H$^+$ accumulation causes peripheral fatigue via inhibition of glycolytic enzymes, slowing calcium reuptake, and interference with cross-bridge cycling properties. For many years, the production of lactate via fast glycolysis was thought to be the major pathway for H$^+$ accumulation. However,

Myths & Misconceptions

Lactate Has No Benefits in the Human Body

Lactate does have benefits. Once produced, lactate will not remain stagnant in skeletal muscles. A large amount is shuttled to adjacent muscle fibers (especially ST) where it can be converted to pyruvate via the reversible LDH catalyzed reaction, or enters circulation (74). Lactate removal is essential for the cell to keep liberating energy via glycolysis. However, a large amount can enter circulation because exercise produces large amounts of lactate that temporarily overwhelm muscle fibers' ability to oxidize it rapidly. The fate of lactate in the blood is short-lived because values typically return to preexercise levels within 1 hour after exercise. Lactate can be taken up by other skeletal (mostly ST fibers) and cardiac muscles and be used as an energy substrate. Lactate in blood can travel to the liver (or kidneys) and be used to form glucose via gluconeogenesis where it can reestablish blood glucose concentrations or replenish liver glycogen. This process is known as the *Cori Cycle*. Lactate is a valuable energy substrate and not a waste product.

The release and uptake of lactate in skeletal and cardiac muscle is dependent upon specific transmembrane transporters known as *monocarboxylate transporters* (MCT). Although eight isoforms have been identified, MCT1 and MCT4 are found in skeletal muscle and MCT1 in the heart (11). The MCTs mediate transport for lactate and H$^+$ and assist in pH balance during exercise (56). Lactate transport capacity is greater in ST than FT fibers and the proportion of ST fibers is related to MCT1 density (56). Lactate uptake from the blood is related to MCT1 content, and training up-regulates MCT1 and MCT4 expression in skeletal muscle (11). An adaptation to training is facilitated lactate removal and uptake mediated by the MCT family of transport proteins. Interestingly, testosterone administration may increase MCT1 and MCT4 content with a concomitant increase in lactate transport capacity (32).

Anaerobic exercise results in an increase in blood lactate concentrations in trained and untrained individuals (Fig. 7.3). At rest, blood lactate values range from 1 to 2 mmol L^{-1}. Because red blood cells only metabolize glucose, there are low levels of lactate in the blood at rest. As exercise intensity increases (and recruitment of FT fibers increases), blood lactate values increase. This corresponding intensity is known as the **lactate threshold**. The lactate threshold typically begins ~50%–60% of Vo$_{2max}$ in untrained individuals and 70%–80% of Vo$_{2max}$ in trained athletes (24). It is thought to reflect the interaction of anaerobic and aerobic energy systems (132). Athletes with high lactate thresholds are capable of excelling at endurance events (132). The blood lactate curve shifts to the right with training at or beyond the lactate threshold indicating that a higher intensity is needed to produce a specific blood lactate level. RT (3–5 sets of 15–20 reps with short rest intervals) and circuit training (8–20 RM with 30-s rest intervals) can increase the lactate threshold (31,71). The second point shown in Figure 7.3 is the **onset of blood lactate accumulation** (OBLA) and represents the point/intensity where blood lactate values exceed 4 mmol L^{-1} and increase exponentially. Blood lactate not only reflects production but also the rate of clearance. Endurance athletes possess a higher rate of lactate clearance (124).

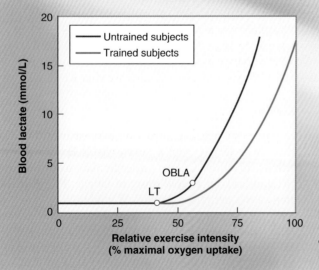

FIGURE 7.3. The lactate threshold. (Reprinted with permission from Cramer JT. Bioenergetics of exercise and training. In: Baechle TR, Earle RW, editors. *Essentials of Strength Training and Conditioning*. 3rd ed. Champaign (IL): Human Kinetics; 2008. pp. 21–39.)

(Continued)

The amount of lactate produced depends on the intensity and duration of exercise with the magnitude less in endurance-trained compared to sprint-trained athletes (77). Blood lactate values in athletes may reach as high as 32 mM immediately following high-intensity exercise (84). During RT, bodybuilding workouts stress the glycolytic system more than strength/power training. Blood lactate increases during resistance exercise (21,63,92,125) with the magnitude greater with high intensities (21,81), large muscle mass exercises (125), high volume (13,92), slow lifting velocities (73), short rest intervals (63), and with augmented ECC loading (81,133). The intensity/volume interaction is critical as larger responses are seen with high-volume, low-to-moderate-intensity (multiple sets of 15 reps with 60% of 1 RM) than low-volume, high-intensity (multiple sets of 4 reps with 90% of 1 RM) workouts (60). A reduced lactate response occurs at absolute workloads, but not relative workloads (96) following RT. Powerlifters and weightlifters (but not bodybuilders) exhibit greater increases in blood lactate at an absolute workload during cycling than untrained individuals (30). Bodybuilders possess the ability to train with a higher percent of their 1 RM for multiple sets when short rest intervals are used. Training targeting the glycolytic system induces favorable changes in lactate kinetics.

H^+ accumulation results from all metabolic systems, and lactate formation may play a limited role (98). Although the lactate molecule may physically inhibit muscle cross-bridge formation (35), other studies have shown no negative effects (88).

Metabolic Acidosis and Buffer Capacity

Blood and muscle pH decrease during and immediately following anaerobic exercise (23,102). Muscle pH may drop from 7.1 to 6.4 during exhaustive exercise (23). The drop in pH is less in endurance-trained athletes (77). Reduced blood pH decreases intracellular H^+ efflux and disturbs muscle acid-base balance (38). Acidosis adversely affects energy metabolism and force production so that the onset of fatigue is rapid. Metabolic acidosis may cause fatigue by negatively affecting sodium and potassium movement, reducing calcium kinetics, reducing cross-bridge formation, and inhibiting glycolytic enzymes (84). PFK may be inhibited at a pH of 6.9 and glycogen breakdown may be completely halted at a pH of 6.4 (132). Maintaining pH relies upon the cells' ability to extrude protons (H^+) and/or accumulated hydroxide (OH^-) and bicarbonate (HCO_3). An acid is a proton donor and a base is a proton acceptor. Buffering capacity is the ability to resist changes in pH (84). Several intracellular and extracellular factors contribute to improved skeletal muscle buffer capacity. These include

- Phosphates (mostly intracellular; *chemical buffer*): Monohydrogen phosphate (HPO_4), CP (~33% of intracellular buffering especially in FT fibers), and P_i.
- Proteins and peptides (intracellular and extracellular; *chemical buffer*): ~50% of intracellular buffering during exercise. Amino acid supplementation results in better buffering capacity during training (126). Associated with protein buffers are the protein-bound histidyl residues, histidine-containing dipeptides, and free histidine. Carnosine accounts for up to 40% of total intracellular buffering capacity (26,84). Elevated carnosine is seen in sprinters and rowers compared to endurance athletes and untrained individuals (83). Carnosine (β-alanyl-l-histidine) and β-alanine are used in supplementation. β-alanine (the rate-limiting precursor of carnosine) supplementation elevates muscle carnosine by >35% (29). Four weeks of β-alanine supplementation (4.5–4.8 g day^{-1}) can augment isokinetic torque, RT volume, muscle endurance, and reduce fatigue (29,49,50). However, 10 weeks of supplementation with 6.4 g day^{-1} increased muscle carnosine by 12% but did not augment performance (61). Lastly, some blood proteins serve as a buffer like hemoglobin.
- Bicarbonate (extracellular, intracellular; *chemical buffer*): the bicarbonate anion (HCO_3) accepts H^+ to form carbonic acid where it is converted to H_2O and CO_2 by the enzyme *carbonic anhydrase*. Sahlin (103) suggested that bicarbonate could contribute as much as 15%–18% of total buffer capacity during exercise. Although bicarbonate's role is to buffer extracellular fluid, it indirectly acts as an intracellular buffer by facilitating H^+ flux out of muscle (108). Bicarbonate loading can be an ergogenic aid during exercise (90).
- Respiratory and renal buffers: both are *physiological buffers*. Because a rise in CO_2 leads to acidosis, respiratory rate increases (hyperventilation) to expel CO_2 at a higher rate. The kidneys can neutralize acid as the renal tubules expel H^+ from the body.

Increasing muscle buffer capacity enables greater tolerance for acidosis. Higher lactate concentrations are seen following anaerobic training with concomitant improvements in performance (54,108). Enhanced buffer capacity prolongs high-intensity exercise. Trained individuals have a greater buffer capacity than untrained individuals (104). Muscle buffer capacity may increase by 16%–44% after 7–8 weeks of sprint training (9,80,108). RT may lessen H^+ accumulation but may not increase buffer capacity (31).

AEROBIC METABOLISM

The aerobic, or oxidative, energy system is highly engaged when adequate oxygen is available. In some ways, the term *aerobic* is misleading because oxygen's role is limited until the end where its presence assists indirectly in ATP production. The majority of energy derived aerobically comes from the oxidation of CHOs and fats, with very little from protein under normal conditions (unless the individual has very low kilocalorie intake or has performed a substantial endurance activity). Oxidation reactions donate electrons whereas reduction reactions accept electrons. The removal of hydrogen is critical as hydrogen atoms possess potential energy stored from food sources and these electrons are transported and used for ATP synthesis. Aerobic metabolism occurs within the cell's mitochondria (powerhouses of the cell).

The mitochondria contain carrier molecules that oxidize electrons from hydrogen and pass them to oxygen via reduction reactions that generate a large amount of ATP (74). The aerobic system provides the primary source of ATP at rest and during low to moderate steady-state exercise. Seventy percent of ATP produced at rest comes from fats whereas 30% comes from CHOs (24). As exercise intensity increases, so does the percent of ATP liberation from CHOs. High-intensity exercise relies predominantly upon CHO metabolism.

Metabolism of CHOs begins with glycolysis. Remember, the fate of pyruvate was twofold: (a) converted to lactate, or (b) converted to acetyl CoA and CO_2 via *pyruvate dehydrogenase*. Acetyl CoA is capable of being oxidized and can be formed from fat and protein sources, which makes it the common link of these fuel sources.

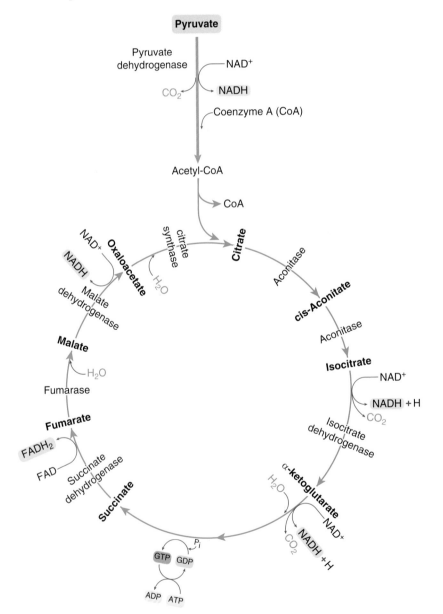

■ **FIGURE 7.4.** The Krebs cycle. (Modified from Kraemer WJ, Fleck SJ, Deschenes MR. *Exercise Physiology: Integrating Theory and Application.* Baltimore (MD): Lippincott Williams & Wilkins; 2012.)

The aerobic system (Fig. 7.4) begins with the **Krebs cycle** (named after Nobel Prize-winning scientist Hans Krebs), which involves reactions (that do not require oxygen) that continue the oxidation of acetyl CoA and produces 2 ATP indirectly. The goals are to oxidize acetyl groups and attach electrons to the carriers NAD^+ and FAD. Acetyl CoA transfers two carbons to oxaloacetate to form the 6-C citrate via *citrate synthase*. Oxaloacetate is further converted into isocitrate (via *aconitase*), α-ketoglutarate (via *isocitrate dehydrogenase*), succinyl CoA (via *α-ketoglutarate dehydrogenase*), and succinate (via *succinyl-CoA-synthetase*). Succinate is converted to fumarate via the enzyme *succinate dehydrogenase (SDH)*. Fumarate is converted to malate (via *fumarase*) and to oxaloacetate (via *malate dehydrogenase [MDH]*). The following reaction describes the Krebs cycle:

$$Acetyl\ CoA + 3\ NAD^+ + FAD + GDP + P_i + 2\ H_2O \rightarrow$$
$$2\ CO_2 + GTP + 3\ NADH + 3\ H^+ + FADH_2 + CoA$$

Remember, two molecules of acetyl CoA enter the Krebs cycle as two pyruvates are produced in glycolysis. The intermediates produced in Figure 7.4 will be doubled. The removal and transport of H^+ via NAD and FAD yields large energy liberation in another part of the mitochondria. Fatty acids can be converted to acetyl CoA via a process known as **beta oxidation**. Amino acids may enter the Krebs cycle at various sites including conversion to acetyl CoA. Branched-chain amino acids are the major source. Some enzymes of the Kreb's cycle are stimulated by ADP concentrations and inhibited by rising ATP and GTP levels.

Overall, six molecules of NADH and two molecules of $FADH_2$ are produced from the Krebs cycle. Most energy is liberated from the *electron transport chain* (Fig. 7.5), which couples reactions between electron donors and acceptors across the inner mitochondrial membrane. ATP synthesis (from ADP) occurs from transferring electrons from NADH and $FADH_2$ to oxygen. Hydrogen atoms are passed along the chain of cytochromes in complexes where they reduce oxygen to form water and a proton-motive gradient to phosphorylate ADP (**chemiosmotic hypothesis**) (59). Uncoupling proteins (UCP1–UCP5) assist and play a role in thermogenesis and energy expenditure (5).

Energy Yield from Carbohydrates

Generally, 3 ATP will be produced per molecule of NADH and 2 ATP from $FADH_2$. From glucose oxidation, 2 (from blood glucose) or 3 (from stored glycogen) ATP will be produced from glycolysis, 2 ATP will be produced from the Krebs cycle, 12 ATP will be produced from 4 NADH produced from glycolysis and pyruvate conversion to acetyl CoA, and 22 ATP will be produced from the electron transport chain totaling 38 or 39 ATP.

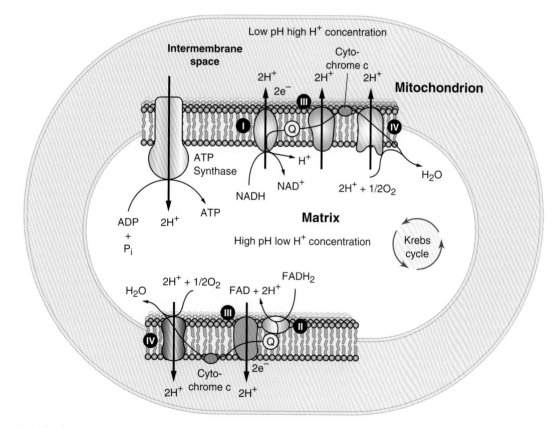

FIGURE 7.5. The electron transport chain. (From Porth CM. *Pathophysiology Concepts of Altered Health States.* 7th ed. Philadelphia (PA): Lippincott Williams & Wilkins; 2005.)

Energy Yield from Fats

Fat provides a concentrated source of energy. Fat metabolism predominates at rest and during low-to-moderate-intensity exercise. Fats, or lipids, are broken down during **lipolysis** by *hormone-sensitive lipase* into glycerol and three free fatty acids. Fatty acids can enter circulation or be oxidized from muscle stores via beta oxidation (Fig. 7.6). Beta oxidation involves the splitting of 2-carbon acyl fragments from a long chain of fatty acids. Protons are accepted, water is added, ATP phosphorylates the reactions, and acyl fragments form with coenzyme A to yield acetyl CoA (74). Acetyl CoA enters the Krebs cycle and hydrogen released enters the electron transport chain. If an 18-carbon fatty acid is examined, ~147 ATP can be generated per fatty acid. Since there are three fatty acids in a triglyceride, 441 ATP (147 × 3) can be generated. Glycerol can be converted to 3-phosphoglyceraldehyde and enter glycolysis that yields 19 ATP. An 18-carbon triglyceride can yield a total of 460 ATP. Fat breakdown and oxidation is highly dependent on oxygen consumption. Beta-oxidation will not proceed if oxygen does not join hydrogen (74). Individuals with high aerobic capacity can oxidize fats at a large rate.

Aerobic Training Adaptations

AT leads to a milieu of adaptations that increases maximal aerobic capacity (Vo_{2max}). AT increases the number of capillaries surrounding each muscle fiber and **capillary density** (number of capillaries relative to muscle CSA) by up to 15% (132). Higher capillary content enables greater nutrient and oxygen exchange during exercise, and favors greater reliance on fat metabolism. AT increases the number of mitochondria and **mitochondrial density** in muscle in proportion to training volume (132). Endurance-trained men may have ~103% greater mitochondrial number and three times greater mitochondrial volume than untrained men (74). Myoglobin

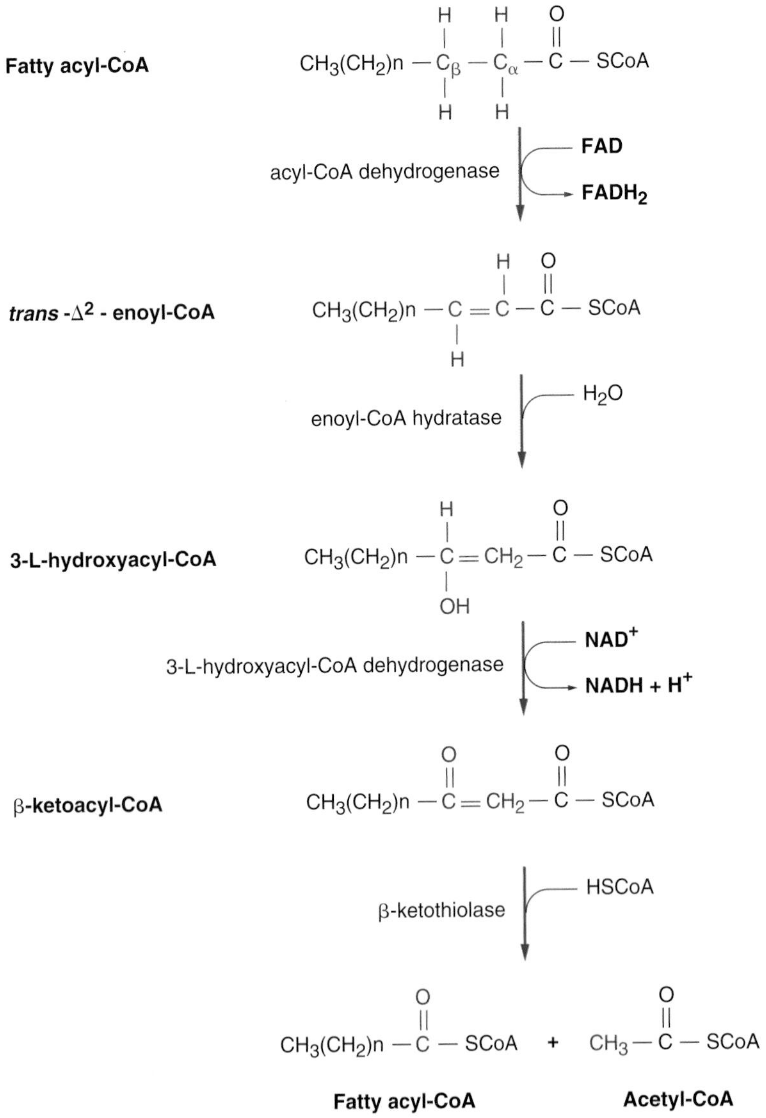

Fatty acyl-CoA

$$CH_3(CH_2)n - \overset{\overset{\displaystyle H}{|}}{\underset{\underset{\displaystyle H}{|}}{C_\beta}} - \overset{\overset{\displaystyle H}{|}}{\underset{\underset{\displaystyle H}{|}}{C_\alpha}} - \overset{\overset{\displaystyle O}{\|}}{C} - SCoA$$

acyl-CoA dehydrogenase — **FAD**
↘ **FADH₂**

***trans*-Δ² - enoyl-CoA**

$$CH_3(CH_2)n - \overset{\overset{\displaystyle H}{|}}{\underset{\underset{\displaystyle H}{|}}{C}} = C - \overset{\overset{\displaystyle O}{\|}}{C} - SCoA$$

enoyl-CoA hydratase — **H₂O**

3-L-hydroxyacyl-CoA

$$CH_3(CH_2)n - \overset{\overset{\displaystyle H}{|}}{\underset{\underset{\displaystyle OH}{|}}{C}} = CH_2 - \overset{\overset{\displaystyle O}{\|}}{C} - SCoA$$

3-L-hydroxyacyl-CoA dehydrogenase — **NAD⁺**
↘ **NADH + H⁺**

β-ketoacyl-CoA

$$CH_3(CH_2)n - \overset{\overset{\displaystyle O}{\|}}{C} = CH_2 - \overset{\overset{\displaystyle O}{\|}}{C} - SCoA$$

β-ketothiolase — **HSCoA**

$$CH_3(CH_2)n - \overset{\overset{\displaystyle O}{\|}}{C} - SCoA \quad + \quad CH_3 - \overset{\overset{\displaystyle O}{\|}}{C} - SCoA$$

Fatty acyl-CoA   **Acetyl-CoA**

■ **FIGURE 7.6.** Beta oxidation and energy yield from fats. (From McArdle WD, Katch FI, Katch VL. *Exercise Physiology: Nutrition, Energy, and Human Performance.* 7th ed. Baltimore (PA): Lippincott Williams & Wilkins; 2010.)

(a protein that binds oxygen in muscle and transports it to the mitochondria) is highest in ST fibers and is important for muscle endurance increases. AT may increase myoglobin content up to 80% (132). Krebs cycle, beta-oxidation, and electron transport system enzyme activity increases during AT. AT increases activities of *SDH, citrate synthase, cytochrome C oxidase,* and *pyruvate dehydrogenase* (87,132). The increased enzyme activity occurs in proportion to the level of training. Substrate metabolic changes occur. AT increases muscle glycogen stores at rest and have a glycogen-sparing effect during exercise (1,74,132). As a result, endurance athletes are better able to utilize free fatty acids for energy during exercise. Endurance athletes have greater intramuscular triglyceride stores at rest, enhanced lipolysis during exercise, and have higher beta-oxidation enzymatic activity all resulting in more efficient fat metabolism at rest and during exercise (1,132).

Anaerobic Training Adaptations

Anaerobic training (resistance, sprint, plyometric, and agility) provides little stimulus to the aerobic energy system as much of the energy demands are met by the ATP-PC and glycolytic systems. An increase in capillary number per fiber may occur after RT (75,110). Bodybuilders (8) and powerlifters (57) have greater capillary number than untrained individuals. However, capillary density is unaffected by RT and decreases in response to hypertrophy (8,52,57,75,128), which could result in a reduced capacity for oxygen delivery to recruited muscle fibers. Bodybuilders have greater capillary density than powerlifters and Olympic lifters but values are similar to untrained men (119). Mitochondrial density decreases up to 26% in response to RT (67,69) although mitochondrial size may increase in women (128). Myoglobin may not change following 8 weeks of RT (72) to perhaps help preserve oxygen transport during hypertrophy. Most studies have shown no change or decreases in Krebs cycle and electron transport chain enzyme activity (citrate synthase, MDH, SDH) during RT (22,39,72,106,115,128). However, some studies have shown increased citrate synthase, MDH, cytochrome oxidase, and β-HAD

(an enzyme of β-oxidation) activities following RT (113,120,128). Bodybuilders have greater citrate synthase and β-HAD activity than powerlifters and weightlifters (117). Sprint training may increase, decrease, and not change citrate synthase activity and not change or increase SDH activity (101). Most studies that found increased aerobic enzyme activity used long-distance sprints, whereas those that did not used repeated short sprints (101).

ENERGY SYSTEM CONTRIBUTION AND ATHLETICS

All energy systems are engaged at all times regardless of the activity (Table 7.1). Each system works together to meet the demands of exercise. However, one may predominate based on the intensity, volume/duration, and recovery intervals of exercise. During a 30-second cycle sprint 28%–40% of energy is liberated from aerobic metabolism, ~45% from glycolysis, and ~17% from ATP-PC system. During a 12-second cycle sprint, 47% of energy is liberated from glycolysis, 22% from ATP-PC, and 31% from aerobic metabolism (109). Table 7.2 depicts the metabolic demands of various sports. Training programs can be designed to target each system by manipulation of the intensity, volume/duration, and rest intervals used. An athlete whose sports require energy from ATP-PC system should target this system specifically with high-intensity, short bouts of explosive exercise to achieve the best results. Metabolic specificity is critical to off-season, preseason, and in-season training of athletes. **Interval training** allows the athlete to train at higher intensities for periods of time using prescribed rest intervals. The athletes can dedicate a greater proportion of time to high intensities as opposed to continuous training that may limit intensity and depends on fatigue. Work-to-rest ratios are prescribed. A 1:10 ratio indicates that athletes rest 10× longer than the work interval. An explosive bout lasting ~8 seconds requires the athlete to rest ~80 seconds. The work-to-rest ratio can target energy systems such that 1:12 to 1:20 ratios target ATP-PC, 1:3 to 1:5 ratios target fast glycolysis, 1:3 to 1:4 ratios target fast glycolysis and aerobic oxidation, and 1:1 to 1:3 ratios target aerobic oxidation (24).

TABLE 7.1 ENERGY SYSTEM USE

DURATION OF EVENT	INTENSITY OF EVENT	PRIMARY ENERGY SYSTEM(S)
0–6 s	Very intense	Phosphagen
6–30 s	Intense	Phosphagen and fast glycolysis
30 s to 2 min	Heavy	Fast glycolysis
2–3 min	Moderate	Fast glycolysis and oxidative system
>3 min	Light	Oxidative system

TABLE 7.2 METABOLIC DEMANDS OF SPORTS

SPORT	PHOSPHAGEN SYSTEM	ANAEROBIC GLYCOLYSIS	AEROBIC METABOLISM
Baseball	High	Low	—
Basketball	High	Moderate to high	—
Boxing	High	High	Moderate
Diving	High	Low	—
Fencing	High	Moderate	—
Field events	High	—	—
Field hockey	High	Moderate	—
Football (American)	High	Moderate	Low
Gymnastics	High	Moderate	—
Golf	High	—	—
Ice hockey	High	Moderate	Moderate
Lacrosse	High	Moderate	Moderate
Marathon	Low	Low	High
Mixed martial arts	High	High	Moderate
Powerlifting	High	Low	Low
Skiing:			
Cross-country	Low	Low	High
Downhill	High	High	Moderate
Soccer	High	Moderate	Moderate
Strength competitions	High	Moderate to high	Low
Swimming:			
Short distance	High	Moderate	—
Long distance	—	Moderate	High
Tennis	High	Moderate	—
Track (athletics):			
Short distance	High	Moderate	—
Long distance	—	Moderate	High
Ultra-endurance events	Low	Low	High
Volleyball	High	Moderate	—
Wrestling	High	High	Moderate
Weightlifting	High	Low	Low

Note: All types of metabolism are involved to some extent in all activities.

Reprinted with permission from Ratamess NA. Adaptations to anaerobic training programs. In: Baechle TR, Earle RW, editors. *Essentials of Strength Training and Conditioning.* 3rd ed. Champaign (IL): Human Kinetics; 2008. pp. 93–119.

Case Study 7.1

Nicole is an aerobic athlete who has predominately trained with traditional, continuous aerobic exercise workouts. She had learned from fellow athletes who incorporated interval training into their programs that these individuals improved their race times and attributed their success, in part, to interval training. Nicole has decided to include interval training in preparation for a 10-km race. She has approached you, a prominent strength and conditioning coach, for advice on how to incorporate interval training into her preparatory training program.

Questions for Consideration: **What work-to-rest ratio would you prescribe to Nicole to enhance her running program? What type of progression strategy would you suggest Nicole follow?**

METABOLIC DEMANDS AND EXERCISE

Exercise metabolism is measured several ways but the most common method involves indirect calorimetry. Indirect calorimetry involves measurement of oxygen consumption via open-circuit spirometry. Changes in oxygen and CO_2 percentages in expired air are compared to normal inspired ambient air, *e.g.*, 20.93% oxygen, 0.03% CO_2, and 79.04% nitrogen (74). A metabolic cart can measure each breath and consists of a flow meter, system to analyze expired air, CO_2 and oxygen analyzers, and a computer interface for calculations. One variable assessed is oxygen consumption. Oxygen consumption data can estimate **energy expenditure.** Energy expenditure can be measured at rest and during exercise. Resting energy expenditure provides an estimate of resting metabolic rate. The **respiratory quotient** (RQ) is a measure of CO_2 produced per unit of oxygen, *e.g.*, RQ = CO_2 produced ÷ O_2 consumed. This gives an indication of fuel usage, *i.e.*, CHO (RQ close to or greater than 1.00), fat (RQ = ~0.70), protein or mixed diet (RQ = ~0.82–0.86). Similar to RQ, the *respiratory exchange ratio* (RER) can be measured. Although RQ assumes that gas exchange results from nutrient breakdown solely, RER reflects more accurately the role of anaerobic exercise metabolism during exhaustive exercise. It is calculated the same way as RQ.

BASAL METABOLIC RATE

Basal metabolic rate (BMR) is the minimal level of energy needed to sustain bodily functions. Control of BMR, and essentially metabolism, is critical to body fat reductions and weight control. BMR represents the individual's total energy expenditure in a day. With aging (especially due to sedentary lifestyles), BMR decreases approximately 2%–3% per decade (74). Total energy expenditure or BMR is comprised of resting metabolic rate (RMR; ~60%–75%), the thermic effect of physical activity (15%–30%), and thermic effect of food consumption (~10%). RMR is the energy required to perform normal bodily functions while the body is at rest and is somewhat similar to BMR although it is measured under less stringent conditions, *e.g.*, does not require a 12-hour fast or 8 hours of sleep. Manipulation of any or all of these components of BMR can increase energy expenditure thereby resulting in greater kilocalories burned per day. BMR is affected by the following factors:

- *Body mass* — the larger the body size, the higher the BMR. Lean body mass (LBM; or fat-free mass) is a strong component of BMR. This is why RT is important to increasing BMR and reducing body fat. RT increases RMR by up to 9% after 24 weeks, with a larger response seen in men (66). An increase in LBM of 1 lb could increase RMR by 7–10 kcal day^{-1} (74). RT may or may not preserve LBM and increases RMR during strict dieting whereas strict dieting alone reduces LBM and RMR (15,36). Because of gender differences in body size, RMR is ~5%–10% higher in men than women (74). Fat tissue has less metabolic activity than muscle mass, so high body fat has a negative impact on BMR.

- *Regular exercise* — regular exercise enhances BMR with the magnitude dependent upon intensity, volume/duration, and muscle mass involvement. AT and RT can increase RMR by 8%–10% (74). Athletes have greater BMR than untrained individuals matched for LBM. A comprehensive progressive program consisting of aerobic and anaerobic exercise is critical to increasing BMR.

- *Diet-induced thermogenesis* — involves the increase in BMR associated with digestion, absorption, and assimilation of nutrients and activation of the sympathetic nervous system in response to meal consumption. Dietary-induced thermogenesis reaches maximum levels ~1 hour after meal consumption (74). Meals higher in protein content elicit a higher increase in BMR and may produce greater muscle anabolism during RT. Diets high in protein (relative to CHOs and fat intake) increase satiety (sense of fullness) and energy expenditure (82). Animal and whey proteins induce a greater thermogenic effect than other proteins (soy) and are thought to increase satiety to a greater extent possibly due to changes in hormones that control hunger (82). High-protein meals are thought to increase thermogenesis by up-regulating uncoupling proteins (82). The BMR increase during exercise is larger when exercise is performed following a meal, showing that exercise can augment diet-induced thermogenesis (74). Light to moderate exercise 1 hour following a meal may be beneficial in individuals trying to lose weight.

- *Environment* — warm environments can produce higher BMRs. Exercise in warm conditions can augment oxygen consumption by ~5% (74). The greater core temperature and physiologic demands of perspiration in the heat poses a stimulus to BMR. Cold temperatures pose a stimulus to BMR. Shivering generates body heat, and BMR can increase to accommodate the cold conditions (74).

- *Other factors* — low kilocalorie diets have the opposite effect. Decreasing kilocalorie intake decreases RMR and leads to weight gain. Stress, and the hormonal response, increases RMR. Catecholamines and thyroid hormones increase BMR. Hormonal control of metabolism is potent and varies based on genetics, nutritional intake, stress levels, and physical activity.

Estimating Resting Energy Expenditure

Estimating resting energy expenditure is important for weight loss/gain programs as direct measurement is impractical. Several (>100) population-specific equations have been developed to estimate resting energy expenditure from predictor variables such as body mass or LBM, height, and age that are based on gender. LBM may be the strongest predictor of RMR (121). The first equation developed and one still commonly used is the Harris-Benedict equation (46). The Cunningham (25)

TABLE 7.3 RESTING METABOLIC RATE (RMR) PREDICTION EQUATIONS

EQUATION	REFERENCE
RMR = 66.47 + 6.23 × BW(lb) + 12.67 × Ht(in) − 6.76 + age (y) in men	Harris and Benedict (45)
RMR = 655.1 + 4.34 × BW(lb) + 4.69 × Ht(in) − 4.68 + age(y) in women	
RMR = 10 × BM(kg) + 6.25 × Ht(cm) − 5 × age(y) + 5 in men	Mifflin-St Jeor (79)
RMR = 10 × BM(kg) + 6.25 × Ht(cm) − 5 × age(y) − 161 in women	
RMR = 500 + 22 × LBM(kg)	Cunningham (25)

and Mifflin and St. Jeor (79) equations have been used (Table 7.3). They have been cross-validated in athletes with many showing RMR underestimation (28). The exception is the Cunningham equation that has shown favorable RMR estimation (28,121).

SIDEBAR BASAL METABOLIC RATE ESTIMATION IN ATHLETES

Estimation of BMR involves estimation of RMR, diet-induced thermogenesis, and physical activity energy expenditure (PAEE). The following example utilizes the Cunningham (25) equation in a very active 22-year-old athlete who weighs 240 lb and has 11% body fat.

1. The first step is to convert 240 lb to kg (1 lb = 2.2 kg). 240/2.2 = **109.1 kg**.
2. LBM must be calculated. Total mass (109.1 kg) is multiplied by the decimal of body fat percentage (0.11) to calculate fat mass. Fat mass = 109.1 kg × 0.11 = **12 kg**. LBM = total mass − fat mass = 109.1 kg−12.0 kg = **97.1 kg**. Another method is to multiply total mass (109.1 kg) × 0.89 (1.00−0.11 for fat percentage) = **97.1 kg**.
3. Equation (25): RMR = 500 + 22 × LBM(kg): RMR = 500 + 22 × (97.1 kg) = **2,636 kcal**.
4. Diet-induced thermogenesis is calculated. This accounts for ~10% of BMR. TEF = 2,636 kcal × 0.10 = **264 kcal**. Note: a higher percentage (up to 15%) may be used if one consumes a high-protein diet (>1.5 g kg^{-1} body mass^{-1}).
5. Determination of PAEE. This could be estimated or the following conversion system can be used:
   1.2–1.3: for bedridden individuals
   1.4–1.5: for sedentary occupation without daily movement
   1.5–1.6: for sedentary occupation with daily movement
   1.6–1.7: for occupation with prolonged standing
   1.9–2.1: for strenuous work and physically-active
   If 1.9 is used for our example: PAEE + RMR = 2,636 kcal × 1.9 = **5,008 kcal**.
6. 5,008 kcal + 264 kcal (TEF) = **5,272 kcal** needed per day to maintain body weight.

Estimating Energy Expenditure during Exercise

At rest, the average individual requires 0.20–0.35 L of O_2 min^{-1} or 1.0–1.8 kcal min^{-1} of energy expenditure (132). A commonly used unit is the MET (metabolic equivalent): 1 MET (resting oxygen consumption) = ~250 mL min^{-1} for men and ~200 mL min^{-1} in women (74). 1 MET = a relative Vo_2 of 3.5 mL kg^{-1} min^{-1}. A man with a Vo_{2max} of 50 mL kg^{-1} min^{-1} exercising at 70% (35 mL kg^{-1} min^{-1}) is equivalent to 10 METS. Exercise increases energy expenditure with the magnitude dependent on intensity, volume, muscle mass involvement, and rest intervals (continuity). Energy cost of sport and exercise is determined via oxygen consumption (Table 7.4). These values are based on a 70-kg man and a 55-kg woman. Larger individuals yield higher values and smaller individuals yield smaller values. Light exercise is considered <5 kcal min^{-1} in men (<4 METS) and <3.5 kcal min^{-1} in women (<2.7 METS), moderate exercise is considered 5.0–7.4 kcal min^{-1} in men (4–6 METS) and 3.5–5.4 kcal min^{-1} in women (2.8–4.3 METS), and heavy exercise is considered >7.5 kcal min^{-1} in men (>6–7 METS) and >5.5 kcal min^{-1} in women (4.5–5.5 METS) (74). Most sports exceed the metabolic classifications of heavy exercise whereas general fitness activities rank light, moderate, or heavy based on intensity. The ACSM has provided several metabolic equations that estimate energy expenditure for walking, running, stepping, and cycling and conversion factors (Table 7.5). Relative VO_2 during exercise is calculated first, converted to absolute VO_2, and converted to kcal min^{-1} by multiplying it by 5. Energy expenditure is higher after exercise cessation. More kilocalories are burned after exercise than would have been if one did not exercise. Estimations of daily energy expenditure are not adequate in factoring the postexercise effects.

OXYGEN CONSUMPTION AND ACUTE TRAINING VARIABLES

Oxygen consumption increases during exercise in proportion to intensity (Fig. 7.7). There is an exponential rise as exercise approaches steady state (within 1–4 min) termed the *fast component of VO$_2$*. Aerobically trained athletes can reach steady state in a shorter time period than untrained individuals (45). At the onset of exercise, the respiratory and cardiovascular systems do not supply enough

TABLE 7.4 ENERGY EXPENDITURE DURING EXERCISE

ACTIVITY	MEN (Kcal min^{-1})	WOMEN (Kcal min^{-1})
Baseball/softball	6.1	4.8
Basketball	8.6	6.8
Boxing (competitive)	14.7	11.6
Hitting bag	7.4	5.8
Cycling		
7.0 mph	5.0	3.9
10.0 mph	7.5	5.9
Football	11.0	8.7
Golf	5.5	4.3
Handball	11.0	8.6
High jump/long jump	7.4	5.8
Judo/jiu jitsu	12.3	9.6
Racquetball	12.3	9.6
Rope jumping	9.8–14.7	7.7–11.2
Rugby	12.3	9.6
Running		
7.5 mph	14.0	11.0
10.0 mph	18.2	14.3
Shot put and discus	4.9	3.9
Soccer	12.2	9.6
Standing	1.8	1.4
Swimming (crawl, 3.0 mph)	20.0	15.7
Tennis	7.1	5.5
Walking		
3.5 mph	5.0	3.9
5.0 mph	9.8	7.7
Weight lifting	8.2	6.4
Wrestling	13.1	10.3

Reprinted with permission from Wilmore JH, Costill DL. *Physiology of Sport and Exercise.* 2nd ed. Champaign (IL): Human Kinetics; 1999; and Ainsworth BE, Haskell WL, Whitt MC, et al. Compendium of physical activities: an update of activity codes and MET intensities. *Med Sci Sports Exerc.* 2000;32(suppl):S498–S516.

oxygen to meet the demands. It takes a few minutes for these systems to catch up, indicating anaerobic systems predominate early in providing energy. The difference between oxygen supply and demand is **oxygen deficit** and is shown in the shaded area in Figure 7.7. Oxygen deficit is larger during anaerobic (Fig. 7.7B) than aerobic exercise (Fig. 7.7A) and is smaller in aerobically trained athletes than untrained individuals and strength/power athletes

(74). Steady state occurs at the VO$_2$ plateau where oxygen supply meets demand and is where aerobic metabolism predominates. Steady state can occur at various levels of VO$_2$ depending on intensity. At higher intensities (above the lactate threshold), VO$_2$ can rise gradually to meet additional energy costs termed the *slow component of VO$_2$* and is attributed to increased core temperature, pulmonary ventilation, and the recruitment of FT muscle fibers (59).

TABLE 7.5 THE ACSM'S METABOLIC EQUATIONS

ACTIVITY	EQUATION
Walking	VO$_2$ = 3.5 + 0.1(walking speed) + 1.8(speed)(percent grade)
Running	VO$_2$ = 3.5 + 0.2(running speed) + 0.9(speed)(percent grade)
Stepping	VO$_2$ = 3.5 + 0.2(step rate) + 2.4(step rate)(step height)
Leg cycling	VO$_2$ = 7 + 1.8(work rate)/body mass
Arm cycling	VO$_2$ = 3.5 + 3(work rate)/body mass

Units: VO$_2$ (mL · min^{-1} · kg^{-1}); Speed (m · min^{-1}); Work rate (kg · m · min^{-1}); Body mass (kg); Step rate (steps per minute); Step height (m)

(Continued)

TABLE 7.5 THE ACSM'S METABOLIC EQUATIONS (*Continued*)

ACTIVITY	EQUATION

Conversion Factors for Metabolic Equations

$$\frac{(\dot{V}O_2 \text{ in } L \cdot min^{-1}) \times 1{,}000}{\text{body mass}} = \dot{V}O_2 \text{ in } mL \cdot min^{-1} \cdot kg^{-1}$$

$$\frac{(\dot{V}O_2 \text{ in } mL \cdot min^{-1} \cdot kg^{-1})(\text{body mass})}{1000} = \dot{V}O_2 \text{ in } L \cdot min$$

$$\dot{V}O_2 \text{ in METs} \times 3.5 = \dot{V}O_2 \text{ in } mL \cdot min^{-1} \cdot kg^{-1}$$

$$\frac{(\dot{V}O_2 \text{ in } mL \cdot min^{-1} \cdot kg^{-1})}{3.5} = \dot{V}O_2 \text{ in METs}$$

$$\dot{V}O_2 \text{ in } mL \cdot min^{-1} \times 5 = \text{energy exp. in kcal} \cdot min^{-1}$$

$$\frac{\text{energy exp. in kcal} \cdot min^{-1})}{5} = \dot{V}O_2 \text{ in } L \cdot min^{-1}$$

$$(\text{speed in mph}) \times 26.8 = \text{speed in } m \cdot min^{-1}$$

$$\frac{\text{speed in } m \cdot min^{-1}}{26.8} = \text{speed in mpho}$$

$$\frac{\text{speed in kph}}{0.06} = \text{speed in } m \cdot min^{-1}$$

$$(\text{speed in } m \cdot min^{-1}) \times 0.06 = \text{speed in kph}$$

$$\frac{\text{work rate in kg} \cdot m \cdot min^{-1}}{6} = \text{power in W}$$

$$(\text{power in W}) \times 6 = \text{work rate in kg} \cdot m \cdot min^{-1}$$

(*Note:* kg m min^{-1} is not technically a unit of power; also conversion with the acceleration of gravity yields a correction factor of 6.12; however, the ACSM uses 6 as a reasonable approximation for exercise prescriptions.)

$$(\text{weight in lb}) \times 2.2 = \text{mass in kg}$$

$$\frac{\text{mass in kg}}{2.2} = \text{weight in lb}$$

(*Note:* Pounds are not a unit of mass but can be converted with the factor 2.2 when the mass in question is subject to earth's gravity; for greater precision, a factor of 2.2046 can be used.)

$$(\text{height in inches}) \times 0.0254 = \text{height in m}$$

$$\frac{\text{height in m}}{0.0254} = \text{height in inches}$$

Reprinted with permission from Swain DP, Leutholtz BC. *Exercise Prescription: A Case Study Approach to the ACSM Guidelines.* 2nd ed. Champaign (IL): Human Kinetics; 2007. pp. 49-69.

Oxygen consumption remains elevated during recovery following exercise. The magnitude depends on exercise intensity and duration, and is proportional to the oxygen deficit accrued at the onset of exercise (74,89). There is little elevated VO_2 after light, short-duration exercise. However, intense aerobic and anaerobic exercise of sufficient duration results in a large rise in VO_2 after exercise. The additional oxygen consumed over baseline levels following exercise is termed **excess postexercise oxygen consumption** (EPOC), or formerly known as oxygen debt. The EPOC period consists of a rapid initial component followed by a slow component. The rapid component elicits recovery in VO_2 within the first few minutes. The slow component may persist for an hour but may take as long as 24 hours to return to homeostatic VO_2 (74) depending on exercise intensity and duration. Several factors contribute to EPOC. The cardiovascular and respiratory systems remain elevated, which results in greater VO_2 needed to resynthesize ATP and PC, oxidize lactate and resynthesize glycogen from lactate, restore oxygen to myoglobin, and increase oxygen content in the blood and other tissues. Tissue repair, elevated protein synthesis, and redistribution of minerals require energy and higher VO_2. Thermogenesis is enhanced due to lingering effects of the sympathetic nervous system and several hormones (catecholamines, thyroid hormones, glucocorticoids, growth hormone superfamily), and the acute rise in body temperature (74). The EPOC period results in greater energy expenditure and is important for body fat reductions and weight loss.

Resistance Exercise and Oxygen Consumption

Resistance exercise increases VO_2 during and after a workout. Several factors influence the response. Studies have shown:

- VO_2 is greater during large muscle-group exercises than smaller muscle-group exercises (58,99,105). A lower-body workout may elicit metabolic responses up to ~60% of Vo_{2max} (119) showing that traditional RT programs (moderate to high intensity, at least 1–2 min rest intervals) have limited effects on increasing Vo_{2max} in fit individuals.
- VO_2 varies based on lifting velocity. One study showed exercises (matched for rep number) performed with slow to moderate velocities yielded greater VO_2 than fast velocities (6). Another study showed greater energy expenditure (7.3 vs. 6.4 kcal min^{-1}) when explosive squats were performed compared to a 2-second squat (60% of 1 RM) (73).
- VO_2 is greater when exercises are performed with high (80%–90% of 1 RM) > moderate (60%–70% of 1 RM) > low (20%–50% of 1 RM) intensity (21,53,131).
- VO_2 is greater when exercises are performed for high rep number compared to low rep number, or multiple sets compared to single sets (41).

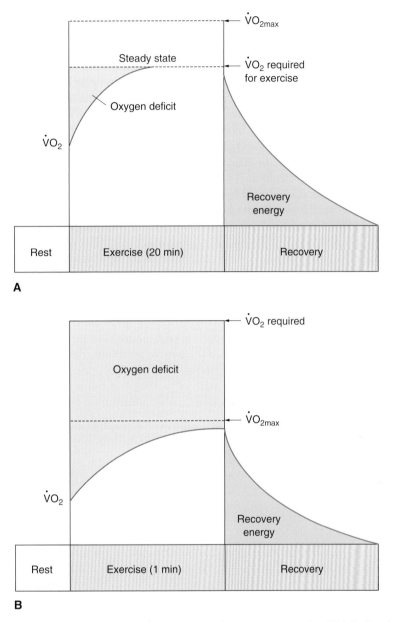

FIGURE 7.7. A,B: Oxygen consumption during exercise and excess postexercise oxygen consumption (EPOC). (Reprinted with permission from National Strength and Conditioning Association. *Essentials of Strength Training and Conditioning.* Champaign (IL): Human Kinetics; 1994. p. 77.)

- VO_2 is greater when exercises are performed with short versus long rest intervals (43,92). The lack of continuity with long rest intervals limits the metabolic response (92,93) and could pose a limitation to increasing Vo_{2max} among fit populations.
- VO_2 and energy expenditure for a workout is not affected by exercise order (34). However, VO_2 may be lower for an exercise when it was performed first versus last (34).

The culmination of these program variables affects the acute metabolic response. Workouts that consist of moderate to high intensity, moderate to high number of repetitions, large muscle mass exercises, with short rest intervals greatly increase VO_2. Circuit weight training

(performing exercises continuously from station to station with minimal rest in between) increases acute VO_2 and Vo_{2max}. A similar effect is seen with endurance training programs consisting of high reps, low weight, and short rest intervals. Strength and power workouts elicit small VO_2 increases due primarily to long rest intervals and low reps. High metabolic demand is important for body fat reductions and muscle endurance enhancement.

Resistance exercise elicits substantial EPOC in men and women (10,12,14,78,92) and the magnitude may be greater than that of aerobic exercise (17). Circuit weight training elicits a greater EPOC than AT in women (14). The magnitude for either modality depends on the degree of disturbance to homeostasis. Greater thermogenesis, hormonal response, glycogen depletion, lactate elevations and reductions in pH, and cardiorespiratory demand yields substantial EPOC. EPOC following resistance exercise is biphasic (with a rapid component <1 h and a slow component) and may last up to 48 hours (10,12,107) especially as protein synthesis increases and muscle damage is present. Resting energy expenditure is greater 72 hours after a workout that produces muscle damage (40). Resistance exercise has the advantage of increasing energy expenditure throughout the day following a workout. Binzen et al. (10) showed an 18.6% increase in EPOC and greater fat oxidation over 2 hours after exercise in women. However, the overall net kilocalorie expenditure may be low despite the elevation in EPOC (78).

BODY FAT REDUCTIONS

Reducing body fat involves proper diet and exercise. Energy expenditure must exceed energy intake so a net kilocalorie deficit is seen. Dietary recommendations include consuming a well-balanced diet from major food groups and high water intake (at least eight glasses per day). Individuals should consume ~55%–60% of kilocalories from CHOs (preferably complex CHOs), at least 15% of kilocalories from protein, and <25% of kilocalories from fats (mostly unsaturated fats). Increasing BMR is important, *i.e.*, eating smaller meals more frequently throughout the day, maintaining a higher protein intake than the RDA values, early morning workouts, and avoiding simple sugars. Aerobic exercise is highly recommended for its role in increasing fat oxidation during exercise and EPOC. Diet appears to be the key factor with aerobic exercise complimentary. RT is beneficial as the higher LBM increases BMR and energy expenditure throughout the day. Similar to AT, RT increases energy expenditure and yields substantial EPOC. The combination of AT and RT augments each other in comprehensively reducing body fat. Total body workouts of moderate to high volume (multiple sets per exercise of at least 10–12 reps), moderate to high intensity, and short rest intervals have profound effects on reducing body fat. Scientific body fat loss (not through crash dieting) is a relatively slow process but one that has a more profound effect on permanent fat loss.

Interpreting Research

Oxygen Consumption and Rest Interval Manipulation

Ratamess NA, Falvo MJ, Mangine GT, et al. The effect of rest interval length on metabolic responses to the bench press exercise. *Eur J Appl Physiol*. 2007;100:1–17.

Ratamess et al. (92) studied the metabolic responses to rest interval manipulation during 5 sets of the bench press using either 10 RM or 5 RM loads with 30-second, 1-minute, 2-minute, 3-minute, or 5-minute rest intervals. Rep number was maintained in each set while weight was reduced when necessary. They found a continuum of effects such that highest VO_2 values were seen with 30-second rest intervals and lowest VO_2 values were seen with 5-minute rest intervals. The acute response pattern was similar between 5 RM and 10 RM loading protocols; however, the VO_2 response was higher in 10 RM than 5 RM for most rest intervals demonstrating a volume/intensity effect. EPOC elevations were shown for all protocols. However, the 30-second and 1-minute protocols elicited greater EPOC during 5 RM protocols but had no substantial effect during 10 RM protocols. The highest relative VO_2 obtained was ~16 mL kg^{-1} min^{-1} (30 s) and the lowest was ~8 mL kg^{-1} min^{-1} (5 min), both of which were below the threshold needed to increase Vo_{2max}. Energy expenditure for 30-second protocols was ~6.8–7.3 kcal min^{-1} whereas 5-minute protocols elicited values of 4.9–5.3 kcal min^{-1}. Figure 7.8 depicts the 30-second and 5-minute VO_2 responses. VO_2 was lower during each set (due to the anaerobic nature of lifting and possible Valsalva maneuvers) but increased during the first 30-seconds to 1-minute of recovery and then rapidly decreased (5-min protocol). The 30-second protocol led to the most pronounced and continuous response, but large levels of recovery were seen with 5-minute rest intervals. A quantitative effect was shown where VO_2 increased from set to set peaking by the fourth set. Figure 7.9 shows that VO_2 area under the curve was highest with short rest (30 s and 1 min) and lowest with 5-minute rest intervals.

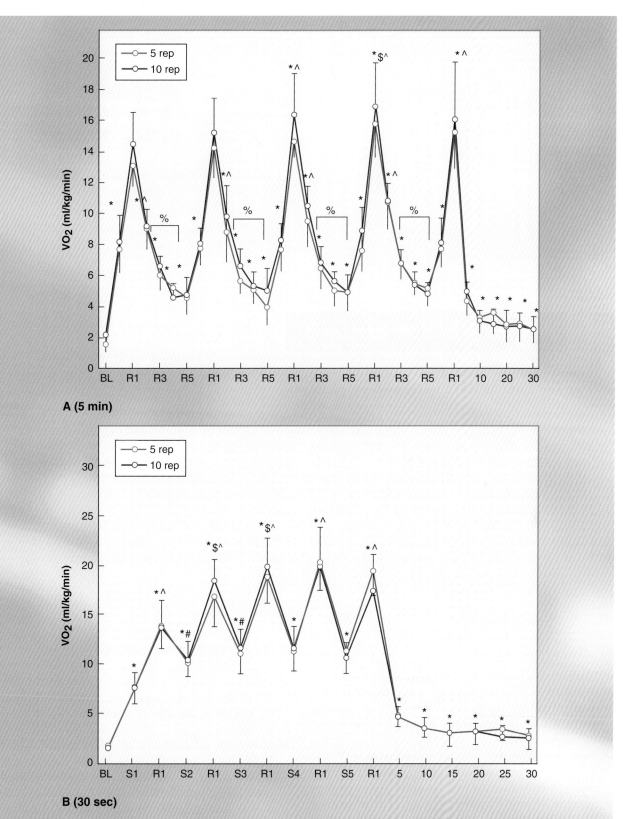

FIGURE 7.8. Metabolic responses to resistance exercise: 30 seconds vs. 5 minutes. BL, baseline; S1, set 1, R1, rest interval 1 minute, and so on. (Reprinted with permission from Ratamess NA, Falvo MJ, Mangine GT, Hoffman JR, Faigenbaum AD, Kang J. The effect of rest interval length on metabolic responses to the bench press exercise. *Eur J Appl Physiol*. 2007;100:1–17.)

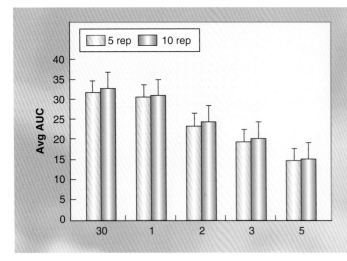

FIGURE 7.9. Total oxygen consumption area under the curve using various rest intervals. (Reprinted with permission from Ratamess NA, Falvo MJ, Mangine GT, Hoffman JR, Faigenbaum AD, Kang J. The effect of rest interval length on metabolic responses to the bench press exercise. *Eur J Appl Physiol.* 2007;100:1–17.)

Myths & Misconceptions

Low-Intensity, Moderate-Duration Exercise is the Single Best Way to Burn Body Fat and Lose Weight Independent of Diet

Some experts have exclusively recommended low-intensity, moderate-duration exercise (30–60 min of leisure walking) as the best way to burn body fat. Fat is the preferred fuel for energy at rest and during low-intensity exercise when oxygen supply meets demand. However, fat is an energy-dense macronutrient. An 18-C fat molecule can generate a total of 460 ATP, >12 times that of glucose. Although fat oxidation prevails during low-intensity exercise, a molecule of fat goes a long way, so very little will be oxidized and low-intensity exercise is not a potent stimulus to increase aerobic capacity. The critical element to fat loss is to increase Vo_{2max}. Fat burning becomes more efficient when Vo_{2max} improves. Prescription including high-intensity training (>60%–70% of Vo_{2max}) in addition to long, slow-duration AT workouts is the best way to lose body fat. Increasing Vo_{2max} is important in building a base by which fat burning becomes easier. So yes, long, slow-duration cardio workouts are beneficial; however, they are more effective when Vo_{2max} is improved with moderate to high intensity AT.

Summary Points

✔ Bioenergetics is the flow of energy change within the human body. The high-energy compound that provides substantial energy for all of the cell's needs from hydrolysis of chemical bonds is known as adenosine triphosphate (ATP).

✔ Three major energy systems resynthesize ATP, the ATP-PC, glycolysis, and oxidative systems. ATP-PC system fuels high-intensity exercise up to ~10 seconds in duration. Glycolysis fuels moderate-to-high-intensity exercise lasting up to a few minutes. The oxidative system resynthesizes ATP aerobically when oxygen supply meets demand.

✔ Anaerobic and AT elicit specific metabolic adaptations that enhance performance via greater substrate storage, altered enzyme activity, or breakdown rates during exercise.

✔ Metabolic acidosis occurs during exercise that stresses glycolysis. Specific training can increase buffer capacity and allow the athlete to tolerate greater levels of acidity.

✔ BMR is the minimal level of energy needed to sustain bodily functions. Control of BMR is critical to body fat reductions and weight control. BMR is affected by body mass, exercise, environment, dietary-induced thermogenesis, and hormonal control.

✔ VO₂ and energy expenditure increase during exercise (and for up to 48–72 h after exercise) with the response in proportion to muscle mass involvement, intensity, volume/duration, and rest interval length.

Review Questions

1. The majority of energy liberation during a 1 RM set of the deadlift exercise will come from
   a. ATP-PC system (phosphagens)
   b. Fast glycolysis
   c. Slow glycolysis
   d. Aerobic system

2. The elevation of oxygen consumption during recovery from exercise is known as
   a. Excess post-exercise oxygen consumption (EPOC)
   b. Oxygen deficit
   c. Vo_{2max}
   d. Oxygen requirement

3. An enzyme that catalyzes the reaction that breaks down glycogen to glucose-6-phosphate is
   a. Hexokinase
   b. Phosphorylase
   c. PFK
   d. Pyruvate kinase

4. Capillary and mitochondrial density typically _____ after traditional RT resulting in substantial muscle hypertrophy
   a. Increase
   b. Decrease
   c. Do not change
   d. None of the above

5. Which of the following does not act as a skeletal muscle/blood buffer?
   a. Creatine phosphate
   b. Bicarbonate
   c. Triglycerides
   d. Carnosine

6. CHO consumption during and immediately following resistance exercise is critical to
   a. Delaying fatigue
   b. Maximizing glycogen repletion during recovery
   c. Sparing muscle glycogen breakdown
   d. All of the above

7. Approximately 65% of PC is replenished within 90 seconds of recovery from exercise.   T F

8. Creatine supplementation has been shown to increase muscle size, strength, and power in several studies.   T F

9. Both aerobic and RT decrease resting glycogen stores over time.   T F

10. The blood lactate response curve to exercise shifts to the right with training at or beyond the lactate threshold.   T F

11. Aerobic and resistance exercises increase energy expenditure acutely but have very limited effects on postexercise metabolism.   T F

12. During resistance exercise, small muscle mass exercises increase oxygen consumption to a greater extent than large muscle mass exercises.   T F

References

1. Abernethy PJ, Thayer R, Taylor AW. Acute and chronic responses of skeletal muscle to endurance and sprint exercise. A review. *Sports Med.* 1990;10:365–389.
2. Ainsworth BE, Haskell WL, Whitt MC, et al. Compendium of physical activities: an update of activity codes and MET intensities. *Med Sci Sports Exerc.* 2000;32(suppl):S498–S516.
3. American College of Sports Medicine, American Dietetic Association, & Dieticians of Canada. Joint Position Stand. Nutrition and athletic performance. *Med Sci Sports Exerc.* 2009;41:709–731.
4. Andrews JL, Sedlock DA, Flynn MG, et al. Carbohydrate loading and supplementation in endurance-trained women runners. *J Appl Physiol.* 2003;95:584–590.
5. Argyropolous G, Harper ME. Uncoupling proteins and thermoregulation. *J Appl Physiol.* 2002;92:2187–2198.
6. Ballor DL, Becque MD, Katch VL. Metabolic responses during hydraulic resistance exercise. *Med Sci Sports Exerc.* 1987;19:363–367.
7. Bell DG, Jacobs I. Muscle fiber-specific glycogen utilization in strength-trained males and females. *Med Sci Sports Exerc.* 1989;21:649–654.
8. Bell DG, Jacobs I. Muscle fibre area, fibre type & capillarization in male and female body builders. *Can J Sport Sci.* 1990;15:115–119.
9. Bell GJ, Wenger HA. The effect of one-legged sprint training on intramuscular pH and nonbicarbonate buffering capacity. *Eur J Appl Physiol.* 1988;58:158–164.
10. Binzen CA, Swan PD, Manore MM. Postexercise oxygen consumption and substrate use after resistance exercise in women. *Med Sci Sports Exerc.* 2001;33:932–938.

11. Bonen A. The expression of lactate transporters (MCT1 and MCT4) in heart and muscle. *Eur J Appl Physiol.* 2001;86:6–11.

12. Borsheim E, Bahr R. Effect of exercise intensity, duration and mode on post-exercise oxygen consumption. *Sports Med.* 2003;33:1037–1060.

13. Brandenburg J, Docherty D. The effect of training volume on the acute response and adaptations to resistance training. *Int J Sports Physiol Perform.* 2006;1:108–121.

14. Braun WA, Hawthorne WE, Markofski MM. Acute EPOC response in women to circuit training and treadmill exercise of matched oxygen consumption. *Eur J Appl Physiol.* 2005;94:500–504.

15. Bryner RW, Ullrich IH, Sauers J, et al. Effects of resistance vs. aerobic training combined with an 800 calorie liquid diet on lean body mass and resting metabolic rate. *J Am Coll Nutr.* 1999;18:115–121.

16. Burgomaster KA, Moore DR, Schofield LM, Phillips SM, Sale DG, Gibala MJ. Resistance training with vascular occlusion: metabolic adaptations in human muscle. *Med Sci Sports Exerc.* 2003;35:1203–1208.

17. Burleson MA, O'Bryant HS, Stone MH, Collins MA, Triplett-McBride T. Effect of weight training exercise and treadmill exercise on post-exercise oxygen consumption. *Med Sci Sports Exerc.* 1998;30:518–522.

18. Cadefau J, Casademont J, Grau JM, et al. Biochemical and histochemical adaptation to sprint training in young athletes. *Acta Physiol Scand.* 1990;140:341–351.

19. Chesley A, Heigenhauser GJ, Spriet LL. Regulation of muscle glycogen phosphorylase activity following short-term endurance training. *Am J Physiol.* 1996;270:E328–E335.

20. Churchley EG, Coffey VG, Pedersen DJ, et al. Influence of preexercise muscle glycogen content on transcriptional activity of metabolic and myogenic genes in well-trained humans. *J Appl Physiol.* 2007;102:1604–1611.

21. Collins MA, Cureton KJ, Hill DW, Ray CA. Relation of plasma volume change to intensity of weight lifting. *Med Sci Sports Exerc.* 1989;21:178–185.

22. Costill DL, Coyle EF, Fink WF, Lesmes GR, Witzmann FA. Adaptations in skeletal muscle following strength training. *J Appl Physiol.* 1979;46:96–99.

23. Costill DL, Barnett A, Sharp R, Fink WJ, Katz A. Leg muscle pH following sprint running. *Med Sci Sports Exerc.* 1983;15:325–329.

24. Cramer JT. Bioenergetics of exercise and training. In: Baechle TR, Earle RW, editors. *Essentials of Strength Training and Conditioning.* 3rd ed. Champaign (IL): Human Kinetics; 2008. pp. 21–39.

25. Cunningham JJ. Body composition and resting metabolic rate: the myth of feminine metabolism. *Am J Clin Nutr.* 1982;36:721–726.

26. Davey CL. The significance of carnosine and anserine in striated skeletal muscle. *Arch Bioch Biophys.* 1960;89:303–308.

27. Dawson B, Fitzsimons M, Green S, Goodman C, Carey M, Cole K. Changes in performance, muscle metabolites, enzymes and fibre types after short sprint training. *Eur J Appl Physiol Occup Physiol.* 1998;78:163–169.

28. De Lorenzo A, Bertini I, Candelaro N, et al. A new predictive equation to calculate resting metabolic rate in athletes. *J Sports Med Phys Fitness.* 1999;39:213–219.

29. Derave W, Ozdemir MS, Harris RC, et al. Beta-alanine supplementation augments muscle carnosine content and attenuates fatigue during repeated isokinetic contraction bouts in trained sprinters. *J Appl Physiol.* 2007;103:1736–1743.

30. Dudley GA. Metabolic consequences of resistive-type exercise. *Med Sci Sports Exerc.* 1988;20(suppl):S158–S161.

31. Edge J, Hill-Haas S, Goodman C, Bishop D. Effects of resistance training on H+ regulation, buffer capacity, and repeated sprints. *Med Sci Sports Exerc.* 2006;38:2004–2011.

32. Enoki T, Yoshida Y, Lally J, Hatta H, Bonen A. Testosterone increases lactate transport, monocarboxylate transporter (MCT) 1 and MCT4 in rat skeletal muscle. *J Physiol.* 2006;577:433–443.

33. Essen-Gustavsson B, Tesch PA. Glycogen and triglyceride utilization in relation to muscle metabolic characteristics in men performing heavy-resistance exercise. *Eur J Appl Physiol.* 1990;61:5–10.

34. Farinatti PT, Simao R, Monteiro WD, Fleck SJ. Influence of exercise order on oxygen uptake during strength training in young women. *J Strength Cond Res.* 2009;23:1037–1044.

35. Favero TG, Zable AC, Colter D, Abramson JJ. Lactate inhibits Ca^{2+}-activated Ca(2+)-channel activity from skeletal muscle sarcoplasmic reticulum. *J Appl Physiol.* 1997;82:447–452.

36. Geleibter A, Maher MM, Gerace L, et al. Effects of strength or aerobic training on body composition, resting metabolic rate, and peak oxygen consumption in obese dieting subjects. *Am J Clin Nutr.* 1997;66:557–563.

37. Goforth HW, Arnall DA, Bennett BL, Law PG. Persistence of supercompensated muscle glycogen in trained subjects after carbohydrate loading. *J Appl Physiol.* 1997;82:342–347.

38. Gordon SE, Kraemer WJ, Pedro JG. Increased acid-base buffering capacity via dietary supplementation: anaerobic exercise implications. *J Appl Nutr.* 1991;43:40–48.

39. Green H, Dahly A, Shoemaker K, Goreham C, Bombardier E, Ball-Burnett M. Serial effects of high-resistance and prolonged endurance training on Na$^+$-K$^+$ pump concentration and enzymatic activities in human vastus lateralis. *Acta Physiol Scand.* 1999;165:177–184.

40. Hackney KJ, Engels HJ, Gretebeck RJ. Resting energy expenditure and delayed-onset muscle soreness after full-body resistance training with an eccentric concentration. *J Strength Cond Res.* 2008;22:1602–1609.

41. Haddock BL, Wilkin LD. Resistance training volume and post exercise energy expenditure. *Int J Sports Med.* 2006;27:143–148.

42. Haff GG, Stone MH, Warren BJ, et al. The effect of carbohydrate supplementation on multiple sessions and bouts of resistance exercise. *J Strength Cond Res.* 1999;13:111–117.

43. Haltom RW, Kraemer RR, Sloan RA, et al. Circuit weight training and its effects on excess postexercise oxygen consumption. *Med Sci Sports Exerc.* 1999;31:1613–1618.

44. Hargreaves M. The metabolic systems: carbohydrate metabolism. In: *ACSM's Advanced Exercise Physiology.* Philadelphia (PA): Lippincott Williams & Wilkins; 2006. pp. 385–395.

45. Harris C, Adams KJ. Exercise physiology. In: *ACSM's Resource Manual for Guidelines for Exercise Testing and Prescription.* 6th ed. Philadelphia, PA: Lippincott Williams & Wilkins; 2010. pp. 45–77.

46. Harris JA, Benedict FG. *A Biometric Study of Basal Metabolism in Man.* Publication number 279. Washington, DC: Carnegie Institution; 1919. pp. 1–266.

47. Hirvonen J, Rehunen S, Rusko H, Harkonen M. Breakdown of high-energy phosphate compounds and lactate accumulation during short supramaximal exercise. *Eur J Appl Physiol.* 1987;56:253–259.

48. Hirvonen J, Nummela A, Rusko H, Rehunen S, Harkonen M. Fatigue and changes of ATP, creatine phosphate, and lactate during the 400-m sprint. *Can J Sport Sci.* 1992;17:141–144.

49. Hoffman JR, Ratamess NA, Faigenbaum AD, et al. Short-duration beta-alanine supplementation increases training volume and reduces subjective feelings of fatigue in college football players. *Nutr Res.* 2008;28:31–35.

50. Hoffman JR, Ratamess NA, Ross R, et al. Beta-alanine and the hormonal response to exercise. *Int J Sports Med.* 2008;29:952–958.

51. Holloszy JO, Kohrt WM, Hansen PA. The regulation of carbohydrate and fat metabolism during and after exercise. *Front Biosci.* 1998;3:D1011–D1027.

52. Hostler D, Schwirian CI, Campos G, et al. Skeletal muscle adaptations in elastic resistance-trained young men and women. *Eur J Appl Physiol.* 2001;86:112–118.

53. Hunter GR, Seelhorst D, Snyder S. Comparison of metabolic and heart rate responses to super slow vs. traditional resistance training. *J Strength Cond Res.* 2003;17:76–81.

54. Jacobs I, Esbjornsson M, Sylven C, Holm I, Jansson E. Sprint training effects on muscle myoglobin, enzymes, fiber types, and blood lactate. *Med Sci Sports Exerc*. 1987;19:368–374.

55. Johansen L, Quistorff B. 31P-MRS characterization of sprint and endurance trained athletes. *Int J Sports Med*. 2003;24:183–189.

56. Juel C. Current aspects of lactate exchange: lactate/H⁺ transport in human skeletal muscle. *Eur J Appl Physiol*. 2001;86:12–16.

57. Kadi F, Eriksson A, Holmner S, Butler-Browne GS, Thornell LE. Cellular adaptation of the trapezius muscle in strength-trained athletes. *Histochem Cell Biol*. 1999;111:189–195.

58. Kalb JS, Hunter GR. Weight training economy as a function of intensity of the squat and overhead press exercise. *J Sports Med Phys Fitness* 1991;31:154–160.

59. Kang J. *Bioenergetics Primer for Exercise Science*. Champaign (IL): Human Kinetics; 2008. pp. 3–104.

60. Kang J, Hoffman JR, Im J, et al. Evaluation of physiological responses during recovery following three resistance exercise programs. *J Strength Cond Res*. 2005;19:305–309.

61. Kendrick IP, Harris RC, Kim HJ, et al. The effects of 10 weeks of resistance training combined with beta-alanine supplementation on whole body strength, force production, muscular endurance and body composition. *Amino Acids*. 2008;34:547–554.

62. Komi PV, Viitasalo JT, Rauramaa R, Vihko V. Effect of isometric strength training on mechanical, electrical, and metabolic aspects of muscle function. *Eur J Appl Physiol*. 1978;40:45–55.

63. Kraemer WJ, Noble BJ, Clark MJ, Culver BW. Physiologic responses to heavy-resistance exercise with very short rest periods. *Int J Sports Med*. 1987;8:247–252.

64. Laursen PB, Jenkins DG. The scientific basis for high-intensity interval training: optimizing training programmes and maximizing performance in highly trained endurance athletes. *Sports Med*. 2002;32:53–73.

65. LeBlanc PJ, Howarth KR, Gibala MJ, Heigenhauser GJ. Effects of 7 wk of endurance training on human skeletal muscle metabolism during submaximal exercise. *J Appl Physiol*. 2004;97:2148–2153.

66. Lemmer JT, Ivey FM, Ryan AS, et al. Effect of strength training on resting metabolic rate and physical activity: age and gender comparisons. *Med Sci Sports Exerc*. 2001;33:532–541.

67. Luthi JM, Howald H, Claassen H, Rosler K, Vock P, Hoppeler H. Structural changes in skeletal muscle tissue with heavy-resistance exercise. *Int J Sports Med*. 1986;7:123–127.

68. MacDougall JD, Ward GR, Sale DG, Sutton JR. Biochemical adaptation of human skeletal muscle to heavy resistance training and immobilization. *J Appl Physiol*. 1977;43:700–703.

69. MacDougall JD, Sale DG, Moroz JR, Elder GCB, Sutton JR, Howald H. Mitochondrial volume density in human skeletal muscle following heavy resistance training. *Med Sci Sports*. 1979;11:164–166.

70. MacDougall JD. Adaptability of muscle to strength training—a cellular approach. In: *Biochemistry of Exercise VI*. Champaign (IL): Human Kinetics; 1986. pp. 501–513.

71. Marcinik EJ, Potts J, Schlabach G, Will S, Dawson P, Hurley BF. Effects of strength training on lactate threshold and endurance performance. *Med Sci Sports Exerc*. 1991;23:739–743.

72. Masuda K, Choi JY, Shimojo H, Katsuta S. Maintenance of myoglobin concentration in human skeletal muscle after heavy resistance training. *Eur J Appl Physiol*. 1999;79:347–352.

73. Mazzetti S, Douglass M, Yocum A, Harber M. Effect of explosive versus slow contractions and exercise intensity on energy expenditure. *Med Sci Sports Exerc*. 2007;39:1291–1301.

74. McArdle WD, Katch FI, Katch VL. *Exercise Physiology: Energy, Nutrition, and Human Performance*. 6th ed. Philadelphia (PA): Lippincott Williams & Wilkins; 2007. pp. 123–228.

75. McCall GE, Byrnes WC, Dickinson A, Pattany PM, Fleck SJ. Muscle fiber hypertrophy, hyperplasia, and capillary density in college men after resistance training. *J Appl Physiol*. 1996;81:2004–2012.

76. McMahon S, Jenkins D. Factors affecting the rate of phosphocreatine resynthesis following intense exercise. *Sports Med*. 2002;32:761–784.

77. Medbo JI, Sejersted OM. Acid-base and electrolyte balance after exhausting exercise in endurance-trained and sprint-trained subjects. *Acta Physiol Scand*. 1985;125:97–109.

78. Melby CL, Tincknell T, Schmidt WD. Energy expenditure following a bout of non-steady state resistance exercise. *J Sports Med Phys Fitness*. 1992;32:128–135.

79. Mifflin MD, St. Jeor ST, Hill LA, Scott BJ, Daugherty SA, Koh YO. A new predictive equation for resting energy expenditure in healthy individuals. *Am J Clin Nutr*. 1990;51:241–247.

80. Nevill ME, Boobis LH, Brooks S, Williams C. Effect of training on muscle metabolism during treadmill sprinting. *J Appl Physiol*. 1989;67:2376–2382.

81. Ojasto T, Häkkinen K. Effects of different accentuated eccentric loads on acute neuromuscular, growth hormone, and blood lactate responses during a hypertrophic protocol. *J Strength Cond Res*. 2009;23:946–953.

82. Paddon-Jones D, Westman E, Mattes RD, et al. Protein, weight management, and satiety. *Am J Clin Nutr*. 2008;87(suppl):1558S–1561S.

83. Parkhouse WS, McKenzie DC, Hochachka PW, et al. The relationship between carnosine levels, buffering capacity, fiber types and anaerobic capacity in elite athletes. In: Knuttgen H, Vogel J, Poortmans J, editors. *Biochemistry of Exercise*. Champaign (IL): Human Kinetics; 1983. pp. 275–278.

84. Parkhouse WS, McKenzie DC. Possible contribution of skeletal muscle buffers to enhanced anaerobic performance: a brief review. *Med Sci Sports Exerc*. 1984;16:328–338.

85. Pascoe DD, Costill DL, Fink WJ, Robergs RA, Zachwieja JJ. Glycogen resynthesis in skeletal muscle following resistive exercise. *Med Sci Sports Exerc*. 1993;25:349–354.

86. Paul DR, Mulroy SM, Horner JA, et al. Carbohydrate-loading during the follicular phase of the menstrual cycle: effects on muscle glycogen and exercise performance. *Int J Sport Nutr Exerc Metab*. 2001;11:430–441.

87. Perry CG, Heigenhauser GJ, Bonen A, Spriet LL. High-intensity aerobic interval training increases fat and carbohydrate metabolic capacities in human skeletal muscle. *Appl Physiol Nutr Metab*. 2008;33:1112–1123.

88. Posterino GS, Dutka TL, Lamb GD. L(+)-lactate does not affect twitch and tetanic responses in mechanically skinned mammalian muscle fibres. *Pflugers Arch*. 2001;442:197–203.

89. Quinn TJ, Vroman NB, Kertzer R. Postexercise oxygen consumption in trained females: effect of exercise duration. *Med Sci Sports Exerc*. 1994;26:908–913.

90. Ratamess NA. *Coaches Guide to Performance-Enhancing Supplements*. Monterey (CA): Coaches Choice Books; 2006.

91. Ratamess NA, Kraemer WJ, Volek JS, et al. Androgen receptor content following heavy resistance exercise in men. *J Steroid Biochem Mol Biol*. 2005;93:35–42.

92. Ratamess NA, Falvo MJ, Mangine GT, Hoffman JR, Faigenbaum AD, Kang J. The effect of rest interval length on metabolic responses to the bench press exercise. *Eur J Appl Physiol*. 2007;100:1–17.

93. Ratamess NA. Adaptations to anaerobic training programs. In: Baechle TR, Earle RW, editors. *Essentials of Strength Training and Conditioning*. 3rd ed. Champaign (IL): Human Kinetics; 2008. pp. 93–119.

94. Rauch LH, Rodger I, Wilson GR, et al. The effects of carbohydrate loading on muscle glycogen content and cycling performance. *Int J Sport Nutr*. 1995;5:25–36.

95. Rehunen S, Naveri H, Kuoppasalmi K, Harkonen M. High-energy phosphate compounds during exercise in human slow-twitch and fast-twitch muscle fibres. *Scand J Clin Lab Invest*. 1982;42:499–506.

96. Reynolds TH, Frye PA, Sforzo GA. Resistance training and the blood lactate response to resistance exercise in women. *J Strength Cond Res.* 1997;11:77–81.

97. Robergs RA, Pearson DR, Costill DL, et al. Muscle glycogenolysis during different intensities of weight-resistance exercise. *J Appl Physiol.* 1991;70:1700–1706.

98. Robergs RA, Ghiasvand F, Parker D. Biochemistry of exercise-induced metabolic acidosis. *Am J Physiol Regul Integr Comp Physiol.* 2004;287:R502–R516.

99. Robergs RA, Gordon T, Reynolds J, Walker TB. Energy expenditure during bench press and squat exercises. *J Strength Cond Res.* 2007;21:123–130.

100. Roberts AD, Billeter R, Howald H. Anaerobic muscle enzyme changes after interval training. *Int J Sports Med.* 1982;3:18–21.

101. Ross A, Leveritt M. Long-term metabolic and skeletal muscle adaptations to short-sprint training: implications for sprint training and tapering. *Sports Med.* 2001;31:1063–1082.

102. Sahlin K, Harris RC, Hultman E. Creatine kinase equilibrium and lactate content compared with muscle pH in tissue samples obtained after isometric exercise. *Biochem J.* 1972;152:173–180.

103. Sahlin K. Intracellular pH and energy metabolism in skeletal muscle of man. *Acta Physiol Scand.* 1978;(suppl): 455.

104. Sahlin K, Henriksson J. Buffer capacity and lactate accumulation in skeletal muscle of trained and untrained men. *Acta Physiol Scand.* 1984;122:331–339.

105. Scala D, McMillan J, Blessing D, Rozenek R, Stone M. Metabolic cost of a preparatory phase of training in weight lifting: a practical observation. *J Appl Sports Sci Res.* 1987;1:48–52.

106. Schantz PG, Kallman M. NADH shuttle enzymes and cytochrome b5 reductase in human skeletal muscle: effect of strength training. *J Appl Physiol.* 1989;67:123–127.

107. Schuenke MD, Mikat RP, McBride JM. Effect of an acute period of resistance exercise on excess post-exercise oxygen consumption: implications for body mass management. *Eur J Appl Physiol.* 2002;86:411–417.

108. Sharp RL, Costill DL, Fink WJ, King DS. Effects of eight weeks of bicycle ergometer sprint training on human muscle buffer capacity. *Int J Sports Med.* 1986;7:13–17.

109. Spencer M, Bishop D, Dawson B, Goodman C. Physiological and metabolic responses of repeated-sprint activities: specific to field-based team sports. *Sports Med.* 2005;35:1025–1044.

110. Staron RS, Malicky ES, Leonardi MJ, Falkel JE, Hagerman FC, Dudley GA. Muscle hypertrophy and fast fiber type conversions in heavy resistance-trained women. *Eur J Appl Physiol.* 1989;60:71–79.

111. Stone MH, Stone M, Sands WA. *Principles and Practice of Resistance Training.* Champaign (IL): Human Kinetics; 2007. pp. 63–86.

112. Swain DP, Leutholtz BC. *Exercise Prescription: A Case Study Approach to the ACSM Guidelines.* 2nd ed. Champaign (IL): Human Kinetics; 2007. pp. 49–69.

113. Tang JE, Hartman JW, Phillips SM. Increased muscle oxidative potential following resistance training induced fibre hypertrophy in young men. *Appl Physiol Nutr Metab.* 2006;31:495–501.

114. Tesch PA, Colliander EB, Kaiser P. Muscle metabolism during intense, heavy-resistance exercise. *Eur J Appl Physiol.* 1986; 55:362–366.

115. Tesch PA, Komi PV, Häkkinen K. Enzymatic adaptations consequent to long-term strength training. *Int J Sports Med.* 1987; 8(suppl):66–69.

116. Tesch PA, Thorsson A, Essen-Gustavsson B. Enzyme activities of FT and ST muscle fibers in heavy-resistance trained athletes. *J Appl Physiol.* 1989;67:83–87.

117. Tesch PA, Thorsson A, Fujitsuka N. Creatine phosphate in fiber types of skeletal muscle before and after exhaustive exercise. *J Appl Physiol.* 1989;66:1756–1759.

118. Tesch PA, Thorsson A, Colliander EB. Effects of eccentric and concentric resistance training on skeletal muscle substrates, enzyme activities and capillary supply. *Acta Physiol Scand.* 1990; 140:575–580.

119. Tesch PA. Short- and long-term histochemical and biochemical adaptations in muscle. In *Strength and Power in Sport.* Boston (MA): Blackwell Scientific Publications; 1992. pp. 239–248.

120. Thibault MC, Simoneau JA, Cote C, et al. Inheritance of human muscle enzyme adaptation to isokinetic strength training. *Hum Hered.* 1986;36:341–347.

121. Thompson J, Manore MM. Predicted and measured resting metabolic rate of male and female endurance athletes. *J Am Diet Assoc.* 1996;96:30–34.

122. Thorstensson A, Hulten B, von Dolben W, Karlsson J. Effect of strength training on enzyme activities and fibre characteristics in human skeletal muscles. *Acta Physiol Scand.* 1976;96:392–398.

123. Thorstensson A, Sjodin B, Tesch P, Karlsson J. Actomyosin ATPase, myokinase, CPK and LDH in human fast and slow twitch muscle fibres. *Acta Physiol Scand.* 1977;99:225–229.

124. Tomlin DL, Wenger HA. The relationship between aerobic fitness and recovery from high intensity intermittent exercise. *Sports Med.* 2001;31:1–11.

125. Volek JS, Boetes M, Bush JA, Putukian M, Sebastianelli WJ, Kraemer WJ. Response of testosterone and cortisol concentrations to high-intensity resistance exercise following creatine supplementation. *J Strength Cond Res.* 1997;11:182–187.

126. Vukovich MD, Sharp RL, Kesl LD, Schaulis DL, King DS. Effects of a low-dose amino acid supplement on adaptations to cycling training in untrained individuals. *Int J Sports Nutr.* 1997;7: 298–309.

127. Walker PM, Brunotte F, Rouhier-Marcer I, et al. Nuclear magnetic resonance evidence of different muscular adaptations after resistance training. *Arch Phys Med Rehabil.* 1998;79:1391–1398.

128. Wang N, Hikida RS, Staron RS, Simoneau JA. Muscle fiber types of women after resistance training—quantitative ultrastructure and enzyme activity. *Pflugers Arch.* 1993;424:494–502.

129. Williams MH. *The Ergogenics Edge.* Champaign (IL): Human Kinetics; 1998.

130. Williams MH, Kreider RB, Branch JD. *Creatine: The Power Supplement.* Champaign (IL): Human Kinetics; 1999.

131. Willoughby DS, Chilek DR, Schiller DA, Coast JR. The metabolic effects of three different free weight parallel squatting intensities. *J Hum Move Studies.* 1991;21:53–67.

132. Wilmore JH, Costill DL. *Physiology of Sport and Exercise.* 2nd ed. Champaign (IL): Human Kinetics; 1999.

133. Yarrow JF, Borsa PA, Borst SE, Sitren HS, Stevens BR, White LJ. Neuroendocrine responses to an acute bout of eccentric-enhanced resistance exercise. *Med Sci Sports Exerc.* 2007;39:941–947.

134. Yeo WK, Paton CD, Garnham AP, Burke LM, Carey AL, Hawley JA. Skeletal muscle adaptation and performance responses to once a day versus twice every second day endurance training regimens. *J Appl Physiol.* 2008;105:1462–1470.

Responses and Adaptations of the Cardiorespiratory System

After completing this chapter, you will be able to:
- Discuss the chambers of the heart and blood flow during cardiac muscle contraction
- Discuss intrinsic and extrinsic regulation of the heart
- Discuss oxygen transport, consumption, and blood flow at rest and during exercise
- Discuss the cardiovascular response to exercise
- Discuss cardiovascular responses at rest and during exercise following training
- Discuss the respiratory system and adaptations to training

The cardiovascular (CV) system consists of three major components: the heart ("pump"), the blood vessels ("transport portals"), and the blood ("fluid medium"). All other systems depend on the CV system, including the lungs, which are essential for blood oxygenation and removal of CO_2, which occurs during **respiration**. The CV system performs a number of critical functions to life including delivery of nutrients, oxygen, and hormones to all tissues; removal of waste products and CO_2; temperature control; pH control; immunity; and hydration. The length of blood vessels within an average-sized man would extend more than 100,000 miles if stretched from end to end (53). This chapter discusses the basic anatomy and physiology of the CV system and the acute responses and chronic adaptations to exercise.

ANATOMY OF THE HEART

The heart acts as a pump circulating blood throughout the body. It consists of four chambers (Fig. 8.1) with approximately two-thirds of its mass located on the left side. On average, the heart weighs ~11 oz in men and 9 oz in women, and its weight is proportional to body size (53). Two of the chambers are receivers (*atria*) whereas the other two chambers (*ventricles*) act to pump blood away from the heart. Blood returns to the heart from the rest of the body through the right atrium (via the superior and inferior vena cava) and then passes through the right ventricle. A *tricuspid valve* opens (between the right atrium and ventricle) as the pressure within the atrium builds up to allow passage of blood to the ventricle and closes to prevent backward flow of blood. Contraction of the right ventricle pumps blood

to the lungs through the pulmonary *semilunar valve* of the pulmonary artery. Blood becomes oxygenated in the lungs and returns to the heart (left atrium) via the pulmonary vein. Contraction of the left atrium pumps blood through the *bicuspid (mitral) valve* into the left ventricle. The left ventricle is the largest chamber as blood is pumped via the aorta to all parts of the circulatory system. The *chordae tendineae* are chord-like tendons that connect the valves to the papillary muscles. They prevent backward flow of blood by preventing the valves from inversion. The *papillary muscles* contract to tighten and stabilize the chordae tendineae. The atria and ventricles are separated by *septum*, the *interatrial* and *interventricular septum*, respectively.

CARDIAC MUSCULATURE

Cardiac muscle, or **myocardium**, is one of three major types of muscle. It contracts on its own and is capable of hypertrophy and adapting to exercise. The thickness of cardiac muscle is affected by stress, and thicker cardiac muscle is stronger. This is particularly true for the left ventricle. The T tubules are fewer in number, larger, broader, and are located along the Z line compared to skeletal muscle. This, in part, allows cardiac muscle to contract forcefully at a lower rate. Cardiac cells, or **cardiocytes**, have the ability to communicate directly with adjacent cells via connective tissue structures known as *intercalated discs*. Intercalated discs enable the rapid spread of action potentials and the synchronized contraction of heart musculature. They enable cardiac muscle in all four chambers to act as one large fiber during contraction. Gap junctions are located within the intercalated disks and act as passages between cells. They allow the

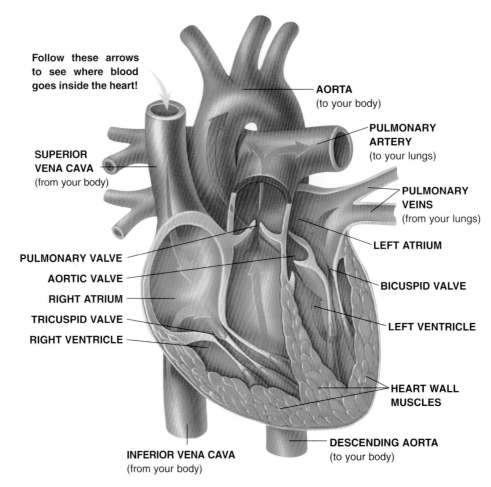

Follow these arrows to see where blood goes inside the heart!

SUPERIOR VENA CAVA
(from your body)

AORTA
(to your body)

PULMONARY ARTERY
(to your lungs)

PULMONARY VEINS
(from your lungs)

LEFT ATRIUM

PULMONARY VALVE

AORTIC VALVE

RIGHT ATRIUM

TRICUSPID VALVE

RIGHT VENTRICLE

BICUSPID VALVE

LEFT VENTRICLE

HEART WALL MUSCLES

INFERIOR VENA CAVA
(from your body)

DESCENDING AORTA
(to your body)

■ FIGURE 8.1. Anatomy of the heart.

heart to contract in a network referred to as a *functional syncytium* that occurs in a squeezing-like fashion thereby ejecting the blood in a fluent manner.

MAJOR BLOOD VESSELS

Blood vessels provide the major routes by which blood is pumped (Fig. 8.2). Because humans have a closed circulatory system, vessels form a large interconnecting network responsible for blood delivery to all tissues, nutrient/waste exchange, and return to the heart. *Arteries* are high-pressure vessels that deliver oxygen-rich blood to tissues. Arteries have walls that contain smooth muscle and elastic fibers. The elastic recoil is large, enabling arteries to forcefully circulate. The aorta is the largest artery and has an ascending and descending branch that exits the left ventricle. It acts as a distributor with many branches. Arteries decrease in size and diameter as they approach the tissue level. Smaller arteries form *arterioles*. Arterioles constrict or relax to regulate blood flow at the tissue level. Approximately 17% of the body's total blood supply circulates through arteries at rest (53). Arterioles branch and form smaller vessels called *metarterioles* that end the arterial side of circulation and form a network of capillaries.

Capillaries are thin (7–10 μm) vessels that serve as the site for nutrient/oxygen exchange at the tissue level. In skeletal muscle, each metarteriole interfaces with ~8–10 capillaries (53). Approximately 8% of total blood supply circulates through capillary beds at rest, and capillaries in skeletal muscle are densely populated, *e.g.*, 2,000–3,000 capillaries per square millimeter of tissue (53). Capillaries have precapillary sphincters that constrict or dilate to regulate blood flow. The opposite side of the capillary bed forms the venous side of circulation. Small veins (*venules*) continue the circulatory route from capillary beds. Venules form larger veins, and all veins circulate blood into the inferior (from lower body) and superior (from upper body) vena cava. Veins are low-pressure structures with extensible walls. Blood is stored in veins when circulatory demands are low and is compelled into circulation when demand necessitates greater activity. Approximately 68% of total blood supply circulates in veins at rest (53).

REGULATION OF THE HEART

Cardiac function stems largely from the heart's force of contraction and rate. Although the heart contracts involuntarily, it operates under the control of intrinsic and

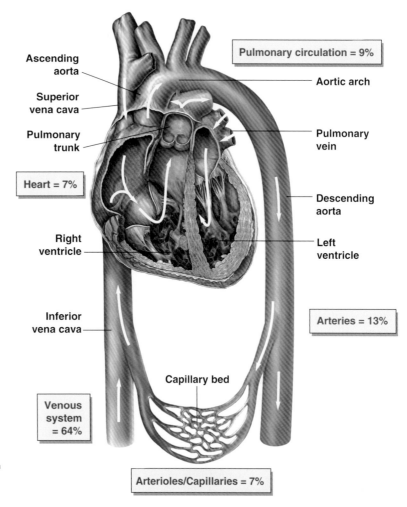

FIGURE 8.2. Circulatory system. Percentages indicate the amount of blood circulating through each region at rest. (Adapted from an asset provided by Anatomical Chart Co.)

extrinsic factors. Intrinsic factors relate to the heart's own conduction system as well as the role venous return to the heart plays in cardiac contractility. Extrinsic factors that control CV function relate to stimuli from other major physiological systems including the nervous and endocrine systems. Both intrinsic and extrinsic factors are critical to mediating CV function at rest and during exercise.

INTRINSIC REGULATION OF THE HEART

The heart has the ability to regulate its own rhythm (Fig. 8.3). The action potential is spontaneously generated in the *sinoatrial node* (SA node). The SA node is located in the right atrium and is the pacemaker of the heart. The wave of depolarization spreads across the atria to the *atrioventricular node* (AV node). The AV node places a delay (~0.10–0.13 s) to allow the atria more time to contract and allow adequate filling time for the ventricles. The AV node gives rise to the *Bundle of His*, which continues the wave of depolarization. Depolarization rapidly spreads through the ventricles via the *left and right bundle branches* and *Purkinje fibers*. The right and left bundle branches send the wave of depolarization toward the heart's apex and then

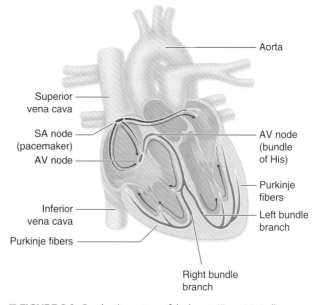

FIGURE 8.3. Conductive system of the heart. (From McArdle WD, Katch FI, Katch VL. *Exercise Physiology: Nutrition, Energy, and Human Performance.* 7th ed. Baltimore (MD): Lippincott Williams & Wilkins; 2010.)

outward. The terminal branches become Purkinje fibers that spread the depolarization throughout the ventricles. Purkinje fibers transmit action potentials at a rate that is approximately six times faster than other cardiac areas (53). The heart's conduction system keeps rate around 60–100 bpm depending on one's conditioning level.

EXTRINSIC REGULATION OF THE HEART

Extrinsic regulation is important to prepare the heart to tolerate stress and exercise. Extrinsic control stems from the nervous and endocrine systems. The medulla oblongata contains a cardiac center that regulates heart rate (HR) and force of contraction, a vasomotor center that controls blood pressure (BP) and vessel diameter, and a respiratory center that controls breathing rate and depth. Feedback from sensory and motor centers in the brain stimulates CV centers to increase HR and force of contraction. The autonomic nervous system plays a substantial role in regulating cardiac function. Sympathetic nervous system stimulation increases cardiac contractility and rate whereas parasympathetic nervous system (mainly through stimulation of the *vagus nerve*) has the opposite effect and returns CV function back toward homeostasis. Catecholamines (epinephrine and norepinephrine) are secreted, bind to receptors on the surface of the heart, and increase HR and force of contraction. They also lead to an anticipatory rise in CV function prior to exercise. Norepinephrine is most effective when it is released as a neurotransmitter from sympathetic nerves whereas epinephrine accounts for most of the catecholamines (~80%) secreted by the adrenal medulla.

BLOOD COMPONENTS

Blood accounts for ~7% of human body weight and is responsible for transportation of several molecules throughout the human body. Molecules such as oxygen, glucose, fatty acids, amino acids, vitamins, minerals, enzymes, antibodies, and hormones travel through the blood to target tissues. Waste products are removed by blood. Blood volume is dependent on body size and level of aerobic conditioning, but is generally around 5–6 L in men and 4–5 L in women (85). The major components of blood include its liquid portion (plasma) and the segment of formed elements. Plasma comprises 55%–60% of blood volume of which ~90% is water, 7% plasma proteins, and the remaining 3% nutrients and waste (85). Formed elements comprise ~40%–45% of total blood volume. The percent of formed elements relative to total blood volume is the **hematocrit**. Hematocrit can change based on hydration levels and is often used to investigate potential blood doping in athletes.

Red blood cells (RBCs, erythrocytes) comprise 99% of the formed elements and up to 1% is comprised of white blood cells and *platelets* (85). The body contains >25 trillion RBCs, and RBC production is increased by testosterone (53).

RBCs lack a nucleus and organelles. They transport oxygen primarily bound to the iron-containing protein **hemoglobin**. Although a small percent of oxygen is transported in plasma (~1.5%), most (98.5%) oxygen is transported via hemoglobin. Approximately 65–70 times more oxygen is transported by hemoglobin than plasma dissolution (53). Each RBC contains ~250–280 million hemoglobin molecules; each contains iron and can bind four oxygen molecules. There are ~15 g of hemoglobin per 100 mL of blood in men and ~14 g per dL of blood in women (53,85).

Oxygen binding to hemoglobin is cooperative because binding of one oxygen molecule increases the affinity of others. However, oxygen must be dissociated before it is taken up into tissues. Figure 8.4 illustrates the oxygen-hemoglobin dissociation curve at normal pH (7.4) and temperature (37°C) and at pHs of 7.6 and 7.2. Cooperative oxygen binding is a factor leading to the S-shaped curve. The x-axis depicts the partial pressure of oxygen (PO_2) and the y-axis depicts the percent of hemoglobin saturated with oxygen. The partial pressure is the pressure generated independent of other gases. It is a measure of the quantity of gas present. The air we breathe is composed of 79.04% nitrogen, 20.93% oxygen, and 0.03% CO_2. At sea level, the atmospheric pressure is 760 mm Hg, which creates a PO_2 of 159 mm Hg (760 mm Hg × 0.21). This PO_2 drops to 100–105 mm Hg when air is inhaled as it mixes with water vapor and CO_2 in the alveoli. Differences in PO_2 between the lungs (100 mm Hg) and alveolar capillaries (40 mm Hg) and between arterial circulation (100 mm Hg) and the tissues (40 mm Hg) allow diffusion of oxygen (Fig. 8.5). The latter is the **arterio-venous oxygen difference** (a-VO$_2$ difference) and

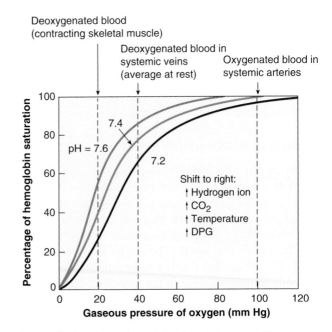

FIGURE 8.4. Oxygen-hemoglobin dissociation curve. (From *Stedman's Medical Dictionary*. 27th ed. Baltimore (MD): Lippincott Williams & Wilkins; 2000.)

is ~4–5 mL of oxygen per dL of blood at rest but may increase up to 15 mL of oxygen per dL of blood during exercise (53). The large PO_2 gradient from the alveoli to the capillaries of 60–65 mm Hg drives oxygen into circulation and is known as the oxygen diffusion capacity. At rest, ~250 mL of oxygen diffuses into pulmonary circulation each minute and this number is far greater in highly trained endurance athletes (53).

In Figure 8.4, hemoglobin saturation remains high (~75%–80%) at PO_2 above 40 mm Hg. Under resting conditions, about 20%–25% of oxygen is unloaded from hemoglobin into capillary beds. This curve can shift to the right or left. A shift to the right and down indicates greater tissue oxygen unloading whereas a shift to the left and up has the opposite effect. Four major factors cause a right/down shift in the curve. A reduction in pH (increased H^+), increased temperature, higher levels of CO_2 (increased partial pressure of CO_2 [PCO_2]), and increased 2,3-*diphosphoglycerate* (2,3-DPG) can increase oxygen dissociation. Exercise has a similar influence. A right/down shift in the curve resulting

from changes in pH and temperature is known as the **Bohr effect** (named after scientist Christian Bohr). 2,3-DPG is found in RBCs and binds to hemoglobin with higher affinity than oxygen. As a result, 2,3-DPG elevations increase oxygen unloading. 2,3-DPG concentrations are higher in athletes than untrained individuals and higher in women than men (53) reflecting greater potential to unload oxygen with training and, in women, a compensatory mechanism to accommodate lower hemoglobin.

CO_2 must be removed while oxygen is consumed. Like oxygen, CO_2 moves via diffusion from high to low PCO_2 values (Fig. 8.5). Blood PCO_2 is 46 mm Hg versus an alveolar PCO_2 of 40 mm Hg. CO_2 travels in the blood by three routes. In plasma, 5%–10% of CO_2 is transported in a dissolved state. Free CO_2 is important for establishing PCO_2 values. Sixty to eighty percent of CO_2 is transported via bicarbonate. In tissues, the reaction catalyzed by the enzyme *carbonic anhydrase* is

$$CO_2 + H_2O \rightarrow H_2CO_3 \rightarrow H^+ + HCO_3^-.$$

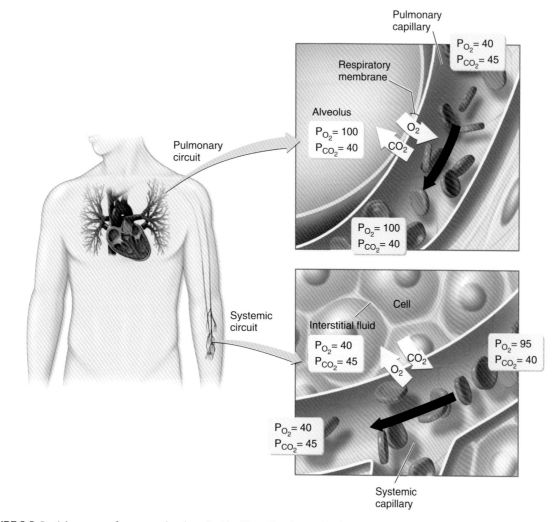

FIGURE 8.5. Partial pressure of oxygen and carbon dioxide. (From Premkumar K. *The Massage Connection Anatomy and Physiology*. Baltimore (MD): Lippincott Williams & Wilkins; 2004.)

The bicarbonate ion (HCO_3^-) buffers pH while transporting CO_2. In the lungs, the carbonic anhydrase/bicarbonate reaction is reversed where CO_2 (and H_2O) is reformed where it is then expired. Lastly, ~20% of CO_2 is transported with hemoglobin (*carbaminohemoglobin*). Oxygenated hemoglobin has less ability to bind CO_2 whereas deoxygenated hemoglobin has higher affinity for CO_2, a concept known as the **Haldane effect**. Dissociation occurs in the lungs leading to CO_2 release via expiration.

RBCs have a lifespan of ~4 months, so they must be replaced adequately. Some RBCs may be destroyed during exercise (*sports anemia*) where mechanical stress via pounding of the feet during running and jarring of kidneys may contribute. Platelets are small molecules required for blood clotting (in addition to several proteins including *fibrin*) whereas white blood cells are critical to immune function. Blood is critical for temperature regulation and pH balance. Blood picks up heat from the body's core and dissipates heat throughout. Skin blood flow increases during exercise, which assists in cooling. Lastly, blood can buffer acids to restore pH.

SIDEBAR   **BLOOD DOPING IN ATHLETES**

Blood doping (dates back to the early 1960s) refers to intravenous infusion of blood or blood products to increase athletic performance. Blood may come from a donor (*homologous infusion*) or the athlete (*autologous infusion*) spaced over weeks, frozen in glycerol, and reinfused 3–5 days before the competition. Blood doping increases RBC (and hemoglobin) content up to ~10% (45) and marked improvements take place within 24 hours. Although this technique was banned by the International Olympic Committee in 1984, the drug *erythropoietin* (EPO) became the new method to boost blood in 1988. EPO is a glycoprotein hormone produced by the kidneys and liver, which stimulates the production of RBCs upon binding to receptors on bone marrow. The synthetic form of EPO (recombinant EPO) is injected to increase RBC count and hemoglobin concentrations. EPO injections (20–50 IU kg body mass^{-1} three times per week) may increase hemoglobin by ~6%–11% and hematocrit by 6%–8.3%, decrease blood lactate during exercise, increase Vo_{2max} by 7% and run time to exhaustion by 17% (2). Blood doping or EPO use enhances endurance performance via increased Vo_{2max}, buffer capacity, blood volume, and heat tolerance. Blood doping increases Vo_{2max} by up to 11%, 5-mile treadmill run time, 10-km race time, and running and cycling time to exhaustion by 13%–26% (2,7,83) and the effects are most notable in athletes with high Vo_{2max} (73).

BLOOD FLOW

Blood flow to working muscles is critical to exercise performance. The body contains ~5 L of blood although the vascular system has the potential to hold four times more than that (53). At rest, skeletal muscle receives ~15%–20% of total blood flow as most blood flows to other organs: 25% to the liver, 20% to the kidneys, 10% to the skin, 14%–15% to the brain, and the remaining ~10%–12% to the heart and other tissues (36). During exercise, blood flow to skeletal muscle may increase to >80% of total flow (via redistribution) to meet the metabolic demands. Blood flow to inspiratory and expiratory muscles during exercise may increase to ~14%–16% of total cardiac output (Q_c) (12). Blood flow is maintained or increased to the brain during exercise. Blood flow to the brain increases as exercise intensity increases to ~60% of Vo_{2max}, where it may plateau or decrease afterward (62). Increased arteriole vasodilation takes place in the brain due to increased PCO_2, decreased PO_2, increased metabolism and activity of muscle mechanoreceptors, and greater mean arterial pressure (62).

Contraction of skeletal muscle is necessary to increase venous blood flow back to the heart. Muscle contraction forces blood against gravity, and venous valves prevent blood from backward flow in healthy veins. Muscle contraction helps create a vibrant circulatory system. Increased muscle blood flow is responsible for the muscle pump associated with resistance training (RT). Muscle blood flow is occluded with contractions >20% of MVC. The mechanical shortening/lengthening of muscle fibers and/or ISOM contraction against a resistance constricts blood vessels and temporarily decreases blood flow. However, greater blood flow circulates to muscle upon relaxation or low-level contractions **(reactive hyperemia)**. During resistance exercise, the lifter may feel blood flow increase to the active muscles in between sets rather than during the set. Ischemia associated with RT is a stimulus for muscle hypertrophy.

Blood flow is tightly regulated. Blood flow follows general principles of hydrodynamics where blood flow is dependent upon the pressure gradient within the vessel (large gradient = greater flow), resistance to flow (lower resistance = greater flow), blood thickness or viscosity (greater viscosity = reduced flow), blood vessel length (greater length = reduced flow), and blood vessel diameter or radius (greater diameter = greater flow) (53). Exercise presents a potent sympathetic nervous system response where blood vessel vasoconstriction is customary. Vasoconstriction increases BP but reduces flow to that specified region. Blood flow can be redirected from other peripheral tissues to skeletal muscle. Local regulatory factors increase blood flow to skeletal muscle during exercise. The metabolic demands cause the release of several vasoactive substances that increase blood vessel vasodilation. CO_2, reduced pH, adenosine, magnesium, potassium, and nitric oxide stimulate local vasodilation (53).

Nitric oxide is a gas produced from its precursor *L-arginine* (with oxygen via the enzyme *nitric oxide synthase*), which is a potent signaling molecule and vasodilatory agent known to produce many functions in the human body. It freely diffuses across cell membranes, is highly reactive, and acts quickly upon arteriole smooth muscle causing relaxation and vasodilation. Nitric oxide regulates skeletal muscle contractility and exercise-induced glucose uptake (6). As a result, nitric oxide (or NO_2) supplements have become popular. Although little research has addressed NO_2 supplementation in athletes, it is thought it may have some potential for muscle strength, hypertrophy, and endurance enhancement.

CARDIOVASCULAR FUNCTION

Several CV variables can be measured and used for health/performance evaluations. These variables include HR, BP, stroke volume (SV) (and ejection fraction), and Q_c.

- **Heart rate** is the frequency the heart beats per minute. Average resting HR values range from 60 to 100 bpm. Resting HR is affected by age, gender (adult women average 5–10 bpm faster than men), posture (standing yields a 10–12 bpm greater HR than lying), food intake (digestion increases metabolism and HR), stress/emotion (increases HR), smoking (increases HR), and environmental and body temperature (HR increases when body temperature increases and during hot and humid weather) (36).
- **Blood pressure** is the pressure in the arteries following contraction of the left ventricle (systole). **Systolic blood pressure** (SBP) is the pressure in the left ventricle during systole and averages ~120 mm Hg. **Diastolic blood pressure** (DBP) represents peripheral resistance to flow during relaxation (diastole) and averages ~80 mm Hg. Mean arterial pressure averages ~93 mm Hg and is calculated as DBP + (0.333[SBP – DBP]).
- **Stroke volume** is the volume of blood ejected from the left ventricle each beat. SV averages ~60–70 mL of blood per beat and is the difference between the blood volume in the left ventricle after filling (*end diastolic volume*; averages ~100 mL of blood) and the blood volume after systole (*end systolic volume*; averages ~40 mL of blood). The proportion of blood pumped from the left ventricle each beat is the *ejection fraction*. It is calculated by (SV/end diastolic volume) × 100. Ejection fraction averages 60% at rest.
- **Cardiac output** (Q_c) is the total volume of blood pumped by the heart per minute. It is the product of HR and SV. Q_c averages 5 L min^{-1} at rest and tends to be higher in a supine position than standing or sitting.

CARDIOVASCULAR RESPONSES TO EXERCISE

Aerobic and anaerobic exercises lead to substantial acute CV responses in men and women. Exercise increases oxygen demand, nutrient usage, waste buildup, and body core temperature that all require augmented CV response to meet the additional needs. Recovery from exercise requires augmented CV system response to return to homeostatic levels. Essentially all components of the CV system are modified during exercise. In this section, HR, SV, Q_c, BP, plasma volume (PV), and oxygen consumption are discussed.

HEART RATE RESPONSE

HR increases during exercise from resting values to rates >195 bpm during maximal exercise (53). The upper limits for HR during exercise can be calculated by taking 220 and subtracting an individual's age in years and target HR for aerobic exercise is calculated based on the maximum predicted HR (see Chapter 16). The magnitude of HR increase depends on muscle mass use, exercise intensity, and the degree of continuity of exercise. At low to moderate to high intensities of exercise, HR will increase linearly up until maximal. If work rate is held constant, HR plateaus after an initial rise at the onset of exercise. The plateau is the *steady-state HR* and is optimal to meet the current workload. For each increase in intensity beyond this point, a new steady-state value will be reached within 1–2 minutes (85). HR may remain at this point if intensity remains constant. However, during prolonged aerobic exercise, HR may subtly increase at the same intensity when it is >15 minutes in duration. This is known as **cardiovascular drift** where the HR increase compensates for reduced SV caused by fluid loss (53). Interval and RT elicit potent increases in HR. Fluctuations are seen due to the breaks in continuity of the exercise modalities. HR increases following each set at the onset of resistance exercise. HR increases progressively after each set for the first 4 sets (of a 5-set protocol) and plateaus (63). During each repetition, HR responds similarly between ECC and CON phases (17).

STROKE VOLUME RESPONSE

SV increases during exercise and physiological factors such as blood volume returning to the heart, arterial pressure, ventricular contractility, and distensibility contribute to the magnitude of SV increase (85). Remember, the venous system acts as a storage site for blood at rest. Exercise increases blood flow in circulation and causes greater venous return to the heart. Greater venous return increases end-diastolic volume in the left ventricle and the heart's force of contraction. Myocardial fibers stretch via greater *preload* and the effect is a stronger force of contraction.

Greater preload-induced stretch places cardiac muscle fibers in a more conducive length to generate force. This is known as the *Frank-Starling mechanism*. Cardiac contractility increases independent of venous return. Sympathetic nervous system stimulation and catecholamines increase cardiac contractility. Vasodilation decreases total peripheral resistance to flow from the heart, which decreases *afterload*. In combination, these factors contribute to greater SV augmentation during exercise.

SV increases linearly up to ~40%–60% of maximal exercise capacity in untrained and moderately trained individuals (85) where a plateau occurs as exercise progresses. However, SV may increase beyond this intensity in highly trained endurance athletes (85). SV may increase to 100–120 mL in untrained individuals but up to 200 mL in highly trained individuals (85). Critical to SV increases is body position. At rest, SV is higher during supine or recumbent positions due to greater venous return. Upright positions yield lower SV due to gravity causing venous pooling in the lower extremities. During exercise, the SV increase is higher in an upright position than supine due to the lower starting value seen in the supine position. SV increases take place despite increases in HR, which decrease chamber filling times. SV increases during resistance exercise (1). When examining each rep, SV does not increase during the CON phase but may increase during the ECC phase (17). In some cases SV is lower during CON actions (17). This may be the result of including a **Valsalva maneuver** (temporary breath-holding) which increases *intrathoracic pressure* (the pressure developed within the chest cavity) and *intra-abdominal pressure*, which increases SBP and DBP. A substantial load (increased BP) is placed on the CV system during lifting (34). The rise in pressure may impede SV temporarily during CON actions. SV rebounds during rest intervals where elevations are seen.

CARDIAC OUTPUT RESPONSE

Q_c is the product of HR and SV. A linear increase in Q_c is seen during aerobic exercise (Fig. 8.6). HR and SV increase during exercise. However, SV may plateau as intensity rises; therefore, an increase in HR is needed at high exercise intensities to reach maximal Q_c. Q_c may increase to 20–40 L min^{-1} depending on the athlete's aerobic fitness level (85). During resistance exercise, Q_c increases over the course of a workout. Similar to SV, the response is limited during CON actions but higher during ECC actions when analyzing individual reps (17). A compensatory increase in Q_c takes place during rest intervals when SV increases.

BLOOD PRESSURE RESPONSE

BP is controlled in different ways. Sympathetic nervous system activity increases vasoconstriction which increases BP and the parasympathetic nervous system has

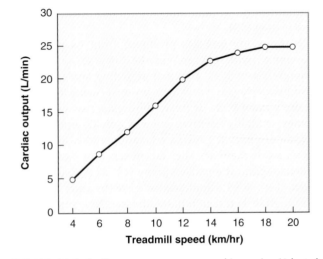

■ **FIGURE 8.6.** Cardiac output response to aerobic exercise. (Adapted with permission from Wilmore JH, Costill DL. *Physiology of Sport and Exercise.* 4th ed. Champaign (IL): Human Kinetics; 2008.)

the opposite effect. Central command of the CV system stimulates the vasomotor center of the brainstem to alter BP. Feedback from sensory and motor centers in the brain stimulates CV centers to increase BP. Stretch-sensitive sensory receptors located in the walls of blood vessels (aortic arch and carotid sinuses) known as **baroreceptors** detect pressure and stimulate the brainstem to modulate BP via negative feedback control. Baroreceptors decrease BP in response to an increase in BP and prevent large elevations in BP during exercise (53). The renin-angiotensin system and the hormone aldosterone (discussed in Chapter 6) regulate BP. Renin leads to the activation of angiotensin II which causes vasoconstriction. Aldosterone increases sodium retention which increases BP.

BP increases during exercise. During steady-state aerobic exercise, SBP increases during the first several minutes but plateaus and/or slightly decreases when steady state is reached (53). Vasodilation reduces peripheral resistance so SBP may decline. DBP does not change much. During progressive aerobic exercise, SBP increases linearly as intensity increases whereas DBP remains constant or decreases (53). SBP values of up to 250 mm Hg are seen in endurance athletes (85). Upper-body exercise increases SBP (by ~18–45 mm Hg) and DBP (by ~20–28 mm Hg) much more than lower-body exercise (53). Smaller muscle mass in the upper body provides greater resistance to blood flow thereby increasing BP to a greater extent. The increase in SBP helps assist in accelerating blood flow and fluid movement through the capillaries (85).

BP increases during resistance exercise with the increase proportional to effort. The response is dependent upon the use of the Valsalva maneuver, muscle mass activation, muscle action, and the intensity/duration of the set (17). Blood flow occlusion during muscle contraction increases BP. The increase is needed to overcome greater peripheral resistance. Mean BPs of 320/250 and 345/245 mm Hg may occur during a high-intensity leg press (48) and squat, respectively, with a peak of 480/350 mm Hg shown (48). Mean SBP of 290–307 mm Hg and DBP of 220–238 mm Hg during the leg press (80%, 95%, and 100% of 1 RM) have been shown (31). Other studies showed SBP values of 198–230 mm Hg and DBP values of 160–170 mm Hg (17). Valsalva maneuvers increase BP response to resistance exercise and may be unavoidable when lifting weights ≥80% of 1 RM (48,49). Breath-holding increases intrathoracic and intra-abdominal pressures, and BP increases proportionally as a result (32,60). Mean BP during a 1 RM leg press was 311/284 mm Hg with a Valsalva maneuver and 198/175 mm Hg without (57). Higher mean BP for the arm curl (166/112 vs. 148/101 mm Hg) and knee extension (166/108 vs. 151/99 mm Hg) occurred when Valsalva maneuvers were used (47).

Muscle mass activation plays a role in the BP response. Mean BPs are greater during the leg press (320/250 mm Hg) than arm curl (255/190 mm Hg) (48). Higher BP is seen during squats than arm curls (60). The BP response is greater during the CON versus ECC phase of each rep and increases nonlinearly with the magnitude of active muscle mass (17,48). BP increases further during the exercise's sticking point (49). Many times the sticking point is where an exaggerated Valsalva maneuver may be used by the lifter. BP increases as sets progress. Gotshall et al. (24) had subjects perform 3 sets of the leg press for 10 reps and showed a progressive rise in SBP and DBP with each successive rep (Fig. 8.7). Peak SBP were 238, 268, and 293 mm Hg, respectively, for each set. Peak BP is higher when a set is performed to failure (31,48,69). Sets performed to failure at 70%–85% 1 RM produced a greater BP response than during a 1 RM leg press (18). BP decreases during rest intervals when blood flow is restored to working muscles.

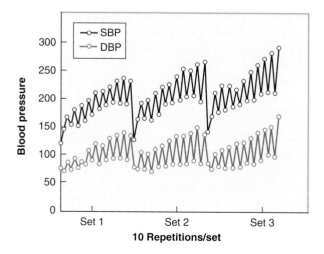

FIGURE 8.7. Blood pressure response to 3 sets of the leg press exercise. SBP, systolic blood pressure; DBP, diastolic blood pressure. (From Gotshall RW, Gootman J, Byrnes WC, Fleck SJ, Valovich TC. Noninvasive characterization of the blood pressure response to the double-leg press exercise. *J Exerc Physiol.* 1999;2:1–6.)

PLASMA VOLUME

PV is reduced during exercise. PV reductions occur as fluid shifts from the blood to the interstitial spaces and intracellular domains. PV shifts take place as the BP increase forces water into the interstitial space and metabolic waste products build up in muscle (increasing *osmotic pressure*) causing a shift of fluid into muscle (85). Fluid loss from perspiration results in additional PV reductions. When PV decreases, RBCs increase via *hemoconcentration* and this increases blood viscosity and reduces oxygen transport. PV reductions of up to 20% occur during endurance exercise. Reduced PV can impair endurance performance and Vo_{2max} (23). SV is reduced as venous return decreases with fluid loss. Consequently, Q_c and Vo_{2max} are reduced. Vo_{2max} correlates to PV (87); therefore, reductions in PV during an endurance exercise bout can lead to reduced performance.

A bout of resistance exercise decreases PV by 7%–14% (9) and in some cases by >20% immediately postexercise (61,63), with the magnitude dependent on intensity and duration (9). PV may almost fully recover within 30–60 minutes after exercise (8,61), especially when fluid intake accompanies the workout. PV reductions begin during the first set of the first exercise with a concomitant change in fluid regulatory factors such as renin, angiotensin II, and atrial peptide (43) and are affected by the type of program used. Craig et al. (10) showed a 22.6% PV reduction after 10 RM workout (3 sets of nine exercises) versus a 13% reduction after a 5 RM workout. Plautz-Snyder et al. (61) examined a 6 × 10 squat protocol with 2-minute rest intervals and showed a 22% PV reduction. Muscle CSA of thigh muscles increased by 5%–10% and correlated highly with PV reductions. Fluid shifts correspond to acute muscle size expansion seen during resistance exercise, *e.g.*, a muscle "pump."

OXYGEN CONSUMPTION

Oxygen consumption, or VO_2, increases proportionally during exercise in relation to intensity, muscle mass activation, and degree of continuity. Oxygen consumption is represented by the **Fick equation,** which states that $VO_2 = Q_c \times$ A-VO_2 difference. The structural hierarchy of the circulatory system is

large arteries → smaller arteries →
arterioles → metarterioles → capillary beds →
venules → small veins → large veins.

Oxygen diffuses through capillary membranes into tissues. The A-VO_2 difference is the amount of oxygen in the arterial side versus the venous side and represents tissue oxygen extraction. At rest, arterial oxygen content is ~20 mL of O_2 per 100 mL of blood (85). However, this value drops to ~15–16 mL of O_2 per 100 mL of blood as

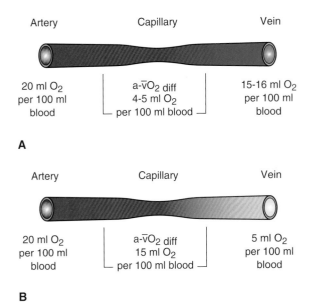

A

B

■ **FIGURE 8.8.** The A-VO$_2$ difference. **A.** The A-VO$_2$ difference at rest. **B.** The A-VO$_2$ difference during exercise. (Reprinted with permission from Wilmore JH, Costill DL. *Physiology of Sport and Exercise.* 2nd ed. Champaign (IL): Human Kinetics; 1999.)

blood passes through capillaries into venules (Fig. 8.8). At rest this value is ~4–5 mL of O$_2$ per 100 mL of blood (85). The A-VO$_2$ difference can increase up to ~15–16 mL of O$_2$ per 100 mL of blood or more during endurance exercise (85). The increase reflects greater oxygen extraction from arterial blood into skeletal muscles. The combination of the increased Q$_c$ and oxygen extraction leads to an increase in VO$_2$ during exercise.

VO$_2$ increases during exercise (Fig. 8.9). A linear rise in VO$_2$ is seen with increasing intensity. Increasing the

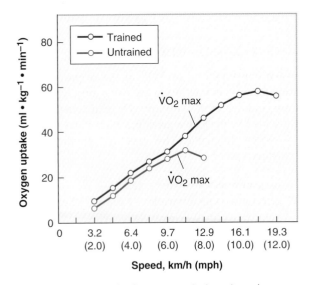

■ **FIGURE 8.9.** Relationship between exercise intensity and oxygen consumption. (Reprinted with permission from Wilmore JH, Costill DL. *Physiology of Sport and Exercise.* 2nd ed. Champaign (IL): Human Kinetics; 1999. p. 140.)

speed of movement, level of inclination (or using a more compliant surface), adding resistance, or increasing the amount of muscular involvement (adding arm exercise to a lower-body exercise modality) during endurance exercise yields proportional increases in VO$_2$. VO$_2$ increases during anaerobic exercise. However, the lower level of continuity produces abrupt fluctuations. VO$_2$ will rise abruptly during and immediately following a maximal sprint but declines soon thereafter during the rest period. VO$_2$ fluctuates during resistance exercise where short rest intervals yield a greater sustained rise; however, long rest intervals yield an initial abrupt increase but a prolonged period of decline during recovery (64). The limited continuity poses great challenges for increasing Vo$_{2max}$. VO$_2$ during resistance exercise increases with higher intensities, short rest intervals, large muscle mass exercises, and slow to moderate repetition velocities. A bodybuilding lower-body workout (multiple sets, squats, leg press and other lower-body exercises, 6–12 reps, with <2 min rest intervals) produces an increase in VO$_2$ to only ~45%–60% of Vo$_{2max}$ (78), usually below the threshold needed to increase Vo$_{2max}$ in trained to highly trained populations.

CHRONIC ADAPTATIONS AT REST AND DURING EXERCISE

Aerobic and anaerobic exercises lead to comprehensive changes to the CV system at rest. Dr. Joel Morganroth was the first to propose in the mid-1970s that training produced two general types of overload, pressure, and volume overload. *Pressure overload* results from the rise in BP and intrathoracic pressure that accompany exercise. Pressure overload can alter several CV variables positively over time in addition to leading to changes in cardiac musculature. *Volume overload* results from greater venous return and blood flow to the heart during exercise. Aerobic exercise is superior for volume overload due to the higher level of continuity. Volume overload leads to positive changes in several CV variables and increases cardiac chamber size. These changes not only alter CV function at rest but also acute responses to exercise.

CARDIAC DIMENSIONS

Training leads to cardiac muscle alterations. Adaptations are thought to be governed by the *Law of Laplace*, which states that wall tension is proportional to pressure and size of the radius of curvature (34). Greater heart size is characterized by greater left ventricular cavity (*eccentric hypertrophy*) and thickening of cardiac walls (*concentric hypertrophy*). Myocardial overload and stretch via exercise stimulates higher rates of protein synthesis leading to hypertrophy (53). Cardiac muscle fibers become more sensitive to calcium and contract stronger when stretched leading to greater contractility (53). Volume overload results in an increase in sarcomeres in series

Myths & Misconceptions

Cardiac Muscle Hypertrophy Only Occurs as a Result of Cardiovascular Disease

Heart size and chamber volume increase during training. These changes are positive; however, at one time they were viewed as negative. Because hypertrophy of cardiac muscle occurs as a consequence of CV disease, some associated all hypertrophy as negative. However, investigations of the hearts of athletes revealed hypertrophy independent of CV disease. This concept of the *athlete's heart* is associated with positive CV effects (greater SV and Q_c). Changes in resting function can be attributed, in part, to cardiac muscle hypertrophy. The size of the heart increases as body size increases. There has been some difficulty in quantifying changes in cardiac hypertrophy independent of body mass changes during RT. Often, cardiac muscle mass changes will be expressed relative to body surface area or body mass. These concerns notwithstanding, aerobic and anaerobic training positively increase cardiac muscle size.

(greater chamber size and end-diastolic volumes) whereas pressure overload increases the number of sarcomeres in parallel (greater wall thickness). The left ventricle is the primary chamber affected by exercise.

Aerobic training leads to comprehensive improvements in cardiac function. In untrained individuals, changes in chamber size occur early with modest changes in wall thickness (58). Cross-sectional comparisons between endurance athletes, strength/power athletes, and nonathletes are difficult because athletes from many sports embark upon endurance, sprint/ plyometric, and RT. That concern notwithstanding, cardiac dimensions in athletes are greater than nonathletes having 10% greater chamber size and 15%–20% greater wall thicknesses (58). Naylor et al. (58) reviewed >40 studies and reported that endurance athletes had greater left ventricular mass (25 of 27 studies), posterior wall thickness (25 of 32 studies), interventricular septal wall thickness (19 of 28 studies), and left ventricular cavity dimensions (27 of 32 studies) than control subjects. Training volume positively increases left ventricular mass in endurance athletes (58). Some studies showed the extent of increase in relative left ventricular mass is augmented during AT more than RT whereas a few have shown greater left ventricular mass in resistance-trained athletes or no differences between strength/power and endurance athletes (58). Female long-distance runners have greater left ventricular wall thickness, mass, and interventricular septal thickness than sprinters (79) showing more comprehensive changes following AT.

RT leads to changes in left-side cardiac muscularity; however, these changes rarely exceed the upper normal levels of cardiac wall thickness/mass and are less in magnitude than individuals with CV disease (17). Resistance-trained individuals have absolute greater left ventricular wall thickness and interventricular septal thickness than untrained individuals (1,17). However, relative changes (to body mass or surface area) are small or nonexistent (17). Elite junior weightlifters have greater absolute

and relative left ventricular wall thickness and mass than untrained controls (19,20). However, other studies showed no such relative changes (31). Although the increased BP and intrathoracic pressure during lifting is attributed to concentric hypertrophy, some have argued that the pressure rise is counterbalanced by reduced *transmural pressure* (left ventricular pressure minus intrathoracic pressure) thereby reducing potential training effects (independent of body size changes) (31,32). Nevertheless, absolute increases in cardiac thickness occur during RT. Bodybuilders have high left ventricular mass and wall thickness (17); however, many bodybuilders perform AT to reduce body fat. Anabolic steroid use was not controlled for in many studies and could have contributed to left ventricular mass changes as steroid users may have greater left ventricular posterior and septal wall thickness than drug-free lifters (13). Most cardiac muscle thickness increases are brought about by changes in LBM. The training program determines potential cardiac changes, *i.e.*, the intensity, volume, muscle mass activation, and rest intervals.

RT elicits very small to no changes in left ventricular cavity size as chamber size increases respond to volume overload. Some studies have shown lifters to have larger chamber size than untrained controls (17,54) whereas others have shown no differences (31). Expression of chamber size relative to body surface area or LBM reduces the increases seen in lifters (17). Bodybuilders, but not weightlifters, may have greater left ventricle chamber volume than controls (11) possibly due to integrated training.

CARDIAC OUTPUT

The CV system adapts by augmenting the Q_c response to exercise. Aerobic training has a profound influence on SV. Resting and exercise-induced SV are enhanced. Untrained individuals possess a SV response of 80–110 mL to exercise; however, trained and highly trained endurance athletes possess a SV response of 130–150 mL and 160 to >220 mL during exercise, respectively (85). Aerobic training leads to greater PV and end-diastolic volume. Coupled with greater cardiac contractility, elastic recoil, and reduced HR (to enhance filling time), SV increases in aerobically trained individuals allowing more blood pumped per beat (85). Ejection fraction during exercise may increase (85). Greater end-diastolic volume with similar end-systolic volume yields a greater SV response.

Aerobic training reduces resting HR. An untrained individual may have a resting HR of 60–80 bpm on average. However, AT reduces resting HR to <60 bpm and some elite endurance athletes have a resting HR of <35 bpm (85). The reduced resting HR is due to greater parasympathetic or reduced sympathetic nervous system stimulation. Aerobic training leads to a reduced HR response to submaximal exercise (Fig. 8.10) and a quicker recovery of HR immediately after exercise. Because SV is increased, HR does not need to increase much to attain a threshold Q_c. However, the HR response to maximal exercise is constant. Although some endurance athletes have maximal HR lower than age-matched controls, often maximal HR remains similar during AT (85). When coupled together (greater SV and similar maximal HR), Q_c increases with improved fitness. Elite endurance athletes have Q_c > 30 L min^{-1} during maximal exercise (85).

Resting SV may slightly increase or not change (expressed relative to LBM) during RT (17). SV is related to body size. Muscle hypertrophy is a stimulus for SV increases, and SV increases during exercise after RT. Strength-trained athletes have greater SV responses and ejection fraction increases during static exercise than controls (1,16). During each rep, SV falls (as intrathoracic pressure increases when a Valsalva maneuver is present)

during the CON and ECC phases by nearly 20 mL but returns to baseline during the intraset rest interval (46). However, SV rises higher than resting level during rest intervals between exercises. The response is augmented in strength athletes but far less than that observed in endurance athletes.

Resting HR may not change or slightly decrease during RT. Short-term RT studies have shown reduced resting HR of 4%–13% (17). The largest effects occur in individuals who have below-average aerobic conditioning. The program is critical as more continuous types of programs, e.g., circuit weight training, reduce resting HR (84), and increase Vo_{2max} (22,27). Nevertheless, any potential HR reduction from RT is much lower than AT. Junior and senior Olympic weightlifters, powerlifters, and bodybuilders had resting HR ranging from 60 to 78 bpm, which was similar to or slightly lower than matched controls (17). Greater reductions in resting HR occur when AT is performed in addition to RT. After RT, the HR response to exercise is decreased for a given submaximal workload (17). The reduction in exercise HR occurs for RT and other exercise modalities such as walking and cycling (17). Bodybuilders have lower HR during submaximal and maximal lifting compared to lesser-trained individuals and controls (18). These data show that RT lessens the stress to the heart during regular physical activity. The culmination of HR and SV data indicate that RT increases the capacity to increase Q_c during exercise but to a lesser extent than AT.

VO$_2$ MAX

Vo_{2max} is the gold standard of aerobic fitness and increases during training due to increases in SV (and Q_c) and a small increase in the A-VO$_2$ difference (up to 20 mL, or 15%) (5,53). Aerobic training is the preferred mode of exercise for increasing Vo_{2max}. Aerobic training leads to Vo_{2max} increases of 10%–30% during the first 6 months (5). Endurance athletes possess higher Vo_{2max} than anaerobic or mixed athletes. Figure 8.11 shows that male endurance athletes (cross-country skiers, distance runners, and cyclists) have higher Vo_{2max} values than do mixed athletes (soccer and basketball players) and strength athletes (bodybuilders, powerlifters, and weightlifters). Elite athletes Bjorn Daehlie (retired Olympic champion cross-country skier), Lance Armstrong (multi Tour de France winner), and Greg LeMond (retired multi Tour de France winner) had Vo_{2max} values of 96, 84, and 92.5 mL kg^{-1} min^{-1}, respectively. Several factors influence Vo_{2max}, such as exercise mode (Vo_{2max} is higher during treadmill tests than cycling or swimming), gender (women have Vo_{2max} values 15%–30% lower than men due to less muscle mass, higher body fat, less testosterone, and lower hemoglobin), age (Vo_{2max} declines with age), body size, and genetics (53). Genetics contribute ~20%–50% to Vo_{2max} (5,53).

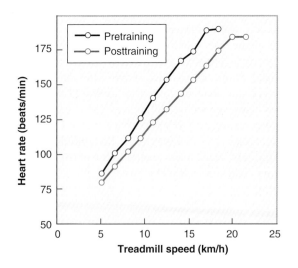

■ **FIGURE 8.10.** Heart rate response during exercise before and after training. (Reprinted with permission from Wilmore JH, Costill DL. *Physiology of Sport and Exercise.* 2nd ed. Champaign (IL): Human Kinetics; 1999.)

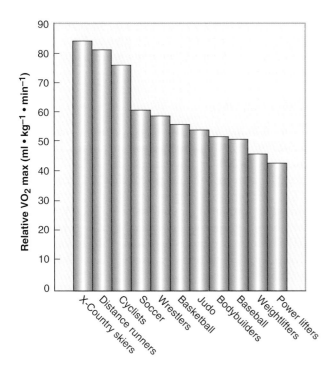

FIGURE 8.11. Comparison of Vo_{2max} data from different male athletes. (Data compiled from McArdle WD, Katch FI, Katch VL. *Exercise Physiology: Energy, Nutrition, and Human Performance.* 6th ed. Philadelphia (PA): Lippincott Williams & Wilkins; 2007. pp. 314–363; Hoffman JR. *Norms for Fitness, Performance, and Health.* Champaign (IL): Human Kinetics; 2006. pp. 67–80; Hakkinen K, Alen M, Komi PV. Neuromuscular, anaerobic, and aerobic performance characteristics of elite power athletes. *Eur J Appl Physiol Occup Physiol.* 1984;53:97–105; MacFarlane N, Northridge DB, Wright AR, Grant S, Dargie HJ. A comparative study of left ventricular structure and function in elite athletes. *Br J Sports Med.* 1991;25:45–48; and Raven PB, Gettman LR, Pollock ML, Cooper KH. A physiological evaluation of professional soccer players. *Br J Sports Med.* 1976;10:209–216.)

Anaerobic training has minimal effects on increasing Vo_{2max}. Weightlifters and powerlifters have Vo_{2max} values similar to or slightly larger than untrained individuals. In comparison, bodybuilders have larger Vo_{2max} values than other lifters (28) because bodybuilders train with short rest intervals and aerobically train. RT with long rest intervals allows HR recovery between sets and rarely reaches a threshold VO_2 level needed to increase Vo_{2max} in trained individuals. RT may increase Vo_{2max} in populations with low levels of aerobic fitness. Olympic weightlifting programs (17,74) and circuit weight training can increase Vo_{2max} by up to 8% (22,27). However, if RT elicits an increased Vo_{2max}, the magnitude is far less than AT. The combination of RT and AT increases Vo_{2max}. Performing RT lessens the volume of AT needed to increase Vo_{2max} (56). Programs of moderate to high intensity, high volume, large muscle mass exercises, and short rest intervals may slightly improve Vo_{2max}. Sprint training can increase Vo_{2max} (50). Sprints that are long in duration with short rest intervals can modestly increase Vo_{2max} but is inferior to AT.

SIDEBAR **LIMITATIONS OF VO$_2$ MAX**

One topic of debate in the exercise sciences is the question, what factors limit Vo_{2max}? Everyone has an upper limit to Vo_{2max} and debate has centered on factors limiting Vo_{2max}. Central and peripheral factors have been identified and some have argued for central whereas some have argued for peripheral limitations (71). Central factors entail limitations in oxygen delivery and include Q_c (estimated to account for ~70%–85% of limitation), SV (due to pericardial restraint), oxygen-carrying capacity, and arterial saturation (14). Oxygen delivery can limit Vo_{2max}. Beginning in the lungs, a limitation with alveolar diffusion of oxygen from the atmosphere to hemoglobin in the blood reduces oxygen delivery to mitochondria. Some highly trained endurance athletes experience arterial desaturation during maximal exercise to ~87%, which is 5% lower than expected. This reduction decreased Vo_{2max} by ~5 mL · kg^{-1} min^{-1} (77) but only accounts for Vo_{2max} limitations in trained athletes. Mechanical limits to ventilation that are reached in conjunction with attainment of Vo_{2max} occur in endurance athletes; the greater the ventilatory response, the greater the degree of mechanical limitation (39). Expiratory flow limitations can reduce hyperventilation and may limit pulmonary function during maximal exercise (26). Limitations on SV and Q_c limit Vo_{2max}. Comparative studies between one- and two-leg and arm exercise showed that muscle blood flow was limited when large amounts of muscle mass were activated (showing Q_c could not keep up with the demand). Blood doping increases Vo_{2max} showing oxygen-carrying capacity and blood volumes are limitations.

Peripheral factors entail oxygen transfer from the capillary bed to the mitochondria and include A-VO2 difference, mitochondrial number and enzyme activity, and capillary density. Oxygen extraction from blood requires dissociation from hemoglobin, diffusion of oxygen from RBCs into muscle fibers, and diffusion and transport of oxygen to the mitochondria. Myoglobin facilitates oxygen dissociation from hemoglobin (in addition to the PO2 gradient) as myoglobin's affinity for oxygen is approximately five times greater than hemoglobin. Some have argued that in highly trained aerobic athletes, blood flow rate is so great that blood passes by muscle too rapidly to allow for optimal oxygen diffusion. This effect may be minimal, however, as capillary density increases, which increases surface area for diffusion and controls blood flow velocity. Lastly, the number and size of mitochondria, as well as mitochondrial enzyme activity, play critical roles (85). Because AT increases mitochondrial size, density, and enzyme activity, the athlete's ability to utilize oxygen increases. It seems that no one single factor limits Vo_{2max}, but all contribute.

BLOOD PRESSURE

Aerobic training may lead to reduced SBP and DBP at rest (85). An individual with normal BP may or may not experience a reduction in BP following endurance training, but a hypertensive individual most likely will see reductions. In the most recent American College of Sports Medicine (ACSM) Position Stand on Exercise and Hypertension (3), it was concluded on an abundance of research that BP decreases following AT although the adaptations are quite variable. These studies reported that SBP drops ~3.4–4.7 mm Hg and DBP drops ~2.4–3.1 mm Hg, with the largest drops seen in hypertensive groups. The mechanisms involved are not completely understood. However, alterations in sodium excretion, decreased peripheral resistance, improved vasodilation, and reduced sympathetic nervous system activity and catecholamine release play substantial roles (3,85). The BP response to submax and maximal exercise may not change or only be slightly reduced by 6–7 mm Hg during submaximal exercise (3). World-class endurance runners have similar acute SBP responses to untrained individuals (~205–210 mm Hg) during maximal exercise but have lower DBP values (~65 vs. 80 mm Hg) (85). The ACSM recommends at least moderate intensity (40%–60% of VO_2 reserve) continuous aerobic exercise for 30 min day^{-1} to reduce BP (3).

RT may not affect or reduce resting BP. Strength-trained athletes have average or below-average resting BP (17). A meta-analysis of the RT literature has shown that SBP and DBP may be reduced by 2%–4% (40,41). The ACSM concludes that RT decreases BP in adults (3). A small 3 mm Hg reduction in BP decreases the risk of CV disease by 5%–9% and stroke by 8%–14% (3). The **rate pressure product** (HR × SBP) is used to estimate myocardial work and decreases after RT (17). This indicates the left ventricle performs less work over time and is a positive adaptation (17). After RT, the acute BP response to exercise is lower (17,34).

BLOOD VOLUME

Aerobic training increases blood volume, or **hypervolemia**, mostly from an increase in plasma (85). PV increases 12%–20% within the first few weeks of AT with noticeable increases taking place after the first workout (53). Endurance athletes have blood volumes ~35% greater than untrained individuals (53). The PV increase is attributed to hormonal changes (aldosterone and ADH) and increased protein content in the blood, which increases the osmotic pressure forcing greater fluid movement (85). RBC content may increase, which contributes to the greater blood volume. PV expands more than the RBC number increases, thereby leading to a decrease in hematocrit (34). The increased blood volume, along with greater capillary density, vasodilation, and more effective blood redistribution, contributes to greater blood flow to working skeletal muscles in endurance-trained athletes (85). Aerobic training reduces blood flow to muscles during submaximal exercise (due to greater oxidative potential and vasodilation of skeletal muscles) and increases blood flow during maximal exercise (due to greater Q_c, redistribution of blood, and increased capillary density and arteriogenesis) (53). The increased blood volume is a critical adaptation that allows SV to increase via the Frank-Starling mechanism. A substantial reduction in PV expansion can be observed within 1 week of detraining (53). Less is known concerning hypervolemia following RT although it is thought that RT may have a limited effect.

Myths & Misconceptions

Resistance Training is Bad for the Heart and Increases Blood Pressure

In the past, some have criticized RT as having negative CV effects on the heart. The evidence overwhelming supports RT as having positive benefits for the heart. Because of the pressure overload, changes in cardiac wall thickness enable individuals to tolerate greater stress. The heart becomes stronger and more resistant to stress. Although the adaptations are less comprehensive than AT, concentric hypertrophy poses health and wellness benefits to the individual. Some feared RT due to the myth that it causes chronic elevated BP or hypertension. As eloquently stated in the ACSM's position stand (3), RT at the very least will cause no change or can decrease resting BP over time. Although an acute rise in BP is observed during a workout (via a rise in intrathoracic pressure and peripheral resistance), the heart adapts to where BP can be reduced following and be lower over time during physical activity. Although BP may increase at rest in individuals who use anabolic steroids or are overtrained, these are exceptions and not the norm. Overwhelming evidence supports RT as safe and beneficial for the CV system and is recommended in some form by the ACSM for essentially all healthy and clinical populations.

BLOOD LIPIDS AND LIPOPROTEINS

Lipids perform several critical functions including energy storage and liberation, protection, insulation, providing structure to cell membranes, vitamin transport, and cellular signaling. Circulating blood lipids and lipoproteins are major factors for CV health. These include triglycerides (glycerol backbone with three fatty acids), cholesterol, low-density lipoprotein cholesterol (LDL-C), very low-density lipoprotein cholesterol (VLDL-C), high-density lipoprotein cholesterol (HDL-C), and lipoprotein A. Cholesterol plays several critical roles including serving as a precursor in steroid synthesis, cell membrane structure, and bile and vitamin D synthesis. However, elevated cholesterol is a risk factor for CV disease. Lipoproteins provide the major means lipids are transported in the blood. Elevations in LDL-C (carry ~60%–80% of total cholesterol) and VLDL-C (transport triglycerides to muscle and adipose tissue and contain the highest lipid component) pose major risk factors whereas elevations in HDL-C lower the risk for CV disease. Lipoprotein A is thought to play a role in coagulation but at high levels is atherogenic. Triglyceride levels of <150 mg dL^{-1}, total cholesterol levels <200 mg dL^{-1}, LDL-C <100 mg dL^{-1}, HDL-C >40 mg dL^{-1}, and lipoprotein A <14 mg dL^{-1} are recommended values for minimizing risk factors for CV disease (53).

Several factors influence blood lipid and lipoprotein content including genetics. Diet is the major factor for increasing HDLs and decreasing LDLs and VLDLs. High dietary fiber intake, mono- and polyunsaturated fats, low saturated and *trans* fat intake, and low alcohol consumption positively affect blood lipid and lipoprotein levels. Reducing stress and eliminating cigarette smoking have substantial positive effects. Blood lipid and lipoprotein levels are coupled with changes in body weight, so weight reduction is critical to lowering blood lipids (85). Exercise produces favorable changes and reduces risk factors for CV disease (independent of weight loss). Reductions in total cholesterol, triglycerides, and LDL-C with concomitant increases in HDL-C occur following AT (85) whereas some studies have shown minimal changes. The increases in HDL-C appear more responsive to AT than LDL-C reductions (53). The ratio of LDL-C to total cholesterol/HDL-C (a major CV risk factor) decreases following AT (85). A dose-response relationship is seen where a threshold of exercise volume/duration is needed. Some suggest the threshold may be ~15–20 miles per week or 1,200–2,200 kcal of energy expenditure per week (15). This exercise level is associated with 2–3 mg dL^{-1} increases in HDL-C and 8–20 mg dL^{-1} reductions in blood triglycerides (15). Higher levels of AT may produce more substantial changes as aerobic athletes (with high Vo$_{2max}$) have much higher HDL-C and lower blood triglycerides than nonathletes (15,85). Lipoprotein A does not change during training or dietary changes; however, distance runners and bodybuilders have shown elevations (52).

RT may have no or very small effects in improving blood lipid and lipoprotein profiles. RT may increase HDL-C by 10%–15%, decrease LDL-C by 5%–39%, decrease total cholesterol by 3%–16%, or produce no changes or slight increases in LDL-C (17). Strength-trained athletes have normal, lower, or higher HDL-C, LDL-C, and total cholesterol (17). Several confounding variables are thought to influence these results. Some studies did not adequately control for diet or weight loss. Cross-sectional studies cannot eliminate other factors such as AT. Bodybuilders have lower total cholesterol, LDL-C, and VLDL-C compared to weight-matched controls (86) and powerlifters have lower HDL-C and higher LDL-C than bodybuilders and runners (37). However, bodybuilders perform AT, so it is difficult to ascertain how much of a role AT played in these results. Anabolic steroid (alone and in combination with human growth hormone) use increases LDL-C by up to 61%, total cholesterol, decrease HDL-C by up to 55%, increase LDL-C to HDL-C ratio by more than 300% (37,72,81,88), and increases coronary artery calcification (72) with the negative effects reversed upon discontinuation in a time frame dependent on the magnitude and duration of steroid use (30,44). Other lipoproteins (lipoprotein-A) and *apolipoprotein* variants (proteins that bind to fats to form lipoproteins) are negatively affected by anabolic steroid use (30). Independent effects of RT do not change or slightly improve blood lipid and lipoprotein profiles. It is thought that RT volume plays a significant role, similar to AT, as reductions have been seen during high-volume phases (17). The best way to improve lipid and lipoprotein profiles is to combine proper diet with AT and RT.

Case Study 8.1

Ben is a high school soccer player who is going to begin an off-season strength and conditioning program. The program consists of total-body RT for 2 days per week and endurance training (running) for 3 days per week. He was told that RT and AT would yield positive benefits to his heart and would increase his stamina on the field. However, Ben is an inquisitive student athlete and was searching for a response that was more specific and physiologically based.

Question for Consideration: How would you describe the CV benefits of strength and endurance training to Ben?

THE RESPIRATORY SYSTEM

The respiratory system is essential for introducing oxygen into the body and removing CO_2. Respiration includes breathing, pulmonary diffusion, oxygen transport, and gas

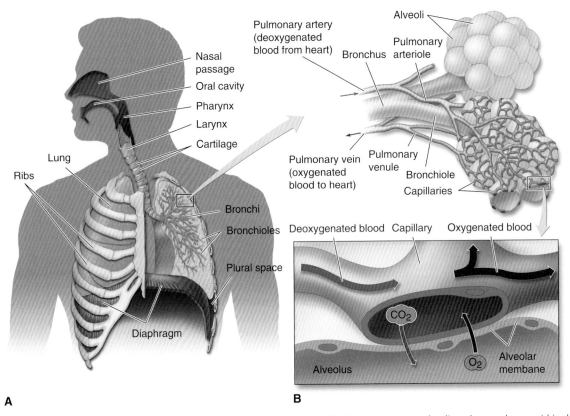

A

B

■ **FIGURE 8.12.** The human respiratory system. **A.** Major pulmonary structures. **B.** Respiratory passages, alveoli, and gas exchange within the alveoli. (From McArdle WD, Katch FI, Katch VL. *Exercise Physiology: Nutrition, Energy, and Human Performance.* 7th ed. Baltimore (MD): Lippincott Williams & Wilkins; 2010.)

exchange (Fig. 8.12). Breathing brings air into and out of the lungs. The average-size adult's lungs weigh ~1 kg and can hold ~ 4–6 L of air (53). Air enters the body through the nose or mouth and travels through the pharynx, larynx, trachea, bronchi, bronchioles, and the alveoli. The alveoli are sites of gas exchange. **Inspiration** is an active event that leads to air entering the lungs. Several muscles contract but inspiration is largely due to contraction of the diaphragm and external intercostal muscles. The diaphragm is a large dome-shaped muscle that provides airtight separation between the thoracic and abdominal cavities. During exercise, several other rib cage and abdominal muscles contract to support forced breathing. Muscle contraction causes the ribs to move up and out thereby expanding the thorax. The diaphragm contracts, flattens, and moves as much as 10 cm (53). The pressure in the lungs decreases (as space increases) causing air from the outside to enter. A pressure gradient is formed where the pressure in the lungs (*intrapulmonary pressure*) is lower than the pressure outside of the body. The pressure gradient allows air to move into the lungs. At the end of inspiration, the pressure in the lungs and outside of the body equilibrates. **Expiration** is a passive process (at rest) where air exits the lungs and the body. During expiration, inspiratory muscles relax, the diaphragm rises (relaxes), and the thorax is depressed as air exits. The lung pressure is greater than the pressure outside

of the body. Air exits and is greatly enhanced by elastic recoil of the lungs. The lungs contain *surfactant*, which reduces surface tension on the alveoli and increases lung compliance. During exercise, other muscles (*e.g.*, abdominal muscles) contract for forced breathing. Air enters the alveoli where gas exchange takes place. Pulmonary diffusion involves the diffusion of oxygen from the alveoli into the pulmonary capillaries across the thin (0.5–4.0 μm) respiratory membrane. The lungs contain >600 million alveoli with a large blood supply and have thin walls that greatly expand the opportunity for gas exchange (53).

LUNG VOLUMES AND CAPACITIES

Several lung volumes and capacities are used to measure lung function. These include

- *Tidal volume:* volume of air inspired or expired every breath (~500 mL in women and ~600 mL in men)
- *Inspiratory reserve volume:* volume of air inspired after normal tidal volume (~1,900 mL in women and ~3,000 mL in men)
- *Expiratory reserve volume:* volume of air expired after normal tidal volume (~800 mL in women and ~1,200 mL in men)
- *Residual volume:* volume of air left in lungs after maximal expiration (~1,000 mL in women and ~1,200 mL in men)

- *Total lung capacity:* volume of air in lungs after maximal inspiration (~4,200 mL in women and ~6,000 mL in men)
- *Forced vital capacity:* maximal volume of air expired after maximal inspiration (~3,200 mL in women and ~4,800 mL in men)
- *Inspiratory capacity:* maximal volume of air after tidal volume expiration (~2,400 mL in women and ~3,600 mL in men)
- *Functional residual capacity:* volume of air in lungs after tidal volume expiration (~1,800 mL in women and ~2,400 mL in men)
- *Forced expiratory volume (FEV$_1$):* volume of air maximally expired forcefully in 1 second after maximal inhalation. Often expressed relative to forced vital capacity and is typically ~85%.
- *Maximum voluntary ventilation (MVV):* maximum volume of air breathed rapidly in 1 minute (~80–120 L min^{-1} in women and 140–180 L min^{-1} in men).
- *Minute ventilation (V$_E$):* volume of air breathed per minute; is the product of breathing rate and tidal volume. At rest, is typically 6 L min^{-1} (12 breaths min^{-1} × 0.5 L). During exercise, breathing rate increase to 35–45 breaths min^{-1} to healthy adults but may increase to 60–70 breaths min^{-1} in elite endurance athletes (53). Tidal volume increases during exercise up to 2.0 L leading to V$_E$ increases of 100 L min^{-1} or more (53). At high exercise intensities, an increase in breathing rate more than tidal volume accounts for the rise in V$_E$ (12). Elite endurance athletes have values of >160–180 L min^{-1} (53,85). V$_E$ increases linearly as VO$_2$ rises. However, V$_E$ increases exponentially after the **ventilatory threshold** (the point at which V$_E$ and CO$_2$ rise exponentially) is reached (53). During resistance exercise, short rest intervals and higher volume produce greater acute increases in V$_E$ (64). Peak value obtained postexercise using 30-second rest intervals for 10 RM sets (5 sets) was 68.2 L min^{-1} compared to 44.8 L min^{-1} when 5-minute rest intervals were used (64), still considerably lower than values seen during endurance exercise. Not all air that enters the body reaches the alveoli. Some air remains in the nose, mouth, trachea, and other areas (*anatomic dead space*) and ranges between 150 and 200 mL (53). The air that reaches the alveoli is known as alveolar ventilation.

CONTROL OF BREATHING

Breathing is an involuntary action but can be controlled voluntarily to some extent. Ventilation is controlled by neural and humoral factors (Fig. 8.13). The medulla oblongata and pons of the brainstem contain respiratory

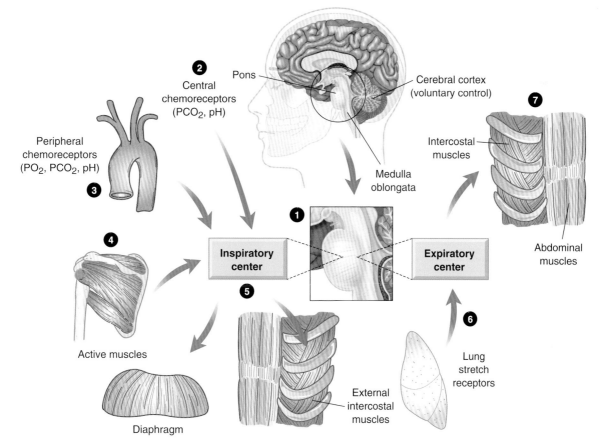

■ **FIGURE 8.13.** Overview of respiratory control. (Adapted with permission from Wilmore JH, Costill DL. *Physiology of Sport and Exercise*. 2nd ed. Champaign (IL): Human Kinetics; 1999:260.)

centers that control inspiration and expiration. Large networks of respiratory neurons conduct action potentials via the spinal cord to the phrenic nerve (stimulates the diaphragm), intercostal, abdominal muscle motor nerves (12) to control rate and depth of breathing. Inspiration results in stretching of the lungs that stimulates stretch receptors and inhibits further inspiration and stimulates expiration. The lack of stretch during deflation stimulates the respiratory neurons to increase inspiration. Inspiratory muscles relax and expiration occurs passively. Precise coordination of motor output to respiratory muscles is critical. Inspiratory and expiratory groups of neurons in the brainstem discharge independently and not simultaneously (12). Inspiratory neuronal discharge inhibits expiratory neuronal discharge and vice versa via reciprocal inhibition which enables full inspiration and expiration to take place, respectively. Proprioceptors located in joints and skeletal muscles stimulate the respiratory centers to alter ventilation during exercise (53). Parallel communication with the motor cortex, cerebellum, and the hypothalamus stimulate the respiratory centers during exercise via a process known as *central command* (12). Rhythmic muscle contraction and frequency of muscular contractions (as seen in AT) provide potent feedback to respiratory centers whereas increased muscle contraction force poses little effect on increasing V_E during exercise (12).

Circulatory (humoral) factors play substantial roles in ventilation. Changes in arterial PO_2, PCO_2, pH, and temperature provide feedback to the medulla to control ventilation. Reduced PO_2 stimulates increased V_E. Oxygen levels (and PCO_2 and pH) are detected by peripheral *chemoreceptors* located in the aorta and carotid bodies, and low PO_2 stimulates respiratory centers to increase V_E at rest and during exercise. However, V_E changes during exercise are more sensitive to reductions in pH, increased temperature, and increased PCO_2. Higher ventilation rates are especially important during exercise to reduce acidity by removing excess CO_2. Hyperventilation decreases PCO_2 and is important for reducing acidity.

During exercise, there is a rapid increase in V_E followed by a slower rise as exercise progresses (Fig. 8.14). A rise in VO_2 and VCO_2 occur in an intensity-dependent manner with a reduction in respiratory dead space (12). The initial steep rise may be produced by feedback from proprioceptors in joints and muscles and the motor cortex that stimulates contraction of inspiratory muscles (85). The increased V_E is proportional to increases in VCO_2 and oxygen demand. The gradual increase as exercise progresses may be due to peripheral feedback from reduced pH and increased PCO_2 (85). Rapid recovery is seen at the completion of exercise.

PULMONARY ADAPTATIONS TO TRAINING

There is little change in lung volumes and capacities with AT. Vital capacity may increase slightly or not change, and

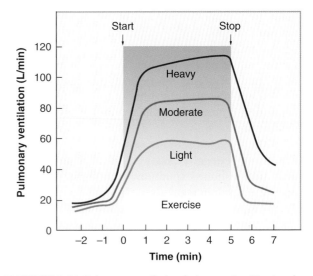

FIGURE 8.14. Pulmonary ventilation during exercise. (Reprinted with permission from Wilmore JH, Costill DL. *Physiology of Sport and Exercise*. 2nd ed. Champaign (IL): Human Kinetics; 1999.)

residual volume may slightly decrease (85). Tidal volume does not change at rest or low-intensity exercise, but will increase during maximal exercise especially in endurance-trained athletes (12,85). Respiratory rate decreases at rest and during submaximal exercise, but increases during maximal exercise (85). Pulmonary V_E (and alveolar ventilation) does not change or may slightly decrease at rest and during submaximal exercise, but increases during maximal exercise to high levels in trained endurance athletes (12,85). Resistance-trained individuals have similar resting V_E values to untrained individuals (64). Pulmonary diffusion does not change at rest or during submaximal exercise but increases during maximal exercise (85). Gender differences exist. Women have pulmonary structural differences than age- and height-matched men that include smaller vital capacity and maximal expiratory flow rates, reduced airway diameter, and a smaller diffusion surface (29). Women have smaller airways and lung volumes, lower resting maximal expiratory flow rates, and have higher metabolic costs of breathing relative to men (75). Female athletes develop expiratory flow limitations more often than men, and have greater increases in end-expiratory and end-inspiratory lung volume at maximal exercise (75). Female athletes have ~7% and 6% greater end-inspiratory and end-expiratory lung volumes, respectively, compared to men (26). Women have a higher work cost of breathing that is twice that of men at ventilations >90 L min^{-1} (26).

VENTILATORY MUSCLE-SPECIFIC TRAINING

Ventilatory muscle-specific training, or *inspiratory muscle training* (IMT), involves RT during respiration. IMT is a technique used to increase respiratory function by improving strength and endurance of inhalation muscles. IMT comprises two popular methods of resistive breathing. One method involves breathing forcefully into a mouthpiece attached to a T-piece with a one-way valve on one side and an inspiratory resistance located on the other side. The valve closes during inspiration so the individual breathes against the resistance (a percent of one's *maximal inspiratory mouth pressure*), and expiration is unimpeded. Another modality includes threshold loading. A mouthpiece connected to a valve is used which is attached to a threshold loading device. IMT increases strength and endurance in respiratory muscles and is used to improve physical function and reduce painful breathing in clinical populations such as those with chronic obstructive pulmonary disease (COPD) (4,21,59). The ACSM recommends IMT for 30 min day^{-1} or two 15-minute sessions daily, 4–5 days per week at at least 30% of one's maximal inspiratory pressure (4). IMT increases respiratory muscle strength and endurance by >28% in athletes (38,42,67,82). However, effects on maximal endurance and Vo_{2max} are limited (38,67,76,82) although some studies have shown small improvements in performance (25) and recovery from sprint exercise (68). Maximal inspiratory mouth pressure does not correlate to Vo_{2max} (42) therefore demonstrating that improvements in respiratory muscle strength may not translate to greater endurance.

■ Summary Points

✔ The cardiorespiratory system includes the heart, blood vessels, lungs, and associated respiratory muscles. Oxygenated blood from the lungs returns to the heart (left atrium) and is pumped to the rest of the body via the left ventricle. Deoxygenated blood returns to the right atrium and is transported to the lungs in a cyclical process.

✔ Aerobic and anaerobic exercises result in pressure overload (rise in BP and intrathoracic pressure) on the heart whereas aerobic exercise increases volume overload (greater venous return and blood flow) to the heart. Pressure overload yields adaptations in cardiac wall muscularity (primarily the left ventricle) whereas volume overload yields increased cardiac chamber size.

✔ Key CV variables include HR, BP, SV (and ejection fraction), and Q_c. AT leads to lower HR, BP, increased SV, and Q_c at rest. RT produces minor changes at rest.

✔ AT and RT can lead to a reduced HR and BP response to submaximal exercise.

✔ Vo_{2max} is most improved via AT whereas anaerobic training only produces small increases at best.

✔ Few changes are observed in pulmonary function at rest and during submaximal exercise following aerobic and anaerobic training. However, acute pulmonary response is enhanced during maximal exercise after AT.

Review Questions

1. As an adaptation to RT
   a. Right ventricular wall increases in thickness and septal wall thickness decreases
   b. BP (systolic and diastolic) increases
   c. Total cholesterol increases
   d. Resting HR and systolic and diastolic BP may decrease slightly

2. The Fick equation states that Vo_{2max} is the product of Q_c and _____
   a. A-VO_2 difference
   b. SV
   c. HR
   d. SBP

3. The part of the heart that pumps blood to the rest of the body is the
   a. Right atrium
   b. Left atrium
   c. Right ventricle
   d. Left ventricle

4. A highly trained endurance athlete may reach a SV of _____ during maximal exercise
   a. 70 mL
   b. 90 mL
   c. 120 mL
   d. 180 mL

5. The volume of air in the lungs after maximal inspiration is known as _____
   a. Residual volume
   b. Tidal volume
   c. Total lung capacity
   d. Minute ventilation

6. Although RT is not the most potent modality to stimulate improvements in Vo_{2max}, which of the following workouts would most likely lead to a higher Vo_{2max}?
   a. 5 exercises for the upper body, 3 sets of 6–8 reps each, 3-minute rest intervals
   b. 8 exercises — total body, 3 sets of 8–10 reps each, 2-minute rest intervals
   c. 5 exercises — lower body, 1 set of 10–12 reps each, 1-minute rest intervals
   d. 10 exercises — total body, 1 set of 10–12 reps performed in a circuit, 3 circuits performed altogether, 15-second rest intervals

7. The rhythm of a healthy heart initiates in the SA node.   T F

8. An increase in pH and decrease in temperature increase oxygen dissociation from hemoglobin during exercise.   T F

9. RT can increase left ventricular wall thickness.   T F

10. A Valsalva maneuver used during weightlifting decreases intra-abdominal pressure and BP and reduces torso rigidity.   T F

11. The volume of air left in lungs after maximal expiration is minute ventilation.   T F

12. The ACSM recommends inspiratory muscle training for 30 min day⁻¹ or two 15-minute sessions per day, 4–5 days per week at least 30% of one's maximal inspiratory pressure for those striving to improve respiratory strength and endurance.   T F

References

1. Adler Y, Fisman EZ, Koren-Morag N, et al. Left ventricular diastolic function in trained male weight lifters at rest and during isometric exercise. *Am J Cardiol.* 2008;102:97–101.

2. American College of Sports Medicine. The use of blood doping as an ergogenic aid. *Med Sci Sports Exerc.* 1996;28:i–viii.

3. American College of Sports Medicine. Position stand: exercise and hypertension. *Med Sci Sports Exerc.* 2004;36:533–553.

4. American College of Sports Medicine. *ACSM's Guidelines for Exercise Testing and Prescription.* 8th ed. Philadelphia (PA): Lippincott Williams & Wilkins; 2010. pp. 262–263.

5. Brawner CA, Keteyian SJ, Saval M. Adaptations to cardiorespiratory exercise training. In: *ACSM's Resource Manual for Guidelines for Exercise Testing and Prescription.* 6th ed. Philadelphia (PA): Lippincott Williams & Wilkins; 2010. pp. 476–488.

6. Bredt DS. Endogenous nitric oxide synthesis: biological functions and pathophysiology. *Free Radic Res.* 1999;31:577–596.

7. Brien AJ, Simon TL. The effects of red blood cell infusion on 10-km race time. *JAMA.* 1987;257:2761–2765.

8. Collins MA, Hill DW, Cureton KJ, DeMello JJ. Plasma volume change during heavy-resistance weight lifting. *Eur J Appl Physiol Occup Physiol.* 1986;55:44–48.

9. Collins MA, Cureton KJ, Hill DW, Ray CA. Relation of plasma volume change to intensity of weight lifting. *Med Sci Sports Exerc.* 1989;21:178–185.

10. Craig SK, Byrnes WC, Fleck SJ. Plasma volume during weight lifting. *Int J Sports Med.* 2008;29:89–95.

11. Deligiannis A, Zahopoulou E, Mandroukas K. Echocardiographic study of cardiac dimensions and function in weight lifters and body builders. *Int J Sports Cardiol.* 1988;5:24–32.

12. Dempsey JA, Miller JD, Romer LM. The respiratory system. In: Tipton CM, editor. *ACSM's Advanced Exercise Physiology.* Philadelphia (PA): Lippincott Williams & Wilkins; 2006. pp. 246–299.

13. Dickerman RD, Schaller F, Zachariah NY, McConathy WJ. Left ventricular size and function in elite bodybuilders using anabolic steroids. *Clin J Sports Med.* 1997;7:90–93.

14. Di Prampero PE. Metabolic and circulatory limitations to Vo_{2max} at the whole animal level. *J Exp Biol.* 1985;115:319–331.

15. Durstine JL, Grandjean PW, Davis PG, et al. Blood lipid and lipoprotein adaptations to exercise: a quantitative analysis. *Sports Med.* 2001;31:1033–1062.

16. Fisman EZ, Embon P, Pines A, et al. Comparison of left ventricular function using isometric exercise Doppler echocardiography in competitive runners and weightlifters versus sedentary individuals. *Am J Cardiol.* 1997;79:355–359.

17. Fleck SJ. Cardiovascular responses to strength training. In: Komi PV, editor. *Strength and Power in Sport.* 2nd ed. Malden (MA): Blackwell Science; 2003. pp. 387–406.

18. Fleck SJ, Dean LS. Resistance-training experience and the pressor response during resistance exercise. *J Appl Physiol.* 1987;63:116–120.

19. Fleck SJ, Henke C, Wilson W. Cardiac MRI of elite junior weight lifters. *Int J Sports Med.* 1989;10:329–333.

20. Fleck SJ, Pattany PM, Stone MH, Kraemer WJ, Thrush J, Wong K. Magnetic resonance imaging determination of left ventricular mass: junior Olympic weightlifters. *Med Sci Sports Exerc.* 1993;25:522–527.

21. Geddes EL, O'Brien K, Reid WD, Brooks D, Crowe J. Inspiratory muscle training in adults with chronic obstructive pulmonary disease: an update of a systematic review. *Respir Med.* 2008;102:1715–1729.

22. Gettman LR, Ward P, Hagan RD. A comparison of combined running and weight training with circuit weight training. *Med Sci Sports Exerc.* 1982;14:229–234.

23. Gledhill N, Warburton D, Jamnik V. Haemoglobin, blood volume, cardiac function, and aerobic power. *Can J Appl Physiol.* 1999;24:54–65.

24. Gotshall RW, Gootman J, Byrnes WC, Fleck SJ, Valovich TC. Noninvasive characterization of the blood pressure response to the double-leg press exercise. *J Exerc Physiol.* (online) 1999;2:1–6.

25. Griffiths LA, McConnell AK. The influence of inspiratory and expiratory muscle training upon rowing performance. *Eur J Appl Physiol.* 2007;99:457–466.

26. Guenette JA, Witt JD, McKenzie DC, Road JD, Sheel AW. Respiratory mechanics during exercise in endurance-trained men and women. *J Physiol.* 2007;581:1309–1322.

27. Haennel R, Teo KK, Quinney A, Kappagoda T. Effects of hydraulic circuit training on cardiovascular function. *Med Sci Sports Exerc.* 1989;21:605–612.

28. Hakkinen K, Alen M, Komi PV. Neuromuscular, anaerobic, and aerobic performance characteristics of elite power athletes. *Eur J Appl Physiol Occup Physiol.* 1984;53:97–105.

29. Harms CA. Does gender affect pulmonary function and exercise capacity? *Respir Physiol Neurobiol.* 2006;151:124–131.

30. Hartgens F, Rietjens G, Keiser HA, Kuipers H, Wolffenbuttel BH. Effects of androgenic-anabolic steroids on apolipoproteins and lipoprotein (a). *Br J Sports Med.* 2004;38:253–259.

31. Haykowsky M, Taylor D, Teo K, Quinney A, Humen D. Left ventricular wall stress during leg-press exercise performed with a brief Valsalva maneuver. *Chest.* 2001;119:150–154.

32. Haykowsky MJ, Dressendorfer R, Taylor D, Mandic S, Humen D. Resistance training and cardiac hypertrophy: unraveling the training effect. *Sports Med.* 2002;32:837–849.

33. Hoffman JR. *Norms for Fitness, Performance, and Health.* Champaign (IL): Human Kinetics; 2006. pp. 67–80.

34. Hoffman JR. The cardiorespiratory system. In: Chandler TJ, Brown LE, editors. *Conditioning for Strength and Human Performance.* Philadelphia (PA): Lippincott Williams & Wilkins; 2008. pp. 20–39.

35. Hoffman JR, Ratamess NA. *A Practical Guide to Developing Resistance Training Programs.* 2nd ed. Monterey (CA): Coaches Choice Books; 2008.

36. Housh TJ, Housh DJ, de Vries HA. *Applied Exercise and Sport Physiology*. 2nd ed. Scottsdale (AZ): Holcomb Hathaway Publishers; 2006. pp. 57–80.

37. Hurley BF, Seals DR, Hagberg JM, et al. High-density-lipoprotein cholesterol in bodybuilders v powerlifters. Negative effects of androgen use. *JAMA*. 1984;252:507–513.

38. Inbar O, Weiner P, Azgad Y, Rotstein A, Weinstein Y. Specific inspiratory muscle training in well-trained endurance athletes. *Med Sci Sports Exerc*. 2000;32:1233–1237.

39. Johnson BD, Saupe KW, Dempsey JA. Mechanical constraints on exercise hyperpnea in endurance athletes. *J Appl Physiol*. 1992; 73:874–886.

40. Kelley GA. Dynamic resistance exercise and resting blood pressure in adults: a meta-analysis. *J Appl Physiol*. 1997;82:1559–1565.

41. Kelley GA, Kelley KS. Progressive resistance exercise and resting blood pressure: A meta-analysis of randomized controlled trials. *Hypertension* 2000;35:838–843.

42. Klusiewicz A, Borkowski L, Zdanowicz R, Boros P, Wesolowski S. The inspiratory muscle training in elite rowers. *J Sports Med Phys Fitness*. 2008;48:279–284.

43. Kraemer WJ, Fleck SJ, Maresh CM, et al. Acute hormonal responses to a single bout of heavy resistance exercise in trained power lifters and untrained men. *Can J Appl Physiol*. 1999;24:524–537.

44. Kuipers H, Wijnen JA, Hartgens F, Willems SM. Influence of anabolic steroids on body composition, blood pressure, lipid profile and liver functions in body builders. *Int J Sports Med*. 1991;12: 413–418.

45. Leigh-Smith S. Blood boosting. *Brit J Sports Med*. 2004;38:99–101.

46. Lentini AC, McKelvie RS, McCartney N, Tomlinson CW, MacDougall JD. Left ventricular response in healthy young men during heavy-intensity weight-lifting exercise. *J Appl Physiol*. 1993; 75:2703–2710.

47. Linsenbardt ST, Thomas TR, Madsen RW. Effect of breathing techniques on blood pressure response to resistance exercise. *Br J Sports Med*. 1992;26:97–100.

48. MacDougall JD, Tuxen D, Sale DG, Moroz JR. Arterial blood pressure response to heavy exercise. *J Appl Physiol*. 1985;58:785–790.

49. MacDougall JD, McKelvie RS, Moroz JR, Sale DG, McCartney N, Buick F. Factors affecting blood pressure during heavy weight lifting and static contractions. *J Appl Physiol*. 1992;73:1590–1597.

50. MacDougall JD, Hicks AL, MacDonald JR, et al. Muscle performance and enzymatic adaptations to sprint interval training. *J Appl Physiol*. 1998;84:2138–2142.

51. MacFarlane N, Northridge DB, Wright AR, Grant S, Dargie HJ. A comparative study of left ventricular structure and function in elite athletes. *Br J Sports Med*. 1991;25:45–48.

52. MacKinnon LT, Hubinger LM. Effects of exercise on lipoprotein(a). *Sports Med*. 1999;28:11–24.

53. McArdle WD, Katch FI, Katch VL. *Exercise Physiology: Energy, Nutrition, and Human Performance*. 6th ed. Philadelphia (PA): Lippincott Williams & Wilkins; 2007. pp. 314–363.

54. Menapace FJ, Hammer WJ, Ritzer TF, et al. Left ventricular size in competitive weight lifters: an echocardiographic study. *Med Sci Sports Exerc*. 1982;14:72–75.

55. Morganroth J, Maron BJ, Henry WL, Epstein SE. Comparative left ventricular dimensions in trained athletes. *Ann Intern Med*. 1975; 82:521–524.

56. Nakao M, Inoue Y, Murakami H. Longitudinal study of the effect of high intensity weight training on aerobic capacity. *Eur J Appl Physiol Occup Physiol*. 1995;70:20–25.

57. Narloch JA, Brandstater ME. Influence of breathing technique on arterial blood pressure during heavy weight lifting. *Arch Phys Med Rehabil*. 1995;76:457–462.

58. Naylor LH, George K, O'Driscoll G, Green DJ. The athlete's heart: a contemporary appraisal of the "Morganroth Hypothesis." *Sports Med*. 2008;38:69–90.

59. Padula CA, Yeaw E. Inspiratory muscle training: integrative review. *Res Theory Nurs Pract*. 2006;20:291–304.

60. Palatini P, Mos L, Munari L, et al. Blood pressure changes during heavy-resistance exercise. *J Hypertens*. 1989;7(suppl):S72–S73.

61. Ploutz-Snyder LL, Convertino VA, Dudley GA. Resistance exercise-induced fluid shifts: change in active muscle size and plasma volume. *Am J Physiol*. 1995:269:R536–R543.

62. Querido JS, Sheel AW. Regulation of cerebral blood flow during exercise. *Sports Med*. 2007;37:765–782.

63. Ratamess NA, Kraemer WJ, Volek JS, et al. Androgen receptor content following heavy resistance exercise in men. *J Steroid Biochem Mol Biol*. 2005;93:35–42.

64. Ratamess NA, Falvo MJ, Mangine GT, Hoffman JR, Faigenbaum AD, Kang J. The effect of rest interval length on metabolic responses to the bench press exercise. *Eur J Appl Physiol*. 2007;100:1–17.

65. Ratamess NA, Hoffman JR, Ross R, et al. Effects of an amino acid/ creatine energy supplement on the acute hormonal response to resistance exercise. *Int J Sport Nutr Exerc Metab*. 2007;17:608–623.

66. Raven PB, Gettman LR, Pollock ML, Cooper KH. A physiological evaluation of professional soccer players. *Br J Sports Med*. 1976; 10:209–216.

67. Riganas CS, Vrabas IS, Christoulas K, Mandroukas K. Specific inspiratory muscle training does not improve performance or Vo_{2max} levels in well trained rowers. *J Sports Med Phys Fitness*. 2008;48:285–292.

68. Romer LM, McConnell AK, Jones DA. Effects of inspiratory muscle training upon recovery time during high intensity, repetitive sprint activity. *Int J Sports Med*. 2002;23:353–360.

69. Sale DG, Moroz DE, McKelvie RS, MacDougall JD, McCartney N. Comparison of blood pressure response to isokinetic and weight-lifting exercise. *Eur J Appl Physiol Occup Physiol*. 1993;67: 115–120.

70. Salke RC, Rowland TW, Burke EJ. Left ventricular size and function in body builders using anabolic steroids. *Med Sci Sports Exerc*. 1985;17:701–704.

71. Saltin B, Strange S. Maximal oxygen uptake: "old" and "new" arguments for a cardiovascular limitation. *Med Sci Sports Exerc*. 1992;24:30–37.

72. Santora LJ, Marin J, Vangrow J, et al. Coronary calcification in body builders using anabolic steroids. *Prev Cardiol*. 2006;9: 198–201.

73. Sawka MN, Young AJ, Muza SR, Gonzalez RR, Pandolf KB. Erythrocyte reinfusion and maximal aerobic power. An examination of modifying factors. *JAMA*. 1987;257:1496–1499.

74. Sentija D, Marsic T, Dizdar D. The effects of strength training on some parameters of aerobic and anaerobic endurance. *Coll Anthropol*. 2009;33:111–116.

75. Sheel AW, Guenette JA. Mechanics of breathing during exercise in men and women: sex versus body size differences? *Exerc Sport Sci Rev*. 2008;36:128–134.

76. Sperlich B, Fricke H, de Marees M, Linville JW, Mester J. Does respiratory muscle training increase physical performance? *Mil Med*. 2009;174:977–982.

77. Sutton JR. Limitations to maximal oxygen uptake. *Sports Med*. 1992;13:127–133.

78. Tesch, PA. Short- and long-term histochemical and biochemical adaptations in muscle. In *Strength and Power in Sport*. Boston, (MA): Blackwell Scientific Publications; 1992. pp. 239–248.

79. Venckunas T, Raugaliene R, Mazutaitiene B, Ramoskeviciute S. Endurance rather than sprint running training increases left ventricular wall thickness in female athletes. *Eur J Appl Physiol*. 2008; 102:307–311.

80. Wagner PD. Gas exchange and peripheral diffusion limitation. *Med Sci Sports Exerc*. 1992;24:54–58.

81. Webb OL, Laskarzewski PM, Glueck CJ. Severe depression of high-density lipoprotein cholesterol levels in weight lifters and

body builders by self-administered exogenous testosterone and anabolic-androgenic steroids. *Metabolism.* 1984;33:971–975.

82. Williams JS, Wongsathikun J, Boon SM, Acevedo EO. Inspiratory muscle training fails to improve endurance capacity in athletes. *Med Sci Sports Exerc.* 2002;34:1194–1198.

83. Williams MH, Wesseldine S, Somma T, Schuster R. The effect of induced erythrocythemia upon 5-mile treadmill run time. *Med Sci Sports Exerc.* 1981;13:169–175.

84. Wilmore JH, Parr RB, Girandola RN, et al. Physiological alterations consequent to circuit weight training. *Med Sci Sports.* 1978;10: 79–84.

85. Wilmore JH, Costill DL. *Physiology of Sport and Exercise.* 2nd ed. Champaign (IL): Human Kinetics; 1999.

86. Yki-Jarvinen H, Koivisto VA, Taskinen MR, Nikkila E. Glucose tolerance, plasma lipoproteins and tissue lipoprotein lipase activities in body builders. *Eur J Appl Physiol Occup Physiol.* 1984;53:253–259.

87. Yoshida T, Nagashima K, Nose H, et al. Relationship between aerobic power, blood volume, and thermoregulatory responses to exercise-heat stress. *Med Sci Sports Exerc.* 1997;29:867–873.

88. Zuliani U, Bernardini B, Catapano A, et al. Effects of anabolic steroids, testosterone, and HGH on blood lipids and echocardiographic parameters in body builders. *Int J Sports Med.* 1989;10:62–66.

9

Principles of Strength Training and Conditioning

Objectives

After completing this chapter, you will be able to:

- Describe the importance of progressive overload in strength training and conditioning and provide examples of how it can be used in program design
- Describe the principle of training specificity and discuss the importance of designing a program most specific to the needs of the athlete
- Describe how the human body adapts specifically to the muscle actions trained, velocity of movement, range of motion, muscle groups trained, energy systems used, and the movement patterns trained
- Describe the importance of variation in program design for continued progression
- Describe the impact proper supervision has on training regarding progression in strength gains

Basic strength training and conditioning (S&C) principles underlie program design. These principles can be applied to all training programs in numerous ways. Ultimately, progression is a long-term goal associated with many S&C practitioners. The advantage of S&C is that there are many ways to design effective programs. Many programs can work effectively provided that guidelines are followed. This is a critical concept for S&C students to understand as one may become bombarded with a spectrum of training advice. This chapter focuses on the three key principles of progressive overload, specificity, and variation (Fig. 9.1). In addition, the principles of individualization and reversibility (detraining) are discussed.

PROGRESSIVE OVERLOAD

Progressive overload refers to the gradual increase in stress placed on the human body during training (17). The concept of progressive overload is not new, and dates back a few thousand years to the ancient Greek strongman and Olympic wrestling champion *Milo of Crotona* (see Chapter 1). The human body has no need to become stronger or more conditioned unless it is forced to meet higher physical demands. The lack of progressive overload in a program is a leading factor for stagnant progress. The use of progressive overload can overcome **accommodation**. Accommodation is the staleness resulting from a lack in change in the training program (37). Adaptations to a training program take place within a few weeks. Proper manipulation of acute program variables alters the training stimulus, and if the stimulus exceeds

the individual's conditioning threshold, then further improvements in muscular fitness can take place. There are several ways to introduce progressive overload during S&C. The following sections discuss resistance training (RT); flexibility; speed, power, and agility; and aerobic training (AT). Brief examples are given but more specific training recommendations and examples are given in subsequent chapters.

RESISTANCE TRAINING

Progressive overload can be incorporated into RT programs in many ways. These include

1. The resistance/loading may be increased. The athlete may train with a higher relative percentage of his or her one-repetition maximum (1 RM) or use greater absolute loading within a constant repetition scheme. For example, during weeks 1–3, the athlete uses 70% of 1 RM for several structural exercises. During weeks 4 and 5, 75% of 1 RM is used. During weeks 6–8, 80% of 1 RM is used. This example applies when a true 1 RM is known for structural exercises and the loading is calculated by taking the 1 RM and multiplying it by 0.70 (and by 0.75 and 0.80, respectively). For an absolute loading example: during weeks 1 and 2, the athlete lifts 220 lb in the bench press for 8 reps. During weeks 3 and 4, the athlete adds weight and performs the bench press with 225 lb for 8 reps (5 lb is added while repetition number stays the same).

2. Repetitions may be added to current workload. For example (8–12 RM loading zone where the athlete

Individualized Training Programs

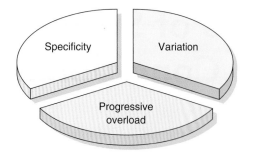

■ **FIGURE 9.1.** Critical components of training program design. The key components to programs targeting progression are progressive overload, specificity, and variation.

performs a range [8–12] of reps for an exercise), during weeks 1 and 2, the athlete lifts 220 lb in the bench press for 3 sets of 8 reps. During weeks 3 and 4, the athlete maintains loading at 220 lb but performs 3 sets of 10 reps. During weeks 5 and 6, the athlete increases rep number to 12 for 3 sets with 220 lb. Once 3 sets of 12 reps are performed over two successive workouts, the athlete adds weight and performs 8 reps and repeats the cycle.

3. Lifting velocity with submaximal loads may be increased to increase the neural response once technique is mastered. The intent is to lift the weight as fast as possible. Because force = mass × acceleration, increasing rep velocity (while mass remains constant) results in higher peak force and greater strength enhancement.

4. Rest intervals may be lengthened to enable greater loading. In combination with previous strategies, lengthening the rest interval will enable more recovery in between sets to tolerate heavier loading. For endurance and hypertrophy training, the rest interval could be reduced, decreasing recovery in between sets.

5. Training volume may be increased within reasonable limits (2%–5%) or varied to accommodate heavier loads (12). From novice to intermediate training, small increases in volume can enhance RT. However, with further progression it is the variation of volume and intensity that becomes most important in program design.

6. Other supramaximal-loading training techniques may be introduced. For example, techniques such as forced repetitions, heavy negatives, partial repetitions in the strongest area of the range of motion (ROM), and variable-resistance devices can be used to load either a segment of the ROM or a muscle action with greater than 100% of 1 RM. These techniques should only be used sparingly by experienced individuals.

FLEXIBILITY

For flexibility training, the intensity, volume, duration, and frequency can be increased for progressive overload. *Intensity* refers to the ROM of the stretch, as higher-intensity stretching expands joint ROM and poses more discomfort to the individual. Volume (number of reps) and duration (length of each stretch) can be increased with progression. Lastly, the frequency of stretching can increase with progression.

POWER, SPEED, AND AGILITY

Similar to RT, intensity, volume (and frequency), and rest intervals can be altered for progressive overload. For plyometric, speed, and agility drills, more complex exercises can be introduced, resistance may be used or increased, longer or higher jumps or throws (drills that require greater power) may be used to increase intensity.

Myths & Misconceptions

The Act of Resistance Training Itself will Build Huge Muscles

Some individuals fear RT because of the misconception they will develop huge muscles. This is primarily a concern in women who appear to believe in this myth to a greater extent. Part of this concern may commence from viewing female bodybuilders in magazines and making the assumption that RT led entirely to the development of their physiques. However, anabolic steroids and other growth agents are mostly responsible for this extreme level of hypertrophy. Anabolic drug-free women have low concentrations of testosterone and it is not physiologically possible to gain extreme amounts of muscle mass. Education is important in debunking this myth. One study showed that women who trained under the supervision of a personal trainer were less likely to believe this myth compared to women who trained on their own (30). This fear is unfounded because it takes a great deal of hard work and dedication and not just simply an act of lifting light weights. Lifting weights does not guarantee increases in size and strength. In order for RT to build size and strength, the stimulus must become gradually more difficult. If one lifts below their threshold of adaptation, then very little will be gained. It takes years of hard training so the fear of excessive hypertrophy is unfounded.

Intensity also increases as athletes increase their speed, jumping ability, power, and agility. Volume may be increased within reasonable limits as conditioning improves. However, caution must be used as volume and intensity are inversely related so proper recovery in between workouts is mandatory. Rest intervals can be manipulated to target power specifically or high-intensity endurance.

AEROBIC ENDURANCE

To progressively overload an AT program, one may increase volume, duration, and intensity and decrease rest intervals. Volume and duration are altered by increasing the distance covered or the length of the exercise bouts. Intensity can be increased modestly by exercising at faster rates, adding resistance, and exercising uphill. It is important to note that intensity cannot increase greatly or the workout can become anaerobic. Interval training can be used to exercise at higher intensities. Decreasing rest intervals in between bouts increases the continuity of exercise and is effective for increasing aerobic endurance.

Case Study 9.1

David is in his second year of RT. For the past 2 months he has not progressed. Upon examination of his training program, David has performed the same exercises, the same number of reps, and has not added weight to any of his exercises. That is, he has followed the same program without altering any variable. At this point David has become discouraged and is considering discontinuing RT.

Question for Consideration: **What advice would you give David regarding his lack of progress?**

SPECIFICITY

The principle of **specificity** entails that all training adaptations are specific to the stimulus applied. Although nonspecific improvements take place, most improvements will take place specific to the stimuli. Training adaptations are specific to the muscle actions involved, velocity of movement and rate of force development (RFD), ROM, muscle groups trained, energy metabolism, movement pattern, and intensity/volume of training (22). Specificity becomes most evident during progression to more advanced RT as many studies have shown a multitude of transfer training effects in untrained and moderately trained individuals. This transfer of training effect applies to

- Strength carryover from unilateral training (to the opposite limb)
- Strength carryover from the trained muscle action to a nontrained action

- Strength carryover from limited-ROM training to other areas of the ROM or full ROM
- Strength carryover from one velocity to another velocity
- Motor performance (jumping ability, sprint speed, and sport-specific movements) improvements resulting from RT

MUSCLE ACTION

RT with eccentric (ECC), concentric (CON), and isometric (ISOM) actions increases muscle strength. Much of the strength gains are specific to the type of muscle action trained (22). Training with CON muscle actions yields the greatest increases in CON muscle strength. However, some transferred training effects occur. When comparing ISOM to dynamic RT, ISOM training can increase dynamic strength (especially when multiple joint angles are trained) and dynamic training can increase ISOM muscle strength (27). Dynamic muscle strength increases are greatest when ECC actions are included (9). Because most training programs include CON and ECC muscle actions, strength will increase mostly in these muscle actions. Although ISOM strength may increase (as there are ISOM actions present during dynamic RT), the most effective way to increase ISOM strength is through specific ISOM training at various joint angles.

VELOCITY OF MOVEMENT

Velocity specificity indicates that greatest strength increases take place at or near the training velocity. Some carryover effects to nontrained velocities may occur as well as carryover velocity effects between muscle actions (ISOM training can increase ISOM RFD and dynamic movement velocity) (22). Research has focused on isokinetic RT where velocity specificity is seen plus some carryover above and below the training velocity (17). Collectively, these studies show training at a moderate velocity (180°–240° per second) produces the greatest strength increases across all testing velocities (12). RT with dynamic muscle actions demonstrates specificity and carryover increases to other nontrained lifting velocities. The greatest carryover effects are seen in untrained or moderately trained individuals. Advanced trainees benefit greatly from training at a velocity specific to their needs. Strength/power athletes benefit most from high-velocity movements (or the intent to maximally accelerate the load) (5,6).

RANGE OF MOTION

Specificity of ROM is seen during limited-ROM dynamic, isokinetic, or ISOM training. Dynamic limited-ROM training can increase strength in the trained ROM, with some carryover increases throughout full ROM (22).

Interpreting Research

The Intent to Lift Weights Rapidly is Critical to Strength Development

Behm DG, Sale DG. Intended rather than actual movement velocity determines velocity-specific training response. *J Appl Physiol*. 1993;74:359–368.

A study was conducted by David Behm and Digby Sale in 1993 (5). In this study, men and women trained 3 days per week for 16 weeks using ISOM or dynamic ballistic ankle dorsiflexions against resistance for 5 sets of 10 reps. Training produced similar velocity-specific strength and RFD increases. Interestingly, the observed training responses previously attributed to high-velocity training also occurred during ISOM ballistic training where the intent was to maximize RFD. The authors concluded that the intent to perform a ballistic, high-velocity action was the key and not the muscle action or resultant velocity per se. The practical application indicates that the major stimulus for strength/power training may be the intent to maximally accelerate the weight.

ISOM-training strength increases are specific to the joint angles trained (**angular specificity**) but may carry over to ±20°–30° of the trained angle (19). The magnitude of carryover is greatest at joint angles at greater muscle lengths. These studies show the importance of training in a full ROM for maximal improvements. There are some exceptions to where dynamic partial ROM repetitions may be beneficial. However, RT is most effective when repetitions are performed in a full ROM. For ISOM training, it is recommended that multiple joint angles are trained corresponding to full joint ROM.

MUSCLE GROUPS TRAINED

Adaptations to training take place predominantly in those muscle groups that were trained (21). Ideally, training will target all major muscle groups. Nevertheless, some areas may be untrained or trained submaximally. Adaptations to training can only take place when muscle group–specific exercises are performed. Training all major muscle groups is important for attaining muscle balance, reducing injuries, and optimizing performance.

ENERGY METABOLISM

Adaptations to training are specific to the energy system involvement. Energy systems adapt mostly by increasing enzyme activity or substrate storage/usage (see Chapter 7). The interaction between volume, intensity, repetition velocity, and rest-interval length is critical to eliciting acute metabolic responses that target different energy systems. Although all metabolic systems are actively engaged, one may predominate based on the training stimulus. Much of the energy demands of resistance exercise are met by the ATP-PC and glycolytic metabolic pathways. Anaerobic glycolysis becomes increasingly important during intense, long-duration sets and when short rest intervals are used.

MOVEMENT PATTERNS

Although a transfer of training effect may occur and is desired when it comes to performing motor skills, specificity in program design relates to movement patterns. Adaptations are specific to the types of movement patterns used during training. Examples of the movement patterns examined include free weights versus machines, open- versus closed-chain kinetic exercises, unilateral versus bilateral training, and movement-specific training.

FREE WEIGHTS VERSUS MACHINES

Specificity of adaptations is seen during training with free weights and machines. Although both are effective for increasing muscle strength, it is difficult to state which modality favors greater strength increases. The testing device is critical as free-weight training leads to greater improvements on free-weight tests and machine training results in greater performance on machine tests (8). When a neutral testing device is used, strength improvement from free weights and machines are similar (36). Free-weight training appears more applicable to motor skill enhancement, *e.g.*, vertical jump performance.

Open- Versus Closed-Chain Kinetic Exercises

A **closed-chain kinetic exercise** is one where the distal segments are fixed (leg press, squat, deadlift), while an **open-chain kinetic exercise** (leg extension, leg curl) enables the distal segment to freely move against loading. Many closed-chain exercises stress multiple joints, while many open-chain exercises are single joint. Moderate-to-high relationships between closed-chain exercise and vertical/long jump performance have been shown (4,7) indicating that performance in closed-chain exercises is strongly related to various motor performance skills.

Augustsson et al. (3) compared 6 weeks of barbell squat training to knee extension and hip adduction exercises on machines and showed that squat training increased vertical jump by 10% whereas no difference was found after open-chain exercise training.

Unilateral Versus Bilateral Training

Unilaterally or bilaterally (one vs. two arms or legs) performed exercises affect the neuromuscular adaptations to training. *Cross education* refers to strength gained in the nontrained limb during unilateral training. The strength increase in the untrained limb may range as high as 22% (mean increase = ~8%) and is thought to occur predominately via neural adaptations (28,32). *Bilateral deficit* refers to the strength produced by both limbs contracting bilaterally, which is smaller than the sum of the limbs contracting unilaterally. Unilateral training (although it increases bilateral strength) contributes to a greater bilateral deficit, whereas bilateral training reduces the bilateral deficit (23). Specificity is observed as unilateral RT results in better performance of unilateral tasks than bilateral training (26). Athletes involved in sports where unilateral strength and power are important and those with glaring weakness on the opposite side may benefit from unilateral training. Unilateral exercises require greater balance and stability. For example, performing a one-arm incline dumbbell press (with only one dumbbell) requires the trunk muscles to contract intensely to offset the torque produced by unilateral loading and enable the athlete to maintain proper posture throughout the exercise. Optimal training may involve the inclusion of both bilateral and unilateral exercises with the ratio of bilateral to unilateral contractions based on the needs of the sport. The American College of Sports Medicine (ACSM) has recommended the inclusion of both into RT programs targeting progression (2).

Movement-Specific Training

Movement-specific training entails the use of exercises that train specific movements. The intent is to improve motor performance through RT and to provide a link between muscular strength gained through traditional RT and movement-specific strength. Training consists of multiplanar movements, sometimes performed in unstable environments to enhance stabilizer-muscle function with various pieces of equipment such as bands, medicine balls, dumbbells, stability balls, kettle bells, ropes, and other devices.

Overweight/Underweight Implements

A common training tool among athletes is to perform sport-specific exercises against a resistance, *e.g.*, overweight implements. Overweight implements allow the athlete to overload a sport-specific motion, thereby eliciting a resisted motor pattern similar to the motion itself. It is thought that the overload enhances the neural response possibly via potentiation and that the enhanced neural responses lead to greater power development with subsequent training. Training with overweight implements targets the force component of the force-velocity relationship. Underweight implements have been used primarily by throwing athletes. Underweight implements target the velocity component of the force-velocity relationship where athletes mimic the motor skill by throwing an object lighter than the ball used for the sport. For throwing athletes, studies have supported the use of over- and underweight implement training to enhance throwing velocity and it has been suggested that the implement used be 5%–20% of normal load for throwing athletes (10). Overweight implements are used for any motor skill but have mostly been studied during overarm throwing in baseball and handball players. Some examples include using a chute, sled, or weighted vest during sprinting and jumping, swinging weighted bats, and using bands during a motor skill. Overweight and underweight implements should be used in conjunction with normal training as the velocity used with heavier implements may be slower.

SIDEBAR | **USE OF OVER/UNDER WEIGHT IMPLEMENTS FOR INCREASING THROWING VELOCITY**

Van den Tillaar R. Effect of different training programs on the velocity of overarm throwing: a brief review. *J Strength Cond Res*. 2004;18:388–396.

Several studies investigated the efficacy of training with overweight and underweight implements. These studies have examined male and female baseball and handball players from high school level to beyond collegiate athletics incorporating a range of 60 to >200 implement throws per week. Van den Tillaar (35) reviewed the literature and reported the following:

- Overweight implements: more than half of studies cited showed throwing velocity was increased (5%–11%) by implement training. Implements ranged from 20% to 25% to >100% of ball weight.
- Underweight implements: most studies cited showed training with underweight (20%–25% less than ball weight) implements increased velocity by 2%–7% with best results found when underweight implements were combined with normal balls during training.
- Over- and underweight implements: most studies cited showed that training with over- and underweight implements increased throwing velocity by 3%–6%.

VARIATION

Training **variation** requires alterations in one or more program variables over time to keep the stimulus optimal. Because the human body adapts rapidly to stress, variation is critical for subsequent adaptations to take place. Studies show the systematic variation of volume and intensity is most effective for long-term progression as compared to programs that did not alter any program variable (11). Workouts can be varied in infinite ways. The S&C practitioner should think of each design characteristic as a tool in the proverbial tool box which provides a wide array of strategies for progression. Many ways exist to increase strength so the trainer benefits by including several methods of variation into program design. Training philosophies that support minimal variation will have limited effectiveness.

PROGRESSION AND PROGRAM DESIGN

TRAINING STATUS AND PROGRESSION

Training status dictates the pattern of progression for a fitness component. Training status reflects a continuum of adaptations such that fitness level, training experience, and genetic endowment each make a contribution. The largest rates of strength improvement occur in untrained individuals as the window of adaptation is greatest during this time. Resistance-trained individuals show a slower rate of progression. In a position stand published by the ACSM in 2002 (1), >150 studies were reviewed and showed strength increases of

- ~40% in untrained individuals
- ~20% in moderately trained individuals
- ~16% in trained individuals
- ~10% in advanced individuals
- ~2% in elite athletes

These studies ranged from 4 weeks to over 2 years in duration, and the training programs and testing procedures varied greatly. It is very difficult if not impossible to accurately classify an individual as trained or moderately trained because each classification comprises an interaction between fitness level and years of experience, e.g., some individuals with many years of experience possess less strength than some with limited experience and vice versa. However, one can see that progression becomes more difficult as one's conditioning improves. Similar results were shown where untrained individuals responded most favorably while less increases were seen in trained individuals (31). Although these studies have focused on muscle strength, the same can be said about any fitness variable. The difficulty in strength progression occurs within as little as several months of training. Each improvement brings the individual closer to his or her

genetic limit. Short-term studies (<16 weeks) show that the majority of strength increases take place within the first 4–8 weeks (16). The rate and magnitude of progression decrease with higher levels of conditioning. Plateaus occur as individuals get closer to their genetic ceiling and it becomes more difficult to improve (*principle of diminishing returns*). Training programs need to incorporate progressive overload, specificity, and variation to progress to a higher level.

GENERAL-TO-SPECIFIC MODEL OF PROGRESSION

Because untrained individuals respond favorably to any training program, less-specific or general program design is all that is needed initially. There is no need for complexity at this stage as most programs will work. This initial phase is characterized by learning proper technique and building a conditioning base for progressive training. The ACSM has recommended general program structures to start (1). However, resistance-trained individuals show a slower rate of progression and demonstrate a cyclical pattern to their training (15). Training cycles provide greater opportunities for variation, and variation is needed in program design. Training progression occurs in an orderly manner from a general, or less-specific, program design initially to a more specific design with higher levels of training (Fig. 9.2). Advanced training targeting progression is more complex and requires great variation specific to training goals. Figure 9.2 is a simplified schematic representing a theoretical continuum of the amount of variation needed, known as a *general-to-specific model* for

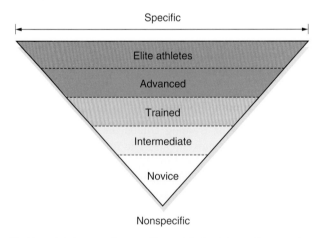

FIGURE 9.2. General-to-specific model of training and progression. The narrow part of the triangle refers to the magnitude of variation needed for beginning trainees. Because beginners progress easily, there is no need for complexity here. General or less-specific programs are recommended during this phase. However, with progression gains take place more slowly. Greater variation is needed in program design (represented by the wide walls of the triangle). Advanced and elite athletes benefit greatly from cycling training. (This theoretical model is proposed based on current literature by the ACSM (1) and Kraemer and Ratamess (22).)

training progression. The narrow segment of the triangle (novice) suggests that limited variation is suitable in this population as it is important to begin gradually. However, the triangle widens as the individual progresses suggesting that more variation (specific training cycles) is necessary.

INDIVIDUALIZATION

All individuals respond differently to training. Figure 9.3 depicts individualized data from a study in our laboratory. Subjects engaged in 10 weeks of combined RT and sprint/plyometric training and individual 1 RM squat and 60-m sprint time improvements are presented. Everyone improved differently despite following the same training program. Genetics, training status, nutritional intake, and the program itself play substantial roles in the level of adaptation. One needs to be aware of individual response patterns and the need for variation if the response is minimal. The most effective programs are those designed to meet individual needs. This can oftentimes be difficult

especially if one is training several athletes at once. When practical, program individualization is beneficial for progression.

DETRAINING (PRINCIPLE OF REVERSIBILITY)

Detraining is the complete cessation of training or substantial reduction in frequency, volume, or intensity that results in performance reductions and a loss of some of the beneficial physiological adaptations associated with training. The length of the detraining period and the training status of the individual dictate the magnitude of performance loss. Performance reductions may occur in as little as 2 weeks, and possibly sooner in trained athletes. In recreationally trained men, muscle strength may be reduced within 4 weeks of detraining (34) whereas other research shows very little change in strength during the first 6 weeks detraining (20). In trained individuals, detraining may result in greater losses in muscle power than strength (18). Strength reductions are related

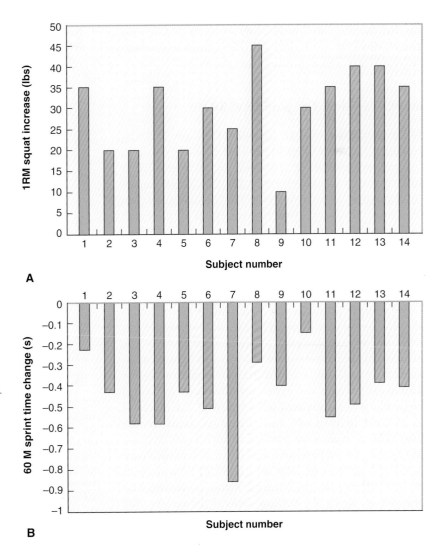

FIGURE 9.3. Individual responses to training. Individual responses to 10 weeks of combined sprint/plyometric and RT. **A.** Increases in 1 RM squat. **B.** Reductions in 60-m sprint times. Both panels show variable magnitudes of improvements for each subject. (Adapted with permission from Ratamess NA, Kraemer WJ, Volek JS, et al. The effects of ten weeks of resistance and combined plyometric/sprint training with the Meridian Elyte athletic shoe on muscular performance in women. *J Strength Cond Res.* 2007;21:882–887.)

Myths & Misconceptions

Detraining will Turn Muscle into Fat

Detraining leads to strength, power, and endurance reductions with the magnitude dependent upon training status and the detraining period duration. Although neural adaptations are mostly responsible for strength reductions initially, detraining periods of at least a few weeks or more result in a loss of muscle mass. The muscle mass lost is, in fact, lost and not directly converted to fat. Muscle mass is critical to enhancing the athlete's metabolism and kilocalorie expenditure on a daily basis. With muscle loss a reduction in basal metabolic rate may ensue. This, coupled with other factors such as dietary kilocalorie intake and lower activity level, increases the likelihood of one increasing his or her body fat. Therefore, an increase in body fat can take place with detraining but not from direct conversion of lost muscle.

to neural mechanisms initially with atrophy of skeletal muscle predominating as the detraining period extends. Detraining leads to other physiological changes such as muscle fiber (IIa to IIx) transitions (34), reduced anaerobic substrate concentrations, and enzyme activity (24). Interestingly, the level of muscle strength, even after detraining, is rarely lower than pretraining levels showing that training has a residual effect when it is discontinued. However, when the individual returns to training, the rate of strength acquisition is high (33).

IMPORTANCE OF SUPERVISION

Supervision is a critical component to any training program. Not only does supervised training result in less injuries and better technique, but performance is enhanced to a greater extent. Athletes who are supervised progress at a higher rate than those training on their own. This was shown by Mazzetti et al. (25) who compared 12 weeks of supervised versus unsupervised RT and found the supervised group increased maximal strength to a greater extent (>10%). Supervised training (in the form of a coach, trainer, or at least a partner) poses several advantages to the athlete targeting progression.

Supervision positively affects the intensities individuals self-select in unsupervised RT. Men and women tend to self-select training loads that are in the range of 40%–56% of their 1 RM per respective exercise (13,14). By many standards these loads can be considered suboptimal or too low for muscle strength and hypertrophy increases in trained populations. We compared self-selected RT intensities of women who trained with and without a personal trainer (30). The women were carefully instructed to select a weight they would perform for 10 repetitions in their own workouts and were subsequently tested for 1 RM strength on four exercises: leg press, leg extension, chest press, and seated row. Figure 9.4 depicts some of the results. The women who trained with a personal trainer had greater 1 RM strength. For self-selected relative intensity, the

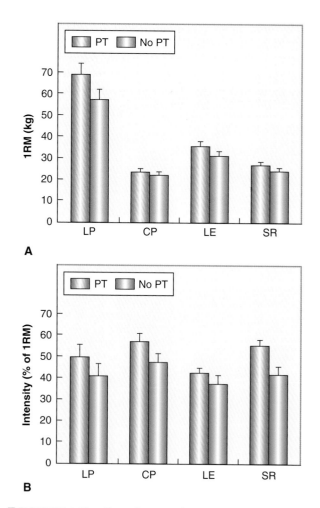

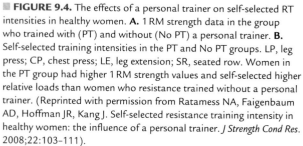

FIGURE 9.4. The effects of a personal trainer on self-selected RT intensities in healthy women. **A.** 1 RM strength data in the group who trained with (PT) and without (No PT) a personal trainer. **B.** Self-selected training intensities in the PT and No PT groups. LP, leg press; CP, chest press; LE, leg extension; SR, seated row. Women in the PT group had higher 1 RM strength values and self-selected higher relative loads than women who resistance trained without a personal trainer. (Reprinted with permission from Ratamess NA, Faigenbaum AD, Hoffman JR, Kang J. Self-selected resistance training intensity in healthy women: the influence of a personal trainer. *J Strength Cond Res.* 2008;22:103–111).

group who trained with a personal trainer selected higher intensities for leg press (50% vs. 41%), chest press (57% vs. 48%), and seated row (56% vs. 42%). Overall, the average self-selected intensity for all exercises was ~51.4% in the personal trainer group and ~42.3% in the unsupervised group showing positive benefits of supervision and an important role for a personal trainer in RT.

Summary Points

✔ The three most important principles in program design are progressive overload, specificity, and variation. A program is effective when these principles are addressed.

✔ Supervised training programs are most effective when they are designed based on individual needs.

✔ Untrained individuals respond favorably to training, provided a threshold volume and intensity are prescribed. It is recommended that general program design be used initially while trainees learn proper technique and build a conditioning base. With training progression, greater specificity is needed to optimally target various training goals.

✔ The effects of RT can be lost upon cessation, or detraining, when the stimulus is removed or the volume and intensity are drastically reduced.

Review Questions

1. Which of the following is not an example of progressive overload?
   a. Increasing the amount of weight for an exercise while keeping the repetition number the same
   b. Maintaining the same amount of weight for an exercise while increasing the repetition number
   c. Decreasing the amount of weight for an exercise while decreasing the number of repetitions
   d. Increasing the amount of weight for an exercise while slightly decreasing the number of repetitions

2. Which of the following exercises is an example of a closed-chain kinetic exercise?
   a. Arm curl
   b. Leg press
   c. Triceps pushdown
   d. Lateral raise

3. The strength gained in a nontrained limb resulting from unilateral training is
   a. Cross education
   b. Bilateral deficit
   c. Detraining
   d. Accommodation

4. An athlete begins an 8-week weight training program. His weights increased substantially during training; however, he was tested using an ISOM device, and his scores only improved minimally. This testing tool appears to have been a violation of the principle of
   a. Specificity
   b. Variation
   c. Progressive overload
   d. Supervision

5. A general-to-specific model of training progression implies that
   a. Novice lifters require great variation in program design
   b. General programs work best in advanced to elite athletes
   c. Advanced to elite athletes require greater specificity in program design for progression
   d. None of the above

6. The staleness resulting from a lack in change in the training program is known as
   a. Specificity
   b. Variation
   c. Accommodation
   d. Progressive overload

7. The principle of diminishing returns entails progression and it becomes more difficult as an athlete gets closer to his or her genetic ceiling.   T F

8. The window of adaptation for strength gains is greatest in an elite strength athlete and least in an untrained individual.   T F

9. Supervised training results in a greater rate of performance improvement.   T F

10. Most studies have shown that training with overweight implements can increase throwing velocity by an average of 5%–11%.   T F

11. ISOM training at one joint angle will not induce a strength carryover to adjacent nontrained areas of the ROM.   T F

12. Detraining can lead to Type IIa to IIx fiber transitions.   T F

References

1. American College of Sports Medicine: Position Stand: Progression models in resistance training for healthy adults. *Med Sci Sports Exerc.* 2002; 34: 364–380.

2. American College of Sports Medicine: Position Stand: Progression models in resistance training for healthy adults. *Med Sci Sports Exerc.* 2009;41:687–708.

3. Augustsson J, Esko A, Thomee R, Svantesson U. Weight training of the thigh muscles using closed vs. open kinetic chain exercises: a comparison of performance enhancement. *J Orthop Sports Phys Ther.* 1998;27:3–8.

4. Augustsson J, Thomee R. Ability of closed and open kinetic chain tests of muscular strength to assess functional performance. *Scand J Med Sci Sports.* 1998;10:164–168.

5. Behm DG, Sale DG. Intended rather than actual movement velocity determines velocity-specific training response. *J Appl Physiol.* 1993;74:359–368.

6. Behm DG, Sale DG. Velocity specificity of resistance training. *Sports Med.* 1993;15:374–388.

7. Blackburn JR, Morrissey MC. The relationship between open and closed kinetic chain strength of the lower limb and jumping performance. *J Orthop Sports Phys Ther.* 1998;27:430–435.

8. Boyer BT. A comparison of the effects of three strength training programs on women. *J Appl Sports Sci Res.* 1990;4:88–94.

9. Dudley GA, Tesch PA, Miller BJ, Buchanan MD. Importance of eccentric actions in performance adaptations to resistance training. *Av Space Environ Med.* 1991;62:543–550.

10. Escamilla RF, Speer KP, Fleisig GS, Barrentine SW, Andrews JR. Effects of throwing overweight and underweight baseballs on throwing velocity and accuracy. *Sports Med.* 2000;29:259–272.

11. Fleck SJ. Periodized strength training: a critical review. *J Strength Cond Res.* 1999;13:82–89.

12. Fleck SJ, Kraemer WJ. *Designing Resistance Training Programs.* 3rd ed. Champaign (IL): Human Kinetics; 2004.

13. Focht BC. Perceived exertion and training load during self-selected and imposed-intensity resistance exercise in untrained women. *J Strength Cond Res.* 2007;21:183–187.

14. Glass S, Stanton D. Self-selected resistance training intensity in novice weightlifters. *J Strength Cond Res.* 2004;18:324–327.

15. Häkkinen K, Pakarinen A, Alen M, Kauhanen H, Komi PV. Neuromuscular and hormonal adaptations in athletes to strength training in two years. *J Appl Physiol.* 1988;65:2406–2412.

16. Hickson RC, Hidaka K, Foster C. Skeletal muscle fiber type, resistance training, and strength-related performance. *Med Sci Sports Exerc.* 1994;26:593–598.

17. Hoffman JR, Ratamess NA. *A Practical Guide to Developing Resistance-Training Programs.* 2nd ed. Monterey (CA): Coaches Choice; 2008.

18. Izquierdo M, Ibanez J, Gonzalez-Badillo JJ, et al. Detraining and tapering effects on hormonal responses and strength performance. *J Strength Cond Res.* 2007;21:768–775.

19. Knapik JJ, Mawdsley RH, Ramos MU. Angular specificity and test mode specificity of isometric and isokinetic strength training. *J Orthop Sports Phys Ther.* 1983;5:58–65.

20. Kraemer WJ, Koziris LP, Ratamess NA, et al. Detraining produces minimal changes in physical performance and hormonal variables in recreationally strength-trained men. *J Strength Cond Res.* 2002; 16:373–382.

21. Kraemer WJ, Nindl BC, Ratamess NA, et al. Changes in muscle hypertrophy in women with periodized resistance training. *Med Sci Sports Exerc.* 2004;36:697–708.

22. Kraemer WJ, Ratamess NA. Fundamentals of resistance training: progression and exercise prescription. *Med Sci Sport Exerc.* 2004;36:674–678.

23. Kuruganti U, Parker P, Rickards J, Tingley M, Sexsmith J. Bilateral isokinetic training reduces the bilateral leg strength deficit for both old and young adults. *Eur J Appl Physiol.* 2005; 94:175–179.

24. MacDougall JD, Ward GR, Sale DG, Sutton JR. Biochemical adaptation of human skeletal muscle to heavy resistance training and immobilization. *J Appl Physiol.* 1977;43:700–703.

25. Mazzetti SA, Kraemer WJ, Volek JS, et al. The influence of direct supervision of resistance training on strength performance. *Med Sci Sports Exerc.* 2000;32:1175–1184.

26. McCurdy KW, Langford GA, Doscher MW, Wiley LP, Malllard KG. The effects of short-term unilateral and bilateral lower-body resistance training on measures of strength and power. *J Strength Cond Res.* 2005;19:9–15.

27. Morrissey MC, Harman EC, Johnson MJ. Resistance training modes: specificity and effectiveness. *Med Sci Sports Exerc.* 1995; 27:648–660.

28. Munn J, Herbert RD, Gandevia SC. Contralateral effects of unilateral resistance training: a meta-analysis. *J Appl Physiol.* 2004; 96:1861–1866.

29. Ratamess NA, Kraemer WJ, Volek JS, et al. The effects of ten weeks of resistance and combined plyometric/sprint training with the Meridian Elyte athletic shoe on muscular performance in women. *J Strength Cond Res.* 2007;21:882–887.

30. Ratamess NA, Faigenbaum AD, Hoffman JR, Kang J. Self-selected resistance training intensity in healthy women: the influence of a personal trainer. *J Strength Cond Res.* 2008;22:103–111.

31. Rhea MR, Alvar BA, Burkett LN, Ball SD. A meta-analysis to determine the dose-response for strength development. *Med Sci Sports Exerc.* 2003;35:456–464.

32. Shima SN, Ishida K, Katayama K, Morotome Y, Sato Y, Miyamura M. Cross education of muscular strength during unilateral resistance training and detraining. *Eur J Appl Physiol.* 2002;86: 287–294.

33. Staron RS, Leonardi MJ, Karapondo DL, et al. Strength and skeletal muscle adaptations in heavy-resistance-trained women after detraining and retraining. *J Appl Physiol.* 1991;70:631–640.

34. Terzis G, Stratakos G, Manta P, Georgladis G. Throwing performance after resistance training and detraining. *J Strength Cond Res.* 2008;22:1198–1204.

35. Van den Tillaar R. Effect of different training programs on the velocity of overarm throwing: a brief review. *J Strength Cond Res.* 2004; 18:388–396.

36. Willoughby DS, Gillespie JW. A comparison of isotonic free weights and omnikinetic exercise machines on strength. *J Hum Mov Stud.* 1990;19:93–100.

37. Zatsiorsky V, Kraemer WJ. *Science and Practice of Strength Training.* 2nd ed. Champaign (IL): Human Kinetics; 2006.

Part Three

Strength Training and Conditioning Program Design

10 Warm-Up and Flexibility

After completing this chapter, you will be able to:

- Discuss the physiological effects of a warm-up and the importance of warming up for injury prevention and performance enhancement
- Design general and specific warm-ups
- Discuss factors that affect flexibility
- Describe different modalities of stretching
- Discuss flexibility training guidelines and design a flexibility training program
- Discuss the importance of including a cooldown following a workout

An athlete can only attain peak performance when he or she has been properly prepared. Preparation can be viewed in terms of chronic and acute. Chronic preparation consists of the athlete's training program, diet, and recovery strategies used over a period of time. Acute preparation focuses on the athlete's strategic plan before a workout or competition. Included in acute preparation are dietary intake and fluid consumption, mental focus and visualization, competition strategy, and the warm-up. The warm-up is used to prepare the body for high-intensity and/or high-volume exercise and reduce the potential risk of injury. A warm-up generally includes some aerobic exercises and/or exercises that increase joint range of motion (ROM) such as very light stretching, dynamic calisthenics, and sport-specific drills. Joint ROM impacts the athlete's flexibility. Flexibility is a health-related fitness component known to affect performance and health. Flexibility training is another critical component to athletic training. In this chapter, the physiological and performance benefits of a proper warm-up and flexibility training are discussed.

WARM-UP

A **warm-up** consists of performing low-intensity exercise to prepare the body for more intense physical activity. Warm-ups precede all exercise modalities when the intensity is at least low-to-moderate to high. The warm-up begins very light but may increase in intensity progressively until the athlete is prepared for the main component of the workout. A warm-up can be passive (one where muscle temperature is increased without exercise via a sauna, hot shower or water immersion, or heat application) or active (via exercise). Both types of

warm-ups increase muscle temperature effectively and augment performance compared to no warm-up (12,13). Active warm-ups tend to result in better short-term performance than passive warm-ups and enhance moderate- and longer-duration exercise provided the active warm-up is not fatiguing (12,13). There are two types of active warm-ups: general and specific. A *general warm-up* consists of low-intensity exercise such as slow jogging and/or stationary cycling that lasts for 5–10 minutes. A *specific warm-up* consists of dynamic or very light static movements similar to the sport/activity and may last between 5 and 15 minutes. Specific warm-ups vary greatly depending on the sport. Often, a general warm-up precedes a specific warm-up. Figure 10.1 depicts a general warm-up followed by two specific warm-ups: one for a sprint workout and the other for a lower-body weight training workout where the first exercise in sequence is the barbell back squat (exercises are described in other chapters).

Many coaches and athletes experiment with different warm-ups and eventually design one individualized to meet their needs. Designing a warm-up is relatively simple. The athlete first selects an activity for the general warm-up, perhaps cycling or light jogging for 5–10 minutes. The intensity should be low and should not fatigue the athlete. A specific warm-up follows. Exercises selected for the specific warm-up vary greatly and may consist of calisthenics, technique drills, resistance exercises, medicine ball exercises, dynamic flexibility exercises (see the Sidebar), and low-to-moderate-intensity plyometric, sprint, and agility preparatory exercises. Several of these exercises are described in other chapters. These are low-to-moderate intensity initially but progress to moderately high intensity if the athlete is preparing for explosive exercise. Some high-intensity exercises may

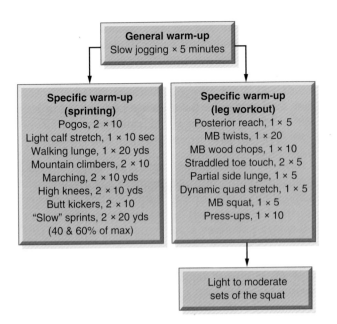

FIGURE 10.1. Examples of general and specific warm-ups.

- Straddled medicine ball rollouts/circles
- Lunge/lateral lunge
- Body weight squats
- Mountain climbers
- Triceps extensions with MB (with posterior reach)
- Stability ball (SB) arm circles (from kneeling, flexed position)
- Press-ups
- SB supine slides (into bridge)
- Overhead claps
- Diagonal reaches
- Rockers (with knees/hips flexed)
- Woodchops

be used for the potentiation of the athletic skills. Five to ten drills can be selected and performed for 1–3 sets totaling 5–15 minutes. For aerobic training, the general warm-up can progress into the main workout or can precede a specific warm-up. For resistance exercise, the specific warm-up may consist of calisthenics and dynamic flexibility exercises and progress into light weight training sets. For sprint, plyometric, and agility training, the specific warm-up may consist of low-intensity drills and progress to high-intensity drills. For sport-specific warm-ups, general drills can be incorporated, which culminate into sport-specific activities, *e.g.*, throwing/hitting for baseball, shooting/layup drills for basketball.

SIDEBAR   **DYNAMIC FLEXIBILITY EXERCISES**

- Arm circles (front and back)
- Neck rotations
- Hip circles
- Overhead medicine ball (MB) lassos
- Toe touches
- Medicine ball front raises
- Medicine ball figure eights
- Arm cross-face circles
- Jumping jacks
- Front/back kicks
- Trunk circles from a straddled position
- Wrist "praying" flexion/extension
- Ankle rolls
- Torso rotations/side bends/bent-over T-rotations
- Knee circles
- Shoulder crossovers (horizontal adduction/abduction)

PHYSIOLOGY OF WARMING UP

A proper warm-up prepares the body for exercise and is thought to reduce the risk of injury. Although very little scientific research supports the contention that a warm-up reduces the incidence of muscular/connective tissue (CT) injury, at the very least a proper warm-up can enhance performance and may reduce injury potential. Several physiological responses occur during an active warm-up. These include (1,12)

- Increased muscle and core temperature
- Increased blood flow
- Increased speed of metabolic reactions
- Increased release of oxygen from hemoglobin and myoglobin (Bohr effect)
- Increased heart rate and cardiac output
- Increased nerve conduction velocity and neural activation
- Increased oxygen consumption
- Decreased joint/CT and skeletal muscle viscosity and resistance
- Increased muscle glycogen breakdown and glycolysis
- Increased mental preparedness and psychological functioning

These acute responses are thought to elicit greater strength, power, ROM, speed, agility, and endurance following a warm-up.

PERFORMANCE EFFECTS

Most studies show an acute warm-up enhances performance more than not performing a warm-up. Vertical jump, swimming time, running time, and cycling power are enhanced after 3–5 minutes of low- to moderate-intensity warm-up (13). Much of the enhancement is attributed to increased muscle temperature. However, some studies have not shown enhancement and a few studies have shown reduced performance, suggesting the warm-up was too intense or did not include enough recovery time before assessment (13). Warm-ups enhance performance of intermediate-duration activities. It is thought that, in addition to higher muscle temperatures, performing a warm-up before an intermediate- or long-duration activity increases the initial VO$_2$ level, thereby reducing oxygen deficit and increasing the contribution of aerobic metabolism throughout the event (13). The longer the duration of the event, the less likely a warm-up will affect performance. *It is recommended that a general warm-up consisting of aerobic exercise at 40%–60% of Vo$_{2max}$ for 10–20 minutes (with ~5 min of recovery before the event begins) be used to enhance athletic performance* (13,60). An endurance-trained athlete may require a higher intensity (70% of Vo$_{2max}$) to adequately increase muscle temperature (9,60). The key elements to the warm-up are to (a) increase muscle temperature, (b) increase VO$_2$, and (c) minimize fatigue (ATP-PC and glycogen depletion, blood lactate).

WARM-UP VERSUS POSTACTIVATION POTENTIATION

One concept of interest is a warm-up versus a potentiation protocol. Many strength and conditioning (S&C) professionals view a warm-up as a low-to-moderate-intensity activity used to prepare the body for more challenging exercises. Some categorize a potentiation protocol as a separate entity and perhaps part of the workout rather than a warm-up. Others view potentiation protocols as high-intensity warm-ups where the warm-up is performed on a continuum that takes place from low to high intensity (while minimizing fatigue) (Fig. 10.2). Notwithstanding the perceptual differences, both are successfully used for competition or training. During postactivation potentiation, activated motor units stay facilitated for a period of time following maximal or near-maximal muscle contractions. During this time, muscle strength, power, and endurance can be enhanced. Studies have shown that: performing back or front squats with 30%–90% of 1 RM enhanced 40-m sprint speed (37,62); performing heavy squats (5 sets of 1 rep with 90% of 1 RM) increased jump power in trained athletes but not recreationally trained individuals (16); performing half squats (20%–90% of 1 RM) increased jump peak force and height and greater improvements were seen in those athletes with higher levels of strength (23,25); performing the bench press (6 reps with 65% of 1 RM) increased bench press peak power (6); and performing a 1 RM back squat protocol increased max vertical jump height by 3% (27). However, some studies have not shown acute potentiation (25).

Potentiation protocols have received some attention. In many cases, they were effective for augmenting maximal strength and power in athletes, especially those who possess higher levels of muscle strength. The acute performance enhancement may persist for several minutes or longer. Most studies examined the potentiating effects of heavy lifting (to maximally recruit fast-twitch [FT] fibers) prior to maximal anaerobic exercise. However, the effects of ballistic exercise prior to maximal anaerobic performance may not produce potentiation (37).

DYNAMIC VERSUS STATIC WARM-UPS

Dynamic warm-ups enhance performance (13). However, a major topic of debate is the decision to include static stretching into the warm-up. For many years, static stretching was widely accepted for use in warm-ups with the intent to increase muscle temperature and ROM, and to reduce injury risk. This was particularly evident for athletes whose sports required high levels of flexibility (gymnastics). However, the last 20 years of research has yielded some interesting findings regarding intense (not light) static stretching prior to strength and power events thereby leaving its use in question.

Muscle strength and power performance, *e.g.*, vertical jump height, power, agility, and sprinting speed, may be limited immediately following a static stretching protocol used as a warm-up compared to a general warm-up absent of stretching (21,28,39,43,50,52,56,63). Performance reductions of ~1%–30% were shown, with prolonged static stretching having the most profound effects. The reduced performance effects linger for up to 2 hours and the strength/power reductions occur while joint ROM is increased following stretching (46). In direct comparison (10 min of static, ballistic, or proprioceptive neuromuscular facilitation stretching), acute vertical jump performance was reduced by 4%, 2.7%, and 5.1%, respectively, but fully recovered after 15 minutes (14).

Reduced electromyographic (EMG) activity of muscles accompanies strength and power deficits following stretching, thereby indicating reduced neural drive (35). Behm et al. (11) tested subjects following 20 minutes of static stretching of the quadriceps and showed a 12% reduction in maximal voluntary contractile force and reduced neural activation ranging from 2% to 20%. It is thought that high-intensity stretching reduces musculotendinous stiffness thereby lessening the ergogenic effects of the stretch-shortening cycle. Musculotendinous stiffness is related to maximal concentric (CON) and isometric (ISOM) force production (58) and decreases following static stretching (48). Dynamic stretching may not produce much of a performance deficit and may be a favorable alternative. Interestingly, upper-body static stretching may not be a limiting factor for upper-body strength and power (55).

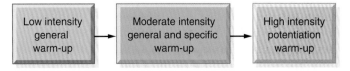

■ **FIGURE 10.2.** The warm-up continuum. Warm-ups exist on an intensity continuum and occur from general to specific. (LI, low intensity; MI, moderate intensity; HI, high intensity.)

Interpreting Research

Acute Static or Ballistic Stretching on Maximal Strength Performance

Bacurau RF, Monteiro GA, Ugrinowitsch C, et al. Acute effect of a ballistic and a static stretching exercise bout on flexibility and maximal strength. *J Strength Cond Res*. 2009;23:304–308.

Bacurau et al. (5) studied three conditions: (a) 20 minutes of static stretching, (b) 20 minutes of ballistic stretching, and (c) control condition. Immediately following each session was the determination of the 1 RM leg press. 1 RM was lower following static stretching (a reduction of ~28 kg) but 1 RM did not decrease after ballistic stretching. These results demonstrate that maximal strength performance can be negatively affected by intense prestatic stretching.

Although performance of dynamic warm-up exercise after static stretching may reduce some of the deficit (52), some studies have shown reductions linger even if dynamic exercise is performed (45,52). The critical element is the intensity and duration/volume of the static stretching protocol. Minimal effects are seen with light stretching only for a few sets (47,64). Many researchers, coaches, and practitioners have opted to include dynamic warm-up protocols in lieu of intense static stretching. The use of light stretching coupled with dynamic warm-up protocols is effective for optimizing performance (18). However, intense stretching is recommended following the workout as part of a cooldown for strength/power athletes. For those strength/power athletes who require high levels of flexibility (gymnasts, martial artists), some static stretching may be necessary but caution must be used to not overstretch and reduce performance. For example, rhythmic gymnasts generally warm up for ~45 minutes, a slow jog initially followed by sport-specific warm-up exercises and static stretching (22) to achieve the high level of ROM needed for the sport. The need for high flexibility trumps the undesirable effects of prolonged static stretching.

FLEXIBILITY

Flexibility is a measure of joint ROM without injury and is an important health-related component of fitness. *Static flexibility* describes ROM about a joint during active (unassisted) or passive (assisted) movement (where the final position is held), whereas *dynamic flexibility (functional flexibility)* describes ROM during movement. Another type of dynamic flexibility, *ballistic flexibility*, has been defined as ROM attained during explosive- or bouncing-type movements.

Having adequate flexibility has many health and performance benefits. Flexibility training helps maintain appropriate muscle lengths. In some cases, muscle shortening can take place over time, and flexibility training helps improve muscle balance. Flexibility training helps improve muscular weaknesses and is thought to reduce the risk of injury. Flexibility training can improve posture and the ability to move, relieve stress, and reduce the risk of low-back pain.

From an athletic standpoint, improved flexibility may increase performance for several athletic skills. For example:

- Increased flexibility of the shoulders helps the Olympic weightlifter attain the proper overhead position in the snatch
- Increased flexibility of the hips helps the gymnast attain proper position during a split
- Increased flexibility of the hips and shoulders is crucial to the ice hockey goalie who needs to block the puck at many difficult angles
- Increased flexibility of the shoulder is crucial to the tennis player for maximizing the velocity and the accuracy of the serve
- Increased flexibility of the shoulders can help the volleyball player block a shot and spike the ball
- Increased flexibility of the hips and hamstrings is essential for the hurdler who must elevate over the hurdle without much deviation from his or her normal stride

Positive relationships exist between ankle flexibility and flutter kicking speed in female swimmers (38) although flexibility may not correlate to sprint performance (40). A 12-week static stretching program (resulting in an 18.1% increase in flexibility) increased long and vertical jump performance by 2.3% and 6.7%, respectively, 20-m sprint speed by 1.3%, maximal strength by 15%–32%, and endurance by 28%–32% (31). The bottom line is that improving flexibility can enhance athletic performance while poor flexibility may limit performance.

FLEXIBILITY AND INJURY PREVENTION

It is generally thought that greater joint flexibility decreases the risk of pain and injury. Stretching, and the increase in flexibility, are thought to increase compliance of the tendon unit, thereby increasing the tendons' ability to absorb energy (59). Acute static stretching and static stretching programs reduce acute tendon stiffness, decrease **hysteresis** (the amount of energy lost as heat during the elastic recoil), and increase tendon compliance (32,33). These changes enhance joint ROM and are thought to reduce the risk of injury. However, studies examining the effects of stretching and injury incidence produced contrasting results (59). In some studies, reduced ankle dorsi flexion ROM was associated with greater incidence of patellar tendinopathy in volleyball players (34), lower incidence rates of low-back pain were shown in military recruits who included static stretching compared to those who did not stretch (2), and an ~12.4% lower injury rate was shown in military basic trainees who stretched the hamstrings regularly than those trainees who did not stretch (24). In contrast, several studies have shown no benefits of stretching on reducing the incidence of lower-body injuries (53). For example, hip abduction flexibility was not associated with reducing the risk of groin injuries in National Hockey League (NHL) hockey players (17) and flexibility was not shown to relate to injury prevention in soccer players (57). The benefits of greater flexibility in injury prevention are unclear but increased flexibility is advantageous for fitness and performance and may lessen the risk of injury under some circumstances.

FACTORS AFFECTING FLEXIBILITY

An individual's joint flexibility is determined by many factors. These factors include (1,30)

- Joint structure—the type of joint will dictate how many planes of motion are possible. Ball-and-socket joints enable motion in three planes, whereas hinge joints predominately allow motion in one plane. The size of the bones at the articulation site plays a critical role. Large bones with convex surfaces that articulate with a deep fossa or concave surface provide more stability and less mobility than smaller bones/fossa.
- Muscular imbalance—muscle strength and length imbalances reduce flexibility. Unequal pull by antagonist muscles or *hypertonic* (shortened) muscles reduce flexibility.
- Muscular control—for some movements (hip abduction from a lying position), a certain degree of strength and balance is needed to reach a certain level of the ROM. A lack of strength and balance can decrease flexibility.
- Age—flexibility decreases with age. Older, sedentary individuals lose motor units and muscle fibers while

fibrous CT expands. The higher collagen content reduces compliance and flexibility.
- Gender—women tend to be more flexible than men in some areas, especially in the hips. Anatomical, structural, and hormonal (estrogen, progesterone) differences between genders account for flexibility differences. Women have larger pelvic girdles and broader and shallower hips than men, which enhances flexibility in the pelvic/hip region.
- CT—tendons, ligaments, fascia, joint capsules, and skin affect flexibility. Collagen and elastin content affects CT elasticity and plasticity. Training alters CT plasticity.
- Bulk—an increase in muscle bulk or percent body fat can limit joint ROM and decrease flexibility scores. The additional tissue mass acts as an obstruction to joint motion limiting bony segment movement with a high degree of ROM. Elite bodybuilders may have less elbow flexion ROM mostly due to large upper-arm mass rather than poor flexibility of the elbow extensors. Similar restrictions are seen with obesity. An overweight or obese person may have difficulty scoring well on the *sit-and-reach flexibility test* (a test of hamstring, gluteal, and lower-back flexibility) partially due to abdominal bulk rather than neuromuscular factors affecting joint ROM. Thus, ROM and flexibility are not exactly equitable as joint flexibility is limited by CT restrictions whereas ROM can be negatively affected by factors (bulk) independent of joint flexibility. In addition, body segment lengths can affect flexibility scores (26,29).
- Training in a limited ROM—training (especially resistance training [RT]) in a limited ROM can reduce flexibility over time. Training in a full exercise-precribed ROM is recommended.
- Activity level—active individuals tend to be more flexible than sedentary adults.

TYPES OF STRETCHING

Stretching requires positioning a body segment to at least a mild level of resistance or discomfort within the joint's ROM. A force is needed to stretch each joint. An *active stretch* is produced when the athlete provides the force, whereas a

Myths & Misconceptions

Flexibility is Mostly Genetic and Very Limited Improvements Can Be Expected with Training

Some have argued that genetics is the primary factor affecting one's flexibility. Although genetics contributes to flexibility to some extent, other trainable factors contribute and can be enhanced with regular flexibility training. Consistent flexibility training consisting of dynamic movements and static stretching can increase flexibility. Studies have shown that 6–12 weeks of static stretching increases joint ROM by more than 10 degrees or more than 18% (20,31,49). Although genetics may pose some limitation, everyone can increase flexibility with training.

passive stretch is produced when a partner or device provides the force. Some research indicates that active stretching is superior to increasing hamstring flexibility than passive stretching over short-term periods (4–6 weeks) of training (19,42), but passive stretching is superior over longer periods (>8 weeks) (19). Four types of stretching are used in training programs: static, dynamic, ballistic, and proprioceptive neuromuscular facilitation stretching.

Static Stretching

Static stretching involves holding a joint position (statically) with some level of discomfort for at least 15–20 seconds. The athlete maintains complete control over the movement and static holding of the joint position. Static stretching is very effective for increasing joint ROM but is most productive postexercise when the goal is to increase flexibility. Several examples of static stretches are presented at the end of this chapter.

Dynamic Stretching

Dynamic stretching involves actively moving a joint through its full ROM without any relaxation or holding of joint positions. These stretches are functional in nature and often replicate sport-specific movements. Specific movements are emphasized rather than individual muscle groups. Some examples include forward and backward arm circles, trunk circles (from a straddled position), and walking knee lifts. Dynamic stretching offers clear advantages to static stretching when included as part of a warm-up (18). Dynamic stretches offer similar physiological responses that assist in preparing the body for exercise yet do not result in the same level of reduced musculotendinous stiffness characteristic of static stretching (which yields reductions in strength and power). Dynamic stretching offers the advantage of warming up several muscle groups simultaneously, which could potentially increase the efficiency of the warm-up. These stretches may be performed as repetitions in place or in series covering a specific distance. In either case, the progression should take place from light, gradual movements to more intense, quicker movements when preparing for strength/power activities (30).

An explosive type of dynamic stretching is **ballistic stretching**. Ballistic stretching involves dynamic movement. However, the movement is ballistic, resulting in a bouncing type of motion where the final position is not held. Ballistic stretching has been controversial in its use. Opponents argue that it may increase the risk of injury and result in greater muscle/CT damage and soreness. Ballistic stretching activates the muscle spindles to initiate the stretch reflex, which facilitates agonist contraction and not relaxation. This may defeat the purpose of stretching for increased flexibility (1). Although ballistic stretching can increase flexibility (1,61), it is believed that the stimulus applied may be too short to optimize increases in flexibility compared to the prolonged lower force application

of static stretching (1). Proponents of ballistic stretching argue it can be effective and safe when performed properly and may help prepare the body for ballistic exercise more effectively. Nevertheless, most S&C coaches and athletes prefer dynamic stretching (without ballistic movements) for warming up. Research shows that acute ballistic stretching results in less vertical jump performance decrement than static and proprioceptive neuromuscular facilitation stretching (14), enhances acute vertical jump height (61), and does not affect acute 1 RM strength while static stretching acutely decreases 1 RM (5).

Proprioceptive Neuromuscular Facilitation Stretching

Proprioceptive neuromuscular facilitation (PNF) stretching was developed in the late 1940s by Herman Kabat as part of rehabilitation for polio patients (1,51). By the late 1970s athletes began to use PNF stretching to increase flexibility. Different from other forms of stretching, PNF stretching incorporates combinations of concentric (CON), eccentric (ECC), and isometric (ISOM) muscle actions, and passive stretching. The physiological rationale is to cause relaxation via muscle inhibition of the agonist muscle group to facilitate greater ROM. In fact, one repetition of a PNF stretch may acutely increase ROM by 3–9 degrees (51). A few neuromuscular mechanisms play critical roles in muscle relaxation. **Autogenic inhibition** involves reflex relaxation that occurs in an agonist muscle group following fatiguing contraction via Golgi tendon organ activation. **Reciprocal inhibition** involves antagonist muscle relaxation resulting from contracting the agonist muscle group. Some have suggested that the ISOM muscle action may slightly alter muscle spindle function to favor relaxation (1). It is thought that PNF stretching enhances an athlete's stretch tolerance or perception thereby enabling greater acute ROM increases and flexibility improvements (51). Various forms of muscle contraction-relaxation cycles are used to expand joint ROM.

PNF stretching offers many benefits to athletes. Studies show PNF stretching increases flexibility by up to 33% (1,51) and some show superiority to static stretching (1,51). PNF and static stretching can alter sprint biomechanics by increasing stride length by 9.1% and 7.1%, respectively (15). Because of its resistive component, PNF stretching can enhance muscle strength, endurance, and joint stability (1). However, PNF stretching performed as a warm-up before strength and power activity has similar negative effects as static stretching (14).

Several variations of PNF stretching may be performed. These variations involve the help of a partner but an athlete may self-apply PNF techniques manually as well. Four commonly used PNF techniques include (a) hold-relax, (b) contract-relax, (c) hold-relax with agonist contraction, and (d) contract-relax with agonist contraction. The term *hold* refers to an ISOM action and *contract* refers to CON contraction of the agonist or antagonist muscle group. *Relax* refers to passive static stretching. It is recommended that PNF stretching be performed 1–2 days per week with the static contraction at least 20% of the maximal voluntary contractile force (51). A 6-second contraction followed by a 10–30-second assisted stretch has been recommended by the American College of Sports Medicine (ACSM) (3).

Hold-Relax

- Technique begins with a passive stretch held at the point of mild discomfort for ~10 seconds
- Partner applies force to the antagonist muscles and instructs athlete to hold the position
- The athlete ISOM contracts and resists the partner's force for ~6 seconds
- Athlete relaxes and partner passively stretches athlete deeper in the ROM for ~20–30 seconds
- Cycle may be repeated until final segment of ROM is reached (Fig. 10.3)

Contract-Relax

- Technique begins with a passive stretch held at the point of mild discomfort for ~10 seconds
- Partner applies force to the agonist muscle group while the athlete CON contracts the agonist group through the joint ROM
- Athlete relaxes and partner applies passive stretch in deeper area of ROM for ~20–30 seconds
- Cycle may be repeated until final segment of ROM is reached

Hold-Relax with Agonist Contraction

- Technique begins with a passive stretch held at the point of mild discomfort for ~10 seconds
- Partner applies force to antagonist muscle group and instructs athlete to hold the position

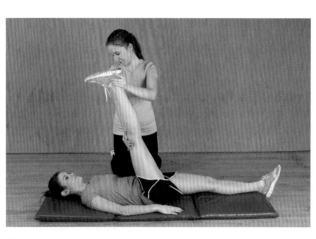

■ FIGURE 10.3. Hold-relax PNF stretching of the hamstrings muscle group.

- A CON action of the agonist muscle group is used against partner resistance
- Passive stretch is applied to athlete and is held for ~20–30 seconds
- Cycle may be repeated until final segment of ROM is reached

Contract-Relax with Agonist Contraction

- Technique begins with a passive stretch held at the point of mild discomfort for ~10 seconds
- Partner applies force to the agonist muscle group while the athlete CON contracts the agonist group through the joint ROM
- Athlete relaxes and partner applies passive stretch in a deeper area of ROM for ~20–30 seconds while the athlete CON contracts
- Cycle may be repeated until final segment of ROM is reached

Myths & Misconceptions

Resistance Training Will Decrease Flexibility

Some have had great concern that RT (muscle hypertrophy) will make one "muscle-bound" and decrease flexibility. This could potentially occur if the athlete does not include any flexibility exercises. Although some athletes with large levels of muscle mass may have poor flexibility, this is most likely the result of initial flexibility deficits or a lack of stretching. It is possible for an athlete who does not resistance train or train for flexibility to lose flexibility regardless of the magnitude of muscle mass. The lack of stretching is the key. RT alone may improve flexibility in some joints especially in sedentary and elderly populations with initial low levels of flexibility (9,54). Although some studies have shown RT may not increase flexibility, RT did not inhibit flexibility increases when a stretching program was used concomitantly with RT (44). Olympic weightlifters have superior shoulder flexibility (from performing the snatch and related lifts) compared to bodybuilders, powerlifters, and football players. The combination of RT and stretching is the most effective method to increase flexibility with concomitant muscle hypertrophy. To enhance flexibility during RT solely, exercises need to be performed in a fully prescribed ROM and the ECC phase of each rep can be emphasized. Several exercises, by design, can increase joint ROM, including the squat, snatch, power clean and front squat, stiff-leg deadlift, and lunge, to name a few. The squat may increase ankle and hip flexibility. The snatch can increase shoulder flexibility. The power clean and front squat can increase wrist flexibility due to the nature of the catch position. The stiff-leg deadlift can increase hamstring flexibility. The lunge (and lateral lunge) can increase hip and ankle flexibility.

Exercises

Static Stretches

The following section illustrates and describes several popular static stretches.

NECK ROTATION

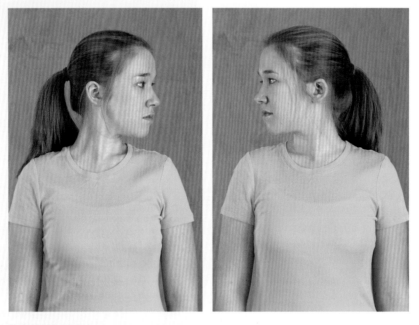

■ **FIGURE 10.4.**

- Athlete maintains a standing or seated position with the head and neck upright and turns head left and holds the position.
- Head returns to the starting position and turns to the right and is statically held.
- Muscles stretched: *neck rotators*

 CAUTION! *A slow and controlled velocity should be used during rotation.*

NECK FLEXION/EXTENSION/LATERAL FLEXION

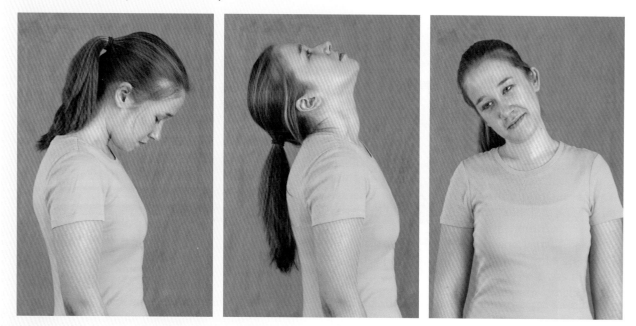

■ **FIGURE 10.5.**

- Athlete stands, sits, or lies supine on a bench with head and neck upright and flexes neck by tucking chin toward chest. The position is held.
- Head returns to starting position and extends and hyperextends back. Position is held.

- Head returns to anatomical position and athlete laterally flexes neck to the right, holds the position, and laterally flexes neck to the left (and holds the position).
- Muscles stretched: *neck extensors*, *flexors*, and *lateral flexors*

PECTORAL WALL STRETCH

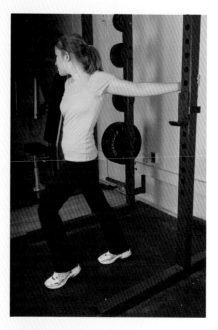

■ **FIGURE 10.6.**

- Athlete stands against an object (open doorway or weight machine) with arms bent at 90° angles with elbows positioned at shoulder level.
- Athlete leans body forward until stretch is felt in upper chest.
- Stretch can be performed with one arm against the wall or weight machine (shown in Fig. 10.6). In this variation, torso rotation helps expand the ROM of the stretch. This stretch can be performed between two benches, chairs, or SBs.
- Another variation is to assume a supine position on a bench with light dumbbells (DB) in hand. Similar to performing a negative fly, the athlete lowers the DBs in an arc fashion until the final position is attained. This position is held.
- Muscles stretched: *pectoralis major*, *shoulder girdle protractors*, and *anterior deltoid*

BENT-OVER SHOULDER/PECTORAL STRETCH

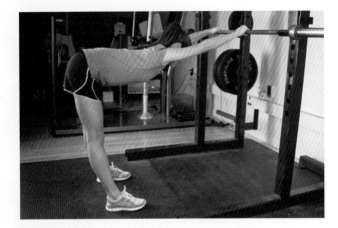

FIGURE 10.7.

- Athlete assumes a shoulder-width grip with shoulders flexed (elbows may be bent as a variation), grasps a bar or bench or power rack, bends over at the waist, and assumes a position where the upper body is parallel to the ground.
- Athlete relaxes the shoulders and continues to bend as far as possible to where the head will be level or lower than the arms.

- This stretch may be performed on the knees with the athlete's hands facing down on the mat or floor.
- Muscles stretched: *shoulder flexors*

POSTERIOR SHOULDER HYPEREXTENSION

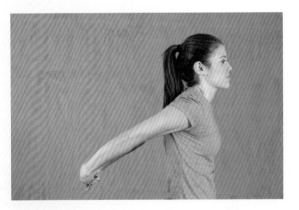

FIGURE 10.8.

- Athlete stands with arms behind back, the elbows are extended and fingers interlocked with palms facing each other. The neck is relaxed and head is upright.
- A variation is to use a broomstick or light bar instead of clasping the fingers together.

- Elbows are fully extended while arms are slowly raised, or shoulders hyperextended.
- Muscles stretched: *shoulder flexors*

SEATED POSTERIOR LEAN

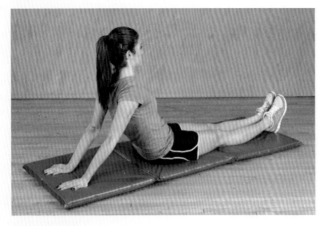

■ FIGURE 10.9.

- Athlete sits with legs straight and arms extended with palms on the floor (pointing away from the body) behind the hips.

- As the hands slide backward, the body leans back.
- Muscles stretched: *shoulder flexors*

ANTERIOR CROSS-ARM STRETCH

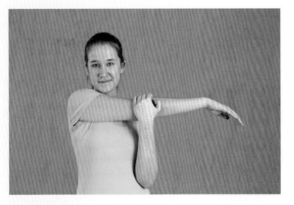

■ FIGURE 10.10.

- Athlete stands or sits with left elbow slightly flexed, arm horizontally adducted across the body, and the right hand pulls the left arm across chest.

- Position is held and repeated for opposite limb.
- Muscles stretched: *upper-back muscles* and *posterior deltoid*

FLEXED ARMS ABOVE HEAD STRETCH

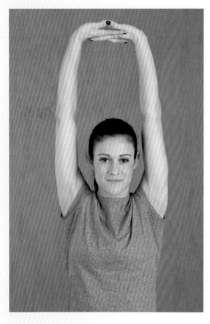

■ FIGURE 10.11.

- Athlete stands with arms stretched in front of the torso, fingers interlocked, and palms facing out.
- Arms straighten (shoulder flexion) above head (palms now face up) and athlete reaches upward and back to expand ROM. This position is held.
- A variation is to hang from a pull-up bar.
- Muscles stretched: *upper-back muscles*

LAT STRETCH

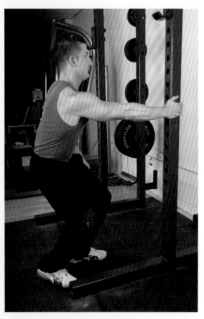

■ FIGURE 10.12.

- Athlete grasps the uprights of a power rack with arms at or near shoulder level.
- Athlete flexes hips/knees, leans back, and stretches upper-back muscles. Position is held.
- Muscles stretched: *upper-back muscles* and *shoulder girdle retractors*

INTERNAL/EXTERNAL SHOULDER ROTATION STRETCH

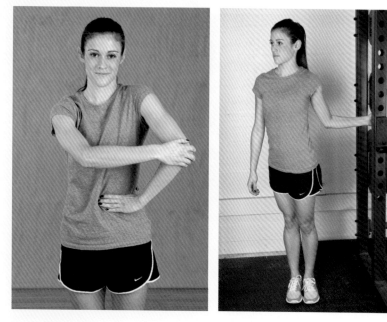

FIGURE 10.13.

- Athlete stands/sits with elbow flexed and hand on hip (Fig. 10.13A). Opposite arm applies force to elbow to facilitate internal rotation. Position is held, stretch is repeated for opposite arm.

- Athlete stands with elbow flexed at 90° against the side of a wall or power rack (Fig. 10.13B). Force is applied by rotating the body to facilitate external rotation. Position is held and stretch is repeated for opposite arm.
- Muscles stretched: *shoulder internal* and *external rotators*

BEHIND-THE-NECK TRICEPS STRETCH

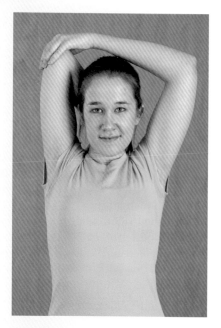

FIGURE 10.14.

- Athlete stands or sits with right shoulder abducted and elbow flexed.
- Left hand grasps right elbow, pulls the elbow behind the head, position is held and repeated for opposite arm.
- Muscles stretched: *triceps brachii*

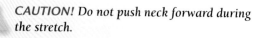 *CAUTION! Do not push neck forward during the stretch.*

FORWARD TRICEPS STRETCH

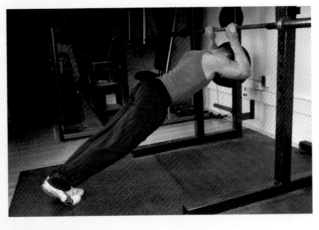

FIGURE 10.15.

- Athlete assumes narrow grip on a bar located in front of the body. Athlete leans the body forward while flexing the elbows, and final position is held.

- Muscles stretched: *triceps brachii*

BICEPS STRETCH

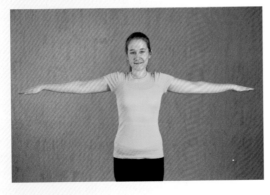

FIGURE 10.16.

- Athlete abducts the shoulders and keeps the elbows extended. The forearm is pronated to stretch the elbow flexors and supinator further. A wall or power rack may be used for support.
- Muscles stretched: *elbow flexors* and *supinator*

PRETZEL

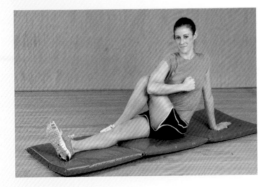

FIGURE 10.17.

- Athlete assumes a seated position, left foot is placed to the side of right knee, and knee is bent. The back part of the right elbow pushes against the left side of knee. Left arm is used for support.
- Left knee is pushed right, while the chest is opened and athlete faces posterior.
- Position is maintained and repeated for opposite side.
- Muscles stretched: *low back*, *abdominals*, and *obliques*

SUPINE HIP FLEXION

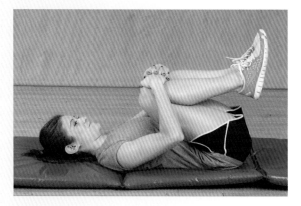

FIGURE 10.18.

- Athlete lies on back with legs straight. Both legs are pulled inward to chest (with hands above knees). Final position is held.
- Muscles stretched: *low back, hip extensors*

> ✔ *VARIATIONS A variation is to stretch one side at a time. Another variation is to roll back onto shoulders (with upper arms assisting in support) while releasing hands from knees. Hands support torso as gravity pulls legs downward to head.*

SEMILEG STRADDLE

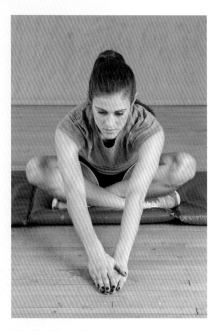

FIGURE 10.19.

- Athlete's knees and hips are flexed with toes pointed outward. Another variation is to sit on a chair rather than the floor.
- Athlete leans forward from the waist as the arms extend forward.
- Muscles stretched: *low back* and *hip extensors*

> ✔ *VARIATIONS A variation is to keep the body upright but to bend the knee to 90° and pull the leg upward at the ankle/lower leg.*

LYING TORSO STRETCH

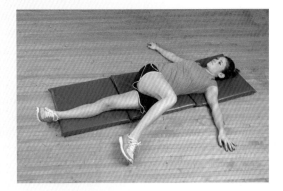

FIGURE 10.20.

- Athlete lies on the mat with shoulders abducted to close to 90° and elbows extended. Hips and knees are flexed.
- Athlete rotates hips all the way to right and position is held. Athlete rotates to the left and position is held. The elbow flexors and shoulder horizontal adductors can be stretched on the ipsilateral side during torso rotation.
- An alternative is to have one leg to rotate while the other remains straight (Fig. 10.20).
- Muscles stretched: *low back, hip extensors/abductors,* and *trunk rotators*

VARIATIONS *A variation is to keep the knees extended while rotating.*

FORWARD LUNGE STRETCH

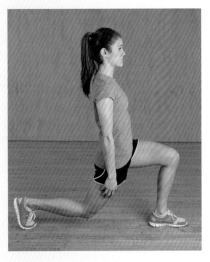

FIGURE 10.21.

- From standing position, athlete takes stride forward with left leg and flexes left knee until it is directly over left foot.
- Left foot is flat on the floor with toes pointed in the same direction and back knee is slightly bent.
- Hips move forward and downward. Position is held and opposite side is stretched.
- Muscles stretched: *hip flexors and opposite side hip extensors*

VARIATIONS *A variation is to perform this stretch from a kneeling position. A torso rotation, flexed arm, or other upper-body stretch can be added.*

PRESS-UP STRETCH

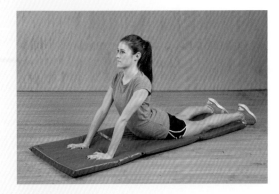

FIGURE 10.22.

- Athlete lies prone on the mat in a push-up position. Athlete pushes upper body upward while keeping hips and lower extremities static. Final position is held.
- Muscles stretched: *hip flexors* and *abdominals*

! CAUTION! *Hips should remain in contact with the ground.*

SIDE BEND STRETCH (STRAIGHT OR FLEXED ARMS)

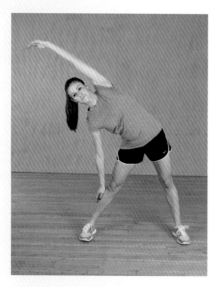

■ **FIGURE 10.23.**

- Athlete stands with feet greater than shoulder width apart, left arm overhead, and right arm down by side (Fig. 10.23).
- Athlete reaches and laterally flexes the trunk to the right side. Position is held and other side is stretched.
- Muscles stretched: *obliques* and *latissimus dorsi*

> ✓ **VARIATIONS** *An alternative is to have the athlete stand with feet hip width apart, and fingers interlaced with palms facing outward and away from torso, or the athlete can perform the stretch from a seated, straddled position.*

PARTNER HIP FLEXOR STRETCH

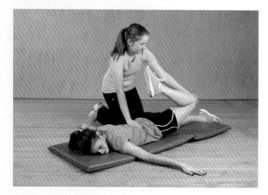

■ **FIGURE 10.24.**

- Athlete lies prone on a bench, floor, or table. A partner is positioned at the side.
- Partner applies pressure to low back and lifts up the flexed leg (under the knee) while athlete contracts the gluteal muscles.
- Position is held and opposite side is stretched. Pressure can be applied to the foot by the partner to assist in stretching the quadriceps simultaneously.
- Muscles stretched: *hip flexors*

SEATED TOE TOUCH STRETCH

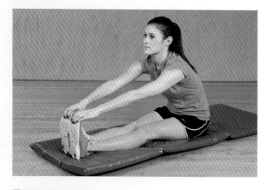

■ **FIGURE 10.25.**

- Athlete is seated with upper body vertical with legs straight. Body leans forward using hip flexors and arms to reach toward toes or ankles (depending on flexibility).
- Legs remain straight and position is held.
- Muscles stretched: *erector spinae, hamstrings,* and *plantar flexors*

SEMISTRADDLE STRETCH

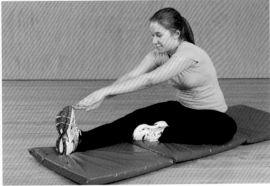

■ **FIGURE 10.26.**

- Athlete is seated with upper body nearly vertical and right leg straight. Sole of left foot is placed on the inner side of right knee.
- Athlete leans forward using hip flexors and arms to reach toward toes. Position is held and opposite side is stretched.
- Muscles stretched: *erector spinae, hamstrings,* and *plantar flexors*

> ⚠ *CAUTION! The nonstretched leg should rotate inward and not outward, which places undue stress on the knees (a variation known as the hurdler's stretch).*

STRADDLE STRETCH

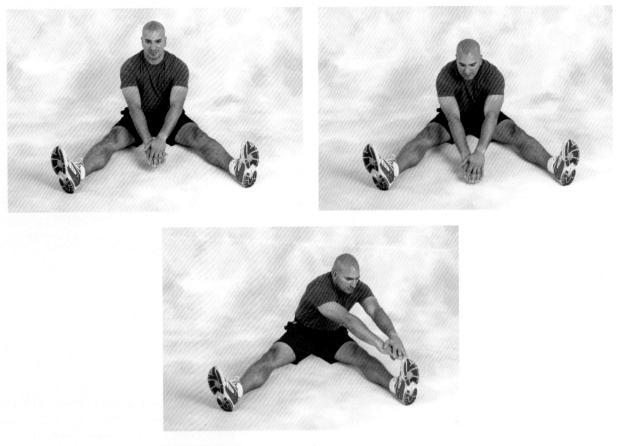

■ **FIGURE 10.27.**

- Athlete assumes a seated position with legs abducted in a wide stance or foot position.
- The athlete bends forward and grasps the ankles or toes while keeping the knees extended. The final position is held.
- Muscles stretched: *erector spinae, hamstrings, hip adductors,* and *plantar flexors*

> ✓ *VARIATIONS A variation is to perform the stretch supine against a wall where the hips are abducted (with knees extended) while touching the wall. A partner could apply pressure to deepen the stretch. This variation targets mostly the hip adductors.*

BUTTERFLY STRETCH

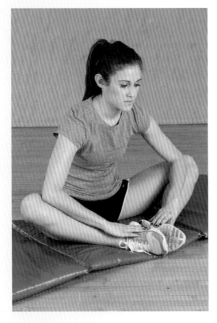

■ **FIGURE 10.28.**

- Athlete assumes an upright position with knees flexed and hips rotated outward with soles of feet touching.
- Athlete attempts to touch knees to floor and leans forward from the waist causing hip abduction.
- Muscles stretched: *hip adductors/internal rotators*

KNEELING HIP ADDUCTOR STRETCH

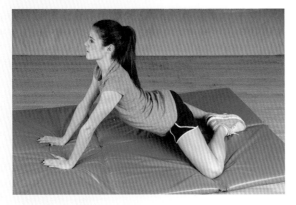

■ **FIGURE 10.29.**

- Athlete assumes a kneeling position on the mat and gradually abducts the hips (widens the base) until the position is attained (Fig. 10.29). Feet can be touching in the rear. This stretch can be performed with the knees extended from a standing position.
- Athlete relaxes and drops body weight downward to stretch the hips.
- Muscles stretched: *hip adductors/internal rotators*

STANDING QUADRICEPS STRETCH

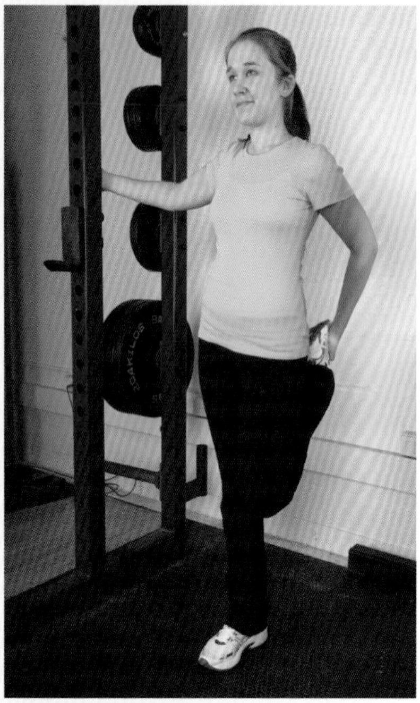

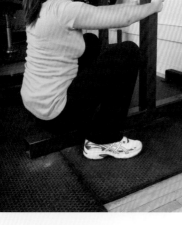

■ **FIGURE 10.30.**

- Athlete stands and supports body weight by holding on to a wall or power rack. This stretch may be performed lying with the legs straight. Front of ankle is grasped with left hand and pulled toward glutes, flexing left knee. Position is held and opposite side is stretched.
- Muscles stretched: *quadriceps*

> ✔ **VARIATIONS** *A variation is to position the foot of the stretched leg against a wall and lean backward.*

SQUAT STRETCH

■ **FIGURE 10.31.**

- Athlete assumes a standing position with shoulder-width stance and squats as low as possible and maintains the final position.
- The athlete may use a power rack for support or may rotate hips forward to deepen the stretch.
- Muscles stretched: *quadriceps* and *hip extensors*

PARTNER QUADRICEPS STRETCH

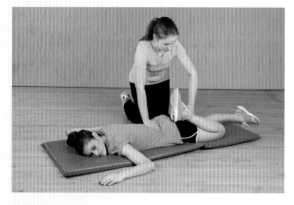

FIGURE 10.32.

- Athlete assumes prone position on bench or floor and flexes one or both knees.
- Partner supplies force to athlete's ankles to enhance ROM. A partner may not be needed for this as the athlete can self-stretch but does benefit the efficacy of the stretch.
- Muscles stretched: *quadriceps*

PIRIFORMIS STRETCH

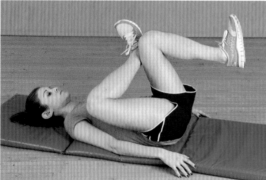

FIGURE 10.33.

- Athlete assumes a standing, seated, or lying position (Fig. 10.33). The left hip and knee are flexed and right leg is crossed over the left leg.
- Pressure is applied to the right knee to stretch the hip external rotators. Left hip flexes to assist in expanding ROM. Athlete can semisquat if in the standing position. Final position is maintained and opposite side is stretched.
- Muscles stretched: *hip external rotators*

STANDING HAMSTRING STRETCH

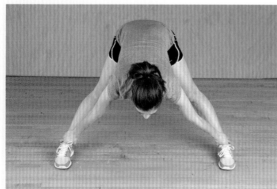

FIGURE 10.34.

- Athlete assumes a wide, straddled stance with upright torso and bends at waist (keeping knees extended) and touches right or left toes (if possible) or flexes toward the center.
- Final position is held and opposite side is stretched.
- Muscles stretched: *hamstrings*, *lower back*, and *glutes*

✔ *VARIATIONS A variation is to narrow the stance and cross one leg over the other where the rear leg is actively stretched. Another variation is to flex one leg forward and elevate it off of the floor onto an object (step, bench). While keeping the toes pointed up, the athlete bends forward (with knee extended) stretching the hamstrings in the process.*

STANDING ADDUCTOR STRETCH

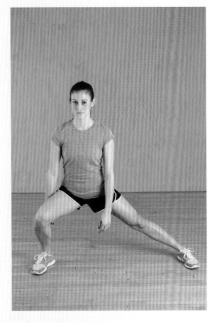

FIGURE 10.35.

- Athlete stands in a straddle stance with feet wider than shoulder width and performs a side lunge until stretch is felt in the athlete's adductors (groin).
- Final position is maintained and opposite side is stretched.
- Muscles stretched: *hip adductors* and *hamstrings*

 CAUTION! Athlete should try to maintain a vertical trunk posture as much as possible.

SUPINE HAMSTRINGS STRETCH

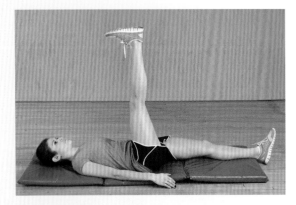

FIGURE 10.36.

- Athlete lies flat on back with legs extended and flexes right hip with knee flexed and extends knee. Final position is held and opposite side is stretched.
- Muscles stretched: *hamstrings*

VARIATIONS A variation is to perform this stretch standing (with hip flexed) or seated in a chair.

WALL CALF STRETCH

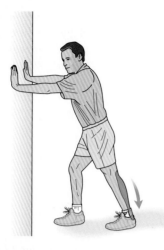

■ FIGURE 10.37.

- Athlete faces the wall with feet shoulder width apart and leans forward with hands on the wall.
- One leg steps back while front leg flexes at knee. Athlete extends back leg trying to lower heel to the floor. Final position is held and opposite side is stretched.
- Muscles stretched: *plantar flexors*

STEP STRETCH

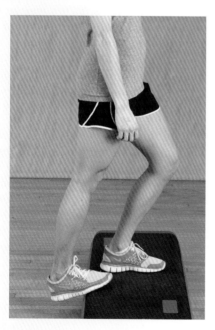

■ FIGURE 10.38.

- Ball of one foot is at the edge of a step with other foot flat on the step. Heel of foot on edge of the step is lowered toward the floor with a straight leg.
- Final position is held and opposite side is stretched.
- Muscles stretched: *plantar flexors*

PRONE HIP ABDUCTOR STRETCH

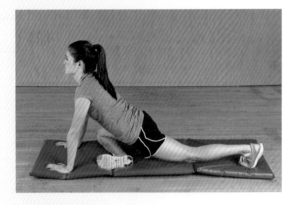

■ FIGURE 10.39.

- Athlete begins in a prone push-up position. Right leg moves forward and inward by hip flexion, internal rotation, and adduction to where it is crosses the body beneath the trunk.
- Athlete gently places weight downward onto leg. Final position is held and opposite side is stretched.
- Muscle stretched: *hip abductors*

FLEXIBILITY TRAINING GUIDELINES

Although dynamic exercise may increase joint flexibility, stretching is the key component to a flexibility training program. Stretching to improve flexibility should be performed following a workout or following a general warm-up (where flexibility exercises are the sole modality) as muscles can be safely stretched to a greater ROM when they are warm. Stretching early or after a workout produces similar increases in flexibility (10) so the latter is preferred if anaerobic exercise is performed during the same workout. Several studies comparing flexibility used program frequencies of 1–6 days per week for individual stretch durations of 15–60 seconds. Studies have shown that: stretching 1–5 days per week increases hamstring flexibility but stretching 3–5 days produces superior results than 1 day (36); stretching once per day for 6 weeks produces similar hamstring flexibility as stretching three times per day (8); 30-second duration stretching produces similar increases in hamstring flexibility as 60-second duration and both are superior to holding each stretch for 15 seconds over 6 weeks of training (7,8); and total stretching duration is critical as similar increases in flexibility were seen when 12 (reps) × 15 seconds, 6 × 30 seconds, and 4 × 45 seconds

stretching exercises were performed over 12 weeks (4). The ACSM (3) has recommended the following flexibility training guidelines:

- Selection of stretches that work each major muscle group.
- The program should be of at least 10-minute duration and should include at least 4 repetitions per muscle group for at least 2–3 days per week.
- Dynamic, static, and PNF stretches may be selected, and ballistic stretching may be suitable for athletes involved in explosive sports.
- Static stretches should be taken to the point of mild discomfort and held for 15–60 seconds. For PNF stretches a 6-second contraction followed by a 10–30-second assisted stretch is recommended.

Table 10.1 depicts a sample progressive 12-week novice flexibility training program. Designing a flexibility training program begins with the selection of exercises and a training frequency. Unlike other modalities, stretching can be performed every day or multiple times per day. Advanced flexibility training may involve higher frequencies. Flexibility training should be performed after the exercise session to maximize joint ROM and minimize performance decrements

TABLE 10.1 A NOVICE, PROGRESSIVE 16-WEEK FLEXIBILITY TRAINING PROGRAM[a]

STRETCH	WEEKS 1–3	WEEKS 4–7	WEEKS 8–10	WEEKS 11–12
Wall Calf Stretch	3 × 30 s	3 × 40 s	4 × 40 s	4 × 50 s
Standing Quadriceps Stretch	3 × 30 s	3 × 40 s	4 × 40 s	4 × 50 s
Butterfly Stretch	3 × 30 s	3 × 40 s	4 × 40 s	4 × 50 s
Semistraddle Stretch	3 × 30 s	3 × 40 s	4 × 40 s	4 × 50 s
Pretzel Stretch	3 × 30 s	3 × 40 s	4 × 40 s	4 × 50 s
Press-Up Stretch	3 × 30 s	3 × 40 s	4 × 40 s	4 × 50 s
Bent-Over Shoulder/Pectoral Stretch	3 × 30 s	3 × 40 s	4 × 40 s	4 × 50 s
Anterior Cross-Arm Stretch	3 × 30 s	3 × 40 s	4 × 40 s	4 × 50 s
Behind-the-Neck Triceps Stretch	3 × 30 s	3 × 40 s	4 × 40 s	4 × 50 s

[a]Each stretch is taken to the point of mild discomfort and held for the designated period of time; the program is performed 3 days per week.

from overstretching during a warm-up. All major muscle groups should be stretched (or at least those trained during the workout). Two to four repetitions (or more can be performed depending on the needs of the athlete) of static stretches are common and each should be held at the point of discomfort. This position may vary especially as one's flexibility increases. The intensity can increase based on the level of stretch or discomfort. Lastly, stretches should be at least 15 seconds initially and then increased. Progression for flexibility training involves increasing stretch ROM, duration, and repetition number gradually.

Case Study 10.1

Dwight is a wrestler who is beginning an off-season training program. Last season Dwight tested well in several assessments. He was at the top or near the top in all strength and power assessments, and he scored well in muscle endurance tests. However, Dwight scored poorly in flexibility. As a result, Dwight has committed himself to increasing his flexibility during the off-season. He would like to increase flexibility for all major muscle groups; however, his emphasis is on increasing his shoulder and hip flexibility. Dwight will be lifting weights 3 days per week and plans on incorporating a stretching program at the conclusion of his weightlifting workouts.

Question for Consideration: **Based on Dwight's goals, what flexibility training advice would you give him?**

THE COOLDOWN

The **cooldown** is a postworkout light exercise activity, which provides an adjustment period between exercise and rest. It helps return the body to homeostasis in a controlled manner. Waste removal is facilitated, cardiovascular responses are reduced appropriately, and a greater sense of well-being is instituted following a cooldown. The cooldown period provides an excellent opportunity for postexercise stretching to increase flexibility. The athlete may perform a light activity such as walking/cycling for 5–10 minutes and include static stretching.

Summary Points

✔ A warm-up consists of a general and specific component. Warm-ups yield several acute physiological changes that help prepare the body for more intense exercise.

✔ A high-intensity warm-up may elicit postactivation potentiation, which can augment strength and power performance.

✔ Dynamic warm-ups are preferred as prolonged high-intensity static stretching can reduce strength and power performance. If stretching is to be performed, it should only be of light-to-moderate intensity. It is acceptable for athletes who require high levels of flexibility to perform prolonged static stretching during the warm-up.

✔ Flexibility is increased by stretching. Factors that influence or limit flexibility include joint structure, muscular imbalance and control, age, genetics, gender, CT, bulk, performing exercises in a limited ROM, and physical activity level.

✔ Stretching may be active or passive. The types of stretching include static stretching, dynamic and ballistic stretching, and PNF stretching.

✔ Recommendations for flexibility training include selection of stretches that work all major muscle groups, 2–3 days per week, at an intensity of mild discomfort, at least 4 repetitions per muscle group, and held for 15–60 seconds.

Review Questions

1. Which of the following is true concerning flexibility?
   A. Males tend to be more flexible than females in the hips
   B. Active individuals are more flexible than sedentary individuals
   C. Training in a limited ROM maximizes flexibility
   D. Tendons and other CT structures play a limited role in joint flexibility

2. The "pretzel" stretch works which major muscle group?
   A. Obliques
   B. Hamstrings
   C. Gastrocnemius
   D. Pectoralis major

3. Reflex relaxation that occurs in an agonist muscle group following fatiguing contraction via Golgi tendon organ activation is known as
   A. Autogenic inhibition
   B. Proprioceptive neuromuscular facilitation
   C. Reciprocal inhibition
   D. Hysteresis

4. A stretch that involves bouncing near the end of the ROM is known as
   A. PNF stretching
   B. Static stretching
   C. Passive stretching
   D. Ballistic stretching

5. A warm-up may
   A. Increase tissue resistance
   B. Reduce muscle blood flow
   C. Increase muscle temperature
   D. Decrease cardiac output

6. The semistraddle stretch works primarily the _____ muscle group
   A. Triceps brachii
   B. Pectoralis major
   C. Hamstrings
   D. Quadriceps

7. Performing a light 5-minute jog is an example of a specific warm-up. T F

8. High-intensity stretching performed as a part of a specific warm-up can maximize vertical jump and sprint performance. T F

9. A potentiation protocol consisting of 3 sets of squats for 1–2 reps with 85% of 1 RM can augment maximal vertical jump performance. T F

10. An athlete who concurrently is involved in an RT and flexibility program will most likely lose flexibility due to muscle hypertrophy. T F

11. The press-up stretch is used to stretch the abdominal and hip flexor muscles. T F

12. The cooldown is a critical segment of the workout because it helps return the body to homeostasis in a controlled manner. T F

References

1. Alter MJ. *Science of flexibility*. 2nd ed. Champaign (IL): Human Kinetics; 1996. pp. 32–142.
2. Amako M, Oda T, Masuoka K, Yokoi H, Campisi P. Effect of static stretching on prevention of injuries for military recruits. *Mil Med*. 2003;168:442–446.
3. American College of Sports Medicine. *ACSM's Guidelines for Exercise Testing and Prescription*. 8th ed. Philadelphia (PA): Lippincott Williams & Wilkins; 2010. pp. 171–174.
4. Ayala F, de Baranda Andujar PS. Effect of 3 different active stretch durations on hip flexion range of motion. *J Strength Cond Res*. 2010;24:430–436.
5. Bacurau RF, Monteiro GA, Ugrinowitsch C, et al. Acute effect of a ballistic and a static stretching exercise bout on flexibility and maximal strength. *J Strength Cond Res*. 2009;23:304–308.
6. Baker D. The effect of alternating heavy and light resistances on power output during upper-body complex power training. *J Strength Cond Res*. 2003;17:493–497.
7. Bandy WD, Irion JM. The effect of time on static stretch on the flexibility of the hamstring muscles. *Phys Ther*. 1994;74:845–850.
8. Bandy WD, Irion JM, Briggler M. The effect of time and frequency of static stretching on flexibility of the hamstring muscles. *Phys Ther*. 1997;77:1090–1096.
9. Barbosa AR, Santarem JM, Filho WJ, Marucci MDFN. Effects of resistance training on the sit-and-reach test in elderly women. *J Strength Cond Res*. 2002;16:14–18.
10. Beedle BB, Leydig SN, Carnucci JM. No differences in pre- and postexercise stretching on flexibility. *J Strength Cond Res*. 2007;21: 780–783.
11. Behm DG, Button DC, Butt JC. Factors affecting force loss with prolonged stretching. *Can J Appl Physiol*. 2001;26:261–272.
12. Bishop D. Warm up I: Potential mechanisms and the effects of passive warm up on exercise performance. *Sports Med*. 2003;33:439–454.
13. Bishop D. Warm up II: Performance changes following active warm up and how to structure the warm up. *Sports Med*. 2003;33:483–498.
14. Bradley PS, Olsen PD, Portas MD. The effect of static, ballistic, and proprioceptive neuromuscular facilitation stretching on vertical jump performance. *J Strength Cond Res*. 2007;21:223–226.
15. Caplan N, Rogers R, Parr MK, Hayes PR. The effect of proprioceptive neuromuscular facilitation and static stretch training on running mechanics. *J Strength Cond Res*. 2009;23: 1175–1180.
16. Chiu LZ, Fry AC, Weiss LW, et al. Postactivation potentiation response in athletic and recreationally trained individuals. *J Strength Cond Res*. 2003;17:671–677.
17. Emery CA, Meeuwisse WH. Risk factors for groin injuries in hockey. *Med Sci Sports Exerc*. 2001;33:1423–1433.
18. Faigenbaum AD, McFarland JE, Schwerdtman JA, Ratamess NA, Kang J, Hoffman JR. Dynamic warm-up protocols, with and without a weighted vest, and fitness performance in high school female athletes. *J Athl Train*. 2006;41:357–363.
19. Fasen JM, O'Connor AM, Schwartz SL, et al. A randomized controlled trial of hamstring stretching: comparison of four techniques. *J Strength Cond Res*. 2009;23:660–667.
20. Ferreira GN, Teixeira-Salmela LF, Guimaraes CQ. Gains in flexibility related to measures of muscular performance: impact of flexibility on muscular performance. *Clin J Sport Med*. 2007;17:276–281.

21. Fletcher IM, Anness R. The acute effects of combined static and dynamic stretch protocols on fifty-meter sprint performance in track-and-field athletes. *J Strength Cond Res.* 2007;21: 784–787.

22. Giudetti L, DiCagno A, Gallotta MC, et al. Precompetition warm-up in elite and subelite rhythmic gymnastics. *J Strength Cond Res.* 2009;23:1877–1882.

23. Gourgoulis V, Aggeloussis N, Kasimatis P, Mavromatis G, Garas A. Effect of a submaximal half-squats warm-up program on vertical jumping ability. *J Strength Cond Res.* 2003;17:342–344.

24. Hartig DE, Henderson JM. Increasing hamstring flexibility decreases lower extremity overuse injuries in military basic trainees. *Am J Sports Med.* 1999;27:173–176.

25. Hodgson M, Docherty D, Robbins D. Post-activation potentiation: underlying physiology and implications for motor performance. *Sports Med.* 2005;35:585–595.

26. Hoeger WW, Hopkins DR. A comparison of the sit and reach and the modified sit and reach in the measurement of flexibility in women. *Res Q Exerc Sport.* 1992;63:191–195.

27. Hoffman JR, Ratamess NA, Faigenbaum AD, Mangine GT, Kang J. Effects of maximal squat exercise testing on vertical jump performance in American college football players. *J Sports Sci Med.* 2007;6:149–150.

28. Holt BW, Lambourne K. The impact of different warm-up protocols on vertical jump performance in male collegiate athletes. *J Strength Cond Res.* 2008; 22: 226–229.

29. Hopkins DR, Hoeger WWK. A comparison of the sit-and-reach test and the modified sit-and-reach test in the measurement of flexibility for males. *J Appl Sport Sci Res.* 1992;6:7–10.

30. Jeffreys I. Warm-up and stretching. In: Baechle TR, Earle RW, editors. *Essentials of Strength Training and Conditioning.* 3rd ed. Champaign (IL): Human Kinetics; 2008. p. 295–324.

31. Kokkonen J, Nelson AG, Eldredge C, Winchester JB. Chronic static stretching improves exercise performance. *Med Sci Sports Exerc.* 2007;39:1825–1831.

32. Kubo K, Kanehisa H, Kawakami Y, Fukunaga T. Influence of static stretching on viscoelastic properties of human tendon structures in vivo. *J Appl Physiol.* 2001;90:520–527.

33. Kubo K, Kanehisa H, Fukunaga T. Effect of stretching training on the viscoelastic properties of human tendon structures in vivo. *J Appl Physiol.* 2002;92:595–601.

34. Malliaris P, Cook JL, Kent P. Reduced ankle dorsiflexion range may increase the risk of patellar tendon injury among volleyball players. *J Sci Med Sport.* 2006;9:304–309.

35. Marek SM, Cramer JT, Fincher AL, et al. Acute effects of static and proprioceptive neuromuscular facilitation stretching on muscle strength and power output. *J Athl Train.* 2005;40:94–103.

36. Marques AP, Vasconcelos AA, Cabral CM, Sacco IC. Effect of frequency of static stretching on flexibility, hamstring tightness, and electromyographic activity. *Braz J Med Biol Res.* 2009;42: 949–953.

37. McBride JM, Nimphius S, Erickson TM. The acute effects of heavy-load squats and loaded countermovement jumps on sprint performance. *J Strength Cond Res.* 2005;19:893–897.

38. McCullough AS, Kraemer WJ, Volek JS, et al. Factors affecting flutter kicking speed in women who are competitive and recreational swimmers. *J Strength Cond Res.* 2009;23:2130–2136.

39. McMillian DJ, Moore JH, Hatler BS, Taylor DC. Dynamic vs. static-stretching warm up: the effect on power and agility performance. *J Strength Cond Res.* 2006;20:492–499.

40. Meckel Y, Atterbom H, Grodjinovsky A, Ben-Sira D, Rotstein A. Physiological characteristics of female 100 metre sprinters of different performance levels. *J Sports Med Phys Fitness.* 1995;35: 169–175.

41. Mediate P, Faigenbaum A. *Medicine Ball for All Kids: Medicine Ball Training Concepts and Program-Design Considerations for School-Age Youth.* Monterey (CA): Coaches Choice; 2007.

42. Meroni R, Cerri CG, Lanzarini C, et al. Comparison of active stretching technique and static stretching technique on hamstring flexibility. *Clin J Sport Med.* 2010;20:8–14.

43. Nelson AG, Driscoll NM, Landin DK, Young MA, Schexnayder IC. Acute effects of passive muscle stretching on sprint performance. *J Sports Sci.* 2005;23:449–454.

44. Nobrega ACL, Paula KC, Carvalho ACG. Interaction between resistance training and flexibility training in healthy young adults. *J Strength Cond Res.* 2005;19:842–846.

45. Pearce AJ, Kidgell DJ, Zois J, Carlson JS. Effects of secondary warm up following stretching. *Eur J Appl Physiol.* 2009;105:175–183.

46. Power K, Behm D, Cahill F, Carroll M, Young W. An acute bout of static stretching: effects on force and jumping performance. *Med Sci Sports Exerc.* 2004;36:1389–1396.

47. Robbins JW, Scheuermann BW. Varying amounts of acute static stretching and its effect on vertical jump performance. *J Strength Cond Res.* 2008;22:781–786.

48. Ryan ED, Herda TJ, Costa PB, et al. Determining the minimum number of passive stretches necessary to alter musculotendinous stiffness. *J Sports Sci.* 2009;27:957–961.

49. Sainz de Baranda P, Ayala F. Chronic flexibility improvement after a 12-week stretching program utilizing the ACSM recommendations: hamstring flexibility. *Int J Sports Med.* 2010;31: 389–396.

50. Samuel MN, Holcomb WR, Guadagnoli MA, Rubley MD, Wallmann H. Acute effects of static and ballistic stretching on measures of strength and power. *J Strength Cond Res.* 2008;22:1422–1428.

51. Sharman MJ, Cresswell AG, Riek S. Proprioceptive neuromuscular facilitation stretching: mechanisms and clinical implications. *Sports Med.* 2006;36:929–939.

52. Taylor KL, Sheppard JM, Lee H, Plummer N. Negative effect of static stretching restored when combined with a sport specific warm-up component. *J Sci Med Sport.* 2008; (ahead of print).

53. Thacker SB, Gilchrist J, Stroup DF, Kimsey CD. Effect of stretching on sport injury risk: a review. *Med Sci Sports Exerc.* 2004;36: 371–378.

54. Thrash K, Kelly B. Flexibility and strength training. *J Appl Sport Sci Res.* 1987;1:74–75.

55. Torres EM, Kraemer WJ, Vingren JL, et al. Effects of stretching on upper-body muscular performance. *J Strength Cond Res.* 2008; 22:1279–1285.

56. Vetter RE. Effects of six warm-up protocols on sprint and jump performance. *J Strength Cond Res.* 2007;21:819–823.

57. Watson AW. Sports injuries related to flexibility, posture, acceleration, clinical defects, and previous injury, in high-level players of body contact sports. *Int J Sports Med.* 2001;22:222–225.

58. Wilson GJ, Murphy AJ, Pryor JF. Musculotendinous stiffness: its relationship to eccentric, isometric, and concentric performance. *J Appl Physiol.* 1994;76:2714–2719.

59. Witvrouw E, Mahieu N, Danneels L, McNair P. Stretching and injury prevention: an obscure relationship. *Sports Med.* 2004;34: 443–449.

60. Woods K, Bishop P, Jones E. Warm-up and stretching in the prevention of muscular injury. *Sports Med.* 2007;37:1089–1099.

61. Woolstenhulme MT, Griffiths CM, Woolstenhulme EM, Parcell AC. Ballistic stretching increases flexibility and acute vertical jump height when combined with basketball activity. *J Strength Cond Res.* 2006;20:799–803.

62. Yetter M, Moir GL. The acute effects of heavy back and front squats on speed during forty-meter sprint trials. *J Strength Cond Res.* 2008;22:159–165.

63. Young WB, Behm DG. Effects of running, static stretching and practice jumps on explosive force production and jumping performance. *J Sports Med Phys Fitness.* 2003;43:21–27.

64. Young W, Elias G, Power J. Effects of static stretching volume and intensity on plantar flexor explosive force production and range of motion. *J Sports Med Phys Fitness.* 2006;46:403–411.

Resistance Training Program Design

After completing this chapter, you will be able to:

· Discuss the importance of designing individualized resistance training programs for obtaining maximal benefits
· Define each acute program variable and identify ways in which to manipulate each one to target specific training goals
· Discuss the ACSM's recommendations for progression during resistance training
· Discuss various advanced resistance training techniques and their potential usage
· Design a phase of a resistance training program from beginning to end

Resistance training (RT) is well known for improving athletic performance. The critical component to optimal RT is the design of the program in addition to the motivation and dedication of the athlete to follow the program consistently. A RT program is a composite of several variables (Fig. 11.1) that interact with each other to provide a stimulus for adaptation. Program design emphasizes the manipulation of these variables to target specific goals and minimize boredom that could accompany training with little variation. Because there are infinite ways to vary programs, many programs can be successful provided that they adhere to general training guidelines. Basic RT guidelines were initially established by the American College of Sports Medicine (ACSM) in 1998 (4). Since then, the ACSM (5,6) has expanded these initial guidelines by providing progression recommendations for strength, power, hypertrophy, and endurance training in healthy young and older individuals. These guidelines and the finer points of program design are discussed in a way to allow the coach/athlete a framework to build a template.

INDIVIDUALIZATION OF RESISTANCE TRAINING PROGRAMS

The most effective RT programs are individualized to the athlete's needs and goals. Training goals (see Chapter 1) serve the basis of the program, and most athletes' programs are based on multiple goals. Goals, in addition to needs of the sport, are obtained by performing a **needs analysis**. A needs analysis consists of answering questions based upon goals and desired outcomes, assessments, access to equipment, health, and the demands of the sport. A sample needs analysis is shown in Table 11.1. Individualized RT programs are most effective because they target the goals and needs of the athlete. The questions a needs analysis may address are (53,95,114)

1. *Are there health/injury concerns that may limit the exercises performed or the exercise intensity?* An injury or health concern may limit some exercises and training intensity until sufficient recovery has ensued. Exercises can be selected to work around an injury.
2. *What type of equipment is available?* Equipment availability is paramount to exercise selection. Although effective programs can be developed with minimal equipment, knowledge of what is available allows one to select appropriate exercises and variations.
3. *What is the training frequency and are there any time constraints that may affect workout duration?* The total number of training sessions per week needs to be derived initially because this will affect all other training variables such as exercise selection, volume, and intensity. Some athletes may be scheduled at specific blocks of time. If this block of time is 1.5 hours, then the program needs to be developed within that time frame. The exercises selected, the number of exercises and total sets performed, and rest intervals between sets and exercises will be affected.
4. *What muscle groups require special attention?* All major muscle groups need to be trained but some may require prioritization based upon strengths/weaknesses or the demands of the sport. It is important to maintain muscle balance especially among those muscles with agonist-antagonist relationships, primary stabilizer roles for large muscle mass exercises, and small muscles often weak in comparison to larger muscle groups.

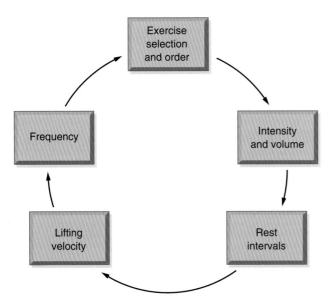

FIGURE 11.1. The acute program variables.

are four to eight times more likely to sustain a tear of their anterior cruciate ligament (ACL) than their male counterparts. Special attention can be given to strengthen the kinetic chain to prevent ACL injuries.

> **SIDEBAR   ANTERIOR CRUCIATE LIGAMENT INJURIES AND FEMALE ATHLETES**
>
> An ACL tear is a severe injury that is costly in rehabilitation time. For noncontact ACL injury, the most common mechanism is deceleration with twisting, pivoting, and/or change of direction (163). ACL injuries are up to eight times more likely to occur in female than male athletes (32). Females have several anatomical and physiological attributes that make them more susceptible to ACL injuries. Females have wider pelvic girdles, a larger angle of pull of the quadriceps muscles, less-developed quadriceps muscle size and strength, increased flexibility (leading to more tibial displacement), more tibial torsion, narrower femoral notch (less space to house the ACL), lower hamstring-to-quadriceps muscle strength ratio, higher estrogen concentrations, generate force more slowly, and have smaller ACLs in comparison to men (32,163). These are factors that decrease knee stability. Women have greater **valgus** stress placed on the knee. A valgus stress is one where abduction (outward angulation) of the joint is seen in a joint where abduction is not a prescribed movement. Valgus stresses increase susceptibility to knee injury and result from some of the aforementioned anatomical factors. The needs analysis for a female athlete may demonstrate that knee injuries

5. *What are the targeted energy systems?* RT programs mostly target the ATP-PC and glycolysis systems. Specific attention can be given to both if they match the metabolic demands of the sport. Although the oxidative system is active during resistance exercise, it is trained more specifically through aerobic training.

6. *What types of muscle actions (CON, ECC, ISOM) are needed?* These are included in all training programs. Some athletes may benefit from targeting one when necessary.

7. *If training for a sport, what are the most common sites of injury?* Special attention can be given to susceptible areas often injured. For example, female athletes

TABLE 11.1 SAMPLE NEEDS ANALYSIS

COLLEGE BASEBALL PLAYER — RIGHT FIELDER
OFF-SEASON STRENGTH AND CONDITIONING PROGRAM

Sport needs	Throwing, hitting, base running, defensive play, sliding, sprinting, occasional diving and jumping
Muscle groups	All major muscle groups are emphasized — special attention for core strength/power, shoulder (rotator cuff), grip strength, and hip/quadriceps strength/power
Common injury sites	Shoulder, knee, hamstrings, elbow, low back
Energy demands	ATP-PC system predominately
Fitness needs	Muscle strength, power, endurance, speed, agility, reaction time and coordination, reduced body fat
Equipment restraints	None
Testing results	Scored well in speed and agility tests; scored fairly well in power assessments; scored fairly well in muscle strength
Desired frequency	3 d per week
Training background	5 yr of resistance training experience. Has good form and technique especially for Olympic lifts. Has built a modest-to-good strength base. Based on examination of training history is considered to be an advanced trainee.
Workout structure	Periodized, total-body workout. Each workout structured in sequence from Olympic/power lifts → basic strength → sport specific needs

Note: This off-season program will strengthen all major muscle groups in a periodized manner to peak strength and power for preseason testing. Speed and agility training will occur separately.

are of concern and special training modifications may be needed to strengthen that area. Prevention of ACL injuries encompasses several concepts and many extend beyond focusing just on the knee. Rather, strengthening the entire kinetic chain (hip, ankle, and core in addition to the knee) is paramount because the knee may be the weak link. Wilk et al. (163) have defined eight areas of concern for female athletes and have proposed exercises to address each area to reduce ACL injuries. These include exercises that target: (a) increased hip strength in three planes (lateral step-over, lunge), (b) strengthened hamstrings to provide greater control of the knee (lateral lunge, slide board), (c) controlled valgus stresses (step-up with band, single-leg squat), (d) controlled knee hyperextension (plyometrics), (e) increased neuromuscular reaction (movement-specific exercises on unstable surfaces), (f) increased thigh musculature (squats, leg press), (g) increased endurance (aerobic training), and (h) increased speed (sprint drills, backward running) (155). Myer et al. have shown knee valgus motion and knee flexion range of motion (ROM) during landing from a jump, body mass, tibia length, and quadriceps-to-hamstrings strength ratio are strong predictors of ACL injury and developed an algorithm to identify athletes at risk using these variables that contribute to high valgus stress (120). Such data can be useful to the coach and athletes to identify early athletes who are at risk.

THE IMPORTANCE OF TRAINING STATUS

Program design differs based on one's level of training. Training status ranges on a continuum from beginner to elite strength/power athlete. Factors to consider include the athlete's history of lifting weights (months and years of experience), level of conditioning (magnitude of strength, power, endurance, and hypertrophy), and sports participation (RT is encountered in several sports and can pose an adaptive stimulus to an athlete independent of weight lifting). Training status is a culmination of these factors and can pose difficulty for the coach to determine in some cases. For example, some individuals have lifted weight for several months to years and only experienced small improvements whereas some individuals with little experience have adapted quickly due to genetics or prior sports participation. Therefore, some difficulty can be encountered in classifying athletes on this continuum. Notwithstanding, a beginner is one who has no or very little experience lifting weights and has a large potential window of adaptation. An intermediate (moderately trained) individual is one who has at least 4–6 months of progressive RT experience and has attained some notable increases in strength. The key is progressive RT experience and not merely working out below one's threshold level

of adaptation. An advanced individual is one with at least 1 year of consistent progressive RT and has experienced a substantial level of adaptation. Those who truly excel in RT may attain elite status in which they rank very highly in one or more components of fitness. Skill level increases as one progresses from beginner to intermediate to advanced.

Training status identification helps determine the rate and magnitude of progression. Untrained individuals respond favorably to any program, thereby making it difficult to evaluate the effects of different RT programs at this stage. Resistance-trained individuals have a slower rate of progression than untrained or moderately trained individuals (95). In the ACSM's 2002 position stand (5), several studies were reviewed and it was estimated that strength increases ~40% in untrained, 20% in moderately trained, 16% in trained, 10% in advanced, and 2% in elite athletes over training periods ranging from 4 weeks to 2 years. Progression in any fitness component becomes more difficult with training. Because of these trends, it was proposed that RT program design be prescribed in an orderly manner from a *general-to-specific progression* (5). This model is illustrated in Figure 11.2. The narrow segment of the pyramid representing novice individuals illustrates that little variation is needed here. Because many programs yield positive results initially, it is recommended that program design be general to begin (keep it simple!). This general phase is characterized by low intensity/volume training where enhancing technique and establishing a conditioning base are primary goals. However, as the window of adaption narrows with conditioning, more variation is needed as illustrated by the wider sides of the pyramid. Greater specificity is needed. A general RT program may improve several components of fitness simultaneously in an untrained individual. However, this same program may only improve one or two components in a trained individual. Advanced training is characterized by greater specificity and this requires greater variation in

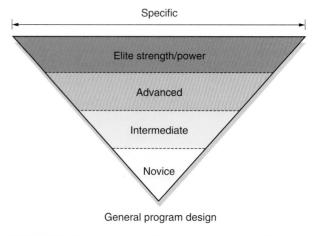

FIGURE 11.2. General-to-specific model of progression. (Adapted with permission from American College of Sports Medicine: Position Stand: Progression models in resistance training for healthy adults. *Med Sci Sports Exerc.* 2002;34:364–380.)

the program. Training cycles are common and each cycle may target a few components of fitness. Training plateaus are encountered at higher levels of training thereby demonstrating the need for variation.

RESISTANCE TRAINING PROGRAM DESIGN

The RT program is a composite of several variables that include (a) muscle actions used, (b) intensity, (c) volume, (d) exercises selected and workout structure, (e) the sequence of exercise performance, (f) rest intervals between sets, (g) repetition velocity, and (h) training frequency. Altering one or several of these variables will affect the training stimuli and increase motivation.

EXERCISE SELECTION

All exercises consist of concentric (CON), eccentric (ECC), and/or isometric (ISOM) muscle actions. Each dynamic repetition consists of ECC, CON, and may include ISOM muscle actions. Physiologically, ECC actions provide greater force per unit of muscle cross-sectional area (CSA), involve less motor unit activation per unit of force, require less energy expenditure per level of tension, result in higher levels of muscle damage, and are more conducive to muscle growth than CON or ISOM muscle actions (6,95). They are important to mediating neuromuscular adaptations to training. Dynamic strength improvements are greatest when ECC actions are emphasized (46). Because dynamic repetitions consist of CON and ECC phases, very little manipulation of these muscle actions occurs. However, each CON or ECC phase can be altered by manipulating the loading, volume, velocity, and rest interval length. Some advanced forms of training involve prioritizing the ECC phase. With traditional RT, most of the effort is applied at the CON sticking region of exercise. The sticking region is the point where bar velocity is minimal. Mechanically, the lifter is in a disadvantageous position when heavy loading is used or fatigue ensues. Weight selection targets the CON sticking region because any more will result in failure, so this limiting factor is present when full ROM repetitions are used. As a consequence, the ECC phase may not receive optimal loading. Accentuated ECC training can provide some additional benefits to the lifter. Acutely, CON strength may be enhanced and it is thought that accentuated ECC training may reduce neural inhibitions leading to greater CON strength. For the bench press, lowering a heavier weight than one's CON 1 RM (105% of 1 RM) yields a greater 1 RM bench press than lowering the CON 1 RM load (43). This was studied by using hooks that became unloaded at the end of the ECC phase. CON 1 RM performance was enhanced by up to ~7 kg (43). Techniques to enhance ECC training include heavy negatives, forced negatives, and unilateral negatives.

ISOM muscle actions exist in many forms during resistance exercise. Stabilizer muscles contract isometrically to maintain posture and stability during an exercise. ISOM actions occur in between ECC and CON actions for the agonist muscles. The action may be prolonged if a pause is instituted. Gripping tasks require ISOM muscle actions. ISOM contraction of finger, thumb, and wrist muscles is paramount to gripping the weights, especially during pulling exercises. Grip strength training greatly depends upon ISOM muscle actions. Lastly, ISOM muscle actions can serve as the primary mode of exercise in a specific area of the ROM. Exercises such as a leg lift and plank are predominantly ISOM. Strong contraction of the trunk is needed to offset the effects of gravity. Another example is the overhead squat. The upper body and trunk isometrically contract to maintain the overhead bar position. The top position of the pull-up exercise can be held for a specific length of time. This involves ISOM contraction of back and arm musculature and may be used to enhance ROM-specific strength and endurance. Lastly, functional ISOM training can be used. The ACSM recommends ISOM muscle actions be included in RT programs targeting strength, hypertrophy, and endurance (6).

Two types of exercises may be selected: single- and multiple-joint. **Single-joint exercises** stress one joint or major muscle group whereas **multiple-joint exercises** stress more than one joint or major muscle group. Both single- and multiple-joint exercises are effective for increasing muscle strength and can be considered sport-specific depending on the athlete. Single-joint exercises, e.g., triceps pushdown, lying leg curl, are used to target specific muscle groups, and may pose a lesser risk of injury due to the reduced level of skill and technique involved. Multiple-joint exercises, e.g., bench press, shoulder press, and squat, are more neutrally complex and are regarded as most effective for increasing strength because of the lifting of a larger amount of weight (53). Multiple-joint exercises may be subclassified as basic strength or total-body lifts. *Basic strength* exercises involve at least two to three major muscle groups whereas *total-body lifts* (Olympic lifts and variations) involve most major muscle groups and are the most complex exercises. These are the most effective exercises for increasing power because they require explosive force production and fast bodily movements.

Muscle mass involvement is important when selecting exercises. Exercises stressing multiple or large muscle groups produce the greatest acute metabolic responses (15). Large muscle mass, multiple-joint exercises such as deadlifts, jump squats, and Olympic lifts augment the acute testosterone and growth hormone response to resistance exercise more than the bench press and shoulder press (94). The ACSM recommends unilateral and bilateral single- and multiple-joint (free weight and machine) exercises be included, with emphasis on multiple-joint exercises for maximizing muscle strength, size, and endurance in novice, intermediate, and advanced

TABLE 11.2 SAMPLE WORKOUTS DEPICTING EXERCISE SELECTION FOR VARIOUS TRAINING GOALS

WEIGHTLIFTER	STRENGTH/POWER ATHLETE	BODYBUILDER	POWERLIFTER
Full snatch 5 × 1–3	Hang clean 4 × 3–5	Back squat 5 × 8–10	Bench press 6 × 3–6
Snatch pull 5 × 1–3	Back squat 4 × 5–8	Leg press 3 × 8–10	Bench press (with pause) 3 × 5
Overhead squat 4 × 5	Bench press 4 × 5–8	Leg extension 3 × 10–12	Wide-grip bench press 3 × 5
Good mornings 3 × 5	Barbell step-up 3 × 8	Stiff-leg deadlift 4 × 10–12	Dumbbell shoulder press 3 × 6
Bench press 3 × 5	Bent-over row 3 × 8	Lying leg curl 3 × 10–12	Front raise 3 × 8
	Standing calf raise 3 × 10		Lying triceps extension 3 × 8
	Internal/external rotation 3 × 10		
	Plyo leg raise 3 × 20		

individuals (6). However, the ACSM recommends the use of predominately multiple-joint exercises for novice, intermediate, and advanced power training (6). Alterations in body posture, grip, and hand width/foot stance and position changes muscle activation to some degree and alters the exercise. Many variations or progressions of single- and multiple-joint exercises can be performed. Table 11.2 illustrates example workouts characteristic of the training of athletes, powerlifters, bodybuilders, and Olympic weightlifters.

SIDEBAR   FREE WEIGHTS VERSUS MACHINES

Free weight and machine exercises are recommended by the ACSM (6). Free weight training leads to greater improvements in free weight test performance, and machine training results in greater performance on machine tests (16,100) although free weight training increases machine-based maximal strength and vice versa. When a neutral testing device is used, strength improvements from free weights and machines appear similar (100,168). The advantages and disadvantages of free weights and machines include (77,114)

- Machines are safe and easy to learn (some have instructions in plain sight to the lifter). Free weights are safe to use but they may require a longer learning phase than machines.
- Machines are more costly than free weights. Free weights enable performance of several exercises with very few pieces of equipment.
- Machines require more maintenance than free weights.
- If the machine uses a weight stack, changing the pin is quick and easy, which is useful if the athlete is performing a circuit training program or if short rest intervals are used.
- Loading differs between free weights and machines. Comparison of free weight bench press and squat versus Smith machine versions showed that lifters have ~5% higher 1 RM performance for Smith

machine squats (than free weight) and ~11% higher free weight bench press (than Smith machine) (37).
- Machines enable the performance of some exercises that are difficult with free weights.
- Some machines provide variable resistance throughout the ROM based on a single-joint ascending/descending strength curve.
- Isokinetic machines control velocity and may be useful for rehabilitation and testing.
- Machines usually do not require the use of a spotter.
- Some machines may hinder development of coordination as stabilizer muscle activity is limited. Machines are fixed or free form. A *fixed machine* is one in which ROM and path are fixed/preset (leg curl). A *free-form machine* is one that allows multiple movement patterns (cable device). Free-form machines are more advantageous for strength and balance enhancement than fixed-form machines (152).
- Free weights enable greater movement potential, require the lifter to control all aspects of the exercise, and require more balance.
- Some machines may not provide enough resistance for very strong athletes.
- Depending on the machine, free weights enable more variability for exercise performance per foot/hand placement, position, and posture.
- Free weights enable performance of Olympic lifts. Although some machines have been developed to use for Olympic lifts, these do not match free weight kinematic patterns and result in less weight lifted and force production (83).
- Free weights enable greater bar velocity for strength/power training.
- Free weights are most effective for enhancing athletic performance although some new machines are designed to mimic sport-specific movements. Machines with braking systems allow the performance of ballistic resistance exercises.

EXERCISE ORDER AND WORKOUT STRUCTURE

The number of muscle groups trained per workout needs to be considered. There are three basic workout structures to choose from: (a) total-body workouts, (b) upper/lower-body split workouts, and (c) muscle group split routines. Total-body workouts involve performance of exercises that work all major muscle groups (1–2 exercises for each major muscle group or several exercises that stress most major muscle groups). They are common among athletes and Olympic weightlifters. With weightlifting, the Olympic lifts and variations are total-body exercises. The first few exercises in sequence are Olympic lifts (plus variations) and the remainder of the workout may be dedicated to basic strength exercises. Upper/lower-body split workouts involve performance of upper-body exercises only during one workout and lower-body exercises only during the next workout. These are common among athletes, powerlifters, and bodybuilders. Muscle group split routines involve performance of exercises for specific muscle groups during a workout (*e.g.*, a "back/biceps" workout where all exercises for the back are performed then all exercises for the biceps are performed). These are characteristic of bodybuilding programs. Compound split routines involve training more than one muscle per group workout. Isolated split routines involve training only one muscle group per workout. Many times these are used within *double splits* where the lifter may train twice per day. For compound split routines, lifters use different strategies for muscle group organization. Agonist-antagonist (chest/back), synergist (chest, triceps), and unrelated muscle group (shoulders, calves) structures may be used. All of these structures can improve performance. Goals, time/frequency, and personal preferences will determine which structure(s) is selected by the coach or athlete. The major differences between structures are the magnitude of specialization present during each workout (related to the number of exercises performed per muscle group) and the amount of recovery in between workouts. One study reported similar improvements in untrained women between total-body and upper/lower-body split workouts (19). In the elderly, similar improvements in lower-body strength between total-body and lower-body workouts (of equal volume and intensity) were shown (20). Table 11.3 illustrates example workouts.

Exercise order affects acute lifting performance and the rate of strength increases during RT. Exercises performed early in the workout generate higher repetition number and weights lifted because less fatigue is present. Multiple-joint exercise performance declines when these exercises are performed later in a workout rather than early (57,145,149,150). Sforzo and Touey (145) investigated bench press and squat performance. Sequence 1 consisted of the squat, leg extension, leg curl, bench press, shoulder press, and triceps pushdown (4 sets × 8 RM, 2–3-min rest intervals) and sequence 2 was the reverse. There were 75% and 22% declines in bench press and squat performance, respectively, when the reverse order was used. Simao et al. (149,150) compared two sequences: bench press, lat pull-down, shoulder press, biceps curl, triceps extension (3 sets of 10 reps); and the reverse order. When the bench press and lat pull-down were performed at the end there was a 28% and 8% reduction in the number of reps performed, respectively (Fig. 11.3). Spreuwenberg et al. (153) examined the squat when it was performed first or last in sequence and reported higher number of repetitions when it was performed first. Interestingly, average power output of the squat was higher when performed after hang pulls, thereby showing an explosive exercise can augment performance of a basic strength exercise. Performance of an exercise may be augmented if the antagonist muscles are stressed in a preceding set (14), thereby providing a basis for agonist-antagonist exercise sequencing. Large muscle

TABLE 11.3 SAMPLE WORKOUTS OF DIFFERENT TRAINING STRUCTURES

TOTAL-BODY WORKOUT	UPPER-BODY WORKOUT	SPLIT ROUTINE (CHEST/TRICEPS)
Squat 3 × 10	Bench press 3 × 6–8	Bench press 3 × 6–8
Bench press 3 × 10	Bent-over row 3 × 6–8	Incline bench press 3 × 8
Lat pull-down 3 × 10	Incline dumbbell press 3 × 8	Dumbbell flys 3 × 10
Leg press 3 × 10	Seated row 3 × 10	Cable cross-over 3 × 12
Shoulder press 3 × 10	Lateral raise 3 × 10	Standing triceps extension 3 × 10
Back extension 3 × 15	Lying triceps extension 3 × 10	Reverse pushdowns 3 × 10
Triceps pushdown 3 × 10	Preacher curl 3 × 10	Reverse dips 3 × 20
Standing curl 3 × 10		
Standing calf raise 3 × 15		
Torso rotations 3 × 25		

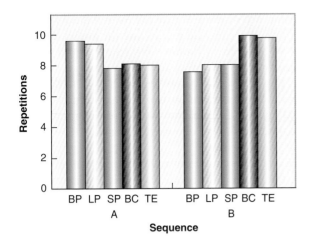

FIGURE 11.3. Resistance exercise performance using two sequences. BP, bench press; LP, leg press; SP, shoulder press; BC, biceps curl; TE, triceps extension. (Adapted with permission from Simao R, Farinatti PTV, Polito MD, Maior AS, Fleck SJ. Influence of exercise order on the number of repetitions performed and perceived exertion during resistive exercises. *J Strength Cond Res.* 2005;19:152–156.)

mass exercises performed in a workout with small-mass exercises can augment ISOM strength gains compared to small-mass exercise training alone (69). Considering that multiple-joint exercises are effective for increasing strength and power, the ACSM recommends giving priority to these exercises early in a workout (6). The Olympic lifts require explosive force production, and fatigue antagonizes the neuromuscular response. They are technically demanding and the quality of each repetition needs to be maximal. These exercises need to be performed early in the workout. Training for endurance and muscle hypertrophy entails using various sequencing schemes. Fatigue is a necessary component of muscle endurance training and

to some extent hypertrophy training. Several exceptions exist when training to maximize muscle growth and endurance. Sequencing strategies for strength and power training are recommended by the ACSM (6,95,114) and examples are illustrated in Table 11.4. They can apply to endurance/hypertrophy training as well. The recommendations/guidelines include

Total-body workout

1. Large muscle exercises should be performed before smaller muscle exercises.
2. Multiple-joint exercises should be performed before single-joint exercises.
3. For power training: total-body exercises (from most to least complex) should be performed before basic strength exercises, *e.g.*, most complex is the snatch (because the bar must be moved the greatest distance) and related lifts, followed by cleans, and presses.
4. Rotation of upper- and lower-body exercises or opposing (agonist-antagonist relationship) exercises can be employed (see the Sidebar: Sample Push-Pull Exercise Pairings). The rationale is to allow muscles to rest while the opposing muscles are trained. This strategy is beneficial for maintaining high training intensities and targeted repetition numbers.
5. Some exercises targeting different muscle groups can be staggered in between sets of other exercises to increase workout efficiency.

Upper/lower-body split

1. Large muscle exercises should be performed before small muscle group exercises.
2. Multiple-joint exercises should be performed before single-joint exercises.
3. Rotation of opposing exercises may be performed.

TABLE 11.4 SAMPLE WORKOUTS ILLUSTRATING VARIOUS EXERCISE ORDERS

TOTAL-BODY WORKOUT SEQUENCING — MUSCLE MASS	UPPER-BODY WORKOUT SEQUENCING — MJ, SJ	SPLIT WORKOUT SEQUENCING — MUSCLE MASS	OLYMPIC LIFTER/ ATHLETE SEQUENCING — OL-BS	BACK WORKOUT SEQUENCING — INTENSITY
Squat	Decline bench press	Bench press	Barbell snatch	Deadlift 4 × 3–5
Stiff-legged deadlift	Close-grip pull-down	Dumbbell incline press	Hang power clean	Bent-over barbell row 3 × 6–8
Lat pull-down	Incline dumbbell press	Decline fly	Clean pull	Reverse lat pull-down 3 × 8–10
Bench press	Upright row	Lying triceps extension	Front squat	Low pulley row 3 × 10
Barbell shrugs	Triceps pushdown	Rope pushdown	Hyperextension	Straight-arm cable pull-down 3 × 12
Triceps extension	Preacher curl			
Seated curl				

MJ, multiple-joint; SJ, single-joint; OL, Olympic lifts; BS, basic strength exercises.

Split routines

1. Multiple-joint exercises should be performed before single-joint exercises.
2. Higher-intensity exercises should be performed before lower-intensity exercises. The sequence can proceed from heaviest to lightest exercises.

SIDEBAR	SAMPLE PUSH-PULL EXERCISE PAIRINGS

- Bench press and bent-over barbell row
- Shoulder press and lat pull-down/pull-up
- Triceps pushdown/extension and curls (and variations)
- Upright row and dips
- Back extension and sit-up
- Leg extension and leg curl
- Squat/leg press and hip flexion
- Hip adduction and hip abduction
- Wrist curl and reverse wrist curl
- Flys and reverse flys
- Lateral raise and cable crossover
- Front raise and pullover

Some exceptions exist to the preceding guidelines for hypertrophy and muscular endurance training. Training to maximize hypertrophy should include strength training so the exercise sequencing recommendations apply. However, muscle hypertrophy is predicated upon mechanical and circulatory factors. Strength training maximizes the mechanical factors whereas training in a fatigued state may potentiate circulatory factors that induce muscle growth. The exercise order may vary considerably. Some bodybuilders use a technique known as **preexhaustion**. Preexhaustion is a technique that requires the lifter to perform a single-joint exercise first to fatigue a muscle group. A multiple-joint exercise is performed after. One example is the sequence of dumbbell flys and bench press. When one examines the bench press, often the triceps brachii may be the primary site of fatigue.

With preexhaustion, the pectoral group is prefatigued that way when the lifter performs the bench press, it is more likely that the targeted muscle, the pectoral muscles, will fatigue earlier. Less weight is used so this technique targets hypertrophy and endurance mostly, with limited strength training effects. A few studies show the targeted muscles are not activated to a greater extent with preexhaustion (10,57). Multiple-joint exercise technique may be altered when performed after the single-joint exercise (26). When training for muscle endurance, fatigue needs to be present for adaptations to take place, thereby leaving numerous sequencing strategies available for use. Warm-up exercises are another exception as some perform a single-joint exercise before a multiple-joint exercise. The key element is the single-joint exercise is performed with light weights and does not cause fatigue.

INTENSITY

Intensity describes the amount of weight lifted during RT and is dependent upon exercise order, volume, frequency, repetition speed, and rest interval length. Intensity has been used to describe the level of exertion during resistance exercise. For clarity, intensity will be used to describe loading whereas *exertion* is the preferred term used to describe the level of difficulty of performing resistance exercise. Intensities range from low to high (Table 11.5) and intensity prescription depends upon the athlete's training status and goals. Intensities of 45%–50% of 1 RM or less increase strength in untrained individuals (8). It is important to stress proper form and technique to beginners, and the intensity prescription must accommodate this. Because light to moderate intensity is effective initially, it is recommended that beginners start light and progress gradually over time. Analysis of the literature has shown that 60% of 1 RM produces the largest strength effects in untrained individuals (135). Strength increases may take place if moderate intensity is accompanied by lifting the weight as rapidly as possible (82). However, high (moderate to very heavy) intensities (≥80%–85% of 1 RM) are needed to increase maximal strength as one progresses

TABLE 11.5 INTENSITY CLASSIFICATION

INTENSITY CLASSIFICATION	PERCENT OF 1 RM	UTILITY
Supramaximal	100–↑	Max strength, partial-ROM, ISOM, and ECC strength, overloads (used cautiously)
Very heavy	95–100	Max strength, hypertrophy, motor unit recruitment
Heavy	90–95	Max strength, hypertrophy, motor unit recruitment
Moderately heavy	80–90	Max strength, power, hypertrophy
Moderate	70–80	Strength, power, hypertrophy, strength endurance
Light	60–70	Power, muscle endurance, hypertrophy
Very light	60–↓	Warm-up, unloading, high endurance, hypertrophy

to advanced training (66,76). Research supports the concept that at least 80%–85% of 1 RM is needed to maximize strength in trained athletes (Fig. 11.4) (126,135). Heavy lifting produces a neural pattern that is distinct from light to moderate loading, and training the nervous system is critical to strength enhancement since neural adaptations tend to take place before muscle hypertrophy occurs. Maximizing strength, power, and hypertrophy may only occur when the maximal numbers of motor units are recruited. High intensity is necessary at times but the periodization of intensity is most critical to strength training. Zatsiorsky (173) reported that ~8% of training encompassed loads of 60% of competition best or less, 24% was dedicated to 60%–70%, 35% was dedicated to 70%–80%, 26% was dedicated to 80%–90%, and only 7% was dedicated to maximal weights (for competition lifts) in elite weightlifters.

An inverse relationship exists between the amount of weight lifted and the number of repetitions that can be successfully performed (141,148). Figure 11.5A, B illustrate the relationship between intensity, velocity, and repetition number. Low numbers of repetitions are performed at high intensities and vice versa. There is a continuum where high intensity and low repetitions are most conducive to strength development. Strength becomes less targeted and endurance becomes the predominant goal as the curve shifts to the right (with an increase in repetition number and decrease in intensity). High-intensity lifting is more conducive to strength increases (82) and a continuum is seen where decreasing the intensity and increasing the volume per set results in a slower rate of strength gains (21). The number of repetitions performed relative to the athlete's 1 RM is variable

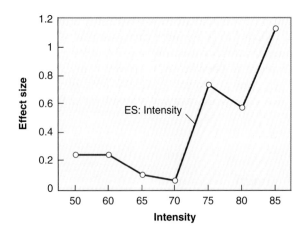

■ **FIGURE 11.4.** Dose-response for resistance training intensity. Examination of literature showed than training at ~85% of 1 RM produced greatest effect size (ES) for strength enhancement. Training with 50%–70% of 1 RM produced the least magnitude of strength gains. (Adapted with permission from Peterson MD, Rhea MR, Alvar BA. Maximizing strength development in athletes: a meta-analysis to determine the dose-response relationship. *J Strength Cond Res.* 2004;18: 377–382.)

depending on the exercise and the level of muscle mass involvement, as large muscle mass exercises yield higher repetitions. Table 11.6 provides a general frame of reference for the relationship between intensity and repetition number. However, as shown in Table 11.7, this relationship is not so simple and depends on factors such as muscle mass involvement, training status, and gender (74,148). These values are based on performance of one set. Fatigue reduces repetition number per intensity zone when multiple sets are performed. Training with loads corresponding to 1–6 RM (>85% of 1 RM) is most effective for increasing maximal strength (95,114) (Fig. 11.6). Although strength increases will occur using 6–12 RM loads (65%–85% of 1 RM), it is believed this range may not be entirely specific to increasing maximal strength in advanced athletes compared to higher intensities. However, this range is ideal for novice to intermediate-trained athletes and is characteristic of programs targeting muscle hypertrophy (6,95). Intensities lighter than this (≤12–15 RM) have only a small effect on maximal strength but are effective for increasing muscular endurance and hypertrophy. The higher the RM, the greater the level of muscle twitch contractile fatigue (17) thereby showing high repetitions poses a potent stimulus for endurance enhancement.

Although each training zone on this continuum has its advantages, an athlete should not devote 100% of training time to one general zone (95). Rather, training cycles should be used that employ each range depending on the training goals. For strength and hypertrophy training, the ACSM recommends that novice to intermediate athletes train with loads corresponding to 60%–70% of 1 RM for 8–12 reps and advanced individuals cycle training loads of 80%–100% of 1 RM to maximize muscular strength (6). For strength training progression in those athletes training at a specific RM load, it is recommended that a 2%–10% (lower percent for small mass exercises, higher percent for large mass exercises) increase in load be applied when the athlete can perform that workload for 1–2 reps over the desired number on two consecutive sessions. For advanced hypertrophy training, the ACSM recommends a loading range of 70%–100% of 1 RM be used for 1–12 reps per set in a periodized manner such that the majority of training is devoted to 6–12-RM and less training devoted to 1–6-RM loading (6). Intensity prescription is exercise-dependent. Some exercises, *e.g.*, multiple-joint structural exercises, benefit greatly from high-intensity strength cycles within the training plan. However, other exercises may have other goals associated with them. The intensity may vary in these cases. The commitment to strength training entails heavy weight lifting but this does not mean every exercise is high in intensity. Rather, those selected as structural exercises are targeted. For novice and intermediate muscle endurance training, the ACSM recommends that relatively light loads be used (10–15 reps). For advanced

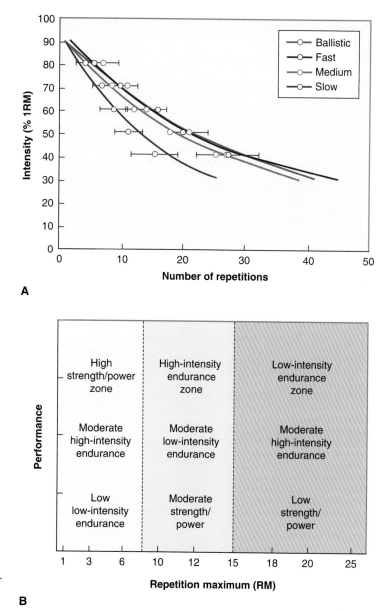

FIGURE 11.5. Relationship between intensity and reps **(A)** and theoretical repetition maximum (RM) continuum **(B)**. (**A** reprinted with permission from Sakamoto A, Sinclair PJ. Effect of movement velocity on the relationship between training load and the number of repetitions of bench press. *J Strength Cond Res.* 2006;20:532–527. **B** adapted with permission from Fleck SJ, Kraemer WJ. *Designing Resistance Training Programs.* 2nd ed. Champaign (IL): Human Kinetics; 1997.)

TABLE 11.6 THE GENERAL RELATIONSHIP BETWEEN INTENSITY AND REPETITIONS PERFORMED

PERCENT OF 1 RM	REPETITIONS PERFORMED
100	1
95	2
93	3
90	4
87	5
85	6
83	7
80	8
77	9
75	10
70	11
67	12
65	15

Source: Baechle TR, Earle RW, Wathen D. Resistance training. In: Baechle TR, Earle RW, editors. *Essentials of Strength Training and Conditioning.* 3rd ed. Champaign (IL): Human Kinetics; 2008. pp. 381–412.

TABLE 11.7 NUMBER OF REPETITIONS PERFORMED AT VARIOUS INTENSITIES RELATIVE TO 1 RM

EXERCISE	40%	60%	70%	75%	80%	85%	90%	95%
Leg press								
UT	80.1	33.9	***	***	15.2–20.3	***	***	***
TR	77.6	45.5	***	***	19.4–21.0	***	***	***
Lat pull-down								
UT	41.5	19.7	***	***	9.8	***	***	***
TR	42.9	23.5	***	***	12.2	***	***	***
Bench press								
UT	34.9	19.7–21.6	***	10.9–10.6	9.1–9.8	***	6.0	***
TR	38.8	21.7–22.6	13.4–14.0	10.0–14.1	9.2–12.2	6.0	4.0	2.2
Leg extension								
UT	23.4	15.4	***	***	9.3	***	***	***
TR	32.9	18.3	***	***	11.6	***	***	***
Sit-up								
UT	21.1	15.0	***	***	8.3	***	***	***
TR	27.1	18.9	***	***	12.2	***	***	***
Arm curl								
UT	24.3	15.3–17.2	***	***	7.6–8.9	***	3.9	***
TR	35.3	19–21.3	***	***	9.1–11.4	***	4.4	***
Leg curl								
UT	18.6	11.2	***	***	6.3	***	***	***
TR	24.3	15.4	***	***	7.2	***	***	***
Squat								
UT	***	35.9	***	***	11.8	***	6.5	***
TR	***	25–29.9	13.5	10.6	8.4–12.3	6.5	4.6–5.8	2.4
Power clean								
UT	***	***	***	***	***	***	***	***
TR	***	***	13.6–17.0	11.5	9.3	7.0	4.6	2.6
Shoulder press								
UT	***	***	***	***	***	***	***	***
TR	***	14.0	***	***	6.0	***	***	***

***Limited data.

UT, untrained; TR, trained

Data obtained from Hoeger WK, Barette SL, Hale DF, Hopkins DR. Relationship between repetitions and selected percentages of one repetition maximum. *J Appl Sport Sci Res.* 1990;1:11–13; Morales J, Sobonya S. Use of submaximal repetition tests for predicting 1-RM strength in class athletes. *J Strength Cond Res.* 1996;10:186–189; Mayhew JL, Ball TE, Arnold MD, Bowen JC. Relative muscular endurance performance as a predictor of bench press strength in college men and women. *J Appl Sport Sci Res.* 1992;6:200–206; Mayhew JL, Ware JS, Bemben MG, et al. The NFL-225 test as a measure of bench press strength in college football players. *J Strength Cond Res.* 1999;13:130–134; Ware JS, Clemens CT, Mayhew JL, Johnston TJ. Muscular endurance repetitions to predict bench press and squat strength in college football players. *J Strength Cond Res.* 1995;9:99–103; Kraemer WJ. A series of studies-the physiological basis for strength training in American football: fact over philosophy. *J Strength Cond Res.* 1997;11:131–142; Kraemer WJ, Fry AC, Ratamess NA, French DN. Strength testing: Development and evaluation of methodology. In: Maud PJ, Foster C, editors. *Physiological Assessments of Human Performance.* 2nd ed. Champaign (IL): Human Kinetics; 2006. pp. 119–150; Ratamess (unpublished); Shimano T, Kraemer WJ, Spiering BA, et al. Relationship between the number of repetitions and selected percentages of one repetition maximum in free weight exercises in trained and untrained men. *J Strength Cond Res.* 2006;20:819–823; Hatfield DL, Kraemer WJ, Spiering BA, et al. The impact of velocity of movement on performance factors in resistance exercise. *J Strength Cond Res.* 2006;20:760–766.

endurance training, it is recommended that various loading strategies be used (10–25 reps or more) in periodized manner (6).

Power training requires two loading strategies. Power is the product of force and velocity so both components must be trained. Figure 11.7 depicts changes in the force-velocity curve as a result of power training. A shift to the right is seen where for a given level of force, velocity is higher. This shift indicates improvement in the athlete's rate of force development (RFD). Moderate to heavy loads are required to increase maximal strength. A second training strategy is to incorporate low to moderate intensities performed at explosive lifting velocities. Lifting velocity is higher at low intensities and decreases in proportion to loading (38). Maximizing velocity is critical to power training.

The intensity may vary depending on the exercise in question and training status of the individual. Peak power is greater for the shoulder throw than shoulder press at both 30% and 40% of 1 RM (40). Most studies show peak power is attained in a range from 15% to 60% of 1 RM for ballistic exercises such as the jump squat and bench press throw (6,12,13,38,86,170). Less resistance (body weight) may maximize power output during jumps (35,36). McBride et al. (110) showed that jump squat training with 30% of 1 RM was more effective for increasing peak power than jump squat training with 80% of 1 RM. With ballistic resistance exercise, the load is maximally accelerated either by jumping or by releasing the weight. However, traditional repetitions result in a substantial deceleration phase that limits power development throughout the complete ROM

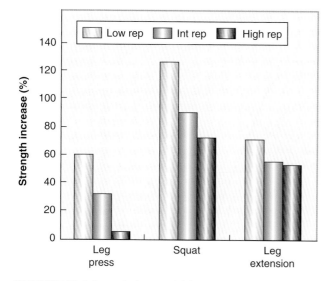

FIGURE 11.6. Strength changes with low reps (4 sets × 3–5 RM, 3-min RI); intermediate reps (3 sets × 9–11 RM, 2-min RI); and high reps (2 sets × 20–28 RM, 1-min RI) for the leg press, squat, and leg extension exercises. (Adapted with permission from Campos GER, Luecke TJ, Wendeln HK, et al. Muscular adaptations in response to three different resistance-training regimens: specificity of repetition maximum training zones. *Eur J Appl Physiol.* 2002;88:50-60.)

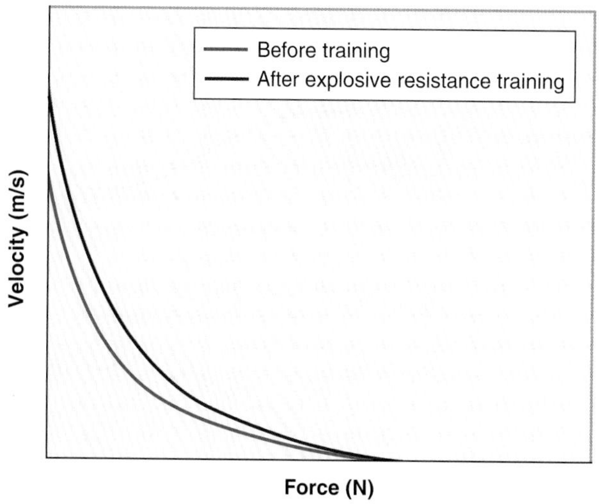

FIGURE 11.7. Shift in the force-velocity curve following training. (Reprinted with permission from Kawamori N, Haff GG. The optimal training load for the development of muscular power. *J Strength Cond Res.* 2004;18:675-684.)

(Fig. 11.8). The length of the deceleration phase depends on the load and average velocity because the load is decelerated for a considerable proportion (24%–40%) of the CON phase (49,123). This percentage increases to 52% when performing the lift with a lower percentage (81%) of 1 RM lifted (49) or when attempting to move the bar rapidly in an effort to train more specifically near the movement speed of the target activity (123). The intensities at which peak power is attained during traditional repetitions are higher than ballistic exercises due to the variance in deceleration, e.g., 40%–60% of 1 RM for the bench press, 40%–70% for

Interpreting Research

Comparison of Three Different Resistance Training Programs

Rana SR, Chleboun GS, Gilders RM, et al. Comparison of early phase adaptations for traditional strength and endurance, and low velocity resistance training programs in college-aged women. *J Strength Cond Res.* 2008;22:119-127.

Rana et al. (131) examined the effects of 3 RT programs over 6 weeks in untrained college-aged women: a strength, endurance, or superslow program. The programs consisted of performing 3 sets of the leg press, leg extension, and Smith machine squats. The strength training group used 6–10 RM loads with 1–2 second CON and 1–2 second ECC velocities. The endurance group trained using 20–30 RM with 1–2 second CON and 1–2 second ECC. The superslow group trained with 6–10 RM with 10-second CON and 4-second ECC. The results showed:

- The strength group experienced the largest increase in strength (62%, 46%, and 54% increases, respectively, for the leg press, squat, and leg extension versus 17%–30% increases seen in other groups).
- The super slow group increased strength 26%–30% versus 17%–23% increases in the endurance group.
- Muscle endurance increased the most in the endurance group ranging from 54% to 72%, the superslow group increased endurance by a range of 17%–47% and the strength group increased endurance by 14%–58%.
- The strength group was the only group to increase power (10%) during the vertical jump.
- Power during cycling increased 9%–10% in the strength and endurance groups but only 1.6% in the superslow group.

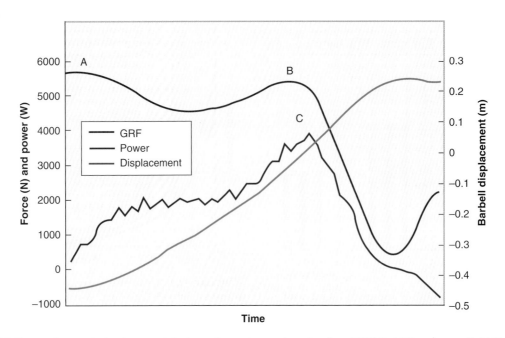

FIGURE 11.8. Force and power during the squat. It is shown that peak ground reaction force (GRF) (*point B*) and power (*point C*) occur well before the repetition is completed. The remaining decline is characteristic of the deceleration phase. (Reprinted with permission from Zink AJ, Perry AC, Robertson BL, Roach KE, Signorile JF. Peak power, ground reaction forces, and velocity during the squat exercise performed at different loads. *J Strength Cond Res.* 2006;20:658–664.)

the squat (147,174). Peak power for the Olympic lifts typically occurs ~70%–80% of 1 RM (85). Although any intensity can enhance muscle power, specificity is needed such that training includes a range of intensities but emphasizes the intensity that closely matches the demands of the sport. The ACSM recommends that a power component consisting of 1–3 sets per exercise using light to moderate loading (30%–60% of 1 RM for upper-body exercises, 0%–60% of 1 RM for lower-body exercises) for 3–6 reps is added concurrently to strength training (6). Progression requires various loading strategies in a periodized manner (for 1–6 reps) where heavy loading (85%–100% of 1 RM) is necessary for increasing the force component and light to moderate loading (30%–60% of 1 RM for upper-body exercises, 0%–60% of 1 RM for lower-body exercises) performed at an explosive velocity is necessary for increasing fast force production.

- Increase 1 RM squat in athletes by 15% and 10.5%, respectively, after 7 weeks of machine jump squat training with either 80% or 20%–43% of 1 RM (70)
- Increase leg press, leg extension, and leg curl strength in untrained individuals after 12 weeks of plyometric training (159)

The addition of ballistic training to traditional RT may augment maximal strength. Mangine et al. (104) compared ballistic plus traditional RT to traditional RT only and showed that the combination group increased bench press 1 RM (but not squat 1 RM) to a greater extent than the traditional-only group. The neuromuscular demand of ballistic training may have some potential transfer effects to increasing 1 RM strength.

SIDEBAR **BALLISTIC TRAINING AND MAXIMAL STRENGTH**

Interest has grown in the potential utility of ballistic RT to enhance maximal strength. In fact, it was shown that loaded sprint training by itself can increase 1 RM squat (140). Ballistic RT alone (not in conjunction with traditional RT) has been shown to

- Not increase 1 RM squat (despite increases in power) in recreationally resistance-trained individuals after 8 weeks of jump squat training with 26%–48% of 1 RM (169)

Methods of Increasing Resistance Exercise Intensity

There are three methods (Fig. 11.9) to increase loading during progressive RT: (a) increase relative percents, (b) train within a RM zone, and (c) increase absolute amounts. Increasing relative percents is common in periodized programs, especially for structural exercises such as the Olympic lifts and variations, squats, and bench press. Percents can be used to vary intensity from set to set, or can be used to quantify a training cycle, *e.g.*, hypertrophy cycle may be characteristic of intensities of 65%–75% of 1 RM versus a strength cycle that may be characteristic of intensities >85% of 1 RM. Over a long training cycle,

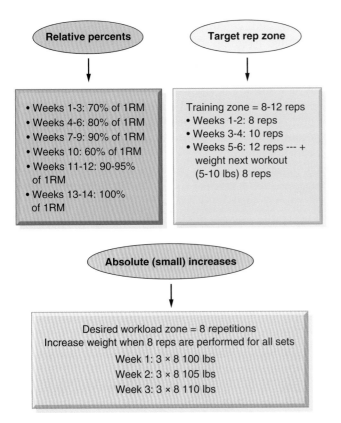

FIGURE 11.9. Examples of ways to increase intensity.

a relative percent can exceed 100% of 1 RM if the coach is factoring in potential strength gains. Relative percents are useful during unloading weeks and may vary as a result of strength testing. Training within a RM zone requires an increase in repetitions with a workload until a target number is reached. In an 8- to 12-RM zone the athlete selects an 8 RM load and performs 8 reps. Within a few workouts, the athlete increases repetitions with that load until 12 reps are performed on consecutive workouts. Loading is increased and the athlete returns to performing 8 reps. Increasing intensity in absolute amounts is common. For example, an athlete completes 6 reps with 100 kg in the bench press. Subsequently, the athlete continues with 6 reps; however, with a greater load (105 kg). When the athlete is stronger, an absolute amount of weight is added. The absolute increase depends on the exercise because a large muscle mass exercise (leg press) can tolerate a 5- to 10-kg increase whereas a small mass exercise may only tolerate 1- to 2-kg increase. All of these methods are effective and it is the preference of the coach/athlete as to which one or combination is used.

TRAINING VOLUME

Training volume is a measure of the total workload and is the summation of the number of sets and repetitions

Myths & Misconceptions

Every Set during Resistance Training Needs to Be Performed to Failure

A concept relating to intensity is when to terminate a set. Should a set conclude when the lifter reaches momentary muscular exhaustion (failure) where another repetition can no longer be performed without assistance using good technique or should a set conclude prior to the lifter reaching failure? Training programs follow a continuum where some athletes conclude many of their sets by reaching failure (bodybuilders) whereas some athletes rarely intentionally encounter muscular failure (Olympic weightlifters) although a missed lift may be viewed as more of a technical breakdown rather than muscular failure. The rationale for training to failure is to maximize motor unit activity and muscular adaptations. It is thought to maximize muscle strength, hypertrophy, and endurance. However, sets performed to failure cause a higher level of fatigue and can limit set performance after (18). It is unclear how many sets in a workout should be performed to failure if any. Analysis of the literature shows that training to failure does not offer any distinct advantages to training to near failure (127). Training to failure may be appropriate under several conditions. However, the challenge is to designate the proper proportion of the total sets performed to failure while still minimizing the risk of overtraining and injury. There is evidence showing fatigue related to training to failure or near exhaustion may enhance strength (139). Drinkwater et al. (44) compared training to failure (4 × 6 reps) or not to failure (8 × 3 reps) with similar loading and found training to failure resulted in a greater increase in 6 RM bench press (9.5%) compared to nonfailure (5%). However, Izquierdo et al. (79) showed similar increases in 1 RM squat (23%) and bench press (22%–23%) strength, and power output (26%–29%) following 16 weeks, although training to failure produced greater improvements in muscle endurance. Although it is unclear how to include sets to failure, evidence supports both philosophies and the goal of the exercise selected may be critical to the decision. Complex exercises that require high force, velocity, power production (high quality of effort), and proper technique, i.e., Olympic lifts, variations, and ballistic exercises, are best performed with minimal fatigue. Consequently, training to failure may be counterproductive. However, strength training with multiple-joint, basic strength, and single-joint exercises to failure, at least part of the time, may be beneficial. Not every set is performed to failure, but it does appear that at least a few sets (perhaps the last 1–2 sets of some exercises) can be performed to failure to maximally increase muscle strength at various points in training.

performed during a workout. Another term used to describe volume is **volume load**. Volume load is calculated by multiplying the load lifted (in kilograms) by the number of sets and repetitions (22). This has greater applicability because it takes into consideration the amount of weight lifted. If two athletes are performing the squat for 4 sets of 8 reps and one lifts 150 kg whereas the second athlete lifts 200 kg, the second athlete would have a greater volume load due to the heavier weight (6,400 kg vs. 4,800 kg, respectively). Volume load is an effective means of quantifying total work in the weight room and is commonly used to quantify training cycles.

Several systems including the nervous, metabolic, hormonal, and muscular systems are sensitive to training volume (95). Manipulating training volume can be accomplished by changing the number of exercises performed per session, the number of repetitions performed per set, or the number of sets per exercise, and the loading (when referring to volume load). There is an inverse relationship between the number of sets per exercise and the number of exercises performed in a workout. There is an inverse relationship between volume and intensity such that volume should be reduced if major increases in intensity are prescribed. Heavy resistance exercise elicits higher neuromuscular fatigue than moderate-intensity resistance exercise (102) and, coupled with high volume, could increase the risk of overtraining. Strength training is synonymous with low to moderate training volume as a low to moderate number of repetitions are performed per set for structural exercises. Hypertrophy and muscle endurance training are synonymous with low to moderate to high intensity and moderate to high volume. These programs are high in total work and stimulate a potent endocrine and metabolic response (61). Interestingly, the addition of a high-volume single set to multiple sets of heavy loads (3–5 RM) for the same exercises enhance muscle hypertrophy to a greater extent than strength training alone (61). Training volumes of athletes vary considerably and depend on other factors besides intensity, *e.g.*, training status, number of muscle groups trained per workout, nutrition practices, practice/competition schedule, etc. Current volume recommendations for strength training include 1–3 sets per exercise in novice athletes. Multiple sets should be used with systematic variation of volume and intensity for progression into intermediate and advanced training. A dramatic increase in volume is not recommended. This was shown in Olympic weightlifters where a moderate training volume was more effective than low or high volumes for increasing strength (60). However, not all exercises need to be performed with the same number of sets, and that emphasis of higher or lower volume is related to the program priorities (6).

Of interest is the number of sets performed per exercise, muscle group, and/or workout. There are few data directly comparing RT programs of varying total sets, thus leaving numerous possibilities for the strength training and conditioning (S&C) professional when designing programs. Most volume studies compared single- and multiple-set training programs, or rather one set per exercise performed for 8–12 reps at an intentionally slow lifting velocity has been compared to both periodized and nonperiodized multiple-set programs. These studies shown untrained individuals respond well to single and multiple sets. However, multiple sets are needed for higher rates of progression in advancing training status. Regarding total sets per workout, one meta-analysis suggested ~4–8 sets per muscle group yielded the most substantial effects in trained individuals (117,126) (Fig. 11.10) whereas 4 sets produced the highest effects in untrained individuals (126). Most studies used 2–6 sets per exercise and found substantial strength increases in trained and untrained individuals (95). Typically, 3–6 sets per exercise are common but more and less can be used successfully.

The following guide may be useful in selecting set number per workout:

- Total-body workouts: 15–40 sets/workout (3–6 sets or 1–2 exercises per muscle group)
- Upper-body workouts: 15–30 sets/workout (6–9 sets or 1–3 exercises per muscle group)
- Lower-body workouts: 15–30 sets/workout (6–9 sets or 1–3 exercises per muscle group)
- Chest workouts: 6–20 sets per workout (3–6 exercises per workout)
- Back workouts: 6–20 sets per workout (3–6 exercises per workout)
- Quadriceps/hamstrings workouts: 8–25 sets per workout (3–7 exercises per workout)
- Calf workouts: 6–15 sets per workout (2–5 exercises per workout)
- Shoulder/trapezius workouts: 6–18 sets per workout (3–6 exercises per workout)

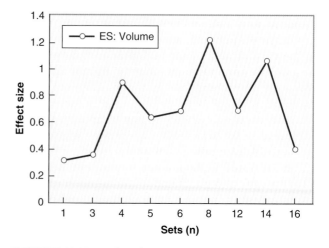

FIGURE 11.10. Number of sets per workout. (Adapted with permission from Peterson MD, Rhea MR, Alvar BA. Maximizing strength development in athletes: a meta-analysis to determine the dose-response relationship. *J Strength Cond Res.* 2004;18:377–382.)

- Biceps workouts: 5–12 sets per workout (2–5 exercises per workout)
- Triceps workouts: 6–15 sets per workout (2–5 exercises per workout)
- Forearm workouts: 6–12 sets per workout (2–4 exercises per workout)
- Core workouts: 6–20 sets per workout (3–6 exercises per workout)

These workouts provide a range of sets commonly used in various RT programs. Ranges are dependent upon training experience, frequency, intensity, nutrition, and recovery factors. Individuals with more training experience can perform more sets in a given workout. Set number depends on intensity because more sets can be performed at low to moderate intensities than high. Frequency is critical. If a muscle group is only trained once per week, then a high number of sets can be performed. However, if a muscle group is trained two to three times per week (within a total-body or upper/lower-body split workout)

then less sets are performed per workout. Nutrition plays a critical role. Protein and carbohydrate (as well as vitamin and mineral) intake must be sufficient to allow athletes to train hard and recover in between workouts. Occasions where athlete's kilocalorie intake is low may require a reduction in the number of sets to prevent overtraining. A factor such as drug usage plays a role. It is not uncommon to read a magazine and view training programs of elite athletes that use higher set numbers than the ranges provided. Anabolic drugs increase recovery ability and enable athletes to train at higher volumes. Thus, a natural athlete must be aware of this when examining various athletic training programs. Lastly, the number of sets per workout depends on other modalities of training. If RT is integrated with sprint/plyometric/agility training or aerobic training, modification of volume may be needed. This is the case for in-season RT programs of athletes where the total number of sets per workout will be lower due to the practice/competition demands of the sport.

Myths & Misconceptions

Single Sets of Resistance Training are Equally as Effective for Maximizing Strength as Multiple Sets

Historically, one long-lasting issue in S&C has been the use of single versus multiple sets per exercise. The issue itself may be the fact that this topic has been an issue in RT when one examines the literature. Nevertheless, the debate began in the 1970s when the company Nautilus popularized single-set training using their weight training equipment. Claims were made stating its efficacy that prompted some investigators to test this program. A common criticism of some studies (as well as some current studies) is that the number of sets per exercise was not separated from other variables. Rather, some of these studies intended to compare programs: one popular single-set program versus various multiple-set programs. That is, one single-set program was compared to other programs where the number of sets was not isolated from other variables. Proponents of single-set training argue these programs are most time efficient, have high exercise adherence rates, are less injurious (slow repetition velocities coupled with machine-based exercises are suggested), and can be as effective as higher volumes of training for all training goals. In their view, much of the improvements in muscle strength take place within the first set; therefore, performing additional sets does not constitute a high benefit:cost ratio. Another way of looking at it is via the *Principle of Diminishing Returns* that entails a reduction in performance improvement (output) despite added time (input) of training (118). Proponents of single-set training argue that increasing the volume yet experiencing less improvement over time is not necessary.

Those who support multiple-set training contend that single-set programs are adequate for beginners or those individuals involved in short-term maintenance training but long-term progression requires more volume and time dedicated to training. For the athlete, this is critical as strength training is incorporated into training for the sport. Examination of training logs of strength athletes or advanced to elite lifters show that nearly all train with multiple sets. A recent survey study concluded that 97% of Division I S&C coaches use multiple-set programs (47). It may be argued that single-set programs limit variation, which is needed during progression. Although more exercises can be performed per workout, variation within each exercise (intensity, volume, rest interval selection) may be limited with performance of only one set. Heavy lifting can be difficult with only one set because many lifters require warm-ups to progress to heavy weights. The feasibility of requiring lifters to perform sets with heavy weights may be limited without proper preparation. Lastly,

(Continued)

other aspects of single-set training such as slow lifting velocities, mostly training in an 8–12 RM zone, and utilizing machine-based exercises do not appeal to all training goals. Although the "less-is-best" argument is attractive philosophically, rarely is it seen that maximal benefit is gained using a minimalistic approach. Both sides of the debate have valid points so the ACSM has recommended single or multiple sets for beginners but periodized multiple-set programs for progression (6).

As a result of this long-term debate, many studies and literature reviews have been published. Some studies have shown similar results in novice individuals (107,144) whereas several studies have shown multiple sets superior in this population (19,23,103,116,133,148). However, periodized, multiple-set programs are superior during progression to intermediate and advanced stages of training in all studies (91,93,97,105,125,135) but one (71). One study (using a crossover design) in resistance-trained postmenopausal women showed that multiple-set training resulted in a 3.5%–5.5% strength increase whereas single-set training resulted in a 1.1%–2.0% reduction in strength (89). Interestingly, several reviews and meta-analyses (a statistical procedure that synthesizes the results of several studies that address similar research hypotheses via calculation of a common measure known as the *effect size*) have been published examining this topic (55,98,125,172). Collectively, these reviews have shown the following:

- Prior to 1998, 13 studies were published; 6 showed similar strength improvements between single and multiple sets and 7 showed multiple sets provided additional benefits (55). Of the studies showing similar strength increases, 4 used untrained subjects and 2 used trained subjects. Of the studies showing multiple-set superiority, 1 used untrained subjects and 6 used trained subjects.
- From 1998 to 2003, 8 studies were published of which 1 (trained subjects) reported similar strength increases whereas the other 7 showed multiple-set superiority (5 studies used untrained subjects, 2 studies used trained subjects).
- From 2003 to the present, 5 studies examined untrained subjects or individuals not currently weight training. Four of these studies demonstrated multiple-set superiority and one showed multiple-set superiority for only one exercise tested out of three using various conditions (99). Munn et al. (120) reported superior increases in strength (48% vs. 25%) using multiple sets versus one set. McBride et al. (111) reported a greater increase in curl 1 RM (22.8% vs. 8.5%) and a trend for greater increase in leg press 1 RM (52.6% vs. 41.2%) following 12 weeks of multiple-set training than single-set. Ronnestad et al. (138) reported greater increases in lower-body strength and hypertrophy with multiple-set RT but similar increases in upper-body strength following 11 weeks of multiple- or single-set training. Kelly et al. (88) compared 1 versus 3 sets of isokinetic leg extensions ($60° \text{ s}^{-1}$) for 8 weeks and showed multiple-set training led to increases in peak torque (mostly during the first 4 weeks) whereas single-set training did not increase peak torque.
- All studies greater than 14 weeks in duration have shown multiple sets superior to single sets for long-term performance enhancement (55,172).
- 2–3 sets per exercise produce ~46% greater gains in strength than single-set training in untrained and trained individuals (98)
- No study has shown single-set training to be superior to multiple-set training in either trained or untrained individuals.

Set Structures for Multiple-Set Programs

When multiple sets are used per exercise, the next decision is to determine the structure, *e.g.*, the pattern of loading and volume prescription from one set to the next. The intensity and volume during each set can increase, decrease, or stay the same. Three basic structures (as well as many integrated systems) can be used (Fig. 11.11). Advantages and disadvantages exist for each one. Because all are effective, use of these may be up to the personal preference of the athlete or coach. The first is a constant load/repetition system. The loading and repetition number remain constant across all sets. A *fixed* system can be used where all exercises are performed for the same number of repetitions (while the loading for each exercise remains constant) or a *variable* system can be used where each exercise can be performed for varying amounts of repetitions (with constant loading). This system is very effective for increasing strength, power, hypertrophy, and muscle endurance. A second system is to work from light to heavy system. Weight is increased each set while repetitions remain the same or decrease. One of the first

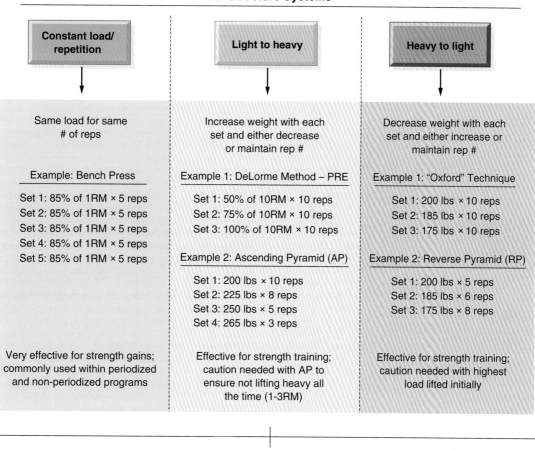

FIGURE 11.11. Set structure systems (Reprinted with permission from McGuigan M, Ratamess NA. Strength. In: Ackland TR, Elliott BC, Bloomfield J, editors. *Applied Anatomy and Biomechanics in Sport.* 2nd ed. Champaign (IL): Human Kinetics; 2009. pp. 119–154.)

known light to heavy systems was the DeLorme method of *Progressive Resistance Exercise.* Ten reps are performed per set. However, 50%, 75%, and 100% of the athlete's 10 RM weight is used for each of the three sets, respectively (41). The first two sets are ramping sets and the third set is the workload set.

Another popular example of a light to heavy system is the *ascending pyramid* where weight is added and repetitions are reduced each set. Ascending pyramids can be used to target any fitness component by manipulating the intensity and volume (Table 11.8) although a classic ascending pyramid is one which targets maximal strength as the athlete progresses toward a 1 RM. This is advantageous in the sense that there is progression prior to lifting the heaviest weight. Classic ascending pyramids have been criticized because there is a wide range of intensity used (70%–100% of 1 RM) and the athletes typically approach a 1 RM, which could lead to overtraining if used too frequently (173). However, ascending pyramids can be modified to target specific intensities with narrower ranges, *i.e.,* a lower peak intensity based on the goals (75%–80% of 1 RM). Some

practitioners suggest ascending pyramids are most effective when a narrow range of intensity is used (10%–20%) (130) as too wide a range (with a corresponding higher repetition number) could result in greater fatigue. Ascending pyramids can be used for any exercise; however, they are more commonly used for multiple-joint basic strength exercises because these exercises typically require at least 3 sets be performed. Not every exercise in a workout may use an ascending pyramid. Rather, a few structural exercises early in the workout are mostly targeted and the remaining exercises may use a different set structure system.

The third basic system structure is to work from heavy to light. This may be accomplished by decreasing weight with each set and either maintaining or increasing repetition number. Some early studies examined a structure known as the *Oxford technique* (175). The Oxford technique requires the lifter to maintain the same number of repetitions for all sets of an exercise but decrease the weight with each set in succession. It is effective for increasing strength and produces similar increases in strength as the DeLorme system

TABLE 11.8 EXAMPLES OF ASCENDING PYRAMIDS

"CLASSIC" ASCENDING STRENGTH PYRAMID		HYPERTROPHY/ENDURANCE ASCENDING PYRAMID	
SET	WEIGHT × REPS	SET	WEIGHT × REPS
1	225 lb × 12 reps	1	135 lb × 20 reps
2	335 lb × 10 reps	2	155 lb × 15 reps
3	415 lb × 8 reps	3	175 lb × 12 reps
4	435 lb × 6 reps	4	185 lb × 10 reps
5	450 lb × 5 reps	5	195 lb × 8 reps
6	485 lb × 1–2 reps		

following 9 weeks of training (52). This system may be effective when short rest intervals are used as loading needs to be reduced to maintain repetition number. Another popular example is the *descending pyramid*. The weight is decreased each set while repetitions increase. The advantage is that the heaviest set is performed first where fatigue may be minimal. Theoretically, this could provide an optimal strength training stimulus. However, critics of this system point out the potential of not being properly warmed up for the heaviest set especially if it is the first exercise in sequence and requires near 1 RM loading. Caution needs to be used. Not every exercise in a workout may be performed using descending pyramids. Rather, the first few exercises may, while other use a different structuring system.

Integrated and/or undulating models (that are based upon constant load/repetition, heavy to light, and light to heavy systems) have been used. Integrated models combine two or more of these systems. A true pyramid system combines ascending and descending pyramids. The lifter increases loading and decreases repetitions on the way up and then decreases loading and increases repetitions on the way down. Proponents suggest that some potentiation may take place on the way down as loading is reduced. Ultimately, many sets need to be performed per exercise. Another integrated model is a *skewed pyramid*. The progression is similar to an ascending period. However, a *down set* (decreased load, higher repetition number) is included at the end rather than the descending portion of a pyramid. Performance of the down set may be enhanced because of the ascending segment of the pyramid via postactivation potentiation (22). Models exist where loading may increase and repetitions decrease (or vice versa) over multiple sets rather than one. Table 11.9 depicts an integrated model for the squat. Intensity is increased and volume is decreased over a span of two sets rather than one so the ascending pyramid has been expanded to increase set number at a specific intensity. This model applies to descending pyramids, and other variations can be applied. Lastly, *undulating models* include heavy and moderate loads alternated across all sets. They are used for multiple-joint exercises comprising several sets (>5 sets). One example is *wave loading*. Although there are many ways to use this system, one requires the athlete perform 3, 2, and 1 repetition, respectively, with 90%, 95%, and 100% of 1 RM in the first wave (ascending pyramid). A second wave is performed for 3, 2, and 1 repetition with 2.5 lb added to each set. The athlete continues until the wave cannot be completed (130). Another undulating example is the double stimulation model. The athlete alternates between single and moderate repetitions with an intensity differential of 10%–15% (22). For example, the athlete may perform 1 rep × 90% for set 1, 5 reps × 80% for set 2, 1 rep × 90% for set 3, 5 reps × 80% for set 4, and this pattern repeats until the sets are completed. Undulating models attempt to maximize potentiation that occurs from performing a lower-intensity set following a higher-intensity set.

TABLE 11.9 AN INTEGRATED MODEL OF SET STRUCTURING: BARBELL SQUAT

SET	WEIGHT × REPS	PERCENT OF 1 RM
1	400 lb × 8 reps	80
2	400 lb × 8 reps	80
3	450 lb × 5 reps	90
4	450 lb × 5 reps	90
5	475 lb × 2 reps	95
6	475 lb × 2 reps	95

Note: Based on a 500-lb 1 RM; excludes warm-up sets.

REST INTERVALS

Rest interval length between sets and exercises is dependent upon training intensity, goals, fitness level, and targeted energy system utilization. Rest intervals between exercises are affected by the muscle groups trained, equipment availability, and the time needed to change weights and relocate to another bench, machine, platform, etc. The amount of rest between sets and exercises affects the metabolic, hormonal, and cardiovascular responses to an acute bout of resistance exercise, as well as performance of subsequent sets and training adaptations (6,95,114). Acute strength and power production is compromised with short rest intervals as minimal recovery is allowed to take place, e.g., ATP-PC resynthesis, lactate removal, muscle buffering, and repayment of the oxygen debt, (6,91) although these short rest intervals are beneficial for hypertrophy and muscle endurance training. Kraemer (91) showed that 10 repetitions with 10 RM loads were performed for 3 sets when 3-minute rest periods were used for the leg press and bench press but only 10, 8, and 7 repetitions were performed, respectively, when rest intervals were reduced to 1 minute. Using 4 sets of the squat and bench press, Willardson and Burkett (164) showed that the highest volume attained was with 5-minute rest intervals, followed by 2 and 1 minute, respectively. Miranda et al. (116) compared two sequences of six exercises performed for 3 sets of 8 RM loading with 1- or 3-minute rest intervals and showed 3-minute rest intervals yielded a range of 4–6 more repetitions performed over 3 sets than 1-minute rest intervals. In this study, exercises that worked similar muscle groups were performed in sequence (wide-grip lat pull-down, close-grip lat pull-down, machine row, barbell row). Interestingly, subjects were not able to perform 8 repetitions on the first set of any exercise after the first, and this effect was exacerbated with 1-minute rest intervals showing exercise performance stressing similar muscle groups may be reduced from prior fatigue.

Figure 11.12 depicts acute lifting performance with various rest intervals. A continuum was shown where greatest reductions in performance were seen with 30-second rest intervals and performance was maintained the best with 5-minute rest intervals (133). Other studies have shown higher repetition numbers performed during the squat and bench press with longer rest intervals, e.g., 5 minute > 3 minute > 2 minute > 1 minute or less (136,165,166). Short rest intervals compromise performance whereas long rest intervals help maintain intensity/volume, and the reductions seen during short rest intervals are inversely related to maximum strength where stronger athletes show a larger reduction.

Long-term studies show greater strength increases with long versus short rest intervals between sets, e.g., 2–3 minutes versus 30–40 seconds (6,114,131). Several studies have collectively shown 2%–8% greater strength increases with longer rest intervals (>2 min) versus short rest intervals (≥1 min) (128,129,137). However, some

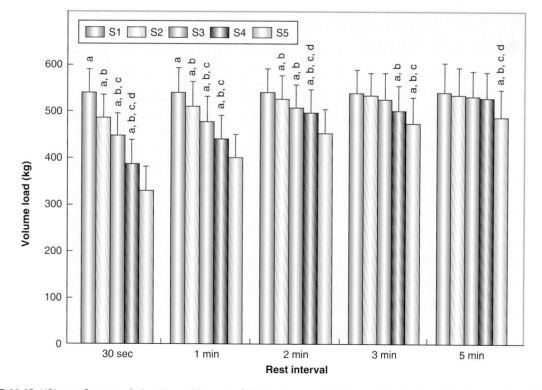

FIGURE 11.12. Lifting performance during 10 repetition sets of the bench press with 30-second, 1-, 2-, 3-, and 5-minute rest intervals. **A.** Significantly less ($P < 0.05$) than set 1. **B.** Less than set 2. **C.** Less than set 3. **D.** Less than set 4. (Reprinted with permission from Ratamess NA, Falvo MJ, Mangine GT, Hoffman JR, Faigenbaum AD, Kang J. The effect of rest interval length on metabolic responses to the bench press exercise. *Eur J Appl Physiol.* 2007;100:1–17.)

studies have shown statistically similar strength increases between rest intervals, *e.g.*, 1 versus 2.5 minutes, 2 versus 4 minutes, and 2 versus 5 minutes (3,27,167). These studies collectively show that strength differentiation mostly occurs when the rest intervals are less than 2 minutes. Rest interval length will vary based on the goals of that particular exercise (not every exercise will use the same rest interval). For novice, intermediate, and advanced strength and power training, the ACSM recommends that rest intervals of at least 2–3 minutes be used for structural exercises using heavier loads and 1–2 minutes of rest for assistance exercises (6). These recommendations extend to training for hypertrophy although shorter rest intervals can be effectively used. Strength and power performance is highly dependent upon the ATP-PC system and it generally takes at least 3 minutes for the majority of repletion to take place. Muscle strength may be increased using short rest intervals but at a slower rate and magnitude. Rest interval selection has a great impact when training for muscular endurance. Training to increase muscular endurance implies the athlete: (a) performs high repetitions (long-duration sets) to enhance submaximal muscle endurance and/or (b) minimizes recovery between sets to enhance high-intensity (or strength) endurance. It is recommended that short rest intervals be used for muscular endurance training, *e.g.*, 1–2 minutes for high-repetition sets (15–20 reps or more), and less than 1 minute for moderate (10–15 reps) sets (6).

SIDEBAR	KINETICS AND KINEMATICS OF LIFTING PERFORMANCE DURING MULTIPLE SETS

Rest interval length affects performance. Reductions in loading and repetitions occur with short rest intervals. However, less noticeable changes can take place with fatigue. Peak muscle force and bar velocity can decrease despite no change in repetition number. Figure 11.13 depicts data collected from our laboratory during a squat protocol consisting of 6 sets of 10 repetitions with 75% of 1 RM using 2-minute rest intervals. Loading was maintained for the first three sets but was reduced to allow performance of 10 repetitions for the last three sets. Although loading was maintained for the first 3 sets, ground reaction force was reduced with each successive set. Repetitions can be performed in a fatigued state; however, they tend to be performed more slowly with less force output. Bar velocity can decrease with each set independent of repetition number. These data have important ramifications for those athletes training for maximal strength and power who require a high quality of repetition performance. Rest interval length needs to be long enough to allow the lifter to maximally perform each repetition for strength and power training.

REPETITION VELOCITY

Repetition velocity affects the neural, hypertrophic, and metabolic responses to training, and is dependent upon loading and fatigue (95). Much of the scientific literature has examined isokinetic resistance exercise. Isokinetic devices possess a dynamometer that maintains the lever arm at a constant angular velocity where slow ($30° \text{ s}^{-1}$), moderate ($180° \text{ s}^{-1}$), and fast ($300° \text{ s}^{-1}$ or more) velocities can be selected. The athlete applies maximal muscle force to the dynamometer; however, the velocity is predetermined and torque or force is displayed. Isokinetic devices account for velocity that is uncontrolled with free weights and machines, act as an accommodating resistance device, and can provide greater ECC loading in a safe environment. However, the cost of an isokinetic

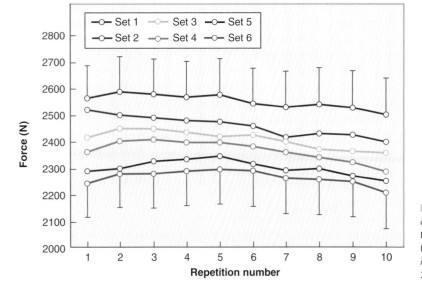

■ **FIGURE 11.13.** Kinetic profile of a squat protocol. (Reprinted with permission from McGuigan M, Ratamess NA. Strength. In: Ackland TR, Elliott BC, Bloomfield J, editors. *Applied Anatomy and Biomechanics in Sport.* 2nd ed. Champaign (IL): Human Kinetics; 2009. pp. 119–154.)

dynamometer is prohibitive so isokinetic training is not as common as free weight/machine RT. Strength increases specific to the velocity trained with some carryover above and below the training velocity (30° s^{-1}) although all velocities result in strength increases (95). Training at moderate velocity (180–240° s^{-1}) produces the greatest strength increases across all testing velocities (84).

Most athletes train in an environment that is not velocity controlled. Rather, *dynamic constant external RT* predominates where the athlete has control over the velocity of the weight to a large extent. For nonmaximal lifts, the intent to control velocity is critical. Since force = mass × acceleration, reductions in force are observed when the intent is to perform the repetition slowly (143). However, there are two types of slow-velocity contractions: unintentional and intentional. Unintentional slow velocities are used during high-intensity repetitions in which either the loading and/or fatigue are responsible for the slower velocity. The athlete exerts maximal force (and attempts to move the weight rapidly) but due to the heavy loading or fatigue, the resultant velocity is slow. These are seen during heavy sets and present a potent stimulus for strength increases. Repetition velocity may decrease during the last few repetitions of a set during the onset of fatigue. During a 5 RM bench press, the CON phase for the first 3 repetitions is approximately 1.2–1.6 seconds in duration whereas the last two repetitions may be ~2.5 and 3.3 seconds, respectively (117). Fatigue plays a critical role in lifting velocity especially near set completion.

Intentional slow-velocity repetitions are used with submaximal weights where the athlete has direct control over the velocity of the weight. These velocities have been used, in part, to increase muscular time under tension. Increasing the time under tension via intentionally slow velocities results in high levels of fatigue (158) that could present a potent stimulus for endurance enhancement. Force production is lower for an intentionally slow velocity (5–10-s CON, 5–10-s ECC) compared to a traditional (moderate) or explosive velocity with a corresponding lower level of muscle fiber activation (72,90). Intentionally lifting a weight slower forces the athlete to reduce the weight and results in fewer repetitions performed per load (Fig. 11.14) (56,72,162), and results in lower force and power output (72). Performing a set of 10 reps using a very slow velocity (10-s CON, 5-s ECC) compared to a slow velocity (2-s CON, 4-s ECC) may result in a 30% reduction in load, and this limits strength gains following 10 weeks of training (87). Intentionally slow velocities may be useful for muscular endurance training but appear counterproductive for intermediate and advanced strength and power training. In untrained individuals, Munn et al. (120) showed an 11% greater strength increase with a faster (1-s CON, 1-s ECC) velocity than a slower one (3-s CON, 3-s ECC). In athletes, training with fast velocities (<0.85-s CON, 1.7-s ECC) produced greater increases in bench press (7.9%) and

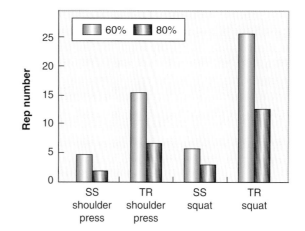

■ **FIGURE 11.14.** Comparison of superslow and traditional repetition velocities. Data show significantly more reps performed for 60% and 80% of 1 RM for the traditional (TR) than super slow (SS) velocities for the shoulder press and squat. (Adapted with permission from Hatfield DL, Kraemer WJ, Spiering BA, et al. The impact of velocity of movement on performance factors in resistance exercise. *J Strength Cond Res.* 2006;20:760-766.)

bench pull (5.5%) strength than a slow velocity (1.7-s CON, 1.7-s ECC) (102). Rana et al. (131) showed slower rate of strength increases with superslow training velocity in untrained women. However, Neils et al. (122) showed similar strength increases for one of two exercises in untrained individuals. Compared to slow velocities, moderate (1–2-s CON, 1–2-s ECC) and fast (<1-s CON, 1-s ECC) velocities are more effective for enhanced muscular performance, *e.g.*, number of repetitions performed, work and power output, volume (119,141), and for increasing the rate of strength gains (73). Sakamoto and Sinclair (141) showed that for a slow velocity lifted for 60%–80% of 1 RM, 3–9 reps were performed; however, for fast or ballistic velocities at the same intensity, 5–15 reps were performed for the Smith machine bench press.

The magnitude velocity has on repetition performance becomes more substantial at low and moderate intensities (141). For strength training, the intent to move the weight as quickly as possible (to optimize the neural response) and the RFD appear to be critical elements (16). The final lifting velocity seen may be viewed as the outcome but the maximal intent to move the bar quickly is critical. This technique has been termed *compensatory acceleration* that requires the athlete to accelerate the load maximally throughout the ROM during the CON phase. A major advantage is that this technique can be used with heavy loads (as well as moderate loads), it is quite effective for multijoint exercises, and it was shown to be more beneficial for strength training than slower velocities (81,82). The ACSM recommends slow and moderate velocities for untrained individuals and moderate velocities for intermediate-trained individuals during strength and hypertrophy training (6). For advanced strength and hypertrophy training, the inclusion of a continuum of velocities from unintentionally slow (for heavy loads) to fast velocities is recommended (6). The velocity selected should correspond to the intensity, and the intent should be to maximize the velocity of the CON muscle action if maximal strength is desired. Power training entails increasing maximal RFD, muscular strength at slow and fast velocities, SSC performance, and coordination or technique (95). Thus, fast/explosive velocities (<1-s CON, <1-s ECC) should be used for power training (6).

Training for muscle endurance, and in some respects hypertrophy, requires a spectrum of velocities with various loading strategies. The critical component to muscle endurance training is to prolong the duration of the set. Two recommended strategies used to prolong set duration are (a) moderate repetitions using an intentionally slow velocity, and (b) high repetitions using moderate to fast velocities. Intentionally slow velocity training with light loads (5-s CON, 5-s ECC and slower) places continued tension on the muscles for an extended period of time. However, it is difficult to perform a large number of repetitions using intentionally slow velocities. When high repetitions are desired, moderate to fast velocities are preferred. Both slow-velocity, moderate repetitions and moderate to fast velocity, high-repetition training strategies increase the glycolytic and oxidative demands of the stimulus, thereby serving as an effective means of increasing muscle endurance. The ACSM recommends intentionally slow velocities be employed for moderate repetitions (10–15) and moderate to fast velocities when performing a large number of repetitions (15–25 or more) (6).

FREQUENCY

The number of training sessions performed during a specific period of time may affect training adaptations. Frequency includes the number of times certain exercises or muscle groups are trained per week and is dependent upon several factors such as volume and intensity, exercise selection, level of conditioning and/ or training status, recovery ability, nutritional intake, and training goals. Heavy training increases the recovery time needed prior to subsequent training sessions especially for multiple-joint exercises involving similar muscle groups. It has been shown that untrained women only recovered ~94% of their strength two days following a lower-body workout consisting of 5 sets of 10 reps with 10 RM loads (68). Numerous studies used frequencies of 2–3 alternating days per week in untrained individuals. In comparison, 2- and 3-day frequencies have produced similar results in untrained individuals when volume is similar (31). This is an effective initial frequency and recommended for beginning lifters (6). In a few studies, 4–5 days per week were superior to 3 days; 3 days per week superior to 1 and 2 days; and 2 days per week superior to 1 day for increasing maximal

strength (62,78). Meta-analysis data show 3 days per week produces the highest effect size in untrained individuals and 2 days per week produces the highest effect size in trained individuals (135). An increase in training experience does not necessitate a change in frequency for training each muscle group, but may be more dependent upon alterations in other acute variables such as exercise selection, volume, and intensity. Increasing frequency may enable greater exercise selection and volume per muscle group.

Frequency for advanced training varies considerably. One study showed football players training 4–5 days per week achieved better results than those who trained either 3 or 6 days per week (75). Advanced weightlifters and bodybuilders use high-frequency training, e.g., four to six sessions per week. The frequency for elite weightlifters and bodybuilders may be even greater. Double-split routines (two training sessions per day with emphasis on different muscle groups) are common, which may result in 8–12 training sessions per week. Frequencies as high as 18 sessions per week have been shown in Olympic weightlifters (173). The rationale is frequent short sessions followed by periods of recovery, supplementation, and food intake allow for a better training stimulus. One study showed greater increases in muscle CSA and strength when training volume was divided into two sessions per day rather than one (67). Elite powerlifters typically train 4–6 days per week. Not all muscle groups are trained specifically per workout using a high frequency. Rather, each major muscle group may be trained 2–3 times per week despite the large number of workouts.

Training frequency affects workout structure. The following guide can be used when matching workout structures to different frequencies:

- 1 day per week: total-body workout
- 2 days per week: total-body or upper/lower-body split workouts
- 3 days per week: total-body, upper/lower-body split, or compound split routine workouts
- 4 days per week: total-body (with split designations),* upper/lower-body split, or compound split routine workouts
- 5 days per week: total-body (with split designations) or compound/isolated split routine workouts
- 6–7 days per week and higher: compound/isolated split routine workouts—when weightlifting total body can be used (with split designations)

---

*Total-body workouts with split designations refer to Olympic lifting type of programs. Because the Olympic lifts are total-body lifts, the workout is considered a total-body workout. However, the split designation refers to the exercises performed after the Olympic lifts. These can be divided into upper- and lower-body exercises.

Case Study 11.1

Lance is a collegiate Division II football player who is ready to begin off-season training. He is a 6′2″ 225-lb linebacker whose goals are to increase maximal strength and power, while gaining some muscle hypertrophy. He has lifted weights for 6 years and is proficient with the Olympic lifts. The athlete's weight room is well-equipped with lifting platforms, racks, benches, and free weight equipment but is limited to only a few machines, *i.e.*, lat pull-down, low pulley row, leg press, and cable/pulley system. He has a history of using total-body workouts and is well balanced in strength through his major muscle groups (he has no glaring weaknesses). Lance asks you to design a 10-week training program.

Question for Consideration: What program would you give Lance?

ADVANCED RESISTANCE TRAINING TECHNIQUES

Some RT techniques better serve trained to advanced individuals. They provide a high degree of overload and can be useful for assisting athletes in overcoming training plateaus. It is not that intermediated-trained individuals cannot benefit from a few of these techniques. Rather, because novice to intermediate individuals progress rapidly with basic programs many suggest incorporating the techniques once a solid strength base has been built. Advanced techniques are based upon most program variables as well as ROM and many are used to train past the point of failure. The techniques covered are

- Muscle actions: heavy negatives, forced negatives, functional ISOMs
- Range of motion: partial repetitions, variable resistance
- Intensity (supramaximal: >100% of CON 1 RM to stimulate nervous system): heavy negatives, forced negatives, overloads, forced repetitions, partial repetitions (strongest ROM)
- Rest intervals and volume: breakdown sets, combining exercises, noncontinuous sets, quality training, spectrum repetition/contrast loading combinations

Heavy and Forced Negatives

Heavy negatives involve loading the bar/machine with >100% of 1 RM (usually by 20%–40%) and only performing the ECC phase with a slow cadence (>3–4 s) in the presence of capable spotters or a power rack with the pins set appropriately. CON phases are performed with spotter assistance. Another form of heavy ECC training involves performing a bilateral exercise with low to moderate weight and then lowering it with only one limb. The athlete can perform a two-legged knee extension but lower the weight with only one leg and then rotate with each repetition or set. Some machines have been developed with multiple loading capacities that enable greater ECC loading. Repetitions during conventional sets can be enhanced with force applied to ECC phase via a spotter (*forced negatives*). Some have thought that supramaximal ECC loading leads to greater muscle hypertrophy and strength gains. Only few studies have investigated heavy negatives in a manner by which athletes may use them. Brandenburg and Docherty (25) compared 9 weeks of traditional (4 × 10 reps, 75% of 1 RM) to accentuated ECC training (3 × 10 reps, 75% of 1 RM for CON phase, 110%–120% of 1 RM for ECC phase) using the preacher curl and triceps extension exercises and found similar strength increases for the preacher curl. However, ECC-accentuated training led to greater strength improvements in the elbow extensors (24% vs. 15%). Heavy ECC training should be used with caution (4–6 week training cycles for only a few sets per workout) to reduce muscle damage and the risk of overtraining and/or injury.

Functional Isometrics

Functional isometrics were first promoted by Bob Hoffman and involve lifting a barbell in a power rack a few inches until it is pressing or pulling up against the rack's pins. The lifter continues to push/pull as hard and as rapidly as possible for the ISOM action for ~2–6 seconds. The pins are set in two places (when not initiating the repetitions from the floor), at the starting position that allows the barbell to rest and at the targeted area of the ROM. Because ISOM strength is greater than CON strength, the rationale is to provide greater force at specific areas of the ROM to increase dynamic strength to a greater extent. Functional ISOMs provide a potent metabolic stimulus when compared to traditional resistance exercise sets (56). Functional ISOMs can be performed in any area of the ROM but are effective when performed near the sticking region of the exercise. This is an effective strength and power training technique that targets the exercise's weak point. Some exercises commonly targeted with functional ISOM are the bench press, deadlift, squat, and clean pull. Jackson et al. (80) found 6-second functional ISOM added to dynamic training increased strength by 19.4% whereas the dynamic-only group increased strength 11.9%. O'Shea and O'Shea (124) compared 6 weeks of functional ISOM to dynamic squat training and showed a greater increase in 1 RM squat strength with functional ISOM than dynamic training (31.8 vs. 13.2 kg, respectively). Giorgi et al. (59) compared dynamic bench press and squat training to dynamic training plus functional ISOM (2–3 s for each repetition) and found similar strength increases (functional ISOM = 13%–25%; dynamic = 11%–16%). However, when the six strongest subjects were analyzed, 5%–10% greater strength increases were seen with functional ISOM. Therefore, functional ISOM training may have potential to enhance dynamic strength in athletes who have already developed a strength base.

Partial Repetitions

Partial repetitions are those performed in a limited ROM. They are useful for those with clinical problems or limited joint ROM in rehabilitation settings. Graves et al. (64) had subjects train using the knee extension for a partial ROM of 120°–60°, 60°–0°, and for full ROM and showed ROM-specific strength gains. In another study, Graves et al. (65) had subjects exercise from 72°–36°, 36°–0°, and full ROM (72°–0°) lumbar extension for 8–12 reps. Strength increased in each respective ROM and training through 36° was effective for increasing strength throughout the full ROM. It was concluded that full ROM strength can be enhanced by training in a partial ROM. Partial repetitions increase strength in a segment of the ROM, and if these changes translate into full ROM strength gains then they may provide useful for athletes during strength training.

Most often the repetitions are performed in the area of maximal strength. Partial repetitions can be used in different ways. Some athletes have used them to extend sets beyond failure (sometimes known as "burns"). Partial repetitions allow more repetitions when the lifter can no longer complete a full CON phase without assistance. This utility of partial repetitions is mostly seen for those training for maximal hypertrophy or endurance (body builders) where training beyond failure may provide additional benefits. Another utility is to integrate partial repetitions into dynamic sets with full ROM repetitions. Bodybuilders have been known to use these techniques in their training. A technique known as "21s" has been used. The lifter selects an exercise and performs 7 reps in the first half of the ROM, 7 reps in the other half of the ROM, and then finishes with 7 full ROM reps. Another example is the 1½ system. The lifter follows a full ROM repetition with a partial ROM repetition until the set is completed.

Many times partial repetitions are performed in the area of maximal strength with larger-than-normal loading. The rationale is to reduce neural inhibitions by applying a supramaximal load and train a ROM that is submaximally trained with conventional loading in a full ROM. Bypassing the weak point and overloading the strongest area of the ROM can be used to stimulate the nervous system for strength gains. Training in a partial ROM where sports performance may be specific (a half squat performed to enhance vertical jump performance) has been performed in athletes and has been called *accentuation* (171). Ascending strength curves are observed for pushing exercises whereas descending curves are seen with pulling exercises. Maximal force production for the bench press occurs near the lockout phase (171). Supramaximal loads may be lifted in this ROM as the sticking region is bypassed. Partial ROM bench press strength may be ~11%–18% greater than full ROM lifts (117), and the

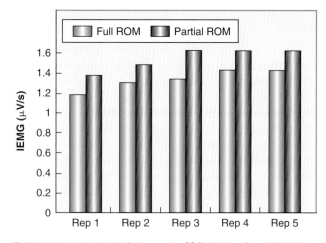

■ **FIGURE 11.15.** IEMG during a set of full ROM and partial ROM bench press.

partial ROM bench presses yield higher integrated EMG (IEMG) data than full ROM lifts (Fig. 11.15). Those unfamiliar with partial repetitions respond favorably by increasing their 1 RM by ~4.5% within a few workouts (117). Clark et al. (33) showed that loads lifted and force production increased as ROM decreased for the bench press, *e.g.*, full versus ¾ versus ½ versus ¼ ROM. Massey et al. (106,107) compared 10 weeks of training consisting of either full ROM bench press, partial ROM bench press, or a combination and showed that all three produced similar 1 RM full ROM bench press increases in untrained men. Interestingly, partial ROM training increased full ROM 1 RM bench press but the combination of both did not augment full ROM strength more than full ROM training alone. Strength athletes such as power-lifters may benefit from enhanced strength in this area as many compete with bench press shirts, and bench press shirts provide greatest support near the lowest and midsegments of the ROM. Partial ROM lifts can be incorporated into strength peaking mesocycles (perhaps sequenced following the full ROM structural exercise but before assistance exercises).

Variable Resistance Training

Variable resistance machines modify the loading throughout joint ROM based on ascending/descending human strength curves. These machines have a cam that varies in length so that loading is modified via altering the distance between the load and pivot point. An advantage to variable RT is loading is reduced through the sticking region and greater in areas of the ROM that are stronger. By reducing the load in this region, variable RT allows other areas of the ROM to be trained to a greater extent.

Variable RT may not be considered an advanced RT technique. However, there are some variations that have become popular among powerlifters and other athletes.

Many athletes have used bands and/or chains to create variable resistance during free-weight training. A recent survey study showed that 39% and 57% of British powerlifters use bands and chains, respectively, in their training programs (157). Both can be used by themselves as forms of variable resistance. Bands and chains come in many sizes and offer various levels of resistance to the user. For the squat, chains applied to both ends of the bar will be suspended in the air (or at least more than half of the chain will be suspended) during lockout (the athlete supports the majority of chain weight in this strong ROM area). As the athlete descends, more links of the chain are supported by the floor thereby reducing weight as the athlete descends to the parallel position. Upon ascent, progressively more weight is applied as the chain links are lifted from the floor. The resistance used depends on the weight and size of the chain and the distance of the bar from the floor (more weight is applied when the bar is higher). A 5- to 7-ft chain can accommodate most athletes. Chains oscillate, which increases the stabilization requirement during the exercise. Figure 11.16 depicts chain sizes. Applying one 5/8 chain to each side of the bar would yield ~40 lb added to the upper segment of the exercise. One 5/8 chain and one ½ chain to each side yields ~60 lb. Chains can provide substantial loading.

A similar effect is gained through stretchable bands attached to the floor and bar. The farther the band is stretched, the more resistance applied to the bar. The ergogenic effects of bands and chains are not well understood from a research perspective although these training tools have been used successfully by competitive athletes and elite powerlifters (151). Cronin et al. (39) compared 10 weeks of jump squat training with or without bungy cords and found similar improvements in strength between the two (although greater EMG activity was seen during the ECC phase when bungy cords were used). Wallace et al. (160) showed that the use of elastic bands added to the back squat increased force and power

output. Bands provide greater neuromuscular loading to barbell exercises but long-term training effects remain to be seen. Ebben and Jensen (48) compared traditional squatting with squatting with either a chain or band (each of which comprised ~10% of 1 RM) and found that all three produced similar muscle activation and mean/peak ground reaction forces. Coker, Berning, and Briggs (20,34) examined chain use during the snatch and power clean in weightlifters (80% and 85% of 1 RM with 5% in chains) and showed no differences in technique or kinetics between conditions. However, all of the lifters perceived working harder with the addition of chains and felt that the oscillations of the chains required greater shoulder, abdominal and back muscle activity to stabilize the bar. Few studies examined training with chains over time. One study examined band and chain use for speed repetitions in the bench press over 7 weeks (chains/bands were only used 1 day per week) and reported no augmentation of strength or power in football players (58). However, Anderson et al. (7) examined 7 weeks of bench press and squat training with free weights only or free weights plus elastic bands (bands provided 20% of load) in athletes and reported greater gains in bench press (8% vs. 4%), squat (16% vs. 6%) strength, and jumping power with band usage. McCurdy et al. (113) compared chain-only versus free weight bench press training over 9 weeks and reported chain-only training increased free-weight and chain 1 RM bench press strength and vice versa similar to free-weight training. Although further research is needed, there are data showing ergogenic effects of band/chain RT.

Overloads

Overloads entail holding a supramaximal load in order to make subsequent sets feel lighter or to engage potential neural inhibiting mechanisms. An athlete preparing to attempt a 1 RM of 375 lb in training/competition may precede this attempt by first loading the bar to ~400 lb

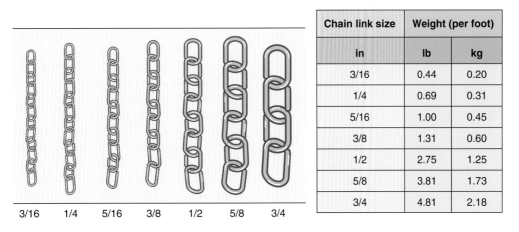

Chain link size	Weight (per foot)	
in	lb	kg
3/16	0.44	0.20
1/4	0.69	0.31
5/16	1.00	0.45
3/8	1.31	0.60
1/2	2.75	1.25
5/8	3.81	1.73
3/4	4.81	2.18

3/16 1/4 5/16 3/8 1/2 5/8 3/4

FIGURE 11.16. Chain size information. Note that chain link sizes and their corresponding rates are displayed per linear foot and can be used to calculate additional weights on the bar.

and holding the weight in the locked-out position. The intent is to potentiate the neural response to the 375-lb attempt. Powerlifters use this technique for the squat as they will walk out with a supramaximal load (after lifting it off of the rack) and stand (without actually performing the squat) to train the neuromuscular system to accommodate the load. The goal is to use postactivation potentiation to enhance the 1 RM attempt.

Forced Repetitions

Forced repetitions are those completed with the assistance of a spotter (although the lifters can spot some exercises themselves like the leg press) beyond failure to increase strength, endurance, and hypertrophy. Minimal assistance is applied to allow movement of the weight for ~1–4 reps. Forced repetitions can be used exclusively as a specific set or can be used to extend a set when muscular failure occurs. For the former, a supramaximal load can be used for a few repetitions in which a spotter assists in all repetitions. For the latter, a spotter can assist the lifter in performing a few additional repetitions beyond fatigue. Forced repetitions produce a greater anabolic hormone response and stress the neuromuscular system to a higher degree. Ahtiainen et al. (1) compared training to failure with a 12 RM versus 12 reps performed with forced repetitions (8 RM load + 4 forced reps) for 8 sets and found both protocols resulted in elevated testosterone, cortisol, and growth hormone. However, the forced repetition workout resulted in greater elevations in cortisol and growth hormone. ISOM strength was reduced by 38.3% following the traditional workout, whereas a 56.5% reduction was seen following the forced repetition workout 3 days after, indicating that forced repetitions provide greater overload to the neuromuscular system and increase the recovery time in between workouts. Training status plays a role in the acute response. Workouts including forced repetitions lead to greater acute elevations in total testosterone (but not free testosterone or growth hormone) in strength-trained athletes compared to untrained individuals (2). One study reported similar strength gains among three training groups regardless of the number of forced repetitions per workout (45). Forced repetitions provide a potent training stimulus and need to be used with caution as greater fatigue may ensue.

Breakdown Sets

Breakdown sets, also known as *descending sets, drop sets,* or *multipoundage system,* involve quickly reducing the load with minimal rest, thereby allowing the lifter to perform additional repetitions. The rationale is when failure occurs, there is still potential to perform more repetitions with less weight. Breakdown sets are another method used to train beyond failure. Single (for one set) or multiple breakdowns (for multiple sets) may be used. Breakdown sets are most effective when a spotter(s) is present to remove weights or change pins on machine weight stacks. Historically, breakdown sets were used to enhance muscle hypertrophy and endurance and predominately used by bodybuilders. However, breakdown sets can be used to target muscle strength as a near maximal weight can be lifted for 1–2 reps, 5% of the load can be reduced and 1–2 additional reps are performed, etc., until the targeted number of repetitions are completed. There are virtually no studies examining this technique over long-term training periods despite it being used successfully in the training of elite athletes (130).

Combining Exercises

Combining exercises involves performing two or more exercises consecutively with minimal to no rest. Multiple exercises can be combined into one exercise (combination lifts). This is common when using Olympic lifts. A combination lift may involve: a clean from the floor, a front squat, and a push press to finish. This sequence is performed for a series of repetitions. Combination exercises have become more common for non-Olympic lifts as well. Another strategy is to perform all repetitions for one exercise followed by consecutive performance of one or more exercises with minimal rest in between exercises. The following terminology describes three different exercise stacking methods:

- *Supersets*—involve consecutive performance of two different exercises (either for the same muscle group or different muscle groups, *i.e.*, agonist-antagonistic, unrelated). Many times the term *compound set* is used to describe supersets of different exercises involving the same muscle groups.
  Example: 10 reps of the incline bench press are immediately followed by 10 reps of the low pulley row. Following a rest interval the sequence is repeated until the targeted numbers of sets have been completed.
- *Tri-Sets*—involve consecutive performance of three different exercises.
  Example: 10 reps of the bench press are immediately followed by 10 reps of body weight dips which are immediately followed by 10 reps of dumbbell flys. Following a rest interval the sequence is repeated until the targeted numbers of sets have been completed.
- *Giant Sets*—involve consecutive performance of four or more different exercises.
  Example: 10 reps of the squat are immediately followed by 10 reps of leg extensions which are immediately followed by 10 reps of leg curls which are immediately followed by 10 reps of barbell setups. Following a rest interval the sequence is repeated until the targeted numbers of sets have been completed.

Combining exercises are primarily used for increasing muscular endurance and hypertrophy, especially if the

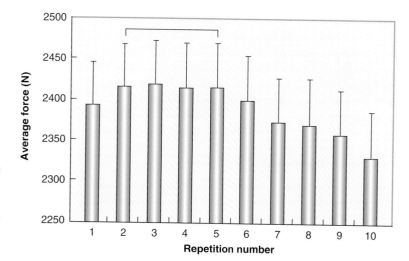

■ **FIGURE 11.17.** Kinetic profile of 10 repetitions of the squat. Data demonstrate reps 2–5 produced highest force values whereas the rest of the reps were significantly lower in progression. (Reprinted with permission from McGuigan M, Ratamess NA. Strength. In: Ackland TR, Elliott BC, Bloomfield J, editors. *Applied Anatomy and Biomechanics in Sport.* 2nd ed. Champaign (IL): Human Kinetics; 2009. pp. 119–154.)

athlete is trying to minimize workout duration. Although strength can increase with these combinations, most strength enhancement is seen in lesser-trained individuals. Combination lifts are used to increase muscular endurance and increase the metabolic demands of a workout as the weight lifted for each exercise is less than what would typically be used if the exercise was performed alone (and dependent on the weakest of the exercises). In our previous example (clean, front squat, press), the weight selected would have to be light enough to accommodate the weakest exercise in sequence (the press) in a fatigued state. Metabolic/endurance goals predominate when using this technique. Many body builders use supersets, tri sets, and giant sets for increasing muscle hypertrophy and the metabolic demands of the workout to aid in body fat reductions. It is common for these athletes to combine exercises stressing the same muscle groups as many body builders use split routines. The largest benefit is enhanced muscle endurance and size due to the large fatigue effect. Some strength athletes

may use super sets to increase muscle strength. Many times the super sets involve opposing or unrelated (upper to lower body) muscle groups so adequate recovery is given and greater loading can be used. This method may be most suitable for strength training out of the methods discussed in this section.

Noncontinuous Sets

Noncontinuous sets involve including an intraset rest interval, or a pause in between repetitions of a set. The rationale is to maximize force and power output of each repetition by minimizing fatigue. Figures 11.17 and 11.18 depict data obtained from our laboratory on 10-repetition sets of the squat and bench press. These data show that the quality of each repetition varies as sets progress. For the squat, peak force occurs in reps 2 through 5 and progressively declines afterward. For the bench press, highest power values were obtained during performance of the first three repetitions. In both cases, the quality of

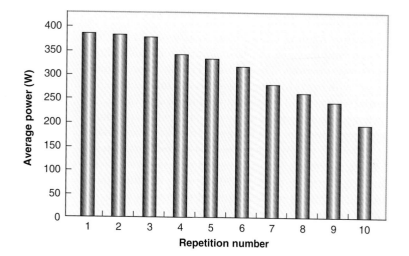

■ **FIGURE 11.18.** Power profile of 10 repetitions of the bench press.

repetitions declined after reps 6 and 3, respectively. This is one reason why many S&C practitioners recommend low repetitions for strength and power training. High quality of repetition performance is critical to several sports including Olympic lifting and power lifting. Inserting a rest interval in between repetitions is thought to minimize fatigue effects so that each repetition is performed at maximal velocity.

Pause between Repetitions

Inserting a rest interval in between repetitions can result in more repetitions performed and higher force/power output (42). It has been suggested that this may be advantageous as each repetition may be performed in a less-fatigued state. Workouts stressing glycolysis stimulate hypertrophy. Light loads (coupled with restricted blood flow and increased metabolites) have produced similar hypertrophy gains to heavier loads (146). However, the role of metabolites in RT is less clear. Rooney et al. (139) trained subjects for 6 weeks and performed repetitions either continuously for 6–10 reps or completed each set with a 30 second rest interval in between repetitions and found strength increased 56.3% when repetitions were performed continuously (vs. a 41.2% increase when rest intervals were used). Lawton et al. (101) compared bench press training with either 4 × 6 reps or 8 × 3 reps (with a 6 RM load) and showed strength increased 9.7% in the continuous (4 × 6) group versus 4.9% in the noncontinuous (8 × 3) group indicating that performing repetitions continuously (inducing more fatigue) was a better strength training stimulus than including intraset rest intervals. However, Folland et al. (54) had untrained subjects train 3 days per week for 9 weeks using either 4 × 10 continuous reps (75% of 1 RM) with a 30-second rest between sets versus performing the same volume with 1 repetition every 30 seconds and showed similar increases in strength. It is unclear as to which is more effective as both have produced substantial strength increases.

Rest-Pause Training and Variations

Rest-pause training allows more repetitions to be performed with maximal or near-maximal weights via short intraset rest periods. The rationale is to increase volume per set with heavy loading. The short rest intervals enable partial recovery and it is thought to increase the quality of each repetition in addition to performing extra repetitions with heavy weights. For example, an athlete may desire to perform 6 reps with a 3 RM load in the bench press. The lifter performs 3 repetitions without assistance, racks the weight, and rests for 15–30 seconds. The lifter then proceeds to perform 1–2 additional repetitions with the same load, rests for 15–30 seconds, and 1–2 additional repetitions are performed, etc. until the targeted number of repetitions are performed. Other rest-pause variations exist. The length of the rest interval can be altered, the loading can be very high (using 100% of 1 RM for single repetitions), and the loads can be slightly reduced with subsequent repetitions. It is suggested that 6–10 reps be performed for only 1 set with several days of recovery in between training sessions.

Rest-pause training variations have been used by elite powerlifters and weightlifters. One training system used by elite powerlifters is the *dynamic method* (151). The dynamic method requires the lifter to perform 8–10 sets of a structural exercise (bench press, squat, box squat) for 2–3 explosive repetitions with ~60% of 1 RM with 45 seconds to 1 minute rest in between sets. Although 2–3 repetitions are performed consecutively, the large set number with substantial rest illustrate a variation of rest-pause training. The use of multiple repetitions is advantageous because some lifters do not attain peak force or power on the first repetition. Rather, some reach their peak during the second or third repetitions.

This rest-pause training method is used successfully in the training of Olympic weightlifters. Inserting intraset rest intervals in between repetitions is called **cluster training**. Generally, 10–45 second rest intervals are used in between repetitions depending on the goals (22,155). Haff et al. (65) studied cluster training in Olympic weightlifters and track and field athletes. They compared it to traditional methods and showed that clusters (with 30-s rest in between repetitions) led to greater bar velocity and displacement during 1 × 5 reps of clean pulls especially during the last 3 reps. Cluster sets can be structured in different ways. The load can be kept constant for all repetitions, or can be increased, decreased, or undulated (22). Clusters can be particularly useful during the Olympic lifts as many times the weight is cautiously dropped to the platform in between repetitions and the intraset rest interval allows for regripping the bar, possibly changing weight, and reestablishing proper body positioning. Clusters are advantageous to advanced lifters because power and velocity can be maintained with the same weight and heavier weights are well-tolerated with short rest intervals (155).

Quality Training

Quality training is a technique used to increase muscle endurance and hypertrophy for the most part, with strength increases secondary. Quality training involves reducing rest interval lengths as training progresses. For example, a lifter is currently training the dead lift for 4 sets of 10 reps with 275 lb using 2.5 minutes in between sets. This lifter would then reduce rest interval length to 2 minutes as training progresses and as he improves his conditioning. Perhaps, the goal may be to be able to perform 4 sets of 10 reps with 275 lb using only 1-minute rest intervals. At that point, training becomes more efficient and the lifter then needs to add weight, increase rest interval length, and begin the process once again. One can see that endurance/conditioning and hypertrophy would be emphasized using the quality training principle.

Spectrum Repetition/Contrast Loading Combinations

Many different repetition patterns have been used over the years. *Spectrum repetitions* refer to targeting low, moderate, and high repetitions within a workout. Accordingly, contrast loading takes places where heavy weights are lifted first followed by light/moderate weights, or are alternated. The repetition variation can occur within an exercise or between exercises. Multiple fitness components are stressed per workout. For example, one system used in some circles was the 6–20 system. The athlete performs 6 sets of an exercise such as the squat. The first 3 sets are performed with heavy weights for 6 repetitions. The last 3 sets are performed with light weights for 20 repetitions. The goal of this contrast loading system is to recruit as many muscle fibers as possible with heavy weights, then stimulate circulatory growth factors with low weight and high repetitions. Another example is the 5-10-20 system. This system involves selecting three exercises that work the same muscle groups. The first exercise is performed with heavy weights for multiple sets of 5 repetitions; the second with moderate weights for multiple sets of 10 repetitions; and the third with light weights for multiple sets of 20 repetitions. A similar rationale is applied here where the lifter begins heavy and proceeds to light to work all areas of the spectrum. Many other variations to these exist. These techniques tend to be used more by bodybuilders where increasing muscle hypertrophy is the primary goal.

KEEPING A TRAINING LOG

A training log is a record or diary of all prescribed workouts. It includes every exercise performed, the weights, and numbers of repetitions, rest intervals, and room for general comments. For example, if an athlete is feeling fatigued or ill, a comment could be left indicating that a poor workout may have been due to confounding variables. Keeping a detailed training log allows the coach and/or athlete to accurately monitor progress and evaluate the efficacy of the RT program. There is little room for error when each workout is accurately recorded.

It provides a valuable assessment tool in addition to regularly scheduled assessments. A training log can be used as a motivational tool for the athlete. Viewing past workouts and drawing comparisons to current workouts can motivate the athlete to train harder.

Summary Points

✔ Manipulation of the acute RT variables is critical to program design as programs must continually be altered to avoid training plateaus.

✔ Individualized training programs are most effective for progression. Performing a needs analysis reveals pertinent information taken into consideration during program design.

✔ Follow these steps for designing RT programs:
  ✔ Make sure athlete has been medically cleared and any known ailments/injuries have been disclosed.
  ✔ Determine training goals, needs of the sport, and strengths/weaknesses of the athlete.
  ✔ Plan out the yearly training schedule, *e.g.*, off-season, preseason, and in-season periods of time, and the training goals associated with each.
  ✔ Determine the training frequency for RT. Also, decide on what other modalities will be trained simultaneously, *e.g.*, sprints, plyometrics, flexibility, aerobic training. The frequency must coincide with other forms of exercise as well as the demands of the sport (practices, games, and competitions).
  ✔ Determine the workout structure based on the frequency, *i.e.*, total-body, upper/lower-body split, or split routine.
  ✔ Determine the exercises to be used in the program and the sequence. These will be the structural and assistance exercises. Many exercises can be selected and a plan can be used to vary or cycle exercises throughout the training year.
  ✔ Determine the intensity and volume for each exercise per training phase. The intensity could be based on a percent of 1 RM if a 1 RM is known via testing or can be used via a trial-and-error approach. The volume will correspond with the phase and accommodate intensity prescription. When multiple sets are used, set structure needs to be determined.
  ✔ Determine the anticipated or intended repetition velocity for each exercise.
  ✔ Determine the rest intervals in between sets and exercises.
  ✔ Decide if any advanced techniques will be used.
  ✔ Keep a training log. Tables 11.10 and 11.11 are examples of RT programs used by athletes.

TABLE 11.10 15-WEEK WRESTLING PROGRAM

MONDAY	SETS × REPS (WEEK NUMBERS)
Power clean	3 × 6 (1–4); 5 (5–8); 4 × 5 (9–12); 5 × 3 (13–15)
Bench press	3 × 10–12 (1–4); 8–10 (5–8); 6–8 (9–12); 3–5 (13–15)
Close-grip bench press	3 × 10–12 (1–4); 8–10 (5–8); 6–8 (9–12); 3–5 (13–15)
Shoulder press	3 × 10–12 (1–4); 8–10 (5–12); 6–8 (13–15)
Pull-up progressions	
Wide-grip pull-ups	3 × 10–25 (1–5)
Towel pull-ups	3 × 10–15 (6–10)
Weighted pull-ups or	3 × 8–10 (11–15)
Unilateral pull-ups	
Internal/external rotations	3 × 10
MB Russian twist	3 × 25–50
Stability ball crunches	3 × 25–50
Manual resistance — neck	2 × 10

WEDNESDAY	SETS × REPS (WEEK NUMBERS)
Back squat	3 × 10–12 (1–4); 8–10 (5–8); 4 × 6–8 (9–12); 5 × 3–5 (13–15)
Overhead squat	3 × 6–8 (1–7)
Front squat	3 × 6–8 (8–15)
Unilateral leg press	3 × 8–10 (1–7)
Split squat/lunge	3 × 8–10 (8–15)
Stiff-leg deadlift	3 × 10–12 (1–6); 8–10 (7–12); 6–8 (13–15)
Back extensions	3 × 15–20
Calf raise	3 × 15–20
Thick bar deadlift	3 × 10
Plyometric leg raise	3 × 15–25
Trunk stabilization ("Plank")	3 × 1 min

FRIDAY	SETS × REPS (WEEK NUMBERS)
Power snatch	3 × 6 (1–4); 5 (5–8); 4 × 5 (9–12); 5 × 3 (13–15)
Bent-over Barbell row	3 × 10–12 (1–4); 8–10 (5–8); 6–8 (9–12); 3–5 (13–15)
Close-grip lat pull-down	3 × 10–12 (1–5); 8–10 (6–10); 6–8 (11–15)
Weighted dips	3 × 12–15 (1–4); 10–12 (5–8); 8–10 (9–15)
Pullovers	3 × 8–10
Push-up progressions	
Basic	3 × 25–50 (1–5)
Stability ball	3 × 15–30 (6–10)
MB Plyo push-ups	3 × 10 (11–15)
Partner plate pass	3 × 25
Weighted curl-ups	3 × 25
Wrist and reverse wrist curls	3 × 10

Intensity: 60%–85% of 1 RM periodized.

Rest Intervals: 2–3 min for structural exercises; 1–2 min for assistance exercises; 30 s–1 min for abs

Adapted with permission from Hoffman JR, Ratamess NA. *A Practical Guide to Developing Resistance Training Programs.* 2nd ed. Monterey (CA): Coaches Choice Books; 2008.

TABLE 11.11 15-WEEK 3-DAY/WEEK TENNIS PROGRAM

MONDAY	SETS × REPS (WEEK NUMBERS)
Hang clean	3 × 6 (1–5); 4 × 5 (6–10); 5 × 3 (11–15)
Back squat	3 × 10–12 (1–4); 8–10 (5–8); 4 × 6–8 (9–12); 5 × 3–5 (13–15)
DB bench press	3 × 10–12 (1–5); 8–10 (6–10); 6–8 (11–15)
Lunge	3 × 8–10
DB lateral raise	3 × 10–12
Pullovers	3 × 10–12
Trunk rotations	3 × 25
Internal/external rotations	3 × 10

WEDNESDAY	SETS × REPS (WEEK NUMBERS)
Leg press	4 × 8–10 (1–5); 6–8 (6–10); 5–6 (11–15)
Stiff-leg deadlift	3 × 10–12 (1–8); 8–10 (9–15)
Front lat pull-downs	3 × 10–12 (1–5); 8–10 (6–10); 6–8 (11–15)
Calf raise	3 × 15–20
Reverse fly	3 × 10
Russian twist	3 × 25–50
Ulnar/radial deviation	2 × 10
Scapula stabilizer circuit	2 × 10

FRIDAY	SETS × REPS (WEEK NUMBERS)
Hang snatch	3 × 6 (1–5); 4 × 5 (6–10); 5 × 3 (11–15)
Front squat	3 × 10–12 (1–5); 8–10 (6–10); 6–8 (11–15)
Unilateral DB row	3 × 10–12 (1–8); 8–10 (9–15)
Incline DB fly	3 × 10–12
Pullovers	3 × 10–12
Wrist/reverse curls	3 × 10
Internal/external rotations	3 × 10
Stability ball crunches	3 × 25–50

Note: Intensity: 60%–85% of 1 RM periodized

Rest Intervals: 2–3 min for structural exercises; 1–2 min for assistance exercises; 30 s–1 min for abs

Modified from Hoffman JR, Ratamess NA. *A Practical Guide to Developing Resistance Training Programs.* 2nd ed. Monterey (CA): Coaches Choice Books; 2008.

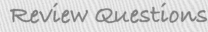

Review Questions

1. A general-to-specific model of RT progression implies that
   a. Novice lifters require great variation in program design
   b. General programs work best in advanced to elite athletes
   c. Advanced to elite athletes require greater specificity in program design for progression
   d. None of the above

2. The program: squat 3 × 6, bent-over row 3 × 10, leg press 3 × 8, bench press 3 × 8, reverse lunge 3 × 6, upright row 3 × 10 is an example of a(n)
   a. "Push/pull" workout
   b. Lower/upper-body exercise sequence
   c. Intensity-based sequence
   d. Muscle group split routine

3. The number of sets performed per workout will be affected by the
   a. Training frequency
   b. Muscle groups trained
   c. Training intensity
   d. All of the above

4. An athlete performs 4 sets of the deadlift exercise in the following manner: 225 × 10; 245 × 8; 265 × 6; 275 × 5. This is an example of
   a. A reverse pyramid
   b. An ascending pyramid
   c. A constant load/repetition system
   d. Progressive resistance exercise (DeLorme technique)

5. Training with an intentionally slow repetition speed is
   a. Most conducive to increasing muscle power
   b. Least effective for increasing muscle hypertrophy
   c. Most effective for increasing maximal muscle strength
   d. Very effective for increasing local muscle endurance

6. An athlete is following a program designed to peak muscle strength. Which of the following loading patterns would be most appropriate for his or her structural exercises?
   a. Weeks 1–12: 80% of 1 RM
   b. Weeks 1–3: 95%–100% of 1 RM, weeks 4–6: 95% of 1 RM, weeks 7–9: 90% of 1 RM, weeks 10–12: 80% of 1 RM
   c. Weeks 1–3: 80% of 1 RM, weeks 4–6: 90% of 1 RM, weeks 7–9: 95% of 1 RM, weeks 10–12: 95%–100% of 1 RM
   d. Weeks 1–4: 70% of 1 RM, weeks 5–8: 75% of 1 RM, weeks 9–12: 80% of 1 RM

7. A needs analysis consists of answering questions based upon goals and desired outcomes, assessments, access to equipment, health, and the demands of the sport.   T F

8. Olympic lifts are examples of basic strength exercises.   T F

9. Performing an exercise such as the barbell squat at the end of a lower-body workout versus first in a workout will not affect the number of repetitions performed or the amount of weight lifted.   T F

10. Volume load is calculated by multiplying the load lifted (in kilograms) by the number of sets and repetitions.   T F

11. Forced repetitions are those completed with assistance of a spotter beyond failure to increase strength, endurance, and hypertrophy.   T F

12. Bands and chains can be added to multiple-joint exercises to be used for variable RT.   T F

References

1. Ahtiainen JP, Pakarinen A, Kraemer WJ, Häkkinen K. Acute hormonal and neuromuscular responses and recovery to forced vs maximum repetitions multiple resistance exercises. *Int J Sports Med.* 2003;24:410–418.
2. Ahtiainen JP, Pakarinen A, Kraemer WJ, Häkkinen K. Acute hormonal responses to heavy resistance exercise in strength athletes versus nonathletes. *Can J Appl Physiol.* 2004;29:527–543.
3. Ahtiainen JP, Pakarinen A, Alen M, Kraemer WJ, Häkkinen K. Short vs. long rest period between the sets in hypertrophic resistance training: influence on muscle strength, size, and hormonal adaptations in trained men. *J Strength Cond Res.* 2005;19:572–582.
4. American College of Sports Medicine. Position Stand: The recommended quantity and quality of exercise for developing and maintaining cardiorespiratory and muscular fitness, and flexibility in healthy adults. *Med Sci Sports Exerc.* 1998;30:975–991.
5. American College of Sports Medicine. Position Stand: Progression models in resistance training for healthy adults. *Med Sci Sports Exerc.* 2002;34:364–380.
6. American College of Sports Medicine. Position Stand: Progression models in resistance training for healthy adults. *Med Sci Sports Exerc.* 2009;41:687–708.
7. Anderson CE, Sforzo GA, Sigg JA. The effects of combining elastic and free weight resistance on strength and power in athletes. *J Strength Cond Res.* 2008;22:567–574.
8. Anderson T, Kearney JT. Effects of three resistance training programs on muscular strength and absolute and relative endurance. *Res. Q.* 1982;53:1–7.
9. Augustsson J, Esko A, Thomee R, Svantesson U. Weight training of the thigh muscles using closed vs. open kinetic chain exercises: a comparison of performance enhancement. *J Orthop Sports Phys Ther.* 1998;27:3–8.
10. Augustsson J, Thomee R, Hornstedt P, et al. Effect of pre-exhaustion exercise on lower-extremity muscle activation during a leg press exercise. *J Strength Cond Res.* 2003;17:411–416.
11. Baechle TR, Earle RW, Wathen D. Resistance training. In: Baechle TR, Earle RW, editors. *Essentials of Strength Training and Conditioning.* 3rd ed. Champaign (IL): Human Kinetics; 2008. pp. 381–412.
12. Baker D, Nance S, Moore M. The load that maximizes the average mechanical power output during explosive bench press throws in highly trained athletes. *J Strength Cond Res.* 2001;15: 20–24.
13. Baker D, Nance S, Moore M. The load that maximizes the average mechanical power output during jump squats in power-trained athletes. *J Strength Cond Res.* 2001;15:92–97.
14. Baker D, Newton RU. Acute effect on power output of alternating an agonist and antagonist muscle exercise during complex training. *J Strength Cond Res.* 2005;19:202–205.
15. Ballor DL, Becque MD, Katch VL. Metabolic responses during hydraulic resistance exercise. *Med Sci Sports Exerc.* 1987;19: 363–367.
16. Behm DG, Sale DG. Intended rather than actual movement velocity determines the velocity-specific training response. *J Appl Physiol.* 1993;74:359–368.
17. Behm DG, Reardon G, Fitzgerald J, Drinkwater E. The effect of 5, 10, and 20 repetition maximums on the recovery of voluntary and evoked contractile properties. *J Strength Cond Res.* 2002;16:209–218.
18. Benson C, Docherty D, Brandenburg J. Acute neuromuscular responses to resistance training performed at different loads. *J Sci Med Sport.* 2006;9:135–142.
19. Berger RA. Comparison of the effect of various weight training loads on strength. *Res Q.* 1963;36:141–146.
20. Berning JM, Coker CA, Briggs DL. The biomechanical and perceptual influence of chain resistance on the performance of the Olympic clean. *J Strength Cond Res.* 2008;22:390–395.
21. Blackburn JR, Morrissey MC. The relationship between open and closed kinetic chain strength of the lower limb and jumping performance. *J Orthop Sports Phys Therapy.* 1998;27: 430–435.

22. Bompa TO, Haff GG. *Periodization: Theory and Methodology of Training.* 5th ed. Champaign (IL): Human Kinetics; 2009.

23. Borst SE, Dehoyos DV, Garzarella L, et al. Effects of resistance training on insulin-like growth factor-1 and IGF binding proteins. *Med Sci Sports Exerc.* 2001;33:648–653.

24. Boyer BT. A comparison of the effects of three strength training programs on women. *J Appl Sports Sci Res.* 1990;4:88–94.

25. Brandenburg JP, Docherty D. The effects of accentuated eccentric loading on strength, muscle hypertrophy, and neural adaptations in trained individuals. *J Strength Cond Res.* 2002;16:25–32.

26. Brennecke A, Guimaraes TM, Leone R, et al. Neuromuscular activity during bench press exercise performed with and without the preexhaustion method. *J Strength Cond Res.* 2009;23: 1933–1940.

27. Buresh R, Berg K, French J. The effect of resistive exercise rest interval on hormonal response, strength, and hypertrophy with training. *J Strength Cond Res.* 2009;23:62–71.

28. Calder AW, Chilibeck PD, Webber CE, Sale DG. Comparison of whole and split weight training routines in young women. *Can J Appl Physiol.* 1994;19:185–199.

29. Campbell WW, Trappe TA, Jozsi AC, et al. Dietary protein adequacy and lower body versus whole body resistive training in older humans. *J Physiol.* 2002;542:631–642.

30. Campos GER, Luecke TJ, Wendeln HK, et al. Muscular adaptations in response to three different resistance-training regimens: specificity of repetition maximum training zones. *Eur J Appl Physiol.* 2002;88:50–60.

31. Candow DG, Burke DG. Effect of short-term equal-volume resistance training with different workout frequency on muscle mass and strength in untrained men and women. *J Strength Cond Res.* 2007;21:204–207.

32. Childs SG. Pathogenesis of anterior cruciate ligament injury. *Orthop Nurs.* 2002;21:35–40.

33. Clark RA, Bryant AL, Humphries B. An examination of strength and concentric work ratios during variable range of motion training. *J Strength Cond Res.* 2008;22:1716–1719.

34. Coker CA, Berning JM, Briggs DL. A preliminary investigation of the biomechanical and perceptual influence of chain resistance on the performance of the snatch. *J Strength Cond Res.* 2006;20:887–891.

35. Cormie, P, McBride JM, McCaulley GO. Validation of power measurement techniques in dynamic lower body resistance exercises. *J Appl Biomech.* 2007;23:103–118.

36. Cormie P, McCaulley GO, McBride JM. Power versus strength-power jump squat training: influence on the load-power relationship. *Med Sci Sports Exerc.* 2007;39:996–1003.

37. Cotterman ML, Darby LA, Skelly WA. Comparison of muscle force production using the Smith machine and free weights for bench press and squat exercises. *J Strength Cond Res.* 2005;19:169–176.

38. Cronin J, McNair PJ, Marshall RN. Force-velocity analysis of strength-training techniques and load: implications for training strategy and research. *J Strength Cond Res.* 2003;17:148–155.

39. Cronin J, McNair PJ, Marshall RN. The effects of bungy weight training on muscle function and functional performance. *J Sports Sci.* 2003;21:59–71.

40. Dalziel WM, Neal RJ, Watts MC. A comparison of peak power in the shoulder press and shoulder throw. *J Sci Med Sport.* 2002; 5:229–235.

41. DeLorme TL, Watkins AL. Technics of progressive resistance exercise. *Arch Phys Med Rehabil.* 1948;29:263–273.

42. Denton J, Cronin JB. Kinematic, kinetic, and blood lactate profiles of continuous and intraset rest loading schemes. *J Strength Cond Res.* 2006;20:528–534.

43. Doan BK, Newton RU, Marsit JL, et al. Effects of increased eccentric loading on bench press 1RM. *J Strength Cond Res.* 2002;16:9–13.

44. Drinkwater EJ, Lawton TW, Lindsell RP, et al. Training leading to repetition failure enhances bench press strength gains in elite junior athletes. *J Strength Cond Res.* 2005;19:382–388.

45. Drinkwater EJ, Lawton TW, McKenna MJ, et al. Increased number of forced repetitions does not enhance strength development with resistance training. *J Strength Cond Res.* 2007;21:841–847.

46. Dudley GA, Tesch PA, Miller BJ, Buchanan MD. Importance of eccentric actions in performance adaptations to resistance training. *Aviat Space Environ Med.* 1991;62:543–550.

47. Durell DL, Pujol TJ, Barnes JT. A survey of the scientific data and training methods utilized by collegiate strength and conditioning coaches. *J Strength Cond Res.* 2003;17:368–373.

48. Ebben WP, Jensen RL. Electromyographic and kinetic analysis of traditional, chain, and elastic band squats. *J Strength Cond Res.* 2002;16:547–550.

49. Elliott BC, Wilson GJ, Kerr GK. A biomechanical analysis of the sticking region in the bench press. *Med Sci Sports Exerc.* 1989; 21:450–462.

50. Fahey TD, Rolph R, Moungmee P, Nagel J, Mortara S. Serum testosterone, body composition, and strength of young adults. *Med Sci Sports* 1976;8:31–34.

51. Faigenbaum AD, Ratamess NA, McFarland J, et al. Effect of rest interval length on bench press performance in boys, teens, and men. *Ped Exerc Sci.* 2008;20:457–469.

52. Fish DE, Krabak BJ, Johnson-Greene D, DeLateur BJ. Optimal resistance training: comparison of DeLorme with Oxford techniques. *Arch Phys Med Rehabil.* 2003;82:903–909.

53. Fleck SJ, Kraemer WJ. *Designing Resistance Training Programs.* 2nd ed. Champaign (IL): Human Kinetics; 1997.

54. Folland JP, Irish CS, Roberts JC, Tarr JE, Jones DA. Fatigue is not a necessary stimulus for strength gains during resistance training. *Brit J Sports Med.* 2002;36:370–374.

55. Galvao DA, Taaffe DR. Single- vs. multiple-set resistance training: recent developments in the controversy. *J Strength Cond Res.* 2004;18:660–667.

56. Gentil P, Oliveira E, Bottaro M. Time under tension and blood lactate response during four different resistance training methods. *J Physiol Anthropol.* 2006;25:339–344.

57. Gentil P, Oliveira E, Junior VAR, Carmo J, Bottaro M. Effects of exercise order on upper-body muscle activation and exercise performance. *J Strength Cond Res.* 2007;21:1082–1086.

58. Ghigiarelli JJ, Nagle EF, Gross FL, Robertson RJ, Irrgang JJ, Myslinski T. The effects of a 7-week heavy elastic band and weight chain program on upper-body strength and upper-body power in a sample of Division 1-AA football players. *J Strength Cond Res.* 2009;23:756–764.

59. Giorgi A, Wilson GJ, Weatherby RP, Murphy AJ. Functional isometric weight training: its effects on the development of muscular function and the endocrine system over an 8-week training period. *J Strength Cond Res.* 1998;12:18–25.

60. Gonzalez-Badillo JJ, Gorostiaga EM, Arellano R, Izquierdo M. Moderate resistance training volume produces more favorable strength gains than high or low volumes during a short-term training cycle. *J Strength Cond Res.* 2005;19:689–697.

61. Goto K, Nagasawa M, Yanagisawa O, et al. Muscular adaptations to combinations of high- and low-intensity resistance exercises. *J Strength Cond Res.* 2004;18:730–737.

62. Graves JE, Pollock ML, Leggett SH, et al. Effect of reduced training frequency on muscular strength. *Int J Sports Med.* 1988;9:316–319.

63. Graves JE, Pollock ML, Jones AE, Colvin AB, Leggett SH. Specificity of limited range of motion variable resistance training. *Med Sci Sports Exerc.* 1989;21:84–89.

64. Graves JE, Pollock ML, Leggett SH, Carpenter DM, Fix CK, Fulton MN. Limited range-of-motion lumbar extension strength training. *Med Sci Sports Exerc.* 1992;24:128–133.

65. Haff GG, Whitley A, McCoy LB, et al. Effects of different set configurations on barbell velocity and displacement during a clean pull. *J Strength Cond Res.* 2003;17:95–103.

66. Häkkinen K, Alen M, Komi PV. Changes in isometric force- and relaxation-time, electromyographic and muscle fibre

characteristics of human skeletal muscle during strength training and detraining. *Acta Physiol Scand.* 1985;125:573–585.

67. Häkkinen K, Kallinen M. Distribution of strength training volume into one or two daily sessions and neuromuscular adaptations in female athletes. *Electromyogr Clin Neurophysiol.* 1994;34:117–124.

68. Häkkinen K. Neuromuscular fatigue and recovery in women at different ages during heavy resistance loading. *Electromyogr Clin Neurophysiol.* 1995;35:403–413.

69. Hansen S, Kvorning T, Kjaer M, Szogaard G. The effect of short-term strength training on human skeletal muscle: the importance of physiologically elevated hormone levels. *Scand J Med Sci Sport.* 2001;11:347–354.

70. Harris NK, Cronin JB, Hopkins WG, Hansen KT. Squat jump training at maximal power loads vs. heavy loads: effect on sprint ability. *J Strength Cond Res.* 2008;22:1742–1749.

71. Hass CJ, Garzarella L, Dehoyos D, Pollock ML. Single versus multiple sets and long-term recreational weightlifters. *Med Sci Sports Exerc.* 2000;32:235–242.

72. Hatfield DL, Kraemer WJ, Spiering BA, et al. The impact of velocity of movement on performance factors in resistance exercise. *J Strength Cond Res.* 2006;20:760–766.

73. Hay JG, Andrews JG, Vaughan CL. Effects of lifting rate on elbow torques exerted during arm curl exercises. *Med Sci Sports Exerc.* 1983;15:63–71.

74. Hoeger WK, Barette SL, Hale DF, Hopkins DR. Relationship between repetitions and selected percentages of one repetition maximum. *J Appl Sport Sci Res.* 1990;1:11–13.

75. Hoffman JR, Kraemer WJ, Fry AC, Deschenes M, Kemp DM. The effect of self-selection for frequency of training in a winter conditioning program for football. *J Appl Sport Sci Res.* 1990;3:76–82.

76. Hoffman JR, Kang J. Strength changes during an in-season resistance-training program for football. *J Strength Cond Res.* 2003;17:109–114.

77. Hoffman JR, Ratamess NA. *A Practical Guide to Developing Resistance Training Programs.* 2nd ed. Monterey (CA): Coaches Choice Books; 2008.

78. Hunter GR. Changes in body composition, body build, and performance associated with different weight training frequencies in males and females. *NSCA.* 1985;7:26–28.

79. Izquierdo M, Ibanez J, Gonzalez-Badillo JJ, et al. Differential effects of strength training leading to failure versus not to failure on hormonal responses, strength, and muscle power gains. *J Appl Physiol.* 2006;100:1647–1656.

80. Jackson A, Jackson T, Hnatek J, West J. Strength development: using functional isometrics in an isotonic strength training program. *Res Q Exerc Sport.* 1985;56:234–237.

81. Jones K, Hunter G, Fleisig G, Escamilla R, Lemak L. The effects of compensatory acceleration on upper-body strength and power in collegiate football players. *J Strength Cond Res.* 1999;13:99–105.

82. Jones K, Bishop P, Hunter G, Fleisig G. The effects of varying resistance-training loads on intermediate- and high-velocity-specific adaptations. *J Strength Cond Res.* 2001;15:349–356.

83. Jones RM, Fry AC, Weiss LW, Kinzey SJ, Moore CA. Kinetic comparison of free weight and machine power cleans. *J Strength Cond Res.* 2008;22:1785–1789.

84. Kanehisa H, Miyashita M. Specificity of velocity in strength training. *Eur J Appl Physiol.* 1983;52:104–106.

85. Kawamori N, Crum AJ, Blumert PA, et al. Influence of different relative intensities on power output during the hang power clean: identification of the optimal load. *J Strength Cond Res.* 2005;19:698–708.

86. Kawamori N, Haff GG. The optimal training load for the development of muscular power. *J Strength Cond Res.* 2004;18:675–684.

87. Keeler LK, Finkelstein LH, Miller W, Fernhall B. Early-phase adaptations of traditional-speed vs. superslow resistance training on strength and aerobic capacity in sedentary individuals. *J Strength Cond Res.* 2001;15:309–314.

88. Kelly SB, Brown LE, Coburn JW, et al. The effect of single versus multiple sets on strength. *J Strength Cond Res.* 2007;21:1003–1006.

89. Kemmler WK, Lauber D, Engelke K, Weineck J. Effects of single- vs. multiple-set resistance training on maximum strength and body composition in trained postmenopausal women. *J Strength Cond Res.* 2004;18:689–694.

90. Keogh JWL, Wilson GJ, Weatherby RP. A cross-sectional comparison of different resistance training techniques in the bench press. *J Strength Cond Res.* 1999;13:247–258.

91. Kraemer WJ. A series of studies-the physiological basis for strength training in American football: fact over philosophy. *J Strength Cond Res.* 1997;11:131–142.

92. Kraemer WJ, Fleck SJ, Maresh CM, et al. Acute hormonal responses to a single bout of heavy resistance exercise in trained power lifters and untrained men. *Can J Appl Physiol.* 1999;24:524–537.

93. Kraemer WJ, Ratamess N, Fry AC, et al. Influence of resistance training volume and periodization on physiological and performance adaptations in college women tennis players. *Am J Sports Med.* 2000;28:626–633.

94. Kraemer WJ, Ratamess NA. Endocrine responses and adaptations to strength and power training. In: Komi PV, editor. *Strength and Power in Sport.* 2nd ed. Malden (MA): Blackwell Science; 2003. pp. 361–386.

95. Kraemer WJ, Ratamess NA. Fundamentals of resistance training: progression and exercise prescription. *Med Sci Sport Exerc.* 2004;36:674–678.

96. Kraemer WJ, Fry AC, Ratamess NA, French DN. Strength testing: Development and evaluation of methodology. In: Maud PJ, Foster C, editors. *Physiological Assessments of Human Performance.* 2nd ed. Champaign (IL): Human Kinetics; 2006. p. 119–150.

97. Kramer JB, Stone MH, O'Bryant HS, et al. Effects of single vs. multiple sets of weight training: impact of volume, intensity, and variation. *J Strength Cond Res.* 1997;11:143–147.

98. Krieger JW. Single versus multiple sets of resistance exercise: A meta-regression. *J Strength Cond Res.* 2009;23:1890–1901.

99. Landin D, Nelson AG. Early phase strength development: a four-week training comparison of different programs. *J Strength Cond Res.* 2007;21:1113–1116.

100. Langford GA, McCurdy KW, Ernest JM, Doscher MW, Walters SD. Specificity of machine, barbell, and water-filled log bench press resistance training on measures of strength. *J Strength Cond Res.* 2007;21:1061–1066.

101. Lawton T, Cronin J, Drinkwater E, Lindsell R, Pyne D. The effect of continuous repetition training and intra-set rest training on bench press strength and power. *J Sports Med Phys Fitness.* 2004;44:361–367.

102. Linnamo V, Pakarinen A, Komi PV, Kraemer WJ, Häkkinen K. Acute hormonal responses to submaximal and maximal heavy resistance and explosive exercises in men and women. *J Strength Cond Res.* 2005;19:566–571.

103. Liow DK, Hopkins WG. Velocity specificity of weight training for kayak sprint performance. *Med Sci Sports Exerc.* 2003;35:1232–1237.

104. Mangine GT, Ratamess NA, Hoffman JR, Faigenbaum AD, Kang J, Chilakos A. The effects of combined ballistic and heavy resistance training on maximal lower- and upper-body strength in recreationally-trained men. *J Strength Cond Res.* 2008;22:132–139.

105. Marx JO, Ratamess NA, Nindl BC, et al. The effects of single-set vs. periodized multiple-set resistance training on muscular performance and hormonal concentrations in women. *Med Sci Sports Exerc.* 2001;33:635–643.

106. Massey CD, Vincent J, Maneval M, Moore M, Johnson JT. An analysis of full range of motion vs. partial range of motion training in the development of strength in untrained men. *J Strength Cond Res.* 2004;18:518–521.

107. Massey CD, Vincent J, Maneval M, Johnson JT. Influence of range of motion in resistance training in women: early phase adaptations. *J Strength Cond Res.* 2005;19:409–411.

108. Mayhew JL, Ball TE, Arnold MD, Bowen JC. Relative muscular endurance performance as a predictor of bench press strength in college men and women. *J Appl Sport Sci Res.* 1992;6: 200–206.

109. Mayhew JL, Ware JS, Bemben MG, et al. The NFL-225 test as a measure of bench press strength in college football players. *J Strength Cond Res.* 1999;13:130–134.

110. McBride, JM, Triplett-McBride T, Davie A, Newton RU. The effect of heavy- vs. light-load jump squats on the development of strength, power, and speed. *J Strength Cond Res.* 2002;16: 75–82.

111. McBride JM, Blaak JB, Triplett-McBride T. Effect of resistance exercise volume and complexity on EMG, strength, and regional body composition. *Eur J Appl Physiol.* 2003;90:626–632.

112. McCurdy KW, Langford GA, Doscher MW, Wiley LP, Mallard KG. The effects of short-term unilateral and bilateral lower-body resistance training on measures of strength and power. *J Strength Cond Res.* 2005;19:9–15.

113. McCurdy K, Langford G, Ernest J, Jenkerson D, Doscher M. Comparison of chain- and plate-loaded bench press training on strength, joint pain, and muscle soreness in Division II baseball players. *J Strength Cond Res.* 2009;23:187–195.

114. McGuigan M, Ratamess NA. Strength. In: Ackland TR, Elliott BC, Bloomfield J, editors. *Applied Anatomy and Biomechanics in Sport.* 2nd ed. Champaign, IL: Human Kinetics; 2009. pp. 119–154.

115. Messier SP, Dill ME. Alterations in strength and maximal oxygen uptake consequent to Nautilus circuit weight training. *Res Q Exerc Sport.* 1985;56:345–351.

116. Miranda H, Fleck SJ, Simao R, et al. Effect of two different rest period lengths on the number of repetitions performed during resistance training. *J Strength Cond Res.* 2007;21:1032–1036.

117. Mookerjee S, Ratamess NA. Comparison of strength differences and joint action durations between full and partial range-of-motion bench press exercise. *J Strength Cond Res.* 1999;13:76–81.

118. Morales J, Sobonya S. Use of submaximal repetition tests for predicting 1-RM strength in class athletes. *J Strength Cond Res.* 1996;10:186–189.

119. Morrissey MC, Harman EA, Frykman PN, Han KH. Early phase differential effects of slow and fast barbell squat training. *Am J Sports Med.* 1998;26:221–230.

120. Munn J, Herbert RD, Hancock MJ, Gandevia SC. Resistance training for strength: effect of number of sets and contraction speed. *Med Sci Sports Exerc.* 2005;37:1622–1626.

121. Myer GD, Ford KR, Khoury J, Succop P, Hewett TE. Biomechanics laboratory-based prediction algorithm to identify female athletes with high knee loads that increase risk of ACL injury. *Br J Sports Med.* 2010; ahead of print.

122. Neils CM, Udermann BE, Brice GA, Winchester JB, McGuigan MR. Influence of contraction velocity in untrained individuals over the initial early phase of resistance training. *J Strength Cond Res.* 2005;19:883–887.

123. Newton RU, Kraemer WJ, Häkkinen K, Humphries BJ, Murphy AJ. Kinematics, kinetics, and muscle activation during explosive upper body movements. *J Appl Biomech.* 1996;12:31–43.

124. O'Shea KL, O'Shea JP. Functional isometric weight training: its effects on static and dynamic strength. *J Appl Sport Sci Res.* 1989; 3:30–33.

125. Paulsen G, Myklestad D, Raastad T. The influence of volume of exercise on early adaptations to strength training. *J Strength Cond Res.* 2003;17:113–118.

126. Peterson MD, Rhea MR, Alvar BA. Maximizing strength development in athletes: a meta-analysis to determine the dose-response relationship. *J Strength Cond Res.* 2004;18:377–382.

127. Peterson MD, Rhea MR, Alvar BA. Applications of the dose-response for muscular strength development: a review of meta-analytic efficacy and reliability for designing training prescription. *J Strength Cond Res.* 2005;19:950–958.

128. Pincivero DM, Lephart SM, Karunakara RG. Effects of rest interval on isokinetic strength and functional performance after short-term high intensity training. *Br J Sports Med.* 1997;31:229–234.

129. Pincivero DM, Campy RM. The effects of rest interval length and training on quadriceps femoris muscle. Part I: knee extensor torque and muscle fatigue. *J Sports Med Phys Fitness.* 2004;44: 111–118.

130. Poliquin, C. *Modern Trends in Strength Training. Volume 1: Reps and Sets.* 2nd ed. QFAC Bodybuilding; 2001.

131. Rana SR, Chleboun GS, Gilders RM, et al. Comparison of early phase adaptations for traditional strength and endurance, and low velocity resistance training programs in college-aged women. *J Strength Cond Res.* 2008;22:119–127.

132. Ratamess NA. Adaptations to anaerobic training programs. In: Baechle TR, Earle RW, editors. *Essentials of Strength Training and Conditioning.* 3rd ed. Champaign (IL): Human Kinetics; 2008. pp. 93–119.

133. Ratamess NA, Falvo MJ, Mangine GT, Hoffman JR, Faigenbaum AD, Kang J. The effect of rest interval length on metabolic responses to the bench press exercise. *Eur J Appl Physiol.* 2007;100:1–17.

134. Rhea MR, Alvar BA, Ball SD, Burkett LN. Three sets of weight training superior to 1 set with equal intensity for eliciting strength. *J Strength Cond Res.* 2002;16:525–529.

135. Rhea MR, Alvar BA, Burkett LN, Ball SD. A meta-analysis to determine the dose response for strength development. *Med Sci Sports Exerc.* 2003;35:456–464.

136. Richmond SR, Godard MP. The effects of varied rest periods between sets to failure using the bench press in recreationally trained men. *J Strength Cond Res.* 2004;18:846–849.

137. Robinson JM, Stone MH, Johnson RL, Penland CM, Warren BJ, Lewis RD. Effects of different weight training exercise/rest intervals on strength, power, and high intensity exercise endurance. *J Strength Cond Res.* 1995;9:216–221.

138. Ronnestad BR, Egeland W, Kvamme NH, et al. Dissimilar effects of one- and three-set strength training on strength and muscle mass gains in upper and lower body in untrained subjects. *J Strength Cond Res.* 2007;21:157–163.

139. Rooney KJ, Herbert RD, Balnave RJ. Fatigue contributes to the strength training stimulus. *Med Sci Sports Exerc.* 1994;26: 1160–1164.

140. Ross RE, Ratamess NA, Hoffman JR, Faigenbaum AD, Kang J, Chilakos A. The effects of treadmill sprint training and resistance training on maximal running velocity and power. *J Strength Cond Res.* 2009;23:385–394.

141. Sakamoto A, Sinclair PJ. Effect of movement velocity on the relationship between training load and the number of repetitions of bench press. *J Strength Cond Res.* 2006;20:532–527.

142. Sanborn K, Boros R, Hruby J, et al. Short-term performance effects of weight training with multiple sets not to failure vs. a single set to failure in women. *J Strength Cond Res.* 2000;14: 328–331.

143. Schilling BK, MJ Falvo, LZF Chiu. Force-velocity, impulse-momentum relationships: implications for efficacy of purposely slow resistance training. *J Sports Sci Med.* 2008;7:299–304.

144. Schlumberger A, Stec J, Schmidtbleicher D. Single- vs. multiple-set strength training in women. *J Strength Cond Res.* 2001;15: 284–289.

145. Sforzo GA, Touey PR. Manipulating exercise order affects muscular performance during a resistance exercise training session. *J Strength Cond Res.* 1996;10:20–24.

146. Shinohara M, Kouzaki M, Yoshihisa T, Fukunaga T. Efficacy of tourniquet ischemia for strength training with low resistance. *Eur J Appl Physiol Occup Physiol.* 1998;77:189–191.

147. Siegel JA, Gilders RM, Staron RS, Hagerman FC. Human muscle power output during upper- and lower-body exercises. *J Strength Cond Res*. 2002;16:173–178.

148. Shimano T, Kraemer WJ, Spiering BA, et al. Relationship between the number of repetitions and selected percentages of one repetition maximum in free weight exercises in trained and untrained men. *J Strength Cond Res*. 2006;20:819–823.

149. Simao R, Farinatti PTV, Polito MD, Maior AS, Fleck SJ. Influence of exercise order on the number of repetitions performed and perceived exertion during resistive exercises. *J Strength Cond Res*. 2005;19:152–156.

150. Simao R, Farinatti PTV, Polito MD, Viveiros L, Fleck SJ. Influence of exercise order on the number of repetitions performed and perceived exertion during resistance exercise in women. *J Strength Cond Res*. 2007;21:23–28.

151. Simmons L. What if? *MILO*. 1996;4:25–29.

152. Spennewyn KC. Strength outcomes in fixed versus free-form resistance equipment. *J Strength Cond Res*. 2008;22:75–81.

153. Spreuwenberg LPB, Kraemer WJ, Spiering BA, et al. Influence of exercise order in a resistance-training exercise session. *J Strength Cond Res*. 2006;20:141–144.

154. Starkey DB, Pollock ML, Ishida Y, et al. Effect of resistance training volume on strength and muscle thickness. *Med Sci Sports Exerc*. 1996;28:1311–1320.

155. Stone MH, Stone M, Sands WA. *Principles and Practice of Resistance Training*. Champaign (IL): Human Kinetics; 2007.

156. Stowers T, McMillian J, Scala D, Davis V, Wilson D, Stone M. The short-term effects of three different strength-power training methods. *Natl Strength Cond Assoc J*. 1983;5:24–27.

157. Swinton PA, Lloyd R, Aqouris I, Stewart A. Contemporary training practices in elite British powerlifters: survey results from an international competition. *J Strength Cond Res*. 2009;23:380–384.

158. Tran QT, Docherty D, Behm D. The effects of varying time under tension and volume load on acute neuromuscular responses. *Eur J Appl Physiol*. 2006;98:402–410.

159. Vissing K, Brink M, Lonbro S, et al. Muscle adaptations to plyometric vs. resistance training in untrained young men. *J Strength Cond Res*. 2008;22:1799–1810.

160. Wallace BJ, Winchester JB, McGuigan MR. Effects of elastic bands on force and power characteristics during the back squat exercise. *J Strength Cond Res*. 2006;20:268–272.

161. Ware JS, Clemens CT, Mayhew JL, Johnston TJ. Muscular endurance repetitions to predict bench press and squat strength in college football players. *J Strength Cond Res*. 1995;9:99–103.

162. Wickwire PJ, McLester JR, Green JM, Crews TR. Acute heart rate, blood pressure, and RPE responses during super slow vs. traditional machine resistance training protocols using small muscle group exercises. *J Strength Cond Res*. 2009;23:72–79.

163. Wilk KE, Arrigo C, Andrews JR, Clancy WG. Rehabilitation after anterior cruciate ligament reconstruction in the female athlete. *J Athl Train*. 1999;34:177–193.

164. Willardson JM, Burkett LN. A comparison of 3 different rest intervals on the exercise volume completed during a workout. *J Strength Cond Res*. 2005;19:23–26.

165. Willardson JM, Burkett LN. The effect of rest interval length on bench press performance with heavy vs. light loads. *J Strength Cond Res*. 2006;20:396–399.

166. Willardson JM, Burkett LN. The effect of rest interval length on the sustainability of squat and bench press repetitions. *J Strength Cond Res*. 2006;20:400–403.

167. Willardson JM, Burkett LN. The effect of different rest intervals between sets on volume components and strength gains. *J Strength Cond Res*. 2008;22:146–152.

168. Willoughby DS, Gillespie JW. A comparison of isotonic free weights and omnikinetic exercise machines on strength. *J Hum Mov Stud*. 1990;19:93–100.

169. Winchester JB, McBride JM, Maher MA, et al. Eight weeks of ballistic exercise improves power independently of changes in strength and muscle fiber type expression. *J Strength Cond Res*. 2008;22:1728–1734.

170. Wilson GJ, Newton RU, Murphy AJ, Humphries BJ. The optimal training load for the development of dynamic athletic performance. *Med Sci Sports Exerc*. 1993;25:1279–1286.

171. Wilson GJ, Murphy AJ, Pryor JF. Musculotendinous stiffness: its relationship to eccentric, isometric, and concentric performance. *J Appl Physiol*. 1994;76:2714–2719.

172. Wolfe BL, LeMura LM, Cole PJ. Quantitative analysis of single- vs. multiple-set programs in resistance training. *J Strength Cond Res*. 2004;18:35–47.

173. Zatsiorsky V. *Science and Practice of Strength Training*. Champaign (IL): Human Kinetics; 1995.

174. Zink AJ, Perry AC, Robertson BL, Roach KE, Signorile JF. Peak power, ground reaction forces, and velocity during the squat exercise performed at different loads. *J Strength Cond Res*. 2006;20:658–664.

175. Zinovieff AN. Heavy-resistance exercises the "Oxford technique". *Br J Phys Med*. 1951;14:129–132.

12

Resistance Training Equipment and Safety

objectives

After completing this chapter, you will be able to:
- Discuss different modalities used in resistance training
- Discuss advantages and disadvantages of free weights and machines
- Review general safety procedures for effective resistance training
- Discuss ways in which resistance training can reduce the risk of injury

Theoretically, any piece of equipment that supplies some degree of resistance can be used for training. In the past 20 years, numerous pieces of resistance training (RT) equipment have been developed. Some equipment is new and innovative, and some manufacturers have expanded upon other pieces used throughout the history of RT. One can design quality RT programs with inexpensive equipment, so the cost should not preclude one from training effectively.

RESISTANCE TRAINING MODALITIES

BODY WEIGHT

The human body is the most basic form of resistance in existence. Exercises such as body weight squats, lunges, push-ups, pull-ups, dips, reverse dips, sit-ups, crunches, leg raises, and hyperextensions all require the athlete to overcome his or her body weight to perform a series of repetitions. Other modalities such as calisthenics, sprint, plyometric, endurance, and agility training all require the athlete to overcome body weight. In the absence of adding external weight, body weight exercises can be made more difficult by changing grip/stance width, leverage (moment arm of resistance), cadence, or by using uni- versus bilateral contractions (one vs. two arms or legs). It is important to note that the basic principles of RT must still be followed even when the resistance is supplied by body weight, *i.e.*, adequate relative intensity must be maintained if strength adaptations are the goal of the training.

The push-up is a prime example (Fig. 12.1). The push-up can be made easier by performing it on the knees (*modified push-up*), which reduces the resistance

arm and allows the ground to support some of the body weight. The difficulty of the push-up can increase when strength and endurance improves. An athlete may widen, narrow, or stagger his or her hand spacing or place hands further in front of the body (head level); elevate the feet on a bench or upper body between chairs, ball, or platform; maintain contact with the floor with only one foot (or cross feet); add a twist to exercise (rotation at the top position), pause, or forward walk with the hands; alter the cadence; and eventually progress to a single-arm push-up. Push-ups can be performed on the fingertips or backs of hands, which increase difficulty as well as require greater hand and wrist strength. The prone push-up position is a potent core exercise so manipulation of limbs while maintaining this position stresses core musculature (one- vs. two-arm plank). All of these variations alter muscle activation and complexity to some degree without adding external resistance to increase difficulty and intensity.

Athletes such as gymnasts who train against body weight possess high levels of muscle strength and power owing to the efficacy of understanding biomechanics and how to use body weight as a training tool. Body weight is a form of resistance that anyone can use for RT at no cost and exercises can be performed in most places. However, it is important for the strength and conditioning (S&C) professional to realize that, due to either a lack of sufficient strength or large amount of weight, some body weight exercises may be impractical for certain populations. For example, some individuals may not be able to complete one dip or pull-up. In these cases, other strengthening exercises (machine dip, lat pull-down) may be used initially until the individual develops the

Myths & Misconceptions

The Best Resistance Training Workouts Involve Costly Equipment

Albeit some popular and effective pieces of RT equipment are expensive, quality RT programs can be developed for free and/or at very low cost. This has large ramifications for training at home, on the road, or training groups of athletes with limited resources. The most basic source of resistance is one's body weight. Body weight exercises can be made more difficult (or easy) by altering biomechanics, intensity, repetition number, exercises selected, and rest intervals. Body weight workouts can be effective for athletes at all fitness levels. Manual RT (self-imposed or partner resistance) is free and can be performed anywhere. Other sources of resistance can be purchased at low cost. Bands, tubing, medicine balls (MBs), dumbbells, and kettlebells (KBs) can be purchased at low cost and are easily transportable. Implements or some items around the home/yard (sledgehammer, cinder blocks, wheelbarrow, couch, etc.) can be used. Larger pieces of free-weight equipment, machines, and gym memberships are more costly and/or prohibitive for home purchase. They also require more space. For example, barbell sets (depending on the amount of plates and weights) are sold per pound and can range in price from $100 to several hundreds of dollars. Free-weight benches can be low in cost but better-quality equipment (equipment designed for more extensive use) can cost hundreds of dollars. Lifting platforms and power racks cost several hundred to a couple of thousand dollars. Machines are quite costly and limit the number of exercises performed. Gym memberships usually cost a few hundred to >$1,000 per year. Cost may preclude some equipment use. However, it is a myth that it is costly to improve physical conditioning.

ability to perform a body weight exercise without assistance. Lastly, some pieces of equipment can be useful for performing some body weight exercises. For example, dip bars can assist in performing dips, bars can be useful for pull-ups, and benches can be used for reverse dips, crunches, sit-ups, and leg raises.

A popular piece of body weight equipment is the TRX® Suspension Trainer (Fig. 12.2). The TRX consists of two straps with adjustable handles and foot attachments that can be suspended or anchored from the ceiling, a door, beams, or from a multipurpose resistance exercise device like a cable unit or power rack. The adjustable straps enable the performance of hundreds of movement-specific body weight exercises. The straps are freely moveable yet supportive, which creates a desirable training stimulus. It is based on a pendulum system where manipulation of the athlete's body position (distance from anchor, body angle relative to floor, height of the starting position and center of gravity [COG], and size of base support) dictates the percent of body weight that

needs to be overcome. For example, the more upright the body (feet back), the easier the exercise is (less weight to support) for some upper body exercises. The closer to the ground (feet closer to anchor), the more difficult the exercise is as a larger percent of body weight must be overcome.

Case Study 12.1

The push-up exercise was discussed in the previous section. Using the same logic, apply biomechanical principles to the basic body weight squat.

Question for Consideration: **Discuss ways an athlete can make the exercise more difficult without adding external weight.**

The body weight of other individuals or partners can be a beneficial RT tool. Exercises such as the squat, bench press, shoulder press, rows, bear hug lifts, and

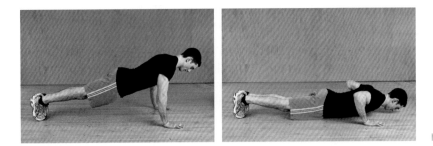

■ **FIGURE 12.1.** Push-up.

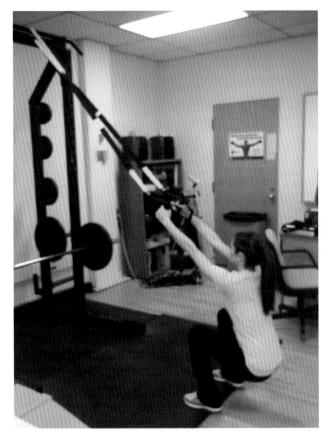

FIGURE 12.2. TRX.

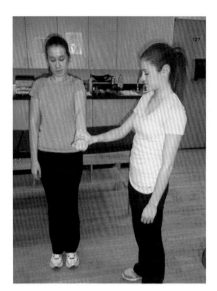

FIGURE 12.3. Manual resistance front raise (with partner assistance).

carries can be performed with the weight of a partner. A partner's weight determines how many repetitions can be performed. It is unique that body weight distribution is not balanced, so performing an exercise with a 150-lb partner will be more difficult than performing the exercise with a 150-lb barbell.

MANUAL OR PARTNER RESISTANCE

An athlete or partner may provide self-resistance for relatively slow repetitions (Fig. 12.3). The advantages of manual or partner dynamic/isometric (ISOM) RT exercises are they can be performed anywhere at very little to no cost, risk of injury is low, high resistance can be applied throughout the range of motion (ROM), many individuals can be trained at once, resistance can be adjusted based on fatigue, and they can add variety to a traditional RT program (23). These exercises can be effective for complete strength development, provided intensity is sufficient. Some examples of manual resistance exercises include unilateral elbow flexion/extension, towel leg press, ISOM chest squeeze and wall push, front raise (held with opposite arm), supine row (with legs) and chest press (on legs), upright row (held with opposite arm), shrug, hip adduction/abduction with arms, ISOM knee extension, knee raise (against arms),

and four-way neck manual resistance exercises. These exercises work best when an exercise is opposed by a muscle group stronger than the agonists (which is not always the case). A partner can supply the resistance directly or with the use of a towel. A partner may be useful for some exercises difficult for one to perform manually, *e.g.*, leg curl, rowing, shoulder press, lateral raise, push-up, and so on. A partner has an advantage of using two arms or his or her whole body for resistance. Thus, loading can be greater than self-resistance. Disadvantages with manual/partner RT include the difficulty in consistently quantifying how much resistance is being used, relatively low exercise selection, and using a partner with a sufficient level of size and strength. Partners (or spotters) must fully communicate with the athlete, watch and monitor technique, and adjust tension when necessary to accommodate fatigue or stronger areas of the ROM.

FREE WEIGHTS

Free weights are aptly named because the athlete must control and can move the weight freely in any direction. Free weights include barbells, dumbbells, plates, collars/clamps, PlateMates (1.25-lb magnetic weights that stick to weights; can be used when 2.5-lb weights are too heavy), and various accessories that enable greater free weight exercise selection. Free weights have many advantages compared to other RT modalities, especially when it comes to ease of loading and the ability to perform a large number of exercises with them.

Barbells

Barbells are bars of various lengths that can be loaded with weights or plates. Typically, barbells are between

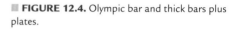

FIGURE 12.4. Olympic bar and thick bars plus plates.

5 and 7 ft in length and may vary in thickness. An Olympic barbell is most commonly used (Fig. 12.4). This is the type used with Olympic weights or plates (those with a larger 2-in. central hole to accommodate an Olympic bar) commonly seen in health clubs, gyms, and weight rooms. They are ~7 ft in length and weigh ~45 lb, although some may be slightly lighter or heavier. They have knurling to increase friction between the hands and bar for better gripping. The bar tends to be ~1 in. in diameter. The bearings, *e.g.*, roller, ball, and needle, allow the weights to freely rotate. Light weight (15-lb) aluminum bars are nice for beginners or young athletes just learning proper technique. A cambered Olympic bar allows the athlete to have more ROM during the bench press or be able to perform shrugs while seated on a bench. Another type of barbell is the thick bar (38). Thick bars come in various diameters, *e.g.*, 2, 2¾, and 3 in., and typically weigh between 20 and 50 lb. Because of the thicker diameter, thick bars are mostly used for grip strength training. Thick bars have minimal effects on pushing exercises such as the bench press and shoulder press (56). However, pulling exercises such as the deadlift, bent-over row, arm curl, and upright row are affected in proportion to the thickness of the bar. For the deadlift and bent-over row, 1 RM lifts are ~28% and 55% lower for the 2- and 3-in. bars, respectively, and ~9% and 37% for the bent-over row. Interestingly, reductions in loading correlate to hand size and maximal ISOM grip strength (56).

Standard barbells have smaller ends than Olympic bars and are used to accommodate standard plates. They weigh less and may accommodate up to ~400 lb. Some gyms have fixed barbells. These are preloaded barbells with a specific weight. Like dumbbells, a range of fixed barbells may be seen, *e.g.*, 10–100 lb or more. These are advantageous because they do not require any loading or unloading so they are nice when performing sets with short rest intervals. Specialty bars may be seen in

many gyms. Curl bars (E-Z bars) are bent in the middle to allow more pronation when gripping. This removes some stress from the wrists when performing exercises such as curls or triceps extensions. These are nearly 4-ft long and weigh 15–25 lb. Triceps bars are narrow but allow the individual to use a midrange hand position for arm curl or extensions exercises. Trap bars have a diamond-shaped middle section that is used for performing shrugs and deadlifts. Safety squat bars have two padded bars extending at 90° angles from the bar base. These can be used as grips but they allow the bar to rest comfortably on the shoulders without support. Some athletes will use their arms to grasp a power rack during the squat for support or assistance during the ascent and descent.

Weights, or plates, are added to bars for loading. Plates typically come in weight sizes of 1.25, 2.5, 5, 10, 25, 35, 45, and 100 lb. Standard plates are used for standard bars and Olympic plates are used for Olympic bars. Many Olympic plates are solid. However, some newer models have grips within that make it easier for loading and, in some cases, to perform an exercise with them. Rubberized plates are common. Because they are rubberized, they can easily be dropped or thrown without causing damage. Some rubberized plates are actually cast iron plates coated in rubber. These plates can potentially damage bars and platforms. However, bumper plates are completely rubberized and are specifically designed to be dropped without damaging platforms and floors and to withstand punishment from explosive lifting. This is important when performing the Olympic lifts/variations because one is taught to drop the weight during an unsuccessful attempt and to drop the weight once the lift is complete. Plates are held in place by collars and clamps. These come in various types, including twist/lock (Muscle Clamp), spin/lock, screw-on, or squeeze/lock (spring). They typically weigh less than 1 lb although some may weigh nearly 6 lb.

Dumbbells

Dumbbells are small versions of barbells designed mostly for single-arm use (although a single dumbbell can be used for several exercises). Many types of dumbbells exist from solid, fixed, one-piece units to adjustable (a bar that can be loaded with different weights and supported by clamps/collars) and nonadjustable weight-loaded units. Some dumbbells have rotating handles. Selectorized dumbbells (PowerBlocks) are dumbbells with blocks that support several stacks of small plates. Poundage is selected and the dumbbell is lifted up off of the block with the targeted weight. As with plates, some dumbbells are rubberized, which assists in dropping them with little to no damage. Dumbbells come in many sizes and are stacked in pairs in order on a tiered rack from the smallest (5 lb) to the largest (125 lb or more) usually in 5-lb increments. Their greatest utility is the large movement potential and ROM they provide. Weight magnets may be attached to dumbbells to add 1.25- or 2.5-lb increments.

Free-Weight Equipment

Many other pieces of equipment are available that enable free weight use. These are commonly found in most weight rooms, gyms, and clubs. They are advantageous for allowing the athlete to alter body posture or position when performing free-weight exercises. The following list outlines many of these key pieces of equipment.

- Olympic benches: flat, incline, and decline
- Portable benches (some which are adjustable up to 90°)
- Shoulder press benches
- Sit-up benches
- Dip/leg raise benches
- Glute-ham raise or hyperextension benches
- Lifting platforms: essential for performing Olympic lifts
- Power racks (with adjustable pins)—for multiple exercises
- Multiple rack units—with benches, dipping, and chinning bars
- Squat racks
- Preacher curl benches (standing and seated)
- Plyo boxes — for stepping up or other ballistic exercises
- Wrist rollers
- Belts — for performing loaded dips or pull-ups
- Head/neck harness

MACHINES

Several types of RT machines may be found in clubs and gyms. Some machines offer the athlete a constant level of tension throughout the ROM. Linear motion is produced as is the case with some types of leg press machines. Another example found in many gyms is the *Smith machine*. The Smith machine (named after Rudy Smith, who improved upon the initial design by fitness legend Jack La Lanne in the 1950s) consists of a barbell that can only move vertically upward and downward on steel runners. The Smith machine is versatile and allows performance of many exercises such as bench press (and variations), shoulder press, squats, rows, and several others. It enhances safety as catches can be used to stop the bar if fatigue sets in and prevents any side-to-side or front-to-back movements of the bar. A series of slots run behind each runner in which the bar can be hooked or secured at various locations.

Cable pulley machines consist of a cable that runs through one or more pulleys connected to a weight stack (Fig. 12.5). Many times the weight is selected by placing a pin at the desired location (as most machine plates range from 5–20 lb). The individual applies a force to the cable, the force is redirected by the pulley, and the plates (at the level of the pin and all of those plates above) are lifted to provide tension. Weight stacks (and pulley arrangements) vary when going from one machine to another. An athlete must adjust load or repetition number accordingly because performing an exercise on one machine may be easy but difficult on another using similar loading. Many cable machines are adjustable so that a multitude of unilateral and/or bilateral exercises can be performed. The pulley can be placed low, high, and at many sites in between. Although cable pulley machines are machines (free-form) per se, they do not provide as much stabilization as other types of machines so the athlete can benefit from stabilizer muscle cocontraction.

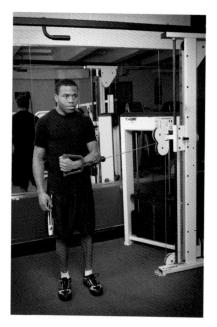

FIGURE 12.5. Cable pulley machine.

Multipurpose cable pulley units are common in gyms and health clubs as many exercises can be performed. Many different types of bars/handles/ropes can be used to vary exercises. Some cable pulley machines are nonadjustable, more specific, and only enable performance of a few exercises, *e.g.*, low pulley row, lat pull-down.

Plate-loaded machines (Fig. 12.6) require the athlete to load weights for resistance. As opposed to a weight stack, plates are loaded to the machine, which offers a few advantages: (a) athletes are provided with a wider range of loading, *i.e.*, 2.5-lb weights can be used to target those desired resistances that may be difficult with weight stacks and (b) greater loading may be used as many weight-stack machines plateau at a resistance that may be insufficient for strong athletes. Some plate-loaded machines, *e.g.*, Hammer Strength, use convergent and divergent arcs of motion and use counterbalanced lever arms to vary the resistance throughout the ROM (a variable resistance machine). At the starting position, the lever is rotated out so the athlete does not have to bear the entire load. However, the lever arm moves toward the horizontal as the weight is lifted, therefore increasing the loading on the individual (50).

Older variable resistance machines used a sliding lever to change the point of application of the resistance on the weight stack. Newer variable resistance machines use a cam to alter the loading throughout the ROM. The cam is an ellipse connected to the machine arm by which the cable or belt is located (62). The shape of the cam dictates the variable resistance to mimic human strength curves. Muscle torque production varies throughout the full joint ROM. Some machines attempt to accommodate these tension variations by altering the shape of the cam to make it more difficult in that segment of the ROM where greater torque is produced and to make it easier in the ROM where less torque is produced. For example, an inverted-U-shaped cam can be used for ascending-descending strength curves (single-joint exercises), an oblong-shaped cam with the largest radius at the distal end can be used for ascending strength curves (multiple-joint pushing exercises), and an oblong-shaped cam with the largest radius at the proximal end can be used for descending strength curves (multiple-joint pulling exercises) (62). Other nonmachine equipment, *e.g.*, elastic bands, springs, tubing, and chains, can provide variable resistance.

Hydraulic resistance machines have a lever arm connected to a hydraulic piston that provides resistance against the oil-filled chamber it is set in (62). Some machines have a flow control, which changes the fluid velocity and the resistance. The resistance matches the effort of the athlete (the faster the individual moves the more resistance). Some machines use a pressure-release valve to allow fluid flow once a force greater than the valve resistance is applied to open the valve (50). This type provides more constant resistance (50). Hydraulic resistance machines utilize a concentric (CON)/CON movement minimizing loaded eccentric (ECC) muscle actions. The machine has a dual-exercise component stressing antagonist muscles.

Pneumatic resistance machines were first designed in the late 1980s and use air pressure for resistance. A ram or piston (similar to a syringe) is preloaded using compressed air. During the lifting phase, the ram compresses the air further providing resistance for CON and ECC phases (50). The athlete can adjust the resistance by letting air out during a set, which can be advantageous. Proponents of pneumatic machines cite smooth, fluid movements and ease of changing resistance as advantages of pneumatic machines compared to those using weight stacks. A pneumatic machine has no inertial effects due to the lack of a weight stack; thus, the resistance is consistent over the entire ROM regardless of the lifting velocity.

We are living in the computer age and computerized resistance machines have been developed. These machines provide variable resistance through gears and belts connected to a motor. A touch screen, button, or foot pedal allows the manipulation of resistance, and some can load the ECC component more than CON.

Isokinetic machines possess a dynamometer that maintains the lever arm at a constant angular velocity for most of the ROM. The utility is that repetition velocity is controlled and acts passively as an accommodating resistance device (35,36). A velocity is selected rather than a resistance. The cost of an isokinetic machine can be prohibitive as isokinetic machines are mostly found in research laboratories, training rooms, and clinical facilities.

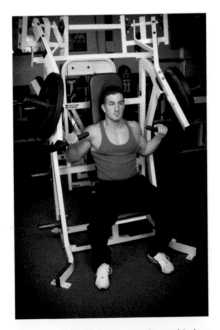

■ **FIGURE 12.6.** A plate-loaded (Hammer Strength) chest press machine.

Isokinetic machines are computerized devices where the velocity is predetermined. They are useful for strength assessment because there are many measures that can be monitored, including peak and mean torque, angle-specific peak torque, total work, time to peak torque, and torque at various time intervals. The variables available depend on the brand and model of dynamometer used, as well as the software package accompanying it.

FREE WEIGHTS VERSUS MACHINES

Several advantages and disadvantages exist when examining RT with free weight and machines. Free-weight exercises (especially multiple-joint exercises) may pose a greater risk of injury because they require the individual to completely control the exercise (maintain body stability and displacement of the resistance) whereas machines may reduce the risk of acute injury because they assist in stabilizing the body and movement of the resistance. However, the risk of developing chronic inflammation in tendons may be greater with machines that limit motion flexibility. One study examined RT-related injuries in 12 athletes and reported that 9 of the injuries occurred using free weights and 3 injuries occurred during machine exercises (66). In either case, the risk of injury during RT is very low. Hamill (21) reported 0.012 and 0.0013 injuries per 100 hours of activity, respectively, for weight training and weightlifting. Although both modalities may cause injury, proper program design and supervision are mandatory.

Free weights and machines offer other advantages/disadvantages (36). The athlete must control repetition velocity, and free-weight training movements are more similar to those found in athletics. Free weights require greater coordination and muscle stabilizer activity than machines (52), because free weights must be controlled through all spatial dimensions, whereas machines generally involve uniplanar control. Thus, stabilization muscles may be more effectively trained with free weights. This can be an advantage or disadvantage depending on the individual's skill level. Some individuals with poor balance and impaired motor function may benefit from machine-based RT initially. Another more practical reason for using free weights is their low cost and availability. Both free weights and machines are effective for increasing strength. Research shows that free-weight training leads to greater improvements in strength assessed with free weights and machine training results in greater performance on machine tests (10). When a neutral testing device is used, strength improvement from free weights and machines are similar (71). The choice to use free weights or machines should be based on the level of training status and familiarity with specific exercise movements, as well as the primary training objective. Both are recommended by the American College of Sports Medicine (ACSM) for progression during RT.

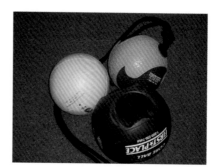

■ FIGURE 12.7. Medicine ball, core ball, and slam ball.

Olympic lifts and variations are performed with free weights as these require large muscle mass recruitment, which cannot be adequately performed within the constructs of machines. Some exercises are difficult to perform with free weights (leg curl, leg extension) so machines are a more favorable alternative. Free weights involve CON and ECC muscle activities. Eccentric muscle activity is not possible on some hydraulic machines or with some isokinetic dynamometers. Free weights allow the desired ROM whereas some machines can be restrictive if it is not possible to get a proper fit between the individual and the machine configuration. Similar to free weights, machines must be closely maintained. This includes checking for lose screws; worn parts; frayed cables, chains, or pulleys; and torn upholstery and grip supports. It is imperative that machines are adjusted properly to the individual and that they are operating smoothly; improper lubrication or a misalignment of the device may add unknown resistance to the machine. This includes making sure that the machine plates do not stick together.

MEDICINE BALLS, STABILITY BALLS, BOSU BALLS, AND OTHER BALANCE DEVICES

Medicine balls are weighted rubber or leather balls that vary in size (Fig. 12.7). They can be used for general RT, calisthenics, and plyometric exercises. Historically, the first so-called MBs (which were merely sand-filled bladders) were used by wrestlers nearly 3,000 years ago. In the 19th and early 20th centuries they were

SIDEBAR	COMPARISON OF FREE WEIGHTS AND MACHINES

Machines
Advantages

- Safe to use and easy to learn. Familiarization is easier and technique is simplified. Higher stability for beginners and special populations.
- Changing resistance is simple by either moving the pin (for weight stack machines) or modifying resis-

(Continued)

tance on other machines (hydraulic, pneumatic). Plate-loaded machines require weight change similar to free weights.

- Some machines provide variable resistance in an attempt to accommodate strength curves. Although strength curves cannot be completely replicated, variable resistance machines provide altered loading, which can be somewhat similar to normal joint mechanics.
- Isokinetic machines control velocity and allow the individual to produce maximal effort and slow, moderate, and fast velocities of muscle action.
- Resistance training can be performed unilaterally or bilaterally.
- Easy to evaluate progress. Monitoring resistance and repetition number is easy. Some machines are computerized and can store training information.
- Allow performance of some exercises that may be difficult with free weights.
- Usually does not require the use of a spotter although spotters can be beneficial with machine-based exercises (especially a Smith machine).
- Hydraulic and pneumatic machines reduce momentum and provide smooth rep cadence.
- Some machines are multiunit and allow performance of several exercises.
- Can be a major attraction for a facility selling memberships.
- Effective for increasing all health- and skill-related components of fitness to some degree, provided the training program is progressive.

Disadvantages

- Are much more costly and require more maintenance than free weights. Machines are large and heavy, making them difficult to move.
- May hinder the development of optimal neuromuscular coordination, and the additional stability lessens the body's need to stabilize itself. Antagonist and stabilizer muscle activities are lower. The machine does some of the work for the individual.
- On some machines, only one or a few exercises may be performed. Some limitations can restrict grip or foot angles/widths.
- Hydraulic/pneumatic machines produce less of an increase in strength and power when compared to free-weight training. Since hydraulic/pneumatic apparatus furnish no preload at the beginning of a

movement, they limit strength increases early in the ROM (28,29).

- Some machines do not provide enough resistance for strong individuals. Loading varies greatly when going from one machine to another when performing the same exercise.
- Can be difficult to thoroughly accommodate individuals of different height, weight, and limb length based on machine setting restrictions.

Free Weights
Advantages

- Less expensive and require less maintenance than machines.
- Require greater antagonist and stabilizer muscle activity to support the body in all planes of motion. Allows multidirectional movement that must be controlled. A better stimulus for balance and coordination is present.
- Allow more variation for hand/foot spacing, etc. to alter the stimulus.
- Can perform a multitude of exercises with little equipment. Exercise selection is greater. Some pieces of equipment can be easily moved.
- Resistance training can be performed unilaterally or bilaterally.
- Can target CON, ECC, and ISOM muscle actions.
- Easy to evaluate progress. Monitoring resistance and repetition number is easy.
- Allow performance of the Olympic lifts. Optimize acceleration for power training. Free weights are more conducive for explosive training and better for developing power and speed.
- Very easy to replicate motions seen in athletics or activities of daily living.
- Effective for increasing all health- and skill-related components of fitness.

Disadvantages

- May potentially pose a greater risk of injury due to the greater stabilization requirements.
- Takes longer to change weights and put them away in between sets and exercises.
- May require more time to learn a proper technique, especially for the Olympic lifts.
- May require a spotter on some exercises (bench press, shoulder press, and squat).
- Line of resistance is vertically downward, thus some exercises performed in a transverse plane (relative to the anatomical position) may not receive maximal resistance.

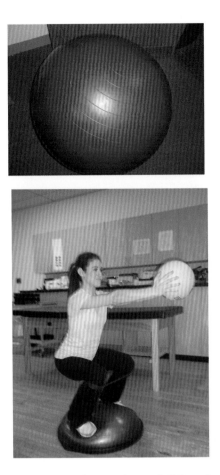

FIGURE 12.8. Stability ball (*top*) and BOSU ball (*bottom*).

commonly used in physical education classes and for gymnastics training. Later they became extensively used for the core training of boxers, *e.g.*, to simulate a body punch. Most MBs today are made of rubber. Rubber MBs are useful because they bounce and can be thrown safely with no damage. An athlete using an MB for an explosive overhead throw could throw the ball against a wall and have the ball rebound back to him or her for multiple reps. MBs come in sizes of 1–30 lb (~5–11 in.) and have developed over the years beyond their initial design. For example, Core Balls are MBs with handles to facilitate better gripping. These balls can be used similar to dumbbells or thrown explosively for plyometric exercises. Slam Balls are MBs with ropes attached. The athlete can grip the rope and throw or slam the ball for power exercises. These are beneficial for rotational core exercises. Some MBs (NRG Ball) have handles on both sides to vary exercise selection. Lastly, rebounding units (that resemble trampolines) have facilitated MB training. These allow the athlete to throw the ball against the unit and a rebound ensues. The athlete may catch the ball in rebound to facilitate the stretch-shortening cycle and enhance plyometric training.

Stability balls (SBs), also known as *Exercise Balls, Physio Balls,* or *Swiss Balls,* are inflatable balls (Fig. 12.8)

that come in many sizes (~30–85 cm). First used for clinical purposes in the mid-1960s, SBs are currently used to train in an unstable environment thereby increasing the activity of stabilizer muscles. SBs are used mostly to target core musculature as stabilizer muscles must contract to a greater extent to keep the athlete from rolling off the ball. SBs can be used with free-weight and body weight exercises and are selected by having the athlete sit on the ball and the hips should flex to ~90°. However, smaller balls pose advantageous for some exercises because they can be used for exercises requiring the athlete to support the ball between the feet/legs, or because a smaller ball is closer to the ground, it can make a basic exercise more challenging, *e.g.*, SB rollout. For some exercises (push-up), an SB that is somewhat deflated may be more beneficial (less stability); however, a ball inflated to a greater extent is more prone to roll and may be more challenging for some exercises (curl-up).

BOSU balls (Balance Trainer) resemble SBs with the exception that the bottom is flat with a stable base (measuring ~21–25 in. in diameter and 12 in. in height when fully inflated). Several exercises can be performed on it, and it has been popular since its invention in 1999. The top portion allows for instability whereas the ball will not roll due to the flat base. BOSU stands for either "Both Sides Utilized" or "Both Sides Up" as the ball can be used

STABILITY BALL EXERCISE AND TRAINING RESEARCH

SB exercise has been a topic of research interest. Electromyography (EMG) studies show conflicting results regarding the chest press exercise where the SB chest press produced similar rectus abdominis muscle activation to a chest press on a bench (2). However, other studies show higher abdominal and lower-back muscle activation when the exercise is performed on an SB (5,41,51). Bench press muscle activation (pectoralis major, triceps brachii, anterior deltoid) is similar when performing the bench press on the ball versus a bench (20), whereas deltoid activity was higher during an SB chest press in one study (41).

SB exercises result in greater trunk muscle activation during core exercises (48). Core exercises performed on SBs increase abdominal muscle activation by 28% compared to a stable surface (5). SB crunches result in greater abdominal muscle activation than crunches performed on a floor primarily when the ball is located under the lower back (as opposed to when the ball is located under the upper-back region) (61). SB curl-ups resulted in 14% and 5% greater activation of the rectus abdominis and external oblique muscles, respectively, compared to a stable surface

(Continued)

(65). In contrast, squats and deadlifts with at least 50%–70% of 1 RM yielded higher lumbar muscle activity than unloaded exercises (bridge, back extension, quadruped) (53). The majority of research indicates performing trunk exercises on an SB provides a novel training stimulus.

Of great importance to RT is the effect performing exercises on SBs has on loading. Reduced loading is used when exercises are performed on an SB. Anderson and Behm (2) showed that maximum ISOM chest press force was ~60% lower on an SB compared to a flat bench. McBride et al. (44) showed that maximum ISOM squat force and rate of force development (and agonist muscle activation) was 40%–46% lower on an unstable surface then on a floor. Work capacity during chest press training on an SB (compared to bench) was 12% lower (15). However, Goodman et al. (20) showed similar 1 RM bench press strength performances between SB and bench. The majority of research supports the concept that loading (and repetition number with a specific load) must be reduced when performing non–body weight exercises on SBs.

Few studies have examined SB training. Cowley et al. (15) showed that 3 weeks of chest press training on an SB or bench in untrained women produced similar increases in strength (assessed both on a bench and SB). However, these were untrained women and the study duration was only 3 weeks so further research is needed.

either way. Dome side down enables the BOSU ball to be used like a wobble board.

Other balance devices have been used in RT. Collectively, these devices provide an unstable environment for training. Balance steps are small vinyl balls filled with air or water that can be used flat side down or up. They can be stepped on during movement or stood upon during exercise to improve balance. Balance discs are small versions of instability equipment that are 14–24 in. in diameter. Likewise, a multitude of exercises can be performed on these. Squatting on a balance disc increases activation of the soleus, erector spinae, and abdominal muscles to maintain stability (3). Balance pads (Airex) (Fig. 12.9) function similarly as they provide instability when stood upon. Balance and wobble boards (Fig. 12.9) possess a circular center with a wooden platform located on top. The platform can move side to side and front to back (or wobble) and requires the individual to balance during exercise. These stress the ankle inversion and eversion muscles nicely in addition to plantar and dorsi flexors.

ELASTIC BANDS, TUBING, CHAINS, AND SPRINGS

Elastic bands and tubing provide variable resistance to the athlete. Resistance increases as the band or tubing is stretched further matching an ascending strength curve. Some band companies provide a chart depicting how many pounds of force are provided at various band lengths. This information is pertinent to the athlete as one can control the tension by positioning the body at a point corresponding to the desired band length/tension. Bands have multiple uses. They can be used to perform conventional RT exercises such as presses, curls, and rows. They can be used to load sport-specific exercises or movements. Bands are used to provide resistance during vertical jumping and sprinting and can be strategically placed to provide resistance to motor skills such as throwing, hitting, striking, kicking, body throwing, etc. Bands can be used to support plates or KBs when attached to a bar to provide oscillations that make the exercise more difficult to perform. The *oscillation bench press* (Figure 12.10) is an exercise used to load the shoulder flexors/adductors and elbow extensors but increases the stabilization muscle activity to control bar path during the lowering and raising of the bar. Bands and tubing are light and portable. They can be transported anywhere and used for home training or for RT while traveling. Many companies make different styles of bands. Usually, they are color-coded based on the amount of resistance they supply and may be labeled anywhere from extra light to super heavy. Bands can be placed under the feet or other bodily region and grasped for tension, or

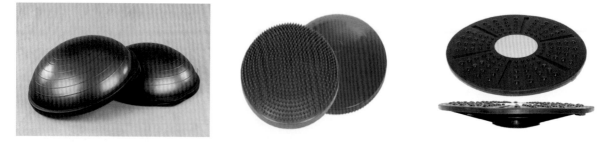

■ **FIGURE 12.9.** Bosu balls and balance discs.

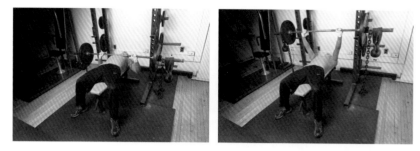

■ **FIGURE 12.10.** The oscillation bench press with chains and kettlebells attached to bar with bands.

placed around a stable object (mounted to wall or post) and grasped for tension. Some short bands can be placed around both legs to resist frontal plane lower-body movements, *e.g.*, side steps, shuffling, lateral movements, or to increase gluteus medius/minimus activity during squats and jumps. The latter has been used as a training tool for ACL injury prevention in female athletes to reduce valgus stress on the knees by increasing hip strength. Elastic band RT is beneficial for increasing muscular strength, endurance, and functional performance (27,37,58).

Another utility of bands (and chains) is to provide variable resistance to a barbell exercise. Bands can be added to barbells especially for exercises such as the bench press and squat. Several elite powerlifters use them quite effectively since their inception of use at the Westside Barbell Club in Columbus, Ohio. Because the squat and bench press are multiple-joint exercises that exemplify ascending strength curves, bands provide greater resistance as the lift progresses (where the athlete is in a stronger area of the ROM). Bands are used for the deadlift exercise. The bands are attached to the upper tiers of a power rack and attached

to the bar in the opposite direction. The band pulls the barbell upward the most when it is on the floor and provides less pull to the bar as the bar ascends. A study by Wallace et al. (70) compared a free-weight squat (85% of 1 RM) to squats using bands, one condition where bands accounted for 20% of the resistance and a second condition where bands accounted for 35% of the resistance. They reported that peak force and power were greater with the use of bands compared to the free-weight squat.

Chains are used in a similar manner for performing the squat, bench press, and variations (Fig. 12.10). Chains are typically 6–7 ft in length, 12 lb and heavier, and attach easily to a clamp on the barbell. Multiple chains can be attached at each side to provide greater resistance. A segment of the chain rests on the floor at the low end of the ROM so the athlete only has to support and lift a fraction of the chain's weight. Less chain weight is supported by the floor during bar ascent (as more links leave the floor), which forces the athlete to produce more tension. The chains oscillate, which increases the stability requirement. Small chains (3/16–5/16 in. links)

Interpreting Research

Comparison of Various Balance Devices

Wahl MJ, Behm DG. Not all instability training devices enhance muscle activation in highly resistance-trained individuals. *J Strength Cond Res.* 2008;22:1360–1370.

A study by Wahl and Behm (69) examined muscle activation to standing and squatting on Dyna Discs, BOSU ball, wobble board, an SB, and the floor. The results showed:

- During standing, soleus muscle activity was highest on the wobble board compared to other modalities, and lower abdominal muscle activity was highest using the wobble board, and second on an SB.
- During standing, the SB increased rectus femoris muscle activity the most, the wobble board increased biceps femoris activity the highest, and the SB and wobble board increased erector spinae muscle activity the most.
- During squatting, soleus activity was highest on the wobble board, and lower abdominal activity was highest on the wobble board and SB.
- Dyna Discs and BOSU balls provided a minimal muscle stimulus in resistance-trained subjects.

The authors concluded that modalities that provided greater instability (SB and wobble board) were more effective for increasing muscle activation than those that provide mild instability (Dyna Discs, BOSU).

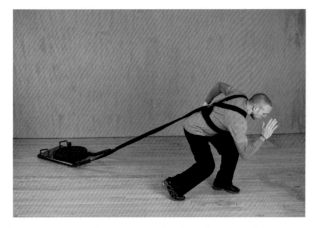

■ FIGURE 12.11. Illustration of resisted running with a sled.

provide 1 lb or less weight per foot of length, whereas larger chains (5/8–3/4 in. links) provide 3–5 lb of weight per foot of length. A few studies examined acute lifting performance using chains. Ebben et al. (17) showed no effects of chains (with chains replacing 10% of the load) on ground reaction force and muscle activation. Coker et al. (14) and Berning et al. (6) showed no difference in ground reaction force and bar velocity of the snatch and clean with chains (replacing 5% of the load) although subjects reported feeling they worked harder with chains. A major consideration is how much of the barbell weight should be replaced by chain weight. Perhaps replacing 5%–10% of the load with chains is too much as this may not stress the lower segment of the exercise maximally (as would be the case if chains were not used).

Springs provide variable resistance. As springs are pulled apart, greater tension is encountered. The use of spring RT was popular in the 1950s and for decades after when strength training entrepreneurs were searching for alternative methods of training to free weights. Some spring devices are still used but they are not as popular.

MOVEMENT-SPECIFIC RESISTANCE DEVICES

Movement-specific resistance devices are those that enable loading to a specific motor skill. For example, power chutes and harnesses are used to resist sprinting. Harnesses may be useful for other acceleration skills for other sports, *e.g.*, resisted take-downs in wrestling or mixed martial arts. Weighted vests are used to resist sprinting, jumping, and numerous other motor skills. Sleds are used to resist sprinting and plyometric drills (Fig. 12.11). New models of treadmills have been developed to resist sprinting without additional loading to the skeletal system. For example, the Woodway Force 3.0 treadmill provides loading within the belt via an electromagnetic braking system of up to 150 lb of resistance. Training on this treadmill has been shown to be effective for increasing land-based speed (59). Many devices are used to resist movements with the intent to increase muscle strength, power, and acceleration ability.

STRENGTH IMPLEMENTS

The use of strength implements in RT has increased in popularity in recent times. However, some of these implements were used for many years in RT. The idea to use these implements stemmed from strength competitions in which various implements were used. As training specificity increased for these events (Strongest Man in the World competition), strength athletes incorporated these implements into their own programs. The efficacy and popularity have carried over to other goals as many strength/power athletes now frequently integrate implements into a general RT program. Implements provide a different stress to the athlete than free weights as many implements provide unbalanced resistance and the gripping may be more difficult. Some exercises with implements cannot be replicated with free weights. The following section discusses some of the more popular implements. It is important to note that other implements not discussed have been used, *e.g.*, trucks for pulling/towing, stones, and other heavy objects.

Kegs

Kegs are fluid-filled drums used in RT. Kegs can weigh as little as 20–30 lb or more than 300 lb. Keg weight is determined by the training status of the athlete, goals of the program, and the targeted exercises. Some facilities have kegs of various weights for training variation. Because kegs are filled with fluids (and sand), there is a greater balance requirement. Fluid moves as the kegs are lifted, thereby requiring the athlete to alter force production and muscle activation for stabilization. As a result, athletes who perform exercises with kegs similar to free-weight exercises need to select lighter kegs to accommodate the stabilization effect. Gripping is important. Although kegs have grip supports, athletes will not have the same strong grip with kegs as they would with a barbell. Many traditional exercises can be performed with kegs including squats, lunges, deadlifts, bench press, and rows (Fig. 12.12). Strength/power-specific exercises such as keg toss, chops, swings, cleans, carries, and throws can be performed.

Kettlebells

Kettlebell lifting has grown in popularity in recent times despite the fact they were used in Russia since the mid-1800s (64). KBs are circular weights with handles attached (Fig. 12.13). They come in sizes similar to dumbbells. KBs provide unique challenges to the athlete separate from the effects of dumbbells. KBs are beneficial for enhancing grip strength because the grips are thicker. The handle is designed to allow the KB to swing freely. Leverage changes as it is lifted, placing greater strength on hand/forearm musculature and requiring greater activation of stabilizer muscles to support the added movement of the KB. As opposed to a dumbbell (which is grasped near the COG

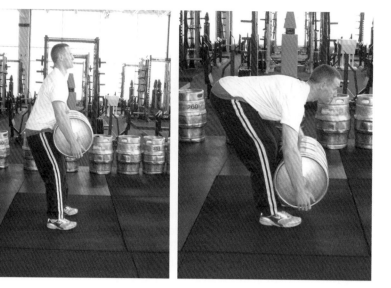

FIGURE 12.12. Illustration of a deadlift with a keg. (Reprinted with permission from Chandler J, Brown L. *Conditioning for Strength and Human Performance*. Baltimore (MD): Lippincott Williams & Wilkins; 2008.)

as the handle is located between the weights), KBs are grasped off of the COG with the handle located on top of the weight. More rotation occurs during some KB exercises forcing the athlete to adapt by greater grip support. Many exercises performed with dumbbells can be performed with KBs. Some popular KB exercises include swings, presses, cleans, snatch, rotations, and Turkish get-ups.

Logs

Logs allow weights to be added to each side. However, they have a midrange grip support, which allows athletes to use them with a pronated forearm position. Some logs are filled with water to add resistance and, similar to kegs, forces the individual to increase stabilizer muscle activity. Many exercises can be performed including cleans, presses, jerks, rows, squats, deadlifts, and lunges.

Farmer's Walk Bars

Farmer's walk bars are implements that allow the athlete to grasp a heavy weight and walk/run with it for a specified distance. Farmer's walk is a popular contested strength competition event. These bars enable training

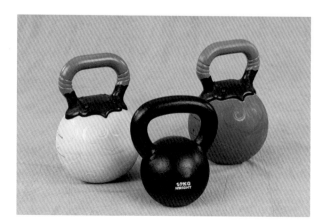

FIGURE 12.13. Illustration of kettlebells.

for this event plus have a carryover effect for improving general strength, power, and fitness. These bars are effective for enhancing grip strength. Because of their design, limited exercise selection is seen compared to some other implements. Various models of Farmer's walk bars have been developed. Nylon webbing (for grasping) can be used in conjunction with dumbbells to replicate the Farmer's walk.

Tires and Sledgehammers

Tires from trucks and heavy equipment provide a great deal of resistance for athletes, primarily for flipping. Tire flipping involves a triple extension of the hips, knees, and ankles that is beneficial for increasing strength and power (Fig. 12.14). The tire is lifted off the ground by pushing the body into it; hands are adjusted and extended to flip the tire. Experienced athletes typically select a tire that is about twice their body weight to start, and with the tire lying flat, that comes to around knee level. Tires can be towed as well. Smaller tires can serve as a target for *sledgehammer training* if a tree stump is not available. Swinging sledgehammers is an excellent exercise that stresses core and grip musculature. Sledgehammers come in various sizes ranging from 8 to 20 lb and are used for vertical, horizontal, and diagonal swings. The athlete explosively strikes the tire with the sledgehammer in a repetitive manner. The athlete must control the rebound of the hammer from the tire, which is less if striking a tree stump. The exercise can be made more difficult by increasing the resistance arm by grasping the hammer closer to the end of the handle or more explosive by grasping the hammer closer to the head.

Sandbags and Heavy Bags

Sandbags have plastic bags filled with sand enclosed within canvas bags. They range in weight from being light to over 100 lb. Smaller bags are filled with sand and then

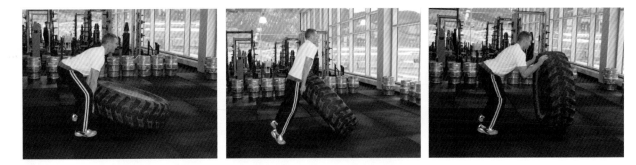

FIGURE 12.14. Illustration of tire flipping.

placed within a larger bag to vary the weight. Sandbags provide the athlete with unbalanced resistance, which forces the athlete to increase stabilizer muscle activation for proper technique (Fig. 12.15). They are effective for increasing grip strength because they must be grasped with very little support. Many exercises can be performed with sandbags including squats, drags, lunges, Turkish get-ups, presses, pulls, cleans, rows, bear hug throws, twists, etc. As with sandbags, heavy bags (punching bags) can be used for RT. These are beneficial for grappling athletes as they mimic an opponent and can be thrown or lifted in multiple directions.

WATER AND THE ENVIRONMENT

Water and the environment are other sources of resistance. Certain properties of water enable it to create resistance to motion. The **buoyancy** of water is defined as the upward force acting in the opposite direction of gravity and is related to the specific gravity of the athlete immersed in the water (63). **Specific gravity** is the ratio of the mass of an object to its mass of water displacement. The specific gravity of the human body is less than the specific gravity of water (1.0); therefore, humans float.

Greater resistance to motion is supplied when athletes move downward against the force of buoyancy. Upward motion encounters less resistance because the buoyancy force supports the movement. Buoyancy forces allow the athlete's limbs to remain parallel to the pool with little effort, *e.g.*, during horizontal abduction (63). Hydrostatic pressure provides resistance to motion in water as depth increases. Resistance in the water is encountered due to the water's viscosity. Human movement through water causes adjacent water molecules to collide, which increases fluid resistance and resists motion. The resistance encountered is increased when the athlete moves at faster rates or uses equipment to increase the amount of surface area exposed to water molecular flow (63).

In addition to swimming, aquatic RT programs are popular. They involve performing exercises in the water against natural water resistance or using aquatic resistance devices, *e.g.*, aqua dumbbells, belts, fan paddles and gloves, wrist and ankle cuffs, and training shoes. Aquatic resistance exercise reduces stress on the joints and skeletal system, which make it attractive for special populations and athletes rehabilitating injuries or general all-purpose training. There is less cardiovascular and thermoregulatory demand. However, there is less

Interpreting Research

Mechanical Analysis of Strongmen Events

McGill SM, McDermott A, Fenwick CMJ. Comparison of different strongman events: trunk muscle activation and lumbar spine motion, load, and stiffness. *J Strength Cond Res.* 2009;23:1148–1161.

McGill et al. (46) analyzed muscle activation and spinal loading characteristics of several strongmen events: farmer's walk, suitcase carry, super yoke walk, tire flip, log lift, Atlas stone lift, and the keg walk. They found:

- Greatest spinal compression was seen during the super yolk walk.
- Greatest L4/L5 vertebrae moments were seen in the tire flip followed by the keg walk and log lift.
- The tire flip and Atlas stone lift produced the greatest activation of rectus abdominis, internal and external obliques, latissimus dorsi, gluteus medius and maximus, biceps femoris, erector spinae, and rectus femoris muscles. The log lift also produced high erector spinae activity.
- All events produced great challenges to the core and hip musculature to stabilize the spine. Carrying events produced differential activation patterns than lifting events.

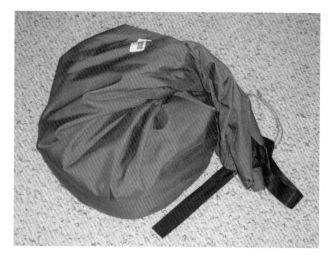

FIGURE 12.15. Illustration of a sandbag.

of an ECC component with aquatic resistance exercise. Aquatic RT is effective for increasing muscle strength, grip strength, hypertrophy, flexibility, endurance, and functional performance in various populations (54,65,68). Plyometric training in the water is effective for increasing vertical jump performance (60).

Environmental factors such as hills (downhill and uphill) and terrain provide added resistance. Running uphill provides a greater neuromuscular and metabolic challenge to the athlete than running on a flat surface. This is evident in athletes who frequently run up (and down) stadium steps. Downhill running has a substantial ECC component and is more likely to result in muscle damage and **delayed onset muscle soreness**. Rougher surfaces are more challenging physiologically and place more strain on the joints then smooth, even surfaces. For example, walking in sand or snow increases metabolic energy expenditure two to three times (43). Terrain can be used to enhance training, especially walking, jogging, and sprinting.

Case Study 12.2

Lisa is a high school student who is considering trying out for the school's basketball team. Although Lisa has been playing some pick-up basketball games with her friends to get in shape, she very much wants to begin RT to increase her chances of making the team. Rather than join a gym or lift weights in the high school weight room, Lisa wants to train in the privacy of her own home. She has limited space in the garage and her father has agreed to purchase some inexpensive equipment for her.

Questions for Consideration: **Based on her situation, what RT modalities would you recommend for Lisa? What type of equipment is reasonably priced and may be of great benefit to her? How would you advise Lisa to begin her RT program?**

VIBRATION DEVICES AND TRAINING

Vibrations are mechanical oscillations that are defined by their frequency (number of cycles per second) and amplitude (half difference between minimum and maximum oscillatory values) (39). The magnitude of vibration can be represented by the acceleration (g or m·s^{-2}) in addition to amplitude (32). Vibrations using different waveforms can be added to the exercise, *i.e.*, *vibration training*, in two ways: (a) applied directly to an exercising muscle via a handheld vibrating unit, or (b) via a vibrating platform (known as *whole-body vibration training*). Although vibration training dates back to the 1960s, the latter has become more popular in recent times not only in athletes but also in elderly and special populations. Whole-body vibration plates have reciprocal vertical displacement (on left and right) or whole-plate uniform up and down oscillations. Most vibration units provide a frequency in the range of 15–60 Hz, displacements of <1–10 mm, and up to 15-g acceleration (11).

Vibrations elicit responses to several physiological systems. The proposed performance improvement effects are thought to occur via enhanced neural responses. Vibrations are thought to stimulate the primary endings of muscle spindles (Ia afferents), which potentiates motoneuron discharge to agonist muscles, called a *tonic vibration reflex* (32). More efficient motor patterns, recruitment, and synchronization result and dynamic muscle force and power production are thought to be enhanced. It has been suggested that vibrations compensate for fatigue by increasing motor unit output (32). Of concern are potential hazards associated with vibrations. In animal and workplace studies, vibrations were associated with cardiovascular stress, lung damage, bone/joint damage, low-back problems, and neurological disorders (32). However, the magnitude of vibrations exposed to athletes appears lower, provided caution is used. Vibration devices have the potential to expose athletes to high levels of vibration that could be injurious; however, training studies have been short term using moderate stimuli.

Vibration devices have been studied during acute exercise and training (Fig. 12.16). Upper-body studies have typically used elbow flexion whereas whole-body vibration studies have mostly used squatting movements (33). Most studies examined vibration training at frequencies of 23–44 Hz with amplitudes ranging from 2 to 10 mm. Vibration training has been shown to enhance strength and power, whereas some studies reported no ergogenic effects. Acute studies using vibrations of 26–44 Hz, 3–10 mm, and 30–170 m · s^{-2} have shown vibrations enhanced muscle power by 5%–12%, jump height by 4%, and produced elevated testosterone and growth hormone and reduced cortisol (7–9,11,30,39). Quadriceps muscle activity was higher during uni- and bilateral ISOM squats on a vibrating platform than with no vibration (54).

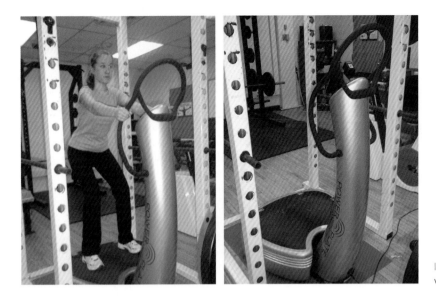

FIGURE 12.16. Illustration of the power plate vibration training system.

Hazell et al. (22) showed vibration exercise resulted in 1%–7% greater lower-body muscle activation and only greater triceps brachii activation in the upper body. However, higher frequencies (>35 Hz) and amplitudes (4 vs. 2 mm) of vibration produced the highest increases in muscle activation. In contrast, some studies did not show any ergogenic potential of vibration training (11,32,39). Chronic vibration training of 1.5–3 weeks may increase muscle strength, power, and flexibility (31,32). Some longer term (6–8 weeks) studies have shown beneficial effects of vibration training on power, velocity, strength, and flexibility (4,18,40,47). However, some studies have shown no effects on strength, power, speed, vertical jump, or agility in athletes (13,16,39), thus leaving some questions on the efficacy of vibration training, especially whether or not it can augment the effects of a traditional RT program.

INJURY PREVENTION

Resistance training is thought to play an important role in reducing the risk of injury—not only injuries encountered in the weight room (which are very low) but also injuries encountered in athletics, recreation, or during performance of activities of daily living. Greater muscular strength increases joint stability, which enables the athlete to offset high levels of force encountered during ballistic activities. Tendons, ligaments, and bone adapt to RT by increasing stiffness (tendons), cross-sectional area, and bone mineral density, which provide greater support to the skeletal system and increase force transmission efficiency. Proper RT, *e.g.*, training all muscle groups and improving weaknesses, increases muscle balance. Increasing muscle balance is thought to reduce injury risk; however, more research is needed

to show a definitive link between muscle balance and injury prevention. Muscle balance should be maintained between muscles of both sides of the body and those that have antagonistic relationships. Muscle balance entails ensuring that muscle strength and length are at comparable levels. Muscle balance training may be important for reducing the risk of overuse injuries (knee ligament sprains/strains, hamstring tears, shoulder injuries, and low-back pain/injury). For example, gender differences (hormonal, anatomical, strength imbalances) make female athletes more susceptible to ACL injuries (24). Strength balance between the internal and external shoulder rotators is important for reducing shoulder injuries in athletes (12). It has been suggested that the ratio of hamstring-to-quadriceps strength be at least 60%, and <10% strength difference be between dominant and nondominant legs. This may be higher in athletes as collegiate female athletes were shown to be at higher risk for leg injury if there was >15% difference in knee flexion strength between right and left legs and hamstrings-quadriceps ratio <75% (34). Lastly, proper strengthening of the abdominal, hamstrings, hip extensors, and spinal muscles is critical to prevention of low-back injuries.

SAFE AND EFFECTIVE RESISTANCE TRAINING

For RT to be safe and effective, general procedures should be followed not only to ensure the safe and effective participation of the athlete, but other athletes working out in the facility. In addition to following general safety (and common sense) procedures, proper gym etiquette should be followed to ensure a productive lifting environment for everyone. The following safety/etiquette checklist can be used to ensure an optimal RT environment.

Myths & Misconceptions

Resistance Training Poses a High Risk of Joint Injury and Damage

Some have stated that RT is highly injurious. However, studies show that RT poses less of a risk of injury compared to other competitive sports when it is performed properly (21,42). For general RT, the most common site of injury is the lower back and the type of injury mostly encountered is a muscle strain (42). The major causes of RT-related injuries are (a) improper lifting technique or poor form, (b) improper loading (increasing load too fast), (c) lack of supervision, (d) overtraining, (e) muscular imbalances, (f) improper warm-up, and (g) weight room accidents. Many of these injury mechanisms stem from inexperience or lack of supervision. A novice individual with poor technique and limited knowledge of program design, and who does not have supervision or an individual (trainer, coach) present for assistance (or spotting), may be at a slightly higher risk. Weight room accidents can occur regardless of experience level, but novice individuals tend to be more susceptible. Experienced athletes are more susceptible to overtraining-related injuries as these individuals train intensively for extended periods of time. Another factor implicated in increasing the injury risk is the use of anabolic steroids (25). Primarily based on some animal data, anabolic steroids increase collagen degeneration (primarily through aromatizing estrogenic effects of anabolic steroid metabolism), thereby placing tendons at greater risk of injury (25). Tendons adapt to loading more slowly than skeletal muscles so an athlete using anabolic steroids who experiences rapid gains in muscular strength and hypertrophy may not have optimal tendinous support at that point in time. As a result, force transmission to bone is compromised and anabolic steroids can be viewed as indirectly increasing the risk of myotendinous injury. However, with proper supervision and exercise prescription there is a very low risk of injury or joint damage resulting from drug-free RT.

There is a higher incidence of injury with advanced RT or competitive lifting. These individuals take themselves to their physical limits regularly, thus exposing themselves to a higher risk of injury. This is inherent to training at a high level. Keogh et al. (33) examined 101 competitive powerlifters and reported an average of 1.2 injuries per year or 4.4 injuries per 1,000 hours of training. In this sample, 36% reported shoulder injuries, 24% reported low-back injuries, and 11% reported elbow injuries. Goertzen et al. (19) examined 358 bodybuilders and 60 powerlifters and reported that 84% reported some type of injury (pulls, sprains, and tendonitis). Shoulder and elbow injuries were most common (>40%) and low-back and knee injuries were common. Powerlifters showed twice the injury rate as bodybuilders. Raske and Norlin (55) reported that weightlifters exhibited higher frequency of low-back and knee injuries whereas shoulder injuries were more prominent in powerlifters.

SIDEBAR SAFETY CHECKLIST

- Obtain medical clearance before initiating RT. Although an individual may appear healthy and the risk of serious illness or death via a cardiovascular event during exercise is very low (<6 individuals per 100,000), it is recommended that screening take place. The ACSM, American Heart Association (AHA), and National Strength and Conditioning Association (NSCA) have published guidelines addressing the procedures used for obtaining medical clearance (1,49). The ACSM and AHA recommend all exercise facilities screen individuals prior to participation with a medical history questionnaire or health appraisal document. All exercise professionals should adhere to the recommendations of these organizations when screening individuals for RT.
- Proper athletic screening. Athletic screening (see Chapter 18) can determine athletes' strengths and weaknesses. Separate from medical clearance, athletic screening can point out glaring motor weaknesses the athlete may have prior to training. Such weaknesses may encompass strength, endurance, flexibility, balance, coordination, and technique deficits that need to be addressed. For example, an athlete with limited flexibility of the hips and ankles who cannot perform a proper squat (posture and depth) with no weight should not begin loaded squat training until motor performance improves. Loading improper motor patterns can be problematic and increase injury risk. Technical (and

(Continued)

perhaps flexibility) training will prepare the athlete for greater loading. Although weaknesses may not preclude the athlete from initiating RT, program design should stress these weaknesses early prior to more advanced RT.

- Proper, nonoffensive clothing should be worn. Nonrestrictive, comfortable clothing (shorts, sweat pants, t-shirts, tank tops, workout pants, sweat shirts, etc.) should be worn to allow optimal joint ROM during resistance exercise. Clothing should reflect ambient temperatures as clothing should be worn to keep the individual cool in hot, humid conditions or warm in cool conditions. Proper athletic shoes should be worn to allow comfort, stability, and ease of movement to the athlete.

- Know how each piece of equipment functions and its proper usage. Prior to RT, each athlete should understand how each exercise is performed and how each piece of equipment works prior to use. Lack of knowledge in this area could lead to injury.

- Practice proper form and technique with each exercise, especially with free weights. Although injury risk is low, improper technique, especially with free weights, can increase the risk of injury. A trainer, supervisor, or coach should be consulted if an individual is unclear as to the correct performance of an exercise.

- Before using machines, check for frayed pulleys, loose screws, loose pads, and proper movement. Damage or wear and tear to machines can be injurious. If damage is present, a staff member should be consulted immediately and the machine should not be used until it is fixed. An "out of order" sign should be placed on the machine subsequently.

- Make sure seat adjustments are correct and pins are all the way through their holes. Each machine will have a proper adjustment point based on the target musculature. For example, in performing a leg extension exercise, the knees should be aligned with the machine's axis of rotation and the seat or back pad should be adjusted accordingly. On a chest press machine, the seat can be adjusted so the grips are positioned at the lower (sternal) chest level. However, positioning the seat above or below this point can shift muscle activation to the upper or lower pectoral muscles, respectively. For machines requiring a pin to change resistance, the pin should be placed all the way through the hole in the weight stack. A partially placed pin may not secure loading appropriately.

- Do not bounce the weight stacks and never put fingers near the stack when someone is using it. Bouncing the weight stack reflects a lack of control, especially during the ECC phase. Weights should be lifted in control and this would negate any loud, clanging bouncing of the weight stack. One should never place fingers or hands near a weight stack while in use. A finger caught in a stack could be very painful or even result in a loss of the finger. Some athletes perform breakdown sets in which a spotter may be located at the weight stack to quickly pull the pin in between sets for an individual to lower the weight. This technique is acceptable; however, spotters must communicate clearly with the individual as to when a set ends and the next set begins. Spotters should keep their hands away from the weight stack except when changing the weight in between sets.

- Never bother anyone while they are in the middle of a set. Common courtesy. Individuals are focused on the task at hand during a set and do not need to be distracted by others in the facility (unless an emergency exists or the individual is placed at great risk for injury where intervention is necessary). Distraction can place the individual at a higher risk for injury or result in poor performance of the exercise. When communicating with someone in the weight room, it is appropriate to do so upon completion of the exercise or in between sets.

- No horseplay in the facility. Common sense but may occur in younger populations. Poor behavior can result in injury or being asked to leave the gym or club.

- Never attempt to lift ultra heavy weights without a spotter or safety rack. For certain exercises such as the squat, bench press and variations, and shoulder press, a spotter is recommended when heavy weights are lifted. Because of the position of the body at the lower point of each exercise, the athlete could be trapped under the bar if unable to complete the repetition. Spotters assist in lifting the weight until completion where the bar can be safely racked. If lifting in a power rack, the weight can be safely placed on the pins. For the squat, multiple spotters can be used depending on the amount of weight.

- Make sure dumbbells are tightened. For dumbbells that are not solid (one-piece) but have plates placed on either side that are fastened in place, it is important that these dumbbells remain tightened. Loose dumbbells can result in plates sliding off of one or both sides, perhaps striking the athlete and causing injury.

- Make sure bars are loaded properly and evenly. When loading barbells, it is important to make sure the same amount of weight is placed on both sides. Improper loading can result in one side being heavier than the other, causing disproportionate lifting technique. Caution must be used when unloading bars or plate-loaded machines. One should not take off weight entirely on one side. This could cause the bar to tip and hit someone, or cause a small machine to tip. It is important to remove plates from bars equally on both sides.

- Use clamps with barbells to prevent slipping of the weights. Clamps or collars keep plates in place on bars, preventing them from slipping off. Although clamps are not used for various reasons, they do increase safety by keeping plates fixed on barbells.

- Make sure there is enough room between you and other people. Space is an important safety consideration. Lifting too close to someone could result in bodily injury via contact with a bar, dumbbell, or any other piece of equipment. The athlete should be aware of extended bars on racks (and other moving parts) to prevent walking into them. Colliding into someone while lifting can disrupt that person's set as well as put him or her at greater risk of injury. Athletes should be aware of the surroundings and always look before moving from one area to the next. This is especially true for lifting platforms where individuals are performing the Olympic lifts. These are explosive lifts and can be dangerous if one gets too close to the bar when another is in the middle of a set. From a weight room perspective, standards have been set by various professional organizations (NSCA) detailing adequate spacing between pieces of equipment. Gym and club owners should be aware of these guidelines and design facilities accordingly.

- Store equipment properly. One should not leave equipment on the floor in another's walkway. This is a safety issue and a measure of etiquette. Leaving free-weight equipment or MBs could result in tripping, loss of balance, and falling, causing injury. It is important for an individual to replace weights when finished. Individuals must share the gym with others and leaving bars loaded and dumbbells at specific stations (away from racks) requires others to house clean in order to use the equipment. Proper gym etiquette mandates individuals return equipment when they have finished using it.

- Exercise using a full ROM. Best results are obtained when individuals perform exercises in a fully-prescribed ROM. Although some advanced techniques require athletes to perform partial ROM exercises, under most conditions it is imperative for athletes to perform each exercise in a full ROM.

- Properly warm-up prior to RT. The benefits of a warm-up are discussed later in this text. It is imperative that athletes properly warm-up before lifting weights to reduce the risk of injury and enhance performance.

- Always make sure the athlete is in a stable position when beginning an exercise. It is important to make sure the athlete is focused, prepared, and ready to begin a set when performing an exercise with a heavy weight. This entails being in the proper body position when initiating an exercise. In some cases, a spotter may be used to help the athlete lift the weight to a starting position (a "liftoff"). This is customary when performing a bench press, behind-the-neck press, and when heavy dumbbells are handed to the athlete for various exercises. Spotters need to make sure the athletes are ready to receive the load so communication is paramount. Handing or lifting off a weight to an athlete unprepared could cause injury.

- Use proper control when lifting weights and placing them down. Athletes should control the weights; the weights should not control the athlete. Proper loading is essential to assisting in controlling weights especially during the ECC phase. A common mistake by beginners is to let gravity control the weight during the ECC phase. Accentuating the ECC phase is critical to maximal strength and hypertrophy development. Not controlling the ECC phase increases the risk of injury and limits performance improvement. In some cases, athletes drop or throw free weights upon completion of a set if they are in a compromised position. For example, some athletes drop dumbbells to the floor after completion of a set of dumbbell bench presses. This is because the athlete must rise off of the bench and it is difficult to do so with heavy dumbbells in hand. Athletes drop weights upon completion of an Olympic lift on a platform using bumper plates. Several examples can be mentioned but the key is to use caution and control in these situations.

- When lifting weights from the floor, use the lower body and proper posture as much as possible. Proper lifting technique is important for reducing the risk of low-back injuries. Low-back injuries stem from different factors (poor extensor muscle endurance and strength, length/strength imbalances, spinal muscle atrophy, reduced neural/muscle activation or coactivation) but improper lifting technique places great stress on lumbar vertebrae, potentially causing injury. Repeated trunk flexion places large amounts of stress on lumbar discs, in some cases enough to cause bulging or

(*Continued*)

herniation. Proper technique involves increasing spinal stability while minimizing spinal loading. This is accomplished in a few ways. First, the athlete must increase spinal stability by increasing IAP. A technique known as abdominal bracing is used. Abdominal bracing involves contraction of all layers of abdominal muscles in unison (45). Lumbar extensor muscles cocontract to increase spine rigidity. This maintains the lordodic arch (flat-back position), which reduces spinal shear stress. It is important to teach athletes the correct posture and bracing technique early in training. It could be described as retracting the shoulder girdle, sticking the chest out, and bracing the core. This position should be maintained for all exercises and not solely for lifting weights off of the ground. A rounded (flexed) spine places the athlete at greater risk of injury. IAP increases in response to a Valsalva maneuver, or temporary breath holding, which compounds the stabilizing effects of bracing. Second, the athlete should lift with the legs as much as possible. This involves strong contraction of the hip extensor muscles especially the gluteus maximus. Contracting the hip musculature reduces spinal loading forcing the hips to do most of the work. Abdominal bracing and correct lifting technique are the best ways to prevent acute low-back injuries.

- Make sure spotters are capable. It is important to select spotters who have experience and know how to spot for a given exercise. Communication with spotters is critical to the type of spot needed by the athlete. Some individuals prefer the spotter to provide no assistance until failure and some individuals prefer to have a spotter assist before failure. Some individuals prefer minimal assistance from the spotter (just enough force to keep the bar moving) while some prefer more assistance. The spotter needs to have sufficient strength. For strong athletes performing a heavy exercise, it is mandatory that the spotter be strong enough to assist if failure occurs. Although spotters many times only need to provide low levels of force, if greater force is needed, the spotter has to be strong enough to accommodate. In rare cases, a poor spotter can increase the risk of injury.

- When perspiring, make sure to carry a towel or clean equipment after use. For proper gym etiquette, it is a good idea to have a towel to prevent excessive perspiration on the equipment. If not, then wiping down the equipment with cleanser after use is recommended. Although perspiration is

desired, leaving a pool of sweat on the equipment is not desirable and inconsiderate to other athletes in the facility. Individuals should make sure to wash their hands or use a hand sanitizer upon completion of a workout. This is important for reducing the risk of catching a cold, flu, or other infection. Although many individuals clean equipment upholstery after perspiration, bars, dumbbells, machine handles, MBs, etc. (pieces of equipment that are gripped with the hands) are rarely cleaned and are the first line by which infections may be passed. Gripping equipment that hundreds of other individuals gripped and placing one's hands on the facial region are easy ways to contaminate oneself.

- Always practice proper breathing. Proper breathing entails exhaling on the positive phase (more difficult segment) and inhaling on the negative (easier phase because muscles are stronger during ECC muscle actions). Under many conditions (low-to-moderate-intensity exercise), proper breathing should be performed during resistance exercise to maximize performance and reduce cardiovascular stress. However, there are exceptions. Holding one's breath (Valsalva maneuver) increases IAP, intrathoracic pressure, and torso rigidity. For example, a powerlifter during a maximal squat may inhale during the decent to the area of the sticking region, temporarily hold his or her breath at the bottom of the descent through early ascent past the sticking region, and then exhale for the completion of the lift. The sticking region is the most difficult part of the exercise and an area that increases vulnerability to a low-back injury. Postural stability is crucial here to develop the force necessary to ascend with a heavy weight while protecting the spine. A temporary Valsalva maneuver can increase IAP and protect the spine at this critical position. Valsalva maneuvers are seen during other explosive activities as well such as the delivery phase of pitching in baseball or during a maximal vertical jump. Postural stability trumps the undesirable effects of the Valsalva maneuver under explosive or heavy-loaded conditions. It is important to note that this is an exception to the breathing principle, and proper breathing should be used under most circumstances.

- If you feel any pain or discomfort while training, stop immediately. It may not be in the best interest of the athlete to attempt to ascertain the cause or nature of the pain at that point; thus, it is wise to stop lifting and prevent further injury from taking place.

- Use proper gym etiquette. Proper gym etiquette should be followed at all times. This includes com-

SIDEBAR SAFETY CHECKLIST (*Continued*)

municating with others when using equipment. When approaching a piece of equipment, make sure no one else is currently using it. If another athlete is using the equipment, then communicating by asking, "can I work in?" or "how many sets do you have left?" is common courtesy. It is not proper to occupy equipment when not using it because other athletes may be waiting to use it. If an athlete needs a spot, the individual should ask politely and the athlete will oblige or decline courteously. It is important to be courteous to others and this includes not using profanity or rude language, cleaning up after oneself and putting equipment away, and not acting like one owns the gym and aggressively trains without concern for others. Distracting others is discouraged. The gym is not a social place per se as many are there to train and not socialize. Sometimes it becomes more difficult to lift when gyms are crowded. Individuals have to wait for equipment and may feel rushed as others are waiting for them to finish an exercise. These can be challenging times for maintaining proper etiquette but it is critical for individuals to identify the congested environment and act accordingly. Communication and courteous behavior is helpful in dealing with crowded gyms. Having a backup plan (other exercises, rest intervals) can help in these situations. Lastly, following the facility's rules is important. Most facilities will have rules posted or provide lifters with a list of rules. Facilities may have policies on dress or attire, music, noise, use of lifting chalk, cleaning equipment, dropping weights or leaning plates on equipment, and how some pieces of equipment are to be used, so it is important to respect and follow the rules.

SIDEBAR BECOMING AN EFFECTIVE SPOTTER

Many athletes (and training partners) provide spots during RT. A spotter is defined as a person who applies assistance to an individual in need. Spotting ability becomes better with repeated exposure. The following is a checklist of items that make one an effective spotter:

- Be familiar with the exercise for which you are spotting.
- Effectively communicate with the athlete about the type of spot preferred, the amount of assistance to apply, when to intervene and assist, if a lift-off is needed, where the athlete prefers to be spotted

(around the waist or shoulders for the squat, under the elbows or stabilizing the wrists for presses), how many reps the athlete is targeting, the potential for forced reps, and if the athlete needs assistance racking the weight upon completion.

- Do not crowd the athlete when spotting and give the athlete adequate space to complete the exercise. For example, when spotting the bench press do not stand too close to the athlete's head to avoid contact during the exercise.
- Make sure you are strong enough to provide assistance for strong athletes.
- When spotting for squats (with only one spotter located behind the athlete), follow the athlete down each repetition to maintain proper position and should avoid accidentally pushing the athlete forward when assisting.
- Make sure you provide just enough force to keep the bar moving. This ensures the athlete is working maximally. Do not take the weight away from the athlete unless it is an emergency situation or a 1 RM test.
- Know when to intervene if the athlete needs assistance. This will occur after a 1–3 second period where the bar is stagnant.
- Be sure to check and clear the area of obtrusive objects before the athlete begins the lift.
- Double-check the bar and make sure the bar is evenly loaded with collars secured. When transferring dumbbells to the athlete, make sure the grips are exposed and easily grasped and hand the weights to the athlete in the starting position of the exercise.
- Maintain proper spotting posture and body position throughout the exercise. Stay focused and do not become distracted by others in the gym.
- Spotting for machine exercises may occur. If so, provide assistance to the athlete's limbs or machine's grip support and use caution if applying pressure to cables.
- Spotting for Olympic lifts is not common and not recommended as athletes are coached to safely release the bar during failed attempts.
- For some exercises, multiple spotters may be needed if heavy weights are used or one spotter alone may be needed in a compromised position to assist.
- For some exercises (leg press, unilateral arm curls or triceps extensions, seated calf raises), an athlete may be able to self-spot himself or herself upon failure.
- In some cases, a spotter may apply resistance for forced negatives or manual resistance exercise. The amount of resistance depends on the strength and goals of the athlete. This must be communicated prior to beginning the exercise.

Summary Points

✔ Several different modalities are used for RT. Free weights and machines are recommended because they enable great exercise selection and are easily quantifiable.

✔ Body weight, manual or partner resistance, and the environment can be used for RT. These are essentially free and can be used independent of one's budget.

✔ Free weights and machines have advantages and disadvantages in direct comparison, and the ACSM has recommended the inclusion of both in an RT program.

✔ MBs come in various sizes and are used for a multitude of exercises. They can be thrown for plyometric training.

✔ Instability equipment increases balance and stabilizer muscle activation. SBs, BOSU balls, wobble boards, pads, and balance discs are commonly used in RT.

✔ Elastic bands, tubing, cables, and chains have increased in popularity because they are portable and can be used for variable RT.

✔ As strength competitions have increased in popularity, so have the training methods used. Strength implements have been successfully incorporated into many RT programs.

✔ RT is very safe provided that general rules and guidelines are followed.

Review Questions

1. Free weights include:
   a. Barbells
   b. Dumbbells
   c. Plates
   d. All of the above

2. Resistance exercise machines that use air pressure for resistance are known as:
   a. Hydraulic machines
   b. Pneumatic machines
   c. Smith machines
   d. Plate-loaded machines

3. Free weights are advantageous because:
   a. They are more costly than machines
   b. Require greater antagonist and stabilizer muscle activity to support the body in all planes of motion
   c. They limit exercise selection
   d. They do not require the use of spotters

4. Variable resistance can be provided solely by:
   a. Medicine balls
   b. Stability balls
   c. Elastic bands
   d. Kettlebells

5. Which of the following is not characteristic of an effective spotter?
   a. Is familiar with the exercise being spotted
   b. Is strong enough to provide adequate assistance if the individual fails during the set
   c. Does not communicate with the individual regarding the set
   d. Checks to make sure area is clear before initiating the exercise

6. Abdominal bracing involves contracting trunk muscles to increase IAP and spinal stability.   T F

7. The risk of injury during a supervised resistance training program is much lower than the injury risk from playing competitive sports.   T F

8. Performing a 1 RM bench press on an SB will yield a higher value than performing the 1 RM on a stable bench.   T F

9. Performing exercises on an SB, a BOSU ball, or a wobble board increases stabilizer muscle activation due to the unstable environment.   T F

10. The use of strength implements is advantageous because some provide unbalanced resistance and some exercises are difficult to replicate with free weights.   T F

11. Chains may be advantageous because they apply variable resistance to a free weight exercise.   T F

12. Proper breathing during resistance exercise entails exhaling on the negative phase and inhaling on the positive phase.   T F

References

1. American College of Sports Medicine & American Heart Association. Joint position stand: recommendations for cardiovascular screening, staffing, and emergency policies at health/fitness facilities. *Med Sci Sports Exerc.* 1998;30:1009–1018.

2. Anderson KG, Behm DG. Maintenance of EMG activity and loss of force output with instability. *J Strength Cond Res.* 2004;18: 637–640.

3. Anderson KG, Behm DG. Trunk muscle activity increases with unstable squat movements. *Can J Appl Physiol.* 2005;30:33–45.

4. Annino G, Padua E, Castagna C, et al. Effect of whole body vibration training on lower limb performance in selected high-level ballet students. *J Strength Cond Res.* 2007;21:1072–1076.

5. Behm DG, Leonard AM, Young WB, Bonsey WA, MacKinnon SN. Trunk muscle electromyographic activity with unstable and unilateral exercises. *J Strength Cond Res.* 2005;19:193–201.

6. Berning JM, Coker CA, Briggs D. The biomechanical and perceptual influence of chain resistance on the performance of the Olympic clean. *J Strength Cond Res.* 2008;22:390–395.

7. Bosco C, Cardinale M, Tsarpela O. Influence of vibration on mechanical power and electromyogram activity in human arm flexor muscles. *Eur J Appl Physiol Occup Physiol.* 1999;79:306–311.

8. Bosco C, Colli R, Introini E, et al. Adaptive responses of human skeletal muscle to vibration exposure. *Clin Physiol.* 1999;19: 183–187.

9. Bosco C, Iacovelli M, Tsarpela O, et al. Hormonal responses to whole-body vibration in men. *Eur J Appl Physiol.* 2000;81: 449–454.

10. Boyer BT. A comparison of the effects of three strength training programs on women. *J Appl Sports Sci Res.* 1990;4:88–94.

11. Cardinale M, Wakeling J. Whole body vibration exercise: are vibrations good for you? *Br J Sports Med.* 2005;39:585–589.

12. Chandler TJ, Kibler WB, Stracener EC, Ziegler AK, Pace B. Shoulder strength, power, and endurance in college tennis players. *Am J Sports Med.* 1992;20:455–458.

13. Cochrane DJ, Legg SJ, Hooker MJ. The short-term effect of whole-body vibration training on vertical jump, sprint, and agility performance. *J Strength Cond Res.* 2004;18:828–832.

14. Coker CA, Berning JM, Briggs DL. A preliminary investigation of the biomechanical and perceptual influence of chain resistance on the performance of the snatch. *J Strength Cond Res.* 2006;20: 887–891.

15. Cowley PM, Swensen T, Sforzo GA. Efficacy of instability resistance training. *Int J Sports Med.* 2007;28:829–835.

16. Delecluse C, Roelants M, Diels R, Koninckx E, Verschueren S. Effects of whole body vibration training on muscle strength and sprint performance in sprint-trained athletes. *Int J Sports Med.* 2005;26:662–668.

17. Ebben WP, Jensen RL. Electromyographic and kinetic analysis of traditional, chain, and elastic band squats. *J Strength Cond Res.* 2002;16:547–550.

18. Fagnani F, Giombini A, Di Cesare A, Pigozzi F, Di Salvo V. The effects of a whole-body vibration program on muscle performance and flexibility in female athletes. *Am J Phys Med Rehab.* 2006;85:956–962.

19. Goertzen M, Schoppe K, Lange G, Schulitz KP. Injuries and damage caused by excess stress in body building and power lifting. *Sportverletz Sportschaden.* 1989;3:32–36.

20. Goodman CA, Pearce AJ, Nicholes CJ, Gatt BM, Fairweather IH. No difference in 1RM strength and muscle activation during the barbell chest press on a stable and unstable surface. *J Strength Cond Res.* 2008;22:88–94.

21. Hamill BP. Relative safety of weightlifting and weight training. *J Strength Cond Res.* 1994;8:53–57.

22. Hazell TJ, Jakobi JM, Kenno KA. The effects of whole-body vibration on upper- and lower-body EMG during static and dynamic contractions. *Appl Physiol Nutr Metab.* 2007;32:1156–1163.

23. Hedrick A. Manual resistance training for football athletes at the U.S. Air Force Academy. *Strength Cond J.* 1999;21:6–10.

24. Henry JC, Kaeding C. Neuromuscular differences between male and female athletes. *Curr Women's Health Rep.* 2001;1:241–244.

25. Hoffman JR, Ratamess NA. Medical issues associated with anabolic steroid use: are they exaggerated? *J Sports Sci Med.* 2006;5: 182–193.

26. Hoffman JR, Ratamess NA. *A Practical Guide to Developing Resistance-Training Programs.* 2nd ed. Monterey (CA): Coaches Choice; 2008.

27. Hostler D, Schwirian CI, Campos G, et al. Skeletal muscle adaptations in elastic resistance-trained young men and women. *Eur J Appl Physiol.* 2001;86:112–118.

28. Hunter G, Culpepper M. Knee extension torque joint position relationships following isotonic fixed resistance and hydraulic resistance training. *Athl Train.* 1988;23:16–20.

29. Hunter G, Culpepper M. Joint angle specificity of fixed masses hydraulic resistance knee flexion training. *J Strength Cond Res.* 1995;9:13–16.

30. Issurin VB, Tenenbaum G. Acute and residual effects of vibratory stimulation on explosive strength in elite and amateur athletes. *J Sports Sci.* 1999;17:177–182.

31. Issurin VB, Liebermann DG, Tenenbaum G. Effect of vibratory stimulation training on maximal force and flexibility. *J Sports Sci.* 1994;12:561–566.

32. Jordan MJ, Norris SR, Smith DJ, Herzog W. Vibration training: an overview of the area, training consequences, and future considerations. *J Strength Cond Res.* 2005;19:459–466.

33. Keogh J, Hume PA, Pearson S. Retrospective injury epidemiology of one hundred one competitive Oceania power lifters: the effects of age, body mass, competitive standard, and gender. *J Strength Cond Res.* 2006;20:672–681.

34. Knapik JJ, Bauman CT, Jones DH, Harris JM, Vaughan L. Preseason strength and flexibility imbalances associated with athletic injuries in female collegiate athletes. *Am J Sports Med.* 1991;19:76–81.

35. Kraemer WJ, Mazzetti SA, Ratamess NA, Fleck SJ. Specificity of Training Modes. In: Brown LE, editor. *Isokinetics in Human Performance.* Champaign (IL): Human Kinetics; 2000. pp. 25–41.

36. Kraemer WJ, Fry AC, Ratamess NA, French DN. Strength testing: development and evaluation of methodology. In: Maud PJ, Foster C, editors. *Physiological Assessments of Human Performance.* 2nd ed. Champaign (IL): Human Kinetics; 2006. pp. 119–150.

37. Kraemer WJ, Keuning M, Ratamess NA, et al. Resistance training combined with bench-step aerobics enhances women's health profile. *Med Sci Sports Exerc.* 2001;33:259–269.

38. Kubik, B. *Dinosaur Training: Lost Secrets of Strength & Development.* 1996.

39. Luo J, McNamara B, Moran K. The use of vibration training to enhance muscle strength and power. *Sports Med.* 2005;35:23–41.

40. Mahieu NN, Witvrouw E, Van de Voorde D, Michilsens D, Arbyn V, Van den Broecke W. Improving strength and postural control in young skiers: whole-body vibration versus equivalent resistance training. *J Athl Train.* 2006;41:286–293.

41. Marshall PW, Murphy BA. Increased deltoid and abdominal muscle activity during Swiss ball bench press. *J Strength Cond Res.* 2006; 20:745–750.

42. Mazur LJ, Yetman RJ, Risser WL. Weight-training injuries. Common injuries and preventative methods. *Sports Med.* 1993; 16:57–63.

43. McArdle WD, Katch FI, Katch VL. *Essentials of Exercise Physiology.* 3rd ed. Philadelphia (PA): Lippincott Williams & Wilkins; 2005. pp. 279–280.

44. McBride JM, Cormie P, Deane R. Isometric squat force output and muscle activity in stable and unstable conditions. *J Strength Cond Res.* 2006;20:915–918.

45. McGill S. *Ultimate Back Fitness and Performance.* 4th ed. Waterloo, Canada: Backfitpro Inc.; 2009. pp. 112–123.

46. McGill SM, McDermott A, Fenwick CMJ. Comparison of different strongman events: trunk muscle activation and lumbar spine motion, load, and stiffness. *J Strength Cond Res.* 2009;23:1148–1161.

47. Mester J, Kleinoder H, Yue Z. Vibration training: benefits and risks. *J Biomech.* 2006;39:1056–1065.

48. Mori A. Electromyographic activity of selected trunk muscles during stabilization exercises using a gym ball. *Electromyogr Clin Neurophysiol.* 2004;44:57–64.

49. National Strength and Conditioning Association. *Strength and Conditioning Professional Standards and Guidelines.* Colorado Springs (CO): NSCA; May 2001.

50. Newton R. Biomechanics of conditioning exercises. In: Chandler TJ, Brown LE, editors. *Conditioning for Strength and Human Performance.* Philadelphia (PA): Wolters Kluwer, Lippincott Williams & Wilkins; 2008. pp. 77–93.

51. Norwood JT, Anderson GS, Gaetz MB, Twist PW. Electromyographic activity of the trunk stabilizers during stable and unstable bench press. *J Strength Cond Res.* 2007;21:343–347.

52. Nosse LJ, Hunter GR. Free weights: A review supporting their use in training and rehabilitation. *Athletic Training.* 1985;20:206–209.

53. Nuzzo JL, McCaulley GO, Cormie P, Cavil MJ, McBride JM. Trunk muscle activity during stability ball and free weight exercises. *J Strength Cond Res.* 2008;22:95–102.

54. Poyhonen T, Sipila S, Keskinen KL, Hautala A, Savolainen J, Malkia E. Effects of aquatic resistance training on neuromuscular performance in healthy women. *Med Sci Sports Exerc.* 2002; 34:2103–2109.

55. Raske A, Norlin R. Injury incidence and prevalence among elite weight and power lifters. *Am J Sports Med.* 2002;30:248–256.

56. Ratamess NA, Faigenbaum AD, Mangine GT, Hoffman JR, Kang J. Acute muscular strength assessment using free weight bars of different thickness. *J Strength Cond Res.* 2007;21:240–244.

57. Roelants M, Verschueren SM, Delecluse C, Levin O, Stijnen V. Whole-body-vibration-induced increase in leg muscle activity during different squat exercises. *J Strength Cond Res.* 2006;20: 124–129.

58. Rogers ME, Sherwood HS, Rogers NL, Bohlken RM. Effects of dumbbell and elastic band training on physical function in older inner-city African-American women. *Women Health.* 2002;36:33–41.

59. Ross RE, Ratamess NA, Hoffman JR, Faigenbaum AD, Kang J, Chilakos A. The effects of treadmill sprint training and resistance training on maximal running velocity and power. *J Strength Cond Res.* 2009;23:385–394.

60. Stemm JD, Jacobson BH. Comparison of land- and aquatic-based plyometric training on vertical jump performance. *J Strength Cond Res.* 2007;21:568–571.

61. Sternlicht E, Rugg S, Fujii LL, Tomomitsu KF, Seki MM. Electromyographic comparison of a stability ball crunch with a traditional crunch. *J Strength Cond Res.* 2007;21:506–509.

62. Stoppani J. *Encyclopedia of Muscle and Strength.* Champaign (IL): Human Kinetics; 2006. pp. 23–37.

63. Thein JM, Brody LT. Aquatic-based rehabilitation and training for the shoulder. *J Athl Train.* 2000;35:382–389.

64. Tsatsouline P. *The Russian Kettlebell Challenge: Xtreme Fitness for Hard Living Comrades.* St. Paul (MN): Dragon Door Publications; 2001.

65. Tsourlou T, Benik A, Dipla K, Zafeiridis A, Kellis S. The effects of a twenty-four-week aquatic training program on muscular strength performance in healthy elderly women. *J Strength Cond Res.* 2006;20:811–818.

66. Van der Wall H, Mc Laughlin A, Bruce W, et al. Scintigraphic patterns of injury in amateur weight lifters. *Clin Nucl Med.* 1999;24:915–920.

67. Vera-Garcia FJ, Grenier SG, McGill SM. Abdominal muscle response during curl-ups on both stable and labile surfaces. *Phys Ther.* 2000;80:564–569.

68. Volaklis KA, Spassis AT, Tokmakidis SP. Land versus water exercise in patients with coronary artery disease: effects on body composition, blood lipids, and physical fitness. *Am Heart J.* 2007; 154:560.e1–e6.

69. Wahl MJ, Behm DG. Not all instability training devices enhance muscle activation in highly resistance-trained individuals. *J Strength Cond Res.* 2008;22:1360–1370.

70. Wallace BJ, Winchester JB, McGuigan MR. Effects of elastic bands on force and power characteristics during the back squat exercise. *J Strength Cond Res.* 2006;20:268–272.

71. Willoughby DS, Gillespie JW. A comparison of isotonic free weights and omnikinetic exercise machines on strength. *J Human Mov Stud.* 1990;19:93–100.

Resistance Training Exercises

Objectives

After completing this chapter, you will be able to:

· Demonstrate proper breathing during resistance exercise
· Describe the proper performance of several barbell, dumbbell, and machine resistance exercises for lower body, upper body, and core musculature
· Describe how exercises can be combined into a single exercise to increase complexity
· Describe methods of grip strength training
· Describe the proper performance of the Olympic lifts and their variations
· Describe the performance of exercises with different modalities including medicine balls, stability balls, BOSU balls, sand bags, kettlebells, and other implements

There are a multitude of exercises that can be performed and incorporated into a resistance training (RT) program. Considering that many devices/pieces of equipment have been developed, the numbers of possible exercises are numerous. Selecting the proper exercises is an important task for the coach and athlete. Exercises need to be selected such that they target specific goals and are similar in movement to motor skills found in the sport. Beginners should focus on a few basic exercises initially and expand to more complex exercises with experience. Technique mastery is important and should be used as a guide to select proper loading and as a prerequisite to advancing to more complex and challenging exercises. This chapter discusses proper performance of more than 70 exercises and lists more than 600 variations. Alteration of an athlete's body position or posture, hand/foot width, and hand/foot position changes muscle activation slightly so each variation must be regarded independently regarding loading and the number of repetitions performed. Several exercises can be performed unilaterally (one arm or leg) as well as bilaterally (two arms or legs). Performing an exercise on one leg, *e.g.*, can be used to enhance muscular strength and balance. Performing an exercise with one arm provides asymmetric loading requiring greater muscle coactivation to maintain balance. The use of a stable or unstable surface affects exercise performance and subsequent adaptation. This chapter describes exercises based on whether they primarily stress upper-body limb muscles, lower-body muscles, the core, or total-body musculature. Exercises performed with free weights (barbells [BBs], dumbbells [DBs], and plates), body weight (BW), stability balls (SBs) and BOSU, medicine balls (MBs), elastic bands/tubing, kettlebells (KBs), sand bags, and other implements (kegs, chains, and strength competition equipment) are described.

EXERCISE KINESIOLOGY

Human motion is described relative to the **anatomical position** (standing erect with joints extended, palms facing forward, and feet parallel) and occurs in three planes of motion (Fig. 13.1). A **sagittal plane** divides the body into right and left segments (Fig. 13.2). Movements occur in a sagittal plane about a transverse (or mediolateral) axis of rotation and take place in a front-to-back manner (flexion, extension) and vice versa. A **frontal plane** divides the body into anterior and posterior regions (Fig. 13.3). Movements occur in a frontal plane about an anteroposterior axis of rotation and take place in a side-to-side manner (adduction, abduction). **Transverse planes** divide the body into upper (superior) and lower (inferior) regions (Fig. 13.4). Movements occur in a transverse plane about a longitudinal axis of rotation and take place in a horizontal manner (rotation, supination, and pronation). Many human movements are multiplanar and take place in two or three planes of motion. Motion planes can vary when a movement is initiated from other postures different than the anatomical position, *e.g.*, elbow flexion can occur in any plane depending on the starting position of the shoulder.

Myths & Misconceptions

An Athlete Should Never Hold His or Her Breath When Lifting

Proper breathing is critical to RT. Under many circumstances, it is recommended that the athlete exhale during the more difficult part (the concentric [CON] or positive phase) and inhale during the easier segment (the eccentric [ECC] or negative phase). However, there are exceptions to this general rule. During the lifting of heavy loads for exercises that require high levels of intra-abdominal pressure (IAP) and lumbar spine support (deadlift, squat, bent-over row, Olympic lifts), many athletes temporarily hold their breath during the most difficult part. During a heavy squat, an athlete may inhale during the decent, temporarily hold his or her breath at the bottom position and during the initial ascent (until the sticking region is surpassed), and then exhale during the upper segment of the ascent. Breath holding helps increase torso rigidity and enables better exercise performance. Valsalva maneuvers are avoided under many circumstances but there are occasions where holding one's breath is advantageous.

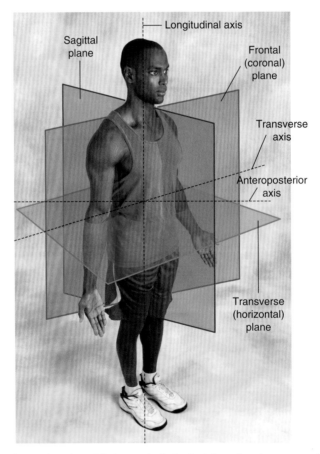

■ **FIGURE 13.1.** Planes of motion and axes of rotation of the human body. Sagittal, frontal, and transverse planes are shown as well as their corresponding axes of rotation (which are perpendicular to the plane). (Reprinted with permission from Thompson W, ed. *ACSM's Resources for the Personal Trainer.* 3rd ed. Baltimore (MD): LWW; 2010.)

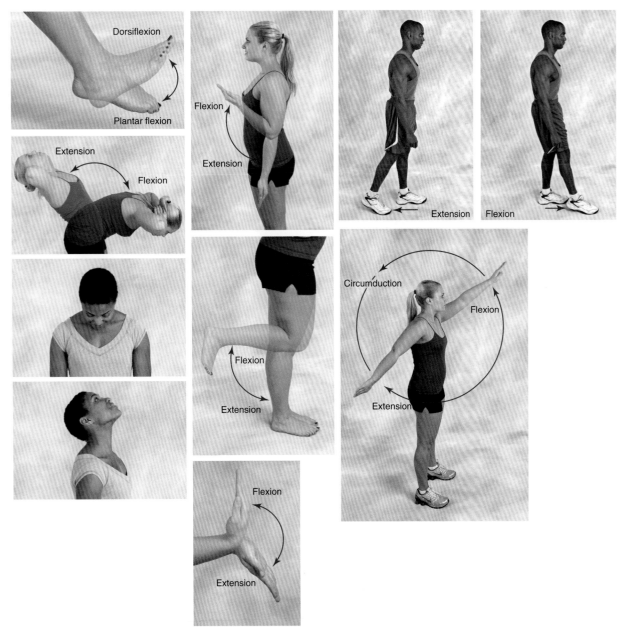

■ **FIGURE 13.2.** Movements in a sagittal plane. The movements flexion, extension, hyperextension, plantarflexion, and dorsiflexion are shown. (Reprinted with permission from Thompson W, ed. *ACSM's Resources for the Personal Trainer*. 3rd ed. Baltimore (MD): LWW; 2010.)

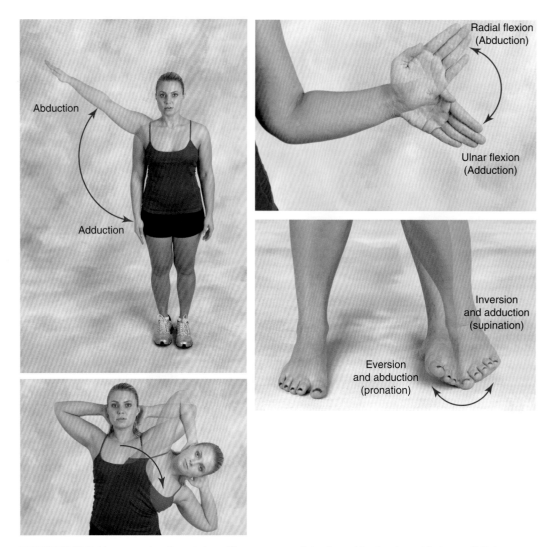

■ **FIGURE 13.3.** Movements in a frontal plane. The movements abduction, adduction, lateral flexion, radial/ulnar deviation, inversion, and eversion are shown. (Reprinted with permission from Thompson W, ed. *ACSM's Resources for the Personal Trainer*. 3rd ed. Baltimore (MD): LWW; 2010.)

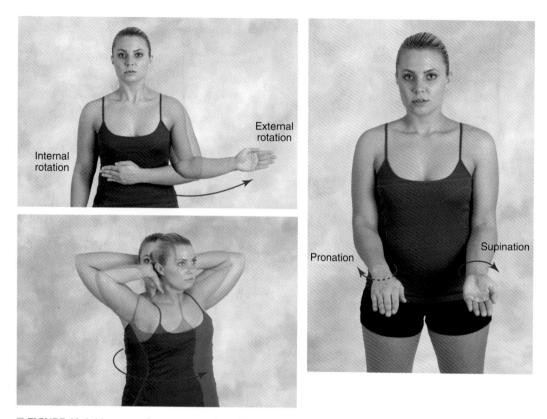

FIGURE 13.4. Movements in a transverse plane. The movements rotation, pronation, and supination are shown. (Reprinted with permission from Thompson W, ed. *ACSM's Resources for the Personal Trainer*. 3rd ed. Baltimore (MD): LWW; 2010.)

Exercise

Resistance Exercises

The following sections discuss many exercises commonly performed in RT. Different modalities may be used. BW, BB, DB, SB, BOSU ball, MB, thick bar (TB), KB, bands/tubing, kegs, sand bags, tires, logs, and other implements are discussed. Each exercise is given a complexity rating allowing the reader to differentiate between simple and challenging exercises to learn. The rating system consists of three classifications: An "A" rating indicates the exercise is simple to perform and has a short learning period. Most exercises with an "A" rating are single-joint with limited balance requirements. Some machine-based multiple-joint exercises are given an "A" rating. A "B" rating indicates the exercise is somewhat challenging to perform and has a longer learning period than an A-rated exercise. These exercises are multiple-joint with sufficient balance requirements. A "C" rating indicates the exercise is very challenging and has either a long learning period or a strong core strength requirement. These exercises are multiple-joint with large balance and coordination requirements.

LOWER-BODY EXERCISES

Lower body exercises encompass motion in three planes (sagittal, transverse, and frontal) about the hip, knee, and ankle joints. Several major muscle groups (Fig. 13.5) produce these motions and must contract isometrically to stabilize the joints when they are not considered to be prime movers. Some are multiarticular or produce motion at multiple joints (Table 13.1).

TABLE 13.1 KINESIOLOGY OF LOWER-BODY MOTION

JOINT	TYPE OF JOINT	JOINT MOVEMENT	MUSCLE INVOLVEMENT
Hip	Ball and socket	Flexion	Psoas major and minor, iliacus, pectineus, rectus femoris, sartorius, tensor fasciae latae, adductor brevis and longus, gracilis
		Extension/hyperextension	Hamstrings (biceps femoris, semimembranosus, semitendinosus), gluteus maximus, adductor magnus
		Abduction	Gluteus medius, minimus, and maximus, sartorius, tensor fasciae latae, piriformis, and hip external rotators
		Adduction	Pectineus, adductors brevis, longus, and magnus, gracilis, gluteus maximus
		Internal and external rotation	IR: gluteus medius, maximus, and minimus, tensor fascia latae, adductors ER: sartorius, piriformis, superior/inferior gamelli, obturator externus/internus, quadratus femoris
Knee[a]	Modified hinge	Flexion	Hamstrings (biceps femoris, semimembranosus, semitendinosus), gracilis, popliteus, sartorius, gastrocnemius
		Extension	Quadriceps (rectus femoris, vastus intermedius, lateralis, and medialis)
Ankle	Hinge	Dorsiflexion	Tibialis anterior, extensor hallucis longus, extensor digitorum longus, peroneus tertius
		Plantar Flexion	Peroneus brevis, peroneus longus, gastrocnemius, soleus, tibialis posterior, flexor digitorum longus, flexor hallucis longus
Subtalar	Plane/Gliding	Inversion	Tibialis anterior, extensor hallucis longus, tibialis posterior, gastrocnemius, soleus, flexor digitorum longus, flexor hallucis longus
		Eversion	Peroneus brevis, peroneus longus, extensor digitorum longus, peroneus tertius

[a]Internal and external rotation of the knee is possible when the hip is flexed.

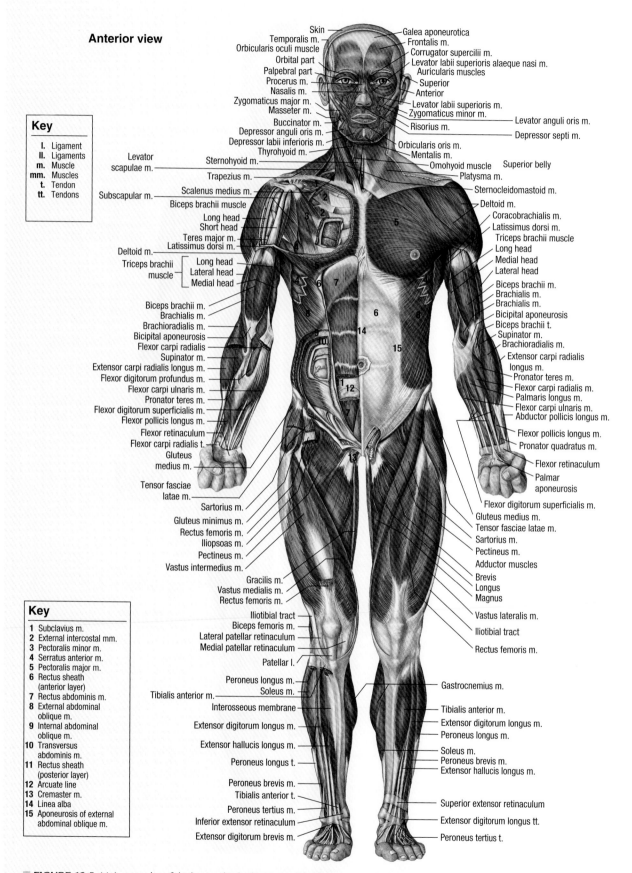

Anterior view

Key

1 Subclavius m.
2 External intercostal mm.
3 Pectoralis minor m.
4 Serratus anterior m.
5 Pectoralis major m.
6 Rectus sheath
  (anterior layer)
7 Rectus abdominis m.
8 External abdominal
  oblique m.
9 Internal abdominal
  oblique m.
10 Transversus
  abdominis m.
11 Rectus sheath
  (posterior layer)
12 Arcuate line
13 Cremaster m.
14 Linea alba
15 Aponeurosis of external
  abdominal oblique m.

■ **FIGURE 13.5.** Major muscles of the human body. (Asset provided by Anatomical Chart Co.)

Posterior view

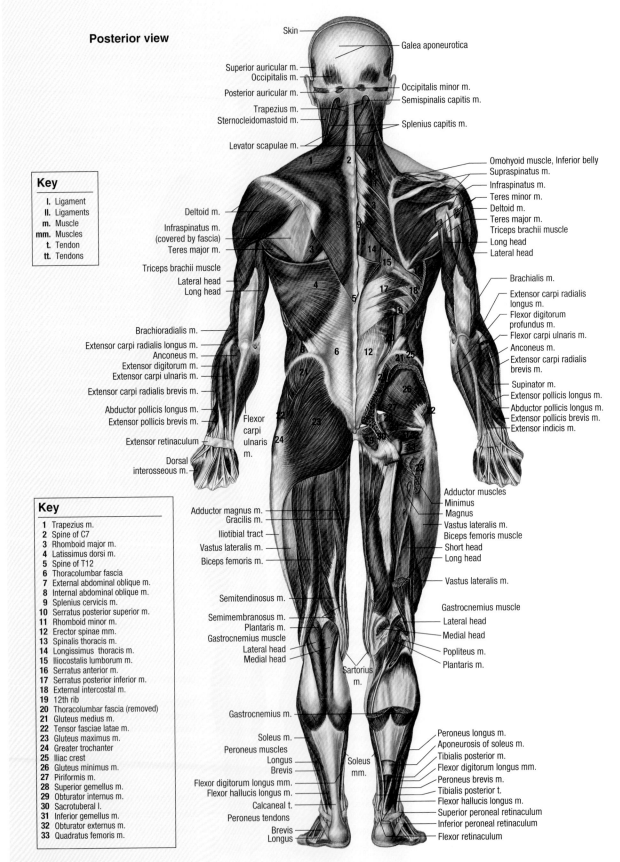

Key

I. Ligament
II. Ligaments
m. Muscle
mm. Muscles
t. Tendon
tt. Tendons

Key

1 Trapezius m.
2 Spine of C7
3 Rhomboid major m.
4 Latissimus dorsi m.
5 Spine of T12
6 Thoracolumbar fascia
7 External abdominal oblique m.
8 Internal abdominal oblique m.
9 Splenius cervicis m.
10 Serratus posterior superior m.
11 Rhomboid minor m.
12 Erector spinae mm.
13 Spinalis thoracis m.
14 Longissimus thoracis m.
15 Iliocostalis lumborum m.
16 Serratus anterior m.
17 Serratus posterior inferior m.
18 External intercostal m.
19 12th rib
20 Thoracolumbar fascia (removed)
21 Gluteus medius m.
22 Tensor fasciae latae m.
23 Gluteus maximus m.
24 Greater trochanter
25 Iliac crest
26 Gluteus minimus m.
27 Piriformis m.
28 Superior gemellus m.
29 Obturator internus m.
30 Sacrotuberal l.
31 Inferior gemellus m.
32 Obturator externus m.
33 Quadratus femoris m.

■ **FIGURE 13.5.** (*Continued*)

SQUAT
Rating: B

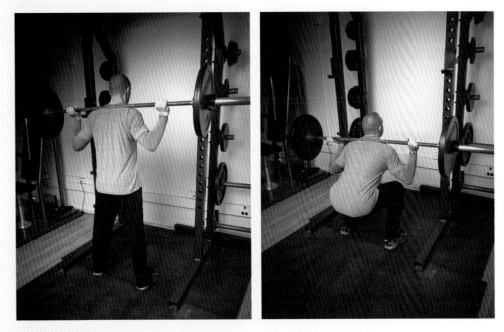

■ **FIGURE 13.6.**

- The bar rests on shoulders in a low bar (across the posterior deltoids and in the middle of the trapezius) or high bar (above the posterior deltoid at the base of the neck) position with shoulders abducted upward and scapula retracted to create a shelf for the bar.
- Bar is grasped with a closed, pronated grip slightly wider than shoulder width.
- Feet are parallel and shoulder width apart or wider with toes pointing slightly outward.
- Head is tilted upward with the eyes focused directly ahead at or above eye level.
- Hips and knees are flexed during descent and bar is lowered in a curvilinear pattern with control while keeping an erect and braced torso (chest out, shoulders back).
- Descent continues until the top of the thighs are parallel to the ground.
- Ascent occurs via extension of the hips and knees.
- May have one spotter on each side of bar or one spotter behind the athlete. It is important to follow the athlete downward during descent. When needed, force may be applied around the athlete's chest/upper torso or to the bar. It is important not to push the athlete forward when applying assistance.
- *Coaching tip:* teaching the bottom position of the exercise is a good place to start for a beginner. Some new lifters have difficulty reaching this position and lack the confidence to squat down and back. Teaching this position first makes it easier for the athlete to descend with proper technique. Using a box or bench as a low-point location marker can be beneficial as the athlete must descend until gluteal contact with the box or bench.

Single-leg versions of squats are common in training and athletic assessment. Because many sports require movements where one leg is pushing off to accelerate the body, single-leg squats force hip, knee, and ankle stabilizers to forcefully contract for stability and assist in sport-specific strength development. They require bodily control over the planted leg, thus reflective of hip/knee strength and postural control. Gender differences are seen in the ability to perform single-leg squats where women display greater motion in the frontal plane and greater valgus forces on the knee (30).

> ⚠ **CAUTION!** *Knees too far ahead relative to toes, excessive forward lean, not performing exercise in a fully-prescribed range of motion (ROM), and head facing downward are common mistakes. The athlete should be instructed to contract the gluteal, hamstring, and quadriceps muscles as forcefully as possible to reduce lower-back strain. Some advocate using a board to elevate the heels in athletes with poor ROM. A board is not needed. Rather, the coach should work on improving the athlete's ROM. A good pair of lifting shoes, by design, slightly elevates the heels.*

✓ **OTHER VARIATIONS AND SIMILAR EXERCISES** *Front squat (arms over bar), hack squat, DB/KB/sand bag squat, DB squat (with shoulders flexed parallel to ground), Smith machine squat, split stance squat, box (or bench) squat, squat with chains or bands, pause squat, lateral squat, staggered (stance) squat, single-leg squat (floor, BOSU), single-leg squat (rear leg supported by SB or bench), single-leg squat (elevated on bench to allow opposite leg to relax downward), TRX single-leg squat, Zercher squat, rack squats, belt squat, sissy squat, machine squat, safety squat, SB wall squats, ISOM wall squats, squats with bands around ankles (to increase hip abductor strength), BW squats, BW squats with TRX, MB squat (with shoulders flexed), knee squats, buddy squat, keg squat, sand bag squats, BOSU or balance board squats, single-DB sumo squat, BW/DB duck walks, balance squat (one-leg support, one-leg hip flexion from BB squat position), KB swing squat, and jump squats (DB, MB, KB, Smith machine, sand bag, weighted vest).*

Interpreting Research

Biomechanical Analysis of Foot Position During the Squat

Escamilla RF, Fleisig GS, Lowry TM, Barrentine SW, Andrews JR. A three-dimensional biomechanical analysis of the squat during varying stance widths. *Med Sci Sports Exerc.* 2001;33:984–998.

Escamilla et al. (9) analyzed the BB squat with a narrow (~107% of shoulder width), medium (~142% of shoulder width), and wide (~169% of shoulder width) stance width and found that in comparison to a narrow stance, the wider stance produced:

- 7–12 degrees greater horizontal thigh position
- 6–11 degrees greater hip flexion
- 6 degrees greater hip external rotation
- 5–9 degrees greater vertical shank (lower-leg) position

These results show that varying stance width affects squat kinematics. Some athletes perform the squat with varying stance widths to alter muscle activation, strengthen muscles in a different way, and add variety to a workout.

LEG PRESS
Rating: A

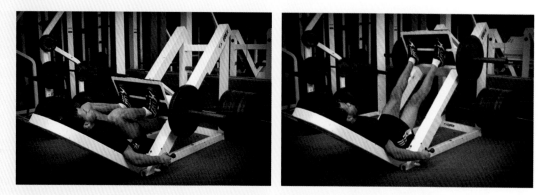

FIGURE 13.7.

- Body is positioned according to machine type (seated, angled, or lying supine).
- Feet are placed on the sled approximately shoulder width apart with knees and hips aligned about 90 degrees when starting from the bottom position.
- The hands grasp the supports firmly at sides or by shoulders (depending on where they are located) while the torso remains straight and flat against the support pads.
- Legs push forward on the sled to extend the knees and hips (without locking out knees).

- It is important to complete a full ROM while maintaining proper foot position.
- Once the repetition is completed, the carriage is returned under control to the starting position.
- One can self-spot by pushing on the legs when assistance is needed or have a spotter located laterally applying pressure to the carriage when assistance is needed.

OTHER VARIATIONS *Supine leg press, vertical leg press, and unilateral leg press. An athlete can alter foot spacing and position.*

DEADLIFT
Rating: B

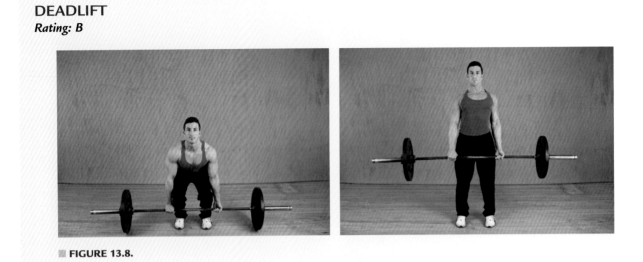

■ FIGURE 13.8.

- Feet are positioned shoulder width apart and flat on the floor with knees inside of arms (for conventional-style deadlift) or arms inside of legs with a wider stance (for sumo-style deadlift). Research has shown that: (a) sumo style yields a more parallel thigh position, greater vertical posture, wider stance with greater hip external rotation, greater muscle activation of the quadriceps and tibialis anterior, and 8%–10% less load shear force at L4/L5 vertebrae position compared to conventional style; and (b) conventional deadlift yields 25%–40% greater bar distance moved, work, and energy expenditure compared to sumo style (4,10,11).
- Grasp bar with a closed grip (pronated or alternated) slightly wider than or close to shoulder width and extend arms fully. The alternated grip allows the athlete more support when grasping the bar and may result in greater weights being lifted.
- Lower body by flexing the knees and hips.
- Position the bar over the feet close to shins with shoulders slightly ahead of bar vertically.
- The back should be maintained flat by hyperextension while holding the chest up and out and pulling the shoulder blades toward each other. Core is braced.
- The bar is pulled upward by extending the knees and moving the hips forward while raising the shoulders. The first third of the movement is predominantly knee extension; the second third is a combination of knee and hip extension; the final segment is predominantly

hip extension. Athlete should forcefully contract hip extensors to lower strain on the lumbar spine.
- With elbows extended, the bar is lifted upward while maintaining close position to the body.
- Upon complete hip and knee extension, the body assumes an erect standing position.
- With control, bar is then lowered to starting position by flexion of hips and knees.
- Although presented in this section, the deadlift stresses several upper-body pulling muscles and is an excellent total-body mass/strength-building exercise.

> **! CAUTION!** *Raising the hips prior to moving the bar (without knee extension) places additional stress on the lower back. The bar should be lifted off of the ground by extension of the knees.*

> **✓ OTHER VARIATIONS AND SIMILAR EXERCISES** *Deadlift (with bands), stiff-legged deadlift, DB/KB (one or two) deadlift, T-bar stiff-legged deadlift, deadlift pulls (in rack), deadlift with a DL bar or thick bar (predominantly a forearm exercise), deadlift from a small elevation, deadlift with keg or sand bag, partner (BW) deadlift, sand bag/heavy bag deadlift with a bear hug (could finish with a throw), cable deadlift pull-through, Renegade deadlift, and DB/KB (one or two) single-leg deadlift (with contralateral leg extended).*

BARBELL LUNGE
Rating: B

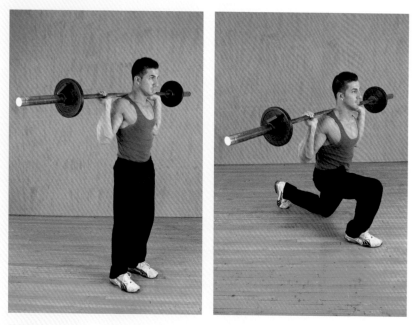

FIGURE 13.9.

- Bar is grasped with a closed, pronated grip slightly wider than shoulder width and is placed on shoulders in a high bar position (above the posterior deltoids at the base of neck) similar to the back squat.
- Feet are placed close to or slightly wider than shoulder width.
- A step forward is taken with a larger than normal step and knees are aligned with toes with the toes pointing straight ahead or slightly inward (Fig. 13.9).
- During the step, the lead knee is flexed under control directly above the lead foot while the training knee is lowered to the floor but no contact is made.
- The torso remains erect throughout and core is braced.
- Athlete pushes off with lead leg and returns to starting position in one large (or two small) step(s).

- The same movement is performed with the opposite leg.

OTHER VARIATIONS (SINGLE OR ALTERNATE LEGS) AND SIMILAR EXERCISES *DB/KB/MB/ BW/sand bag lunge, reverse lunge (DB, KB, and BB), side lunge, Smith machine lunge, box lunge, walking lunge, lunge or reverse lunge with keg or sand bag, buddy lunge, lunge onto BOSU, power lunge, star lunge, lunge/reverse lunge with torso rotation (MB), lunge from an overhead squat BB position, DB/KB (one or two) overhead lunge, DB/MB reaching lunge (front, side), DB lunge with shoulder press or lateral raise, mountain climbers (BW).*

STEP-UPS
Rating: B

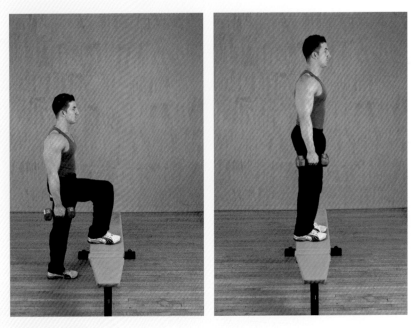

■ **FIGURE 13.10.**

- Athlete stands erect 30–45 cm from a box or bench that is 30–45 cm high (or a height that will create a 90-degree angle at the knee joint when foot is on box) with a DB in each hand (or BB placed on shoulders).
- Athlete steps up with the lead leg onto the top of the bench, placing the foot in the center.
- Without leaning forward, BW is shifted to the lead leg and the body ascends unilaterally into a standing position on the top of the bench.
- The trailing leg is not used to push off but just follows to the top of the bench.
- Athlete steps off the bench with trailing leg to starting position (or if a cycle is used, the lead leg steps off first). As trailing foot is placed on the floor, BW shifts to trailing leg.
- Athlete steps off bench with lead leg and returns to starting position and repeats.

> ✔ **OTHER VARIATIONS (SINGLE OR ALTERNATE LEGS)** *BB/KB/MB/BW step-ups, step-ups with keg or sand bag, side step-up (with or without crossover), partner step-ups, overhead step-ups, step-ups with a curl and press, and plyometric step-ups.*

Several other single-joint hip exercises can be performed with machines, cable devices, bands/tubing, or ankle weights. These include machine and cable hip abduction/adduction, machine and cable hip flexion and extension, cable straight-leg hip extension, lying hip extension, flexion, abduction/adduction, prone kneeling bent-leg hip extension, supine bent-leg hip extension (on the floor with contralateral hip flexion), and "clamshell."

LEG CURL
Rating: A

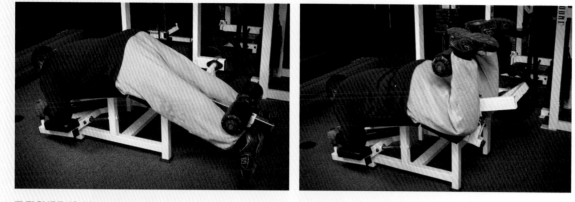

■ **FIGURE 13.11.**

- Athlete lies face down on a bench or machine with hips and chest flat against pads.
- Knees are positioned below the bottom edge of the thigh pad and are aligned with the axis of rotation of the machine and ankles under heel pads while hands grasp the grips.
- Hips remain in contact with bench as knees flex (heels curl close to buttocks).
- Ankle position is important. Knee flexion torque generated is higher when the ankle is dorsiflexed than plantar flexed (12). The gastrocnemius is a multiarticular muscle, which assists in flexing the knee. Performing a leg curl with the ankles dorsiflexed puts the gastrocnemius at a length more conducive to producing force.

- Legs are slowly lowered with control to starting position.
- A spotter could apply pressure to the ankles during knee flexion if assistance is needed.

✔ **OTHER VARIATIONS AND SIMILAR EXERCISES** *Standing unilateral leg curl, seated machine leg curl, DB/KB/MB leg curl, cable leg curls, reverse leg curl (with legs supported), reverse leg curl (with bands), leg curl with bands/tubing or partner, SB (one or two legs) leg curls, and TRX leg curl (one or two legs).*

LEG EXTENSION
Rating: A

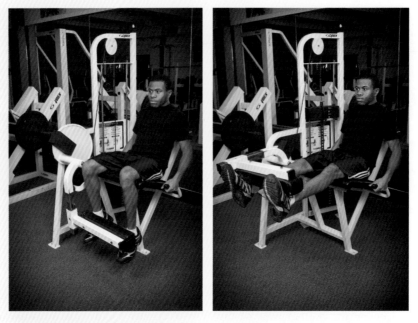

■ **FIGURE 13.12.**

- Athlete sits with back flat against the back support, knees aligned with the machine's axis of rotation, ankles in contact with the roller pads, and hands firmly grasping the handles (to keep hips on the seat when heavy loading is used).
- Buttocks and back should maintain their position on the machine while fully extending knees.
- The athlete slowly lowers the resistance arm to starting position.

- Mistakes include performing the exercise in a limited ROM and not firmly grasping the hand supports. Greater torque and power can be produced when the body is stabilized.

✓ **OTHER VARIATIONS** *Unilateral leg extension, DB/KB/band leg extension, ISOM leg extension, and performing the exercise with varied seat angles.*

CALF (TOE) RAISE
Rating: A

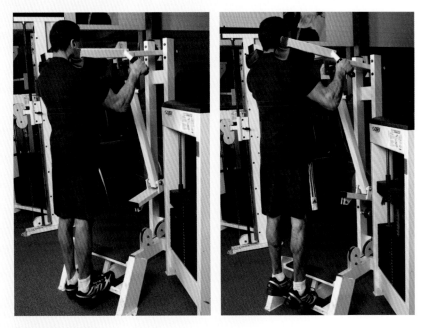

FIGURE 13.13.

- Grip bar with a closed, pronated grip slightly wider than shoulder width or place shoulders under pad if using a machine (Fig. 13.13).
- Stance is shoulder width and knees are fully extended.
- To increase ROM and extend fully, the balls of the feet are near the edge of a raised surface. Pointing the toes inward, outward, or maintaining a neutral position shifts emphasis to different regions of the muscle.
- The athlete ascends (plantar flexion) onto toes as high as possible while maintaining fully extended knees, and toes are kept in a plantar-flexed position for a brief time.
- The weight is lowered until heels are below the level of the toes at the starting position.
- Performing the exercise in a limited ROM is a common mistake.

- Training the ankle dorsiflexors, inverters, and everters is important for balance. Dorsiflexion exercises can be performed with bands, a plate placed over the feet, or a device known as the DARD (dynamic axial resistance device). Balance equipment (wobble board, BOSU) and single-leg exercises train these muscles as well.

> ✓ **OTHER VARIATIONS AND SIMILAR EXERCISES** *Calf raise on leg press (angled, horizontal, or vertical), Smith machine (or BB) calf raise, DB/KB/keg/sand bag calf raise, DB/BW unilateral calf raise, donkey calf raise, calf squats, partner calf raise, seated calf raises (machine, BB, or DB), and ankle dorsiflexion.*

UPPER-BODY EXERCISES

Upper-body exercises encompass motion in three planes (sagittal, transverse, and frontal) about the shoulder, shoulder girdle, elbow, radioulnar, and wrist joints. Several major muscle groups produce these motions and must contract isometrically to stabilize the joints when they are not considered to be prime movers. Some are multiarticular or produce motion at multiple joints (Table 13.2).

TABLE 13.2 KINESIOLOGY OF UPPER-BODY MOTION

JOINT	TYPE OF JOINT	JOINT MOVEMENT	MUSCLES
Sternoclavicular	Saddle	Elevation	Serratus anterior, levator scapulae, rhomboid major/minor, trapezius
		Depression	Pectoralis minor, subclavius, lower trapezius
		Protraction	Serratus anterior, pectoralis minor
		Retraction	Levator scapulae, rhomboid major/minor, trapezius
		Upward rotation	Serratus anterior, trapezius
		Downward rotation	Levator scapulae, rhomboid major/minor
Acromioclavicular	Gliding	—	—
Glenohumeral	Ball and socket	Flexion	Pectoralis major, coracobrachialis, anterior/medial deltoid, biceps brachii
		Extension/hyperextension	Subscapularis, posterior deltoid, latissimus dorsi, teres major, long head of triceps brachii
		Adduction	Pectoralis major, coracobrachialis, biceps brachii, latissimus dorsi, teres major/minor, long head of triceps brachii
		Abduction	Supraspinatus, medial deltoid, infraspinatus
		Medial rotation	Pectoralis major, subscapularis
		Lateral rotation	Infraspinatus, teres minor
Elbow (humeroulnar)	Hinge	Flexion	Biceps brachii, brachialis, brachioradialis, pronator teres
		Extension	Triceps brachii, anconeus
		Pronation	Pronator teres, pronator quadratus
Radioulnar	Pivot	Supination	Biceps brachii, supinator
Radiocarpal (wrist)	Condyloid	Extension	Extensor carpi radialis brevis/longus, extensor carpi ulnaris, extensor digitorum, extensor digiti minimi, extensor pollicis brevis/longus, extensor indicis
		Flexion	Flexor carpi radialis, flexor carpi ulnaris, palmaris longus, flexor digitorum superficialis and profundus, flexor/abductor pollicis longus
		Ulnar deviation	Flexor carpi ulnaris, extensor carpi ulnaris
		Radial deviation	Flexor carpi radialis, flexor digitorum superficialis, extensor carpi radialis brevis/longus

BENCH PRESS
Rating: B

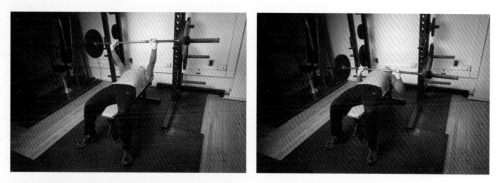

■ **FIGURE 13.14.**

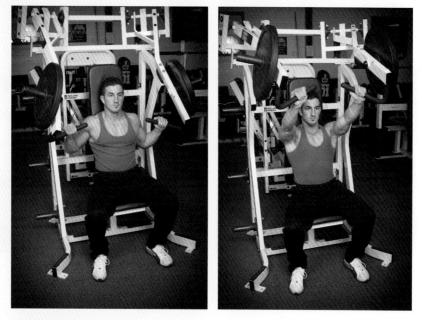

■ **FIGURE 13.15.**

- The athlete lies supine on a bench with feet flat on the floor. The scapulae are retracted and the chest is forced out.
- Bar is grasped with a closed, pronated grip slightly wider than shoulder width. Starting with the palms on the rear of the bar and rotating the hands help place the palms under the bar when lifting off and help lock the shoulders into the bench.
- Bar is removed from the rack and positioned directly over the chest with elbows fully extended.
- With control, the bar is lowered until it touches the lower chest near the nipples.
- Bar is lifted upward in a curvilinear manner until elbows are fully extended. The body remains flat on the bench.

- Bar is returned to the rack after completion of set.
- A spotter is located at the head of the bench and can apply enough force to keep the bar moving slowly when assistance is needed.
- This exercise can be performed on a chest press machine (Fig. 13.15) in an upright position. Similar technique applies to this variation. There are several machines that can be used that alter the grip position (midrange and pronated) and width (narrow, medium, wide). Seats may be adjusted to target different areas of the chest, *e.g.*, adjusting the seat high (with grips near the lower chest) to target lower chest musculature and vice versa.

⚠️ **CAUTION!** *Bouncing the bar off of the chest and excessive arching of the back off of the bench are common mistakes. A mild-to-moderate arch with buttocks still in contact with the bench is a technique commonly used by powerlifters to increase performance by improving leverage. Some lifters like to place their feet on the bench during the bench press. This reduces stability and alters the technique. It is not recommended when lifting heavy weights.*

✅ ***OTHER VARIATIONS AND SIMILAR EXERCISES*** *DB bench press (unilateral or bilateral), close-grip bench press (especially effective for triceps development), decline bench press, reverse-grip bench press, wide-grip bench press, Smith machine bench press, keg, mastiff bar, or sand bag bench press, floor press, board press, bench press with pause, SB DB/KB bench press (with body parallel to ground, incline, decline), bench press in rack (functional isometrics, partial ROM, negatives), bench press with chains/bands, bench press to neck, oscillation bench press (with bands, KBs, and/or plates), machine chest press.*

INCLINE BENCH PRESS
Rating: B

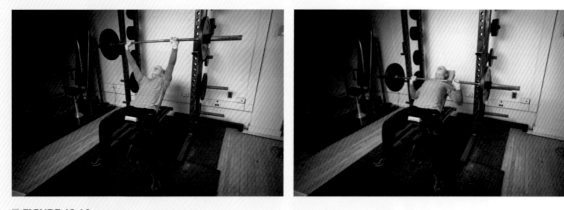

■ **FIGURE 13.16.**

- Athlete lays ~45 degrees (angle can vary) on an incline bench with feet flat on the floor similar to the bench press.
- The bar is grasped with a closed, pronated grip slightly wider than shoulder width.
- Bar is removed from the rack and positioned directly over the upper chest with elbows fully extended.
- With control, bar is lowered until it touches the upper chest near the clavicles.
- Bar is lifted upward in a curvilinear manner until arms are fully extended. Body remains on the bench without excessive back arching or bouncing of weight off the chest.
- Bar is returned to the rack after completion of set.
- A spotter is located at the head of the bench and can apply enough force to keep the bar moving slowly when assistance is needed.

✅ ***OTHER VARIATIONS*** *Similar to many of those listed for the flat bench press. Variations can be performed on a decline bench.*

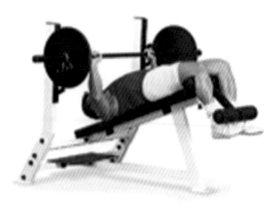

■ **FIGURE 13.17.**

Interpreting Research

Muscle Activation During Variations of the Bench and Shoulder Press

Barnett C, Kippers V, Turner P. Effects of variations of the bench press exercise on the EMG activity of five shoulder muscles. *J Strength Cond Res.* 1995;9:222–227.

Barnett et al. (1) studied muscle activity and strength during the decline, flat, incline, and shoulder press with wide and narrow grips (Fig. 13.18). Body position affected maximum strength as the shoulder press yielded the lowest 1 RM and the decline bench press the highest. The middle (sternocostal) portion of the pectoralis major was most active during the flat bench press whereas similar activity was seen between flat and incline bench presses for the upper (clavicular) pectoralis major. Anterior deltoid activity increased in proportion from the decline press to the shoulder press. Triceps brachii activity was highest during the decline and flat bench presses. Latissimus dorsi activity was greatest during the decline press.

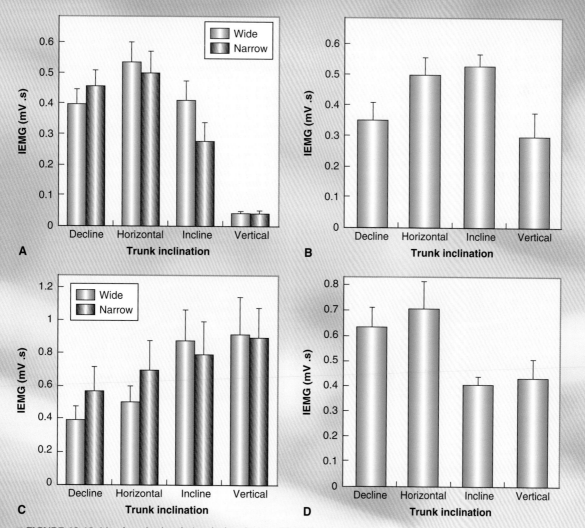

FIGURE 13.18. Muscle activation during the bench press. These figures show that trunk inclination and grip width affect muscle activity during the bench press. **A** shows the mid-sternal segment of the pectoralis major activity is highest during the flat bench press. **B** shows the clavicular (upper) part of the pectoralis major is most active during the incline and flat bench presses. **C** shows the anterior deltoid is most active during the shoulder press (and incline bench press). **D** shows triceps brachii activity is highest during the flat bench press (followed by the decline press).

(Continued)

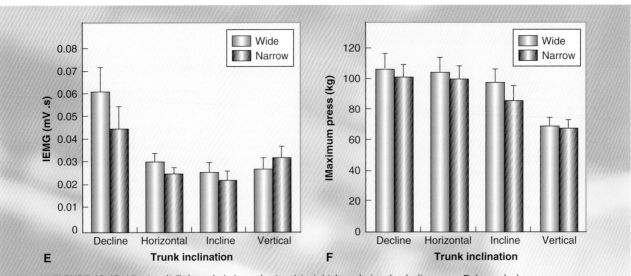

FIGURE 13.18. (*Continued*) **E** shows latissimus dorsi activity is highest during the decline press. **F** shows the largest amount of weight is lifted during the decline press, followed by the flat bench press, incline press, and shoulder press. (Reprinted with permission from Barnett C, Kippers V, Turner P. Effects of variations of the bench press exercise on the EMG activity of five shoulder muscles. *J Strength Cond Res.* 1995;9:222–227.)

DUMBBELL FLY
Rating: A

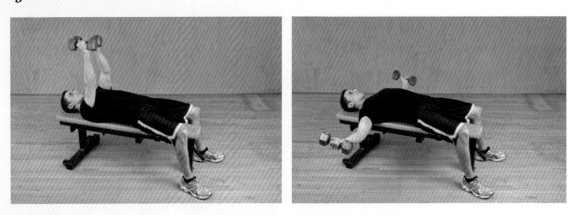

■ **FIGURE 13.19.**

- Athlete lies flat on a bench (or can be inclined or declined) with feet flat on the floor.
- DBs are grasped with a closed, pronated grip above the chest with arms fully extended and are rotated so that the palms of the hands face each other and the elbows point out (elbows are slightly flexed).
- DBs are lowered with control in a wide arc with elbows slightly flexed.
- Arms horizontally adduct a wide arc until they return to the starting arm position above the chest. (Performance note: flexing the elbow during the up phase decreases the moment arm of resistance and makes the exercise

easier. Thus, elbow position should be maintained as best as possible throughout the ROM).
- One can spot by applying pressure medially to the wrist/forearms.

> **OTHER VARIATIONS AND SIMILAR EXERCISES** *Incline DB/KB fly, decline DB/KB fly, machine (pec-deck) fly, cable fly, rotation fly, SB DB fly, SB cable fly, MB fly, TRX fly, standing cable crossover (with multiple postures and arm positions), supine DB/KB arm bar (with trunk rotation).*

PARALLEL BAR DIPS
Rating: B

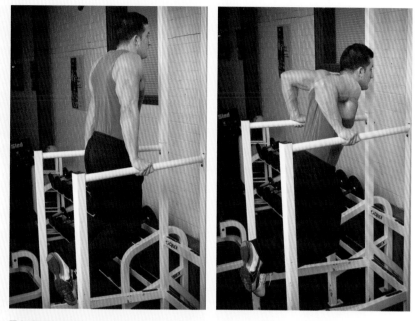

■ **FIGURE 13.20.**

- Body is positioned and supported on the bars with the arms fully extended and knees flexed. Arms are shoulder width apart; torso is erect with a slight forward lean (to increase chest muscle activity).
- In control the body is lowered until the upper arms are parallel to the ground and then lifted back to the starting position.

> **OTHER VARIATIONS AND SIMILAR EXERCISES** *Reverse dips (primarily for the triceps), SB reverse dips, ring (gymnastic rings) dips and stabilization, and machine dips (with support).*

PUSH-UP
Rating: B

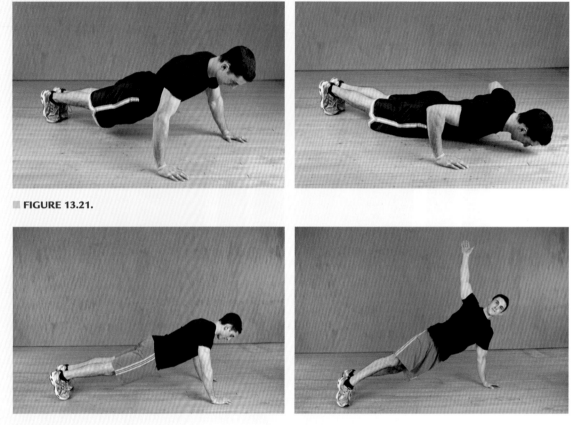

■ **FIGURE 13.21.**

■ **FIGURE 13.22.** T-rotation.

- Athlete begins in prone position with wrists below shoulders, weight supported by arms vertical to the floor, legs extended, toes tucked under, and core contracted.
- With control the athlete flexes elbows (~90 degrees) and horizontally abducts shoulders to where chest is located just above the floor.
- Athlete extends elbows and horizontally adducts shoulders to elevate body back up to the starting position.

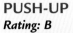 **OTHER VARIATIONS AND SIMILAR EXERCISES** *Modified push-up (on knees), push-ups with various grip widths and hand positions (wide, narrow), push-ups with staggered hand positions, push-ups on finger tips/wrists/fists, push-ups with feet elevated, one-arm push-ups, push-ups on MB (two hands, one hand on ball), MB push-up with shuffle or cross-over, plyo push-up (floor, MB, SB), push-up between chairs/benches, push-up on SB (arms on ball, feet on ball [shins, toes, one leg on SB]), core board, and BOSU (both sides), push-ups with walkout, push-up with T rotation (Fig. 13.22), Spiderman push-up, TRX push-up, push-up with unilateral shoulder flexion at top (single-arm support works core), ISOM half push-up, army crawls, bear crawls, side crawls, wheelbarrows, wheelbarrow drags (dragging plate on floor with feet), push-up walks, push-ups with various stances (feet together, apart, on top of one another, one leg with other extended), wall push-up, and push-ups on DB/KB/bars.*

BENT-OVER BARBELL ROW
Rating: B

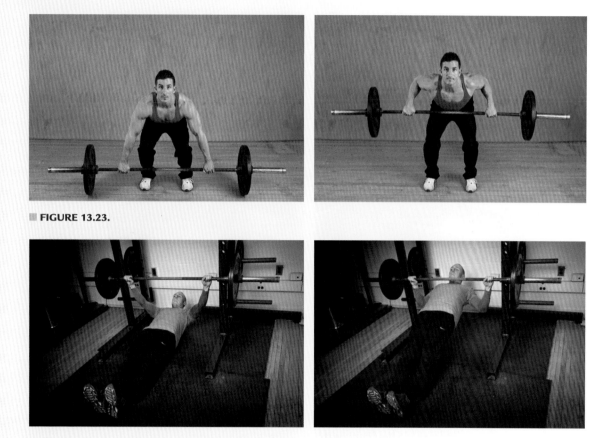

■ **FIGURE 13.23.**

■ **FIGURE 13.24.** Inverted row.

- Athlete stands with feet shoulder width apart and knees flexed.
- Bar is grasped from the floor with a closed, pronated grip wider than shoulder width while the back is flat, chest out, shoulders retracted, head is tilted forward, elbows are fully extended, and torso is flexed forward 10–30 degrees above horizontal.
- Athlete should remain flexed forward throughout the exercise.
- Bar is pulled upward (using back muscles mostly and not the elbow flexors) touching the upper abdomen.
- The elbows are pointed up with a rigid torso and the back should remain hyperextended (straight) throughout the movement.
- Bar is lowered with control until elbows are fully extended.

! *CAUTION! Standing too upright greatly limits ROM and muscle development. A common mistake is to see this exercise performed with the athlete maintaining nearly an upright posture.*

✓ *OTHER VARIATIONS AND SIMILAR EXERCISES Reverse-grip bent-over row, bent-over DB row (with various grip positions), BB bench row, T-bar row, Smith machine row, rows with keg, mastiff bar, or sand bag, one-arm DB/core ball/band/tubing row, one-arm cable row, DB/KB row (single leg for balance), renegade row with DB or KB, one-arm bench row, and inverted row (BW with bar or TRX and feet elevated on bench/SB or placed on the floor, pronated or supinated grip).*

LAT PULL-DOWN
Rating: B

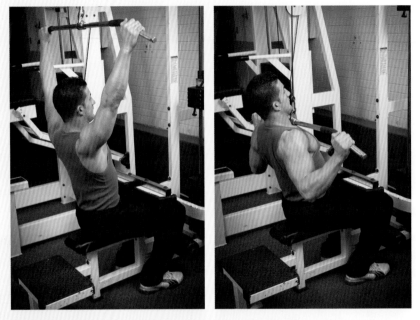

■ FIGURE 13.25.

- The bar (several lat bars to choose from) is grasped with a closed, pronated grip wider than shoulder width (but may vary depending on the variation performed).
- Athlete is seated on the bench with arms fully extended, back hyperextended slightly, chest out, shoulders retracted, and thighs secured under the properly adjusted thigh/hip pad.
- The bar is pulled downward in control to touch the upper chest or below chin level and then the bar is returned to the starting position. Athlete should avoid using momentum generated by the core to complete the lift.

- A spotter may apply downward pressure to the bar if assistance is needed.

✔ OTHER VARIATIONS AND SIMILAR EXERCISES *Wide-grip lat pull-down, parallel grip lat pull-down, close-grip lat pull-down, reverse lat pull-down, machine pull-down (with various machines), rear lat pull-down, straight-arm pull-down, cable double pull-down.*

PULL-UP
Rating: B

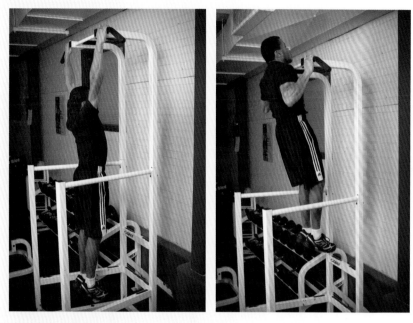

■ **FIGURE 13.26.**

- Using a chinning bar about 6 in. higher than an extended arm overhead position, the bar is held with an overhand grip with hands wider than shoulder width as the body hangs (chest out, back hyperextended) motionless (with knee flexed or straight).
- The body is pulled upward to where the chin surpasses the bar and returns in control to the starting position. The athlete should minimize sway as much as possible. A machine may be used if the athlete cannot lift his or her BW for the desired number of repetitions.

- A spotter may apply pressure to the hips or under the feet for assistance.

> ✓ **OTHER VARIATIONS AND SIMILAR EXERCISES** *Chin-up (supinated grip), sternum chin-ups, weighted pull-ups (with different grips and grip widths), towel chin-ups, single-arm pull-up, rear pull-up, pull-up and press, rope pulls or climbs, and rope pulls on a Marpo Kinetics device.*

Interpreting Research

Muscle Activation During Variations of the Lat Pull-down

Signorile JF, Zink AJ, Szwed SP. A comparative electromyographical investigation of muscle utilization patterns using various hand positions during the lat pull-down. *J Strength Cond Res*. 2002;16:539–546.

Signorile et al. (25) examined muscle activation during the wide-grip lat pull-down (front and rear), reverse grip pull-down, and narrow grip (parallel bar) pull-down and showed that the wide-grip lat pull-down to the front increased latissimus dorsi and teres major activity the most. Posterior deltoid activity was greatest during the close-grip lat pull-down (Fig. 13.27).

(*Continued*)

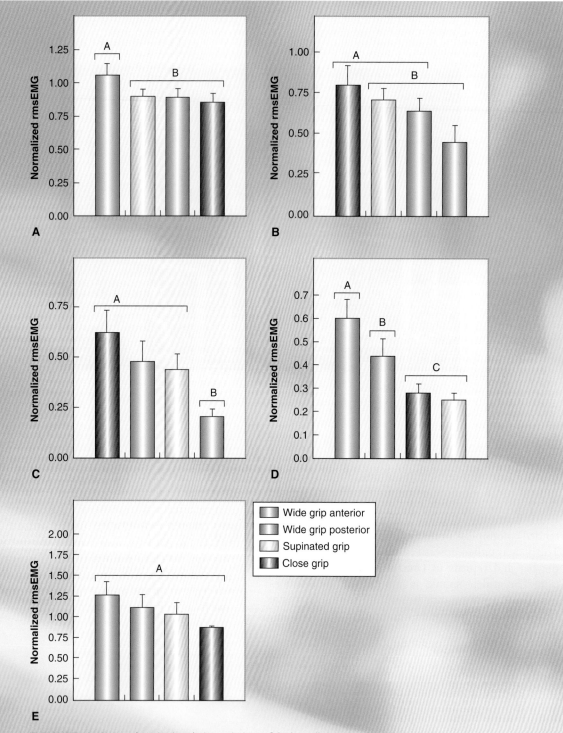

FIGURE 13.27. Muscle activation during variations of the lat pull-down. **A**, **D**, and **E** show latissimus dorsi, triceps brachii, and teres major activity were highest during the wide-grip front lat pull-down. **B** and **C** show pectoralis major and posterior deltoid muscle activity were highest during the close-grip lat pull-down. (Data from Signorile JF, Zink AJ, Szwed SP. A comparative electromyographical investigation of muscle utilization patterns using various hand positions during the lat pull-down. *J Strength Cond Res*. 2002;16:539–546.)

LOW-PULLEY ROW
Rating: A

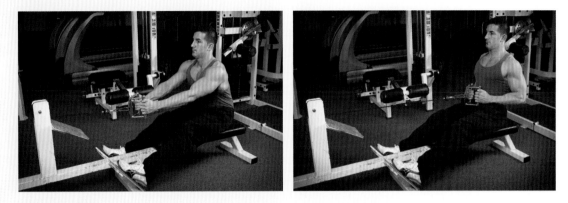

■ **FIGURE 13.28.**

- Athlete sits facing the machine with torso perpendicular to the floor, chest out, shoulders retracted, and knees slightly flexed with feet against foot support.
- The handles are grasped with a closed grip and elbows fully extended.
- With an erect torso, the bar is pulled toward the upper abdomen with control and then returned to the starting position.

> ✅ **OTHER VARIATIONS AND SIMILAR EXERCISES** *Machine rows (with various types of machines), cable rows with various grips and bars (reverse, wide, narrow grip, pronated and supinated grips), and rowing with bands/tubing.*

PULLOVER
Rating: A

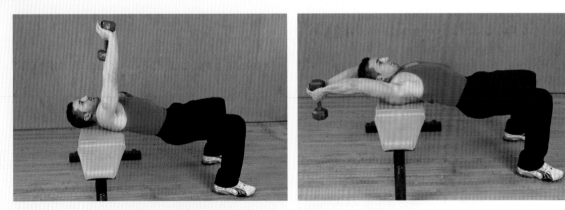

■ **FIGURE 13.29.**

- Athlete lies on the side of a flat bench (cross bench) with the shoulders aligned over the bench and the rest of the body off. The hips should be descended lower than the level of the bench with flexed knees and feet flat on the floor.
- The chest is out, neck is straight, and arms are extended straight over the chest with a DB in between.
- The shoulders are flexed until the upper arm is at the level of the head and then the shoulders extend back to the starting position in control.

> ✅ **OTHER VARIATIONS AND SIMILAR EXERCISES** *BB pullover, machine pullover, MB pullover, DB/KB/MB/sand bag pullover (one or two arms) on SB, and pullover and press.*

STANDING SHOULDER PRESS (MILITARY PRESS)
Rating: B

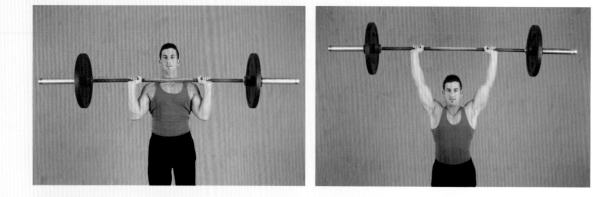

■ **FIGURE 13.30.**

- Bar is grasped with a closed, pronated grip slightly wider than or at shoulder width at shoulder height.
- The elbows are kept under the bar with the wrists hyperextended. Feet should be slightly wider than shoulder width and knees are slightly flexed.
- The bar is lifted upward until elbows are fully extended and then lowered to shoulder level with control.
- The body is kept upright throughout the movement.

> ✔ **OTHER VARIATIONS AND SIMILAR EXERCISES** *Standing DB/KB shoulder press (with pronated or midrange grip; one or two arms), MB/core ball press, Neider press, keg or sand bag press, mastiff bar press, press with bands/tubing, standing DB Arnold press (with rotation), standing DB/KB rotation press, MB/DB "Y" press, shoulder press on BOSU or wobble board, plate/MB squat rotation press, KB side press, Renegade shoulder press.*

SEATED SHOULDER PRESS
Rating: B

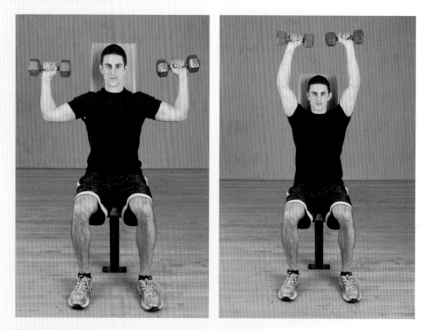

■ **FIGURE 13.31.**

- Athlete sits on a bench with back support (head faces forward and back supported by the bench), chest out, back hyperextended, and feet are flat on the floor.
- The bar is grasped with a closed, pronated grip wider than shoulder width.
- The bar is lifted from the rack to an extended elbow position above the head.
- With control, the bar is lowered to below chin level and pressed overhead until elbows are fully extended.
- When DBs are used (Fig. 13.31), the athlete begins with a pronated grip at or near shoulder level, presses the DBs upward, and returns to the starting position. The exercise can be adapted to target balance by performing it on one leg (see the sidebar below).

OTHER VARIATIONS AND SIMILAR EXERCISES Seated behind-the-neck BB shoulder press, seated KB shoulder press (using pronated or midrange hand positions), SB shoulder press, seated DB Arnold press, Smith machine shoulder press, seated shoulder press rack work (partial ROM, negatives, functional isometrics), machine shoulder press (various types of machines), and DB press out on a hyperextension bench.

SIDEBAR | **ALTERING A BASIC EXERCISE TO IMPROVE BALANCE**

Muscle force production is greater when the body is in a most stable position. For example, athletes can lift large amounts of weight in the shoulder press when performing seated on a stable bench or when standing with proper posture and a large base support. However, when an athlete performs an exercise in a less stable bodily position, other stabilizer muscles are recruited to keep the body still and less weight is lifted. The goal becomes improving balance (and stabilizer muscle activity) rather than improving maximal strength. In our previous example, if one trained specifically for balance when performing the shoulder press, then some variations can be used. The athlete can perform the exercise while sitting on an SB; standing on a BOSU ball, wobble board, or Airex pads; or standing on one leg (one- or two-arm presses), which narrows the base support (Fig. 13.32); the athlete can close his or her eyes, and/or add a reaction component to the exercise. Balance exercises have increased in popularity over the past several years. These exercises should be used specifically to enhance balance and stabilize muscle activity; the great weight reductions needed create an inferior stimulus for maximal strength training.

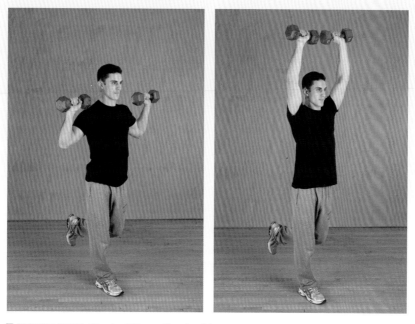

FIGURE 13.32. One-leg DB standing shoulder press.

SHRUG
Rating: A

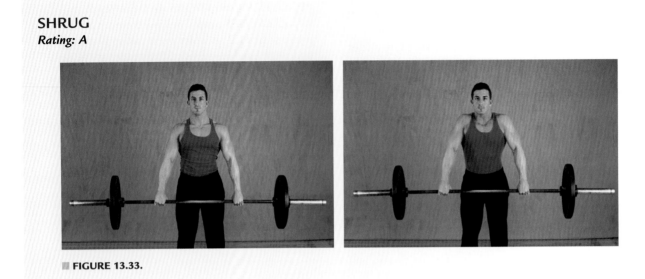

FIGURE 13.33.

- The bar (Fig. 13.33) or DBs are grasped with a closed, pronated grip resting at arm's length at side of thighs (for DBs) or in front of the upper thighs (for BB).
- Feet are slightly wider than shoulder width and knees are slightly flexed.
- The weight is lifted by elevating shoulders while maintaining the body in an upright position with elbows fully extended. Shoulders are shrugged or elevated as high as possible and returned to the starting position (depressed) in control.

OTHER VARIATIONS AND SIMILAR EXERCISES Power shrugs, machine shrugs, cable shrugs, keg/sand bag shrugs, seated DB/KB shrugs, seated trap bar shrugs, DB overhead shrug, and behind-the-back BB shrugs.

UPRIGHT ROW
Rating: A

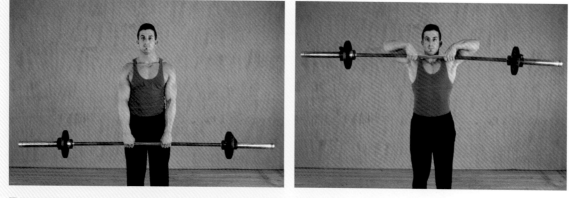

FIGURE 13.34.

- Bar is grasped with a closed, pronated grip with hands about 20–30 cm apart.
- The feet are kept slightly wider than shoulder width, knees are slightly flexed, and the bar rests with elbows fully extended on the thighs.
- The bar is lifted upward close to the body toward the chin (the elbows should be higher than the wrist and above the shoulders). A common mistake is to use the lower body or back to generate momentum to lift the weight. The weight should be lifted with an isolated effort from the upper-body musculature.

- With control, the bar is lowered to the starting position.

> **OTHER VARIATIONS AND SIMILAR EXERCISES** *DB/KB/MB upright row, wide-grip upright row, cable upright row, partner manual resistance towel upright row, one-arm upright row, upright row on BOSU or wobble board, DB step-up with upright row, and upright row with bands/tubing.*

DUMBBELL LATERAL RAISE
Rating: A

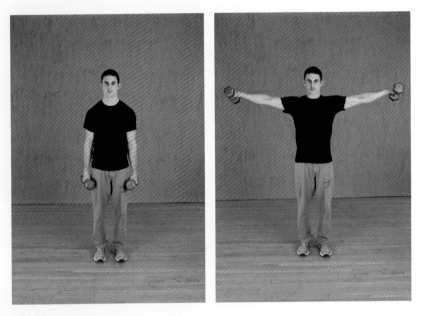

FIGURE 13.35.

- DBs are grasped with a closed, pronated grip in front of the hips with the elbows slightly flexed and are rotated so that the palms face each other with the elbows pointed outward.
- Feet are kept slightly wider than shoulder width, knees are slightly flexed, and back is straight with eyes focused straight ahead.
- DBs are raised laterally until the elbows and wrists are parallel to the floor and in line with the shoulders. A common mistake is to use momentum to swing DBs.
- With control, DBs are lowered to the starting position. This exercise can be added to other exercises (lunge, squat, side plank, push-up) to form a combo exercise.

OTHER VARIATIONS AND SIMILAR EXERCISES *Seated lateral raise, ISOM lateral hold/front raise, cable side laterals, machine lateral raise, rear lateral raise (DB or cable), bent-over lateral raise, kneeling lateral raise on SB, machine reverse fly, cable reverse fly, SB reverse fly, cross-cable laterals, BB front raise, lateral/front raise with core ball, DB/KB/MB front raise, alternate arm front raise, cable front raise, 45 degrees front raise (with arm internally rotated), angled front raise, standing plate front raise (with a twist, steering wheel), standing lateral/front raise on BOSU, DB punches (jabs, upper cuts, with rotation), DB arm swings, and prone/seated/standing shoulder extensions.*

INTERNAL/EXTERNAL SHOULDER ROTATIONS
Rating: A

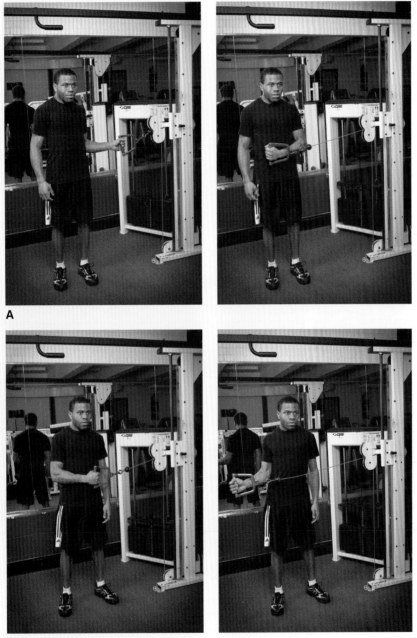

A

B

■ **FIGURE 13.36.** Internal (**left**) and external (**right**) shoulder rotation.

- Athlete stands with feet shoulder width apart near a cable pulley system or bands/tubing. The pulley is aligned with the elbow as the arms are relaxed at the sides.
- Arm is flexed ~90 degrees and externally rotated ~60–80 degrees to the starting position.
- The arm is rotated medially through complete ROM (while maintaining proper body position) while the upper arm remains at the side and then returns to the starting position.
- Weight is changed (internal shoulder rotators are stronger than external rotators) and body is rotated 180 degrees.
- Elbow is flexed to ~90 degrees and shoulder medially rotated ~90 degrees.

- The arm is rotated externally through complete ROM (while maintaining proper body position) and then returns to the starting position.

OTHER VARIATIONS AND SIMILAR EXERCISES *Machine internal/external rotations, standing DB internal/external rotations, lying cross-bench T crucifix, internal/external rotations with bands, standing internal/external rotations (with upper arm parallel to the floor) with bands, prone external rotations on bench or SB, and lying internal/external rotations (on side midrange between supine and prone).*

SCAPULA RETRACTION/PROTRACTION
Rating: A

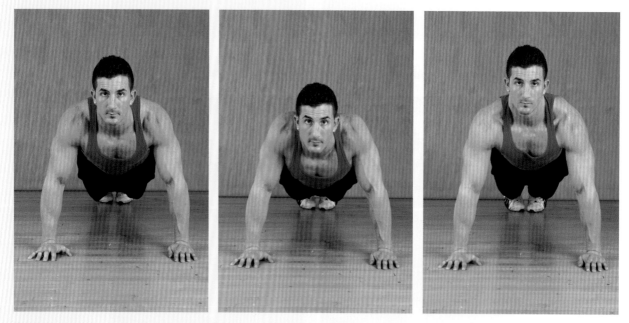

■ **FIGURE 13.37.**

- Athlete lies prone in a push-up position with a slightly wider than shoulder width hand position.
- The shoulder blades (scapulae) are retracted or pulled back while keeping arms extended in a push-up position, and then returned to the starting position.
- From here, scapulae are protracted or pulled forward while keeping arms extended in a push-up position and then returned to the starting position.

OTHER VARIATIONS AND SIMILAR EXERCISES *Prone DB retractions (with arms parallel to the floor and elbows bent at 90 degrees), prone circuit. Same exercise can be performed from a bench press position, on SB/BOSU, with DB, or leaning against a wall.*

STABILITY BALL SLAPS
Rating: A

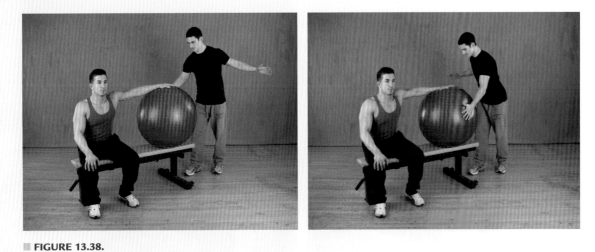

FIGURE 13.38.

- An SB is held in place at the side of the athlete (or in front) supported on a bench. The ball is maintained in a stable position by the athlete isometrically contracting shoulder musculature to hold the ball still.
- A partner slaps the ball at different locations with different intensities with altered timing. This forces the individual to react to the slaps by strongly contracting shoulder muscles.

- Athlete switches arms and supports the SB with the opposite arm while reacting to the partner's slaps.

 OTHER VARIATIONS *Exercise can be performed while standing, lying prone or supine, or kneeling.*

TRICEPS PUSHDOWN
Rating: A

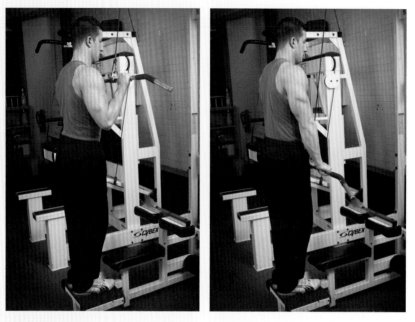

■ FIGURE 13.39.

- The bar on a cable unit is grasped with a closed, pronated grip 10–15 cm apart with thumbs over the top of the bar and feet placed shoulder width apart with knees slightly flexed.
- Body is kept upright throughout movement with elbows positioned next to torso.
- The bar is pushed down until the elbows reach full extension and then, with control, the bar is lowered to the starting position. A common mistake is to use the trunk to generate momentum to lift the weight or to perform the exercise in a limited ROM.

OTHER VARIATIONS AND SIMILAR EXERCISES *Rope pushdowns, V-bar pushdowns, power pushdown, cross-body pushdown (one arm), reverse pushdown (with various bars), and incline bench pushdown (with various bars).*

SEATED TRICEPS EXTENSION
Rating: A

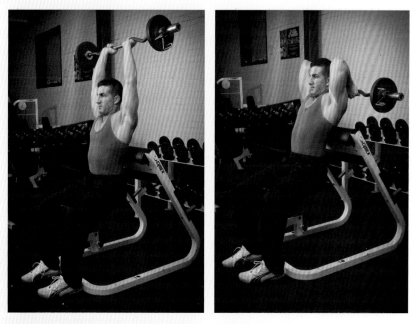

FIGURE 13.40.

- Athlete is seated on a bench with feet flat on the floor and back supported.
- Bar or DB(s) is grasped with a closed, pronated grip and lifted to a position above the head with the elbows fully flexed and pointed outward.
- The weight is extended upward until elbows are fully extended (while proper posture is maintained) and returned to the starting position under control.

OTHER VARIATIONS AND SIMILAR EXERCISES *Bilateral or unilateral triceps extension (with one DB), seated BB triceps extension (with straight or EZ curl bar), incline BB or DB triceps extension, machine triceps extension, seated reverse-grip BB triceps extension, DB extensions (with hand rotation), seated (or incline) cable triceps extension (with various bars or rope), bent-over prone cable triceps extension, BB, cable, or DB kickbacks (bent-over or lying).*

LYING TRICEPS EXTENSION (SKULL CRUSHERS)
Rating: A

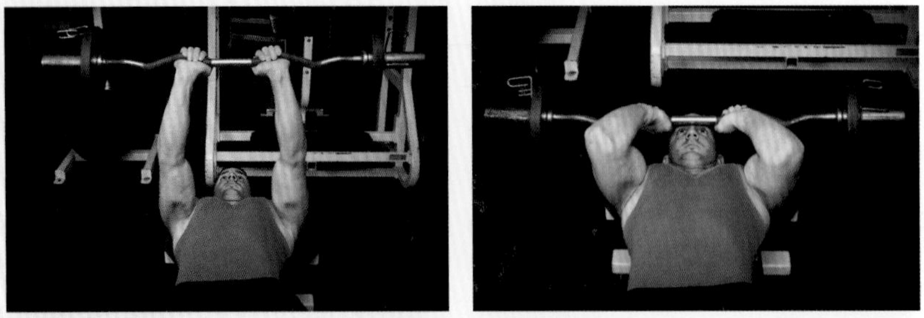

■ **FIGURE 13.41.**

- Athlete lies supine on the bench with feet flat on the floor.
- The bar is grasped with a closed, pronated grip with hands 15–25 cm apart and elbows are extended above the upper chest.
- With control, the bar is lowered to the forehead, and upper arms remain perpendicular to the floor.
- The bar is pushed upward until elbows return to the fully extended position.

✔ **OTHER VARIATIONS AND SIMILAR EXERCISES** *Lying reverse-grip BB extension, lying DB triceps extension (midrange hand position), cross-face DB extensions, cable triceps extension (with various bars or rope), lying BB, cable, or DB extensions with upper arm at 45-degree angle to the floor, and fixed-bar body extension.*

STANDING BICEPS CURL (OLYMPIC/EZ CURL BAR)
Rating: A

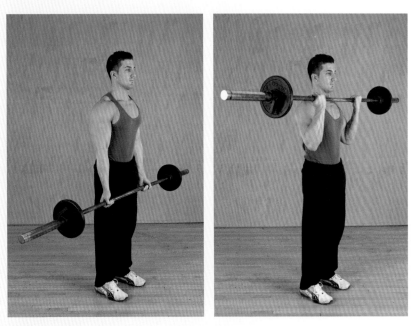

■ **FIGURE 13.42.**

- The bar is grasped shoulder width or slightly wider with a closed, supinated (palms facing forward) grip with elbows extended.
- Feet are shoulder width apart, knees are slightly flexed, back is straight, eyes are focused straight ahead, and upper arms are positioned against trunk perpendicular to the floor.
- Bar is lifted in an arc toward the anterior deltoids by flexing the elbows and then lowered in control to the starting position. DB variations can be added to exercises (lunge, squat) to form combo exercises.

- Common mistake includes using momentum to lift the weight up or not using a full ROM.

> ✔ **OTHER VARIATIONS AND SIMILAR EXERCISES** *Wide-grip curl, cheat curls, slide curl, DB curls, alternate DB curls, cable curls, standing concentration curl, crucifix cable curls, curls (one leg), and DB rotation curls.*

SEATED DUMBBELL BICEPS CURL
Rating: A

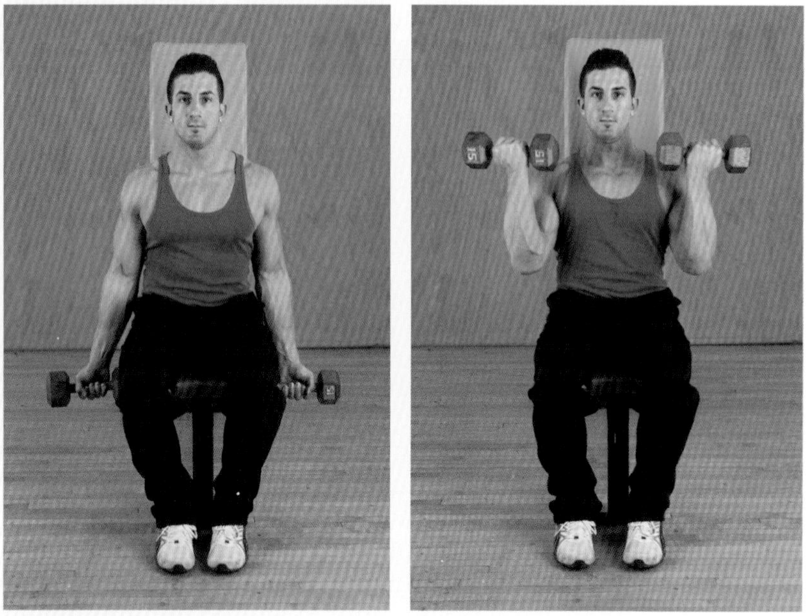

■ FIGURE 13.43.

- Athlete sits on the bench with feet flat on the floor and the back supported by pad.
- DBs are grasped with the elbows extended at the sides with a closed, supinated grip.
- DBs are lifted in an arc toward the anterior deltoid by flexing the elbows and then lowered in control to the starting position.
- May be performed by alternating each arm unilaterally or simultaneously bilaterally.

OTHER VARIATIONS AND SIMILAR EXERCISES *Seated cable curls, incline DB curls, incline cable curls, DB concentration curl, prone bench curl (DB, cables, or BB), machine curls, supine cable curls, supine DB curl.*

HAMMER CURL
Rating: A

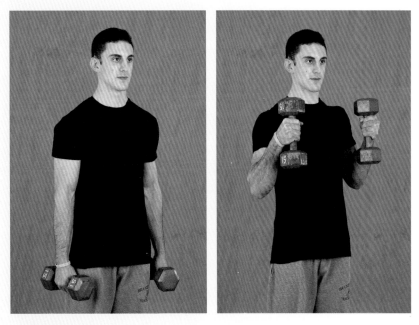

FIGURE 13.44.

- DBs are grasped with elbows extended at the sides in closed, supinated midrange grip (palms of the hands are facing the body) with feet shoulder width apart and knees slightly flexed. Back is straight and eyes are focused straight ahead.
- DBs are raised in an arc toward the anterior deltoid by flexing the elbows and then lowered with control to the starting position.

- Exercise can be performed by alternating each arm unilaterally or bilaterally.

 OTHER VARIATIONS *Cross-body hammer curls and cable hammer curls.*

PREACHER CURL (OLYMPIC/EZ CURL BAR)
Rating: A

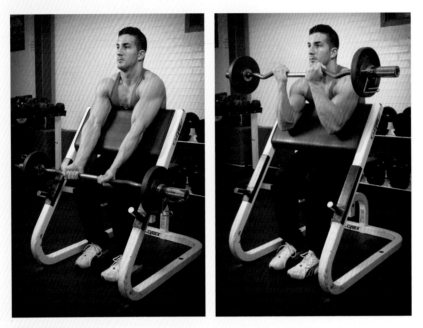

■ **FIGURE 13.45.**

- A preacher bench is used. The bar is grasped with a narrow, closed, supinated grip while athlete is seated.
- Back is straight, eyes are focused straight ahead, and upper arms rest against support pad.
- Bar is lifted in an arc toward the anterior deltoids by flexing the elbows and lowered in control to the starting position.

- A spotter can apply force to the bar during the upward movement if necessary.

> **OTHER VARIATIONS** *DB preacher curl, one-arm DB preacher curl, cable preacher curl, Scott curls, and machine preacher curls.*

WRIST CURL
Rating: A

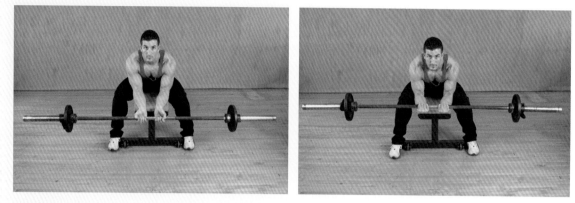

■ **FIGURE 13.46.**

- Athlete sits on the end of a bench and grasps the bar (straight or EZ curl bar) with an open, supinated grip with hands 20–30 cm apart. Wrists are hyperextended.
- Feet are flat on the floor with the torso leaning forward and elbows and forearms resting on the thighs (or bench) throughout the movement.
- The bar is lifted by flexing fingers and wrist and then returning to the starting position.

> ✔ **OTHER VARIATIONS AND SIMILAR EXERCISES** *DB wrist curl, cable wrist curls, behind-the-back BB wrist curls (standing or seated), behind-the-back DB or cable wrist curls, machine wrist curls, wrist curls on a preacher bench, and wrist rolls (with a roller).*

REVERSE WRIST CURL
Rating: A

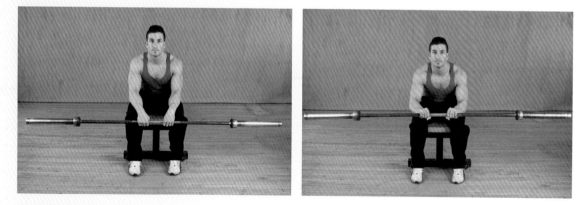

■ **FIGURE 13.47.**

- Athlete sits on the end of a bench and grasps the bar with a closed, pronated grip, wrists flexed, and hands held 20–30 cm apart.
- Feet are flat with the torso leaning forward and elbows and forearms resting on the thighs (or bench) throughout the movement.
- The bar is raised by extending and hyperextending the wrists.

> ✔ **OTHER VARIATIONS AND SIMILAR EXERCISES** *DB or cable reverse wrist curl, machine reverse wrist curl, wrist rows, and reverse wrist rolls (with a roller).*

REVERSE CURL
Rating: A

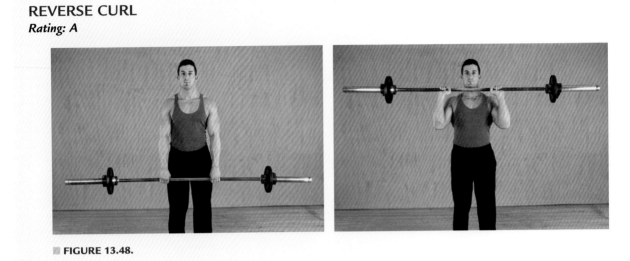

■ **FIGURE 13.48.**

- Bar is grasped shoulder width or slightly wider with a closed, pronated grip with elbows extended.
- Feet are shoulder width apart, knees are slightly flexed, back is straight, eyes are focused straight ahead, and upper arms are positioned against trunk perpendicular to the floor.

- Bar is lifted in an arc toward the anterior deltoids by flexing the elbows (and extending wrists) and then lowered in control to the starting position.

OTHER VARIATIONS *Standing reverse curl (DB, cables) and machine reverse curl.*

CORE EXERCISES

Core exercises encompass motion in three planes about the spinal column and pelvic girdle. Several major muscle groups produce these motions and must ISOM contract to stabilize the joints when they are not considered to be prime movers (Table 13.3). Flexion occurs when anterior muscles contract bilaterally (both sides of vertebral column). Extension occurs when posterior muscles contract bilaterally. Lateral flexion and/or rotation occur when muscles contract unilaterally. Stability when the athlete is standing (while externally loaded), bridged supine on ground with shoulders and feet (knees bent), and prone on all fours (plank) is trained. There are a large number of exercises and variations that develop a strong, durable core.

TABLE 13.3 KINESIOLOGY OF CORE MOTION

JOINT	TYPE OF JOINT	JOINT MOVEMENT	MUSCLES
Cervical	Hinge, pivot (C1-C2)	Lateral flexion Rotation	Rectus capitis (lateralis, anterior), longus capitis and colli, sternocleidomastoid, splenius capitis and cervicis, suboccipital group, levator scapulae, semispinalis capitis and cervicis, multifidus, longissimus capitis, trapezius, rotatores cervicis
		Flexion	Rectus capitis (lateralis, anterior), longus capitis and colli, hyoid muscles, sternocleidomastoid, scalenes
		Extension/ hyperextenision	Splenius capitis and cervicis, suboccipital group, semispinalis capitis and cervicis, erector spinae, multifidus, levator scapulae, longissimus capitis, trapezius, scalenes, sternocleidomastoid, rotatores cervicis
Thoracic lumbar		Flexion	Rectus abdominis, external/internal oblique, quadratus lumborum
		Extension	Spinalis, iliocostalis, and longissimus thoracis, semispinalis thoracis, multifidus, iliocostalis lumborum, rotatores thoracis
		Rotation and lateral flexion	Semispinalis thoracis, erector spinae, multifidus, external/internal oblique, rectus abdominis, psoas major/minor, iliocostalis lumborum, quadratus lumborum
		Abdominal hollowing	Transversus abdominis
Rib cage[a]		Elevation, inspiration	Diaphragm, serratus posterior superior, internal intercostals, levator costarum, transversus thoracis
		Depression, expiration	Serratus posterior inferior, external intercostals

[a]Primary respiration muscles.

PROPER POSITION FOR CORE EXERCISES

Contraction of abdominal and spinal muscles is essential to maintaining spine stability. One muscle, the transversus abdominis, resembles an internal girdle. Its major function is hollowing (or compression) where the abdominal wall is drawn in toward the spine (28) and is activated before other muscles during movement. Special attention has been given to this muscle because of its role in low-back pain. Many therapists, coaches, and trainers teach athletes to draw in the abs by contracting the transversus abdominis. It is assessed by having the athlete lie supine and contract the transversus abdominis with the trainer's hand under the lumbar spine to measure pressure. The exercise is practiced from other positions, *e.g.*, prone, seated, and standing (3). A complex variation is the dead bug (Fig. 13.49) where the arms and legs are elevated off of the floor. Other core muscles need to contract to generate high IAP via bracing (29). Bracing involves ISOM contraction of the transversus abdominis as well as the internal and external obliques, rectus abdominis, and quadratus lumborum, and increases lumbar stability (29). The Sidebar below discusses some ways in whcih core exercises can be made more difficult once proper position is attained.

> **SIDEBAR** **MAKING CORE EXERCISES MORE DIFFICULT**
>
> Several core exercises can be made more difficult by altering the position of the limbs, thereby increasing the moment arm of resistance. For example, a curl-up is more difficult when the arms are extended overhead rather than crossed across the chest. For some SB exercises, less BW can be supported by the ball or one leg can be used instead of two. Bending the knees during the leg raise makes it easier than with extended knees. Several progressions can be developed to increase the difficulty of an exercise without adding additional loading.

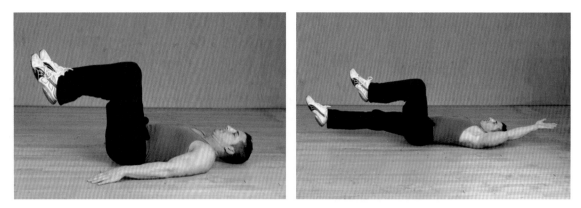

■ **FIGURE 13.49.** "Dead bug."

Core Exercises

CRUNCH (CURL-UP)
Rating: A

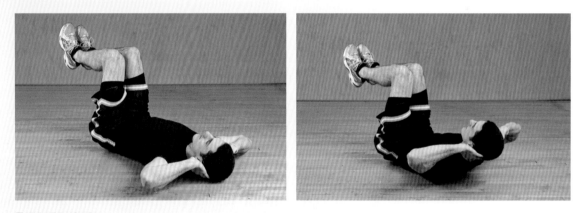

■ **FIGURE 13.50.**

- Athlete lies supine on a mat or floor with hips and knees elevated to form a 90-degree angle.
- Hands are placed at the sides of the head or folded across the chest with chin tucked into the chest.
- Torso is flexed (curled) toward the thighs until shoulders are off the floor and returned in control to the starting position.

> *OTHER VARIATIONS (WITH PLATES, DB, MACHINES, MB, KB, SAND BAG) AND SIMILAR EXERCISES Ab crunches (with feet straight, bent knees, pike position), decline crunches, machine crunches, cable crunches (standing or kneeling), reverse crunch (with SB or MB), hip thrust, ISOM crunch, side (oblique) crunches, SB oblique crunch, cable side crunches, partner (base, bottom man down) crunches, SB crunches, BOSU crunches, crunches with arms overhead (DB/MB), hanging side crunches.*

BENT-KNEE SIT-UP
Rating: A

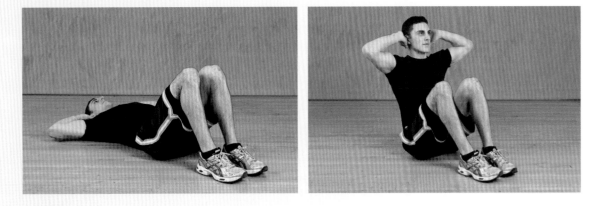

■ FIGURE 13.51.

- Athlete lies supine on the floor with knees flexed and heels close to buttocks.
- Hands are placed at the sides of the head or folded across the chest with chin tucked into the chest.
- Trunk and hips are flexed toward thighs until trunk is off the floor and returned in control to the starting position.

OTHER VARIATIONS (WITH PLATES, DB, MACHINES, MB, KB, SAND BAG) AND SIMILAR EXERCISES Sit-ups on decline bench, Roman chair sit-ups, sit-ups with MB toss, straight-leg sit-ups, sit-ups with straight arms, suspended sit-ups, and sit-ups with BB, DB, or MB press, Janda sit-up.

BENT-KNEE TWISTS
Rating: A

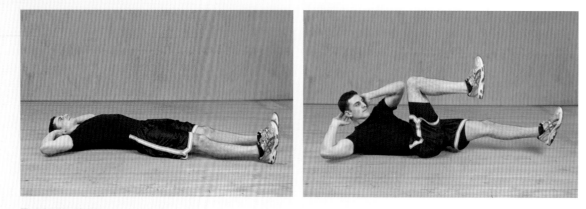

■ **FIGURE 13.52.**

- Athlete lies supine on the floor with knees flexed, heels close to buttocks, and hands placed on the side of the head with elbows pointed forward.
- Torso is flexed and rotated during ascent off of the floor as the elbow approaches the opposite knee (right elbow to left knee) and then returns in control to the starting position.
- Next repetition is performed using the opposite elbow to knee.

OTHER VARIATIONS AND SIMILAR EXERCISES Roman chair twisting sit-ups, decline twisting sit-ups, twisting crunches (flat, decline, Roman chair, with knee raise), cable twisting crunches, reverse trunk twists, SB reverse trunk twist (windshield wiper), SB trunk rotations, machine trunk rotations, Russian twists (flat, sit-up bench, decline with DB, plate, MB), SB/BOSU twisting knee-ups, SB/ BOSU twisting crunches (with bands), partner plate pass, MB side throws, standing/seated twists (with BB, DB, or MB), and bent-over trunk rotations (with stick, BB, DB, or MB).

SIDE BENDS
Rating: A

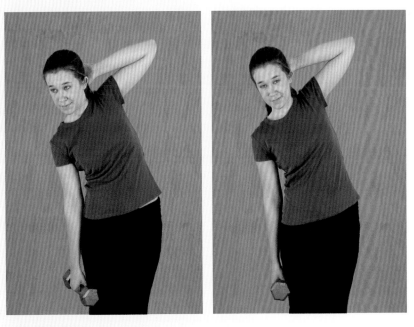

FIGURE 13.53.

- Athlete stands with shoulder width stance grasping a DB in one hand and opposite arm positioned on the side of the head.
- Athlete laterally flexes (bends) to the side grasping the DB and returns in control to the starting position.
- After the required number of repetitions is performed, individual grasps DB with opposite hand and repeats the exercise. A common mistake is to use two DBs for this exercise. The second DB acts as a counterbalance and reduces loading on the core.

OTHER VARIATIONS AND SIMILAR EXERCISES Cable, BB, SB, or stick side bends, lateral flexion (on hyperextension bench), arms overhead, lying side bends.

PLANK
Rating: A

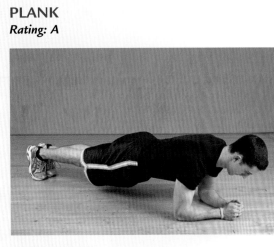

■ **FIGURE 13.54.**

- Athlete begins in a push-up postural position with BW supported by the feet and hands or elbows (which are in contact with the floor).

- Torso remains in a straight line with the hip level for the duration of the exercise.
- Athlete maintains this ISOM hold position with proper body alignment and requires trunk musculature to contract strongly against the force of gravity. A common mistake is to allow the hips to drop too low or rise too high during fatigue.

✔ **OTHER VARIATIONS AND SIMILAR EXERCISES** *SB plank (hands on ball — push-up position; SB under feet — push-up position), MB plank, plank with one leg elevated, one-arm plank, one-arm plank with contralateral arm movement, ISOM side plank (on elbows or hands), side plank with hip abduction or contralateral shoulder lateral raise, angled plank (with BB or bench), TRX plank, TRX side plank, TRX plank with leg scissors, side glide (against wall), dynamic side bridge, prone twist.*

STABILITY BALL ROLL-OUT
Rating: B

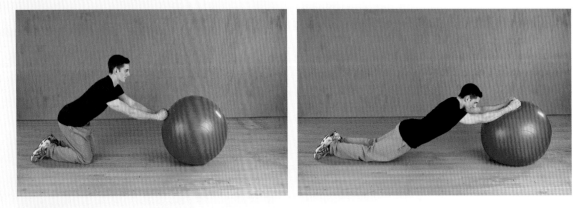

■ **FIGURE 13.55.**

- Athlete begins on knees in an upright position (with slight forward lean) with forearms/wrists near the side of SB.
- Athlete leans forward as ball rolls. Forearms stay in contact with ball (and roll over the ball to elbow level) as the shoulders flex.
- Core muscles contract to maintain posture. Athlete continues to roll the ball until trunk, arms, and shoulders are aligned. With control, the ball is rolled back to starting position via shoulder extension with core muscles contracting to maintain proper position.

- Exercise is more difficult with the body closest to the ground (with a BB, DB, or Ab Roller) or when it is performed from a standing or elevated body position.
- Because of upper-body involvement, shoulder extensors are worked.

✔ **OTHER VARIATIONS** *Ab Roller, standing SB roll-out, elevated SB roll-out, BB/DB roll-out, MB roll-out.*

LYING LEG RAISE
Rating: A

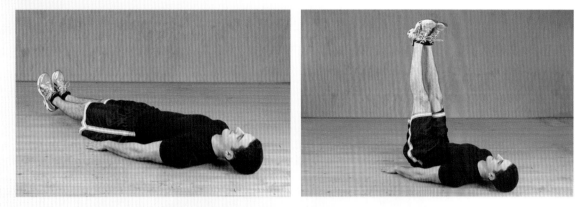

■ **FIGURE 13.56.**

- Athlete lies supine on the floor with hips and knees extended in front.
- Trunk is kept tight, legs are raised with knees slightly bent until they are perpendicular to the floor, and returned in control to the starting position.
- May use BW, SB, or MB for resistance.

✔ *OTHER VARIATIONS AND SIMILAR EXERCISES Plyometric leg raise (with partner), vertical (dip) bench straight- or bent-leg raise, hanging straight- or bent-leg raise (BW or MB), circular (360 degrees) straight leg raise, bent knee-ups (floor,* bench, seated, and decline), cable knee-ups, alternate leg knee-ups, knee-ups + abdominal crunch, lying V-ups, side V-ups, lying flutter kicks, lying scissors, ISOM leg raise holds (6 in.), lying side knee-ups, side flutter kicks, side jackknife, SB prone knee-ups (ball under shins, toes, or one leg), SB twisting knee-ups, SB prone pike knee-up, TRX knee-up and twisting knee-up, TRX pike knee-up, TRX windshield wiper, KB/MB/DB L-sit, and kips.*

STABILITY BALL EXCHANGE
Rating: B

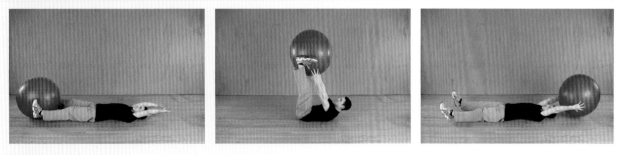

■ **FIGURE 13.57.**

- Athlete begins in a supine position with legs and arms extended in opposite directions. An SB is placed between hands and held in an overhead position.
- Shoulders extend, trunk flexes, and hips flex bringing arms and legs toward the center of the body.
- At the top of the movement, the SB is exchanged from hands to feet (ball is held between the legs near the ankles) and arms and legs are returned in control to the starting position.

✔ *OTHER VARIATIONS MB exchange.*
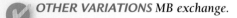

MEDICINE BALL WOODCHOP
Rating: B

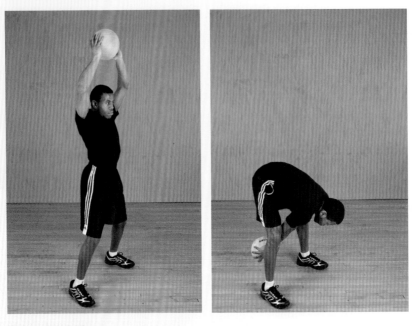

■ **FIGURE 13.58.**

- Feet are placed wider than shoulder width. MB is held with both hands above the head.
- MB is swung forcefully downward between the legs flexing the trunk, hips, and extending the shoulders.
- The movement is reversed back to the starting position.

✓ **OTHER VARIATIONS** DB woodchop, rotational woodchop, diagonal woodchop, cable woodchop, chop and lift, reverse woodchop.

CABLE ROTATIONS
Rating: A

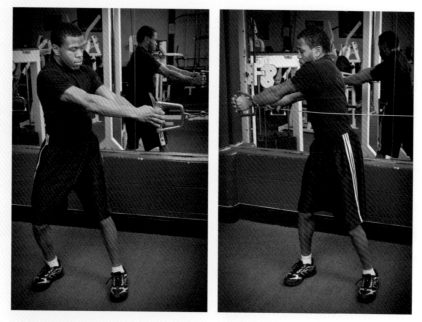

FIGURE 13.59.

- Athlete adjusts a cable pulley system to shoulder height and assumes a position facing away from the machine at a 90-degree angle a few feet away.
- A shoulder width stance is used. With feet planted securely, the athlete rotates the trunk to grasp the handle with both hands.
- Keeping the lower body still, the athlete rotates 180 degrees with arms in an extended position. The exercise is most difficult with the arms straight. Bending the arms decreases the moment arm of resistance.

- In control, the athlete returns to the starting position. Once the required number of repetitions is performed, athlete switches sides and repeats.

OTHER VARIATIONS AND SIMILAR EXERCISES *Cable diagonal (low-to-high) rotation, DB/KB/MB low-to-high rotation, MB rotations (standing, seated, kneeling), plate squat rotation press, band/tubing rotations.*

BAR ROTATION
Rating: B

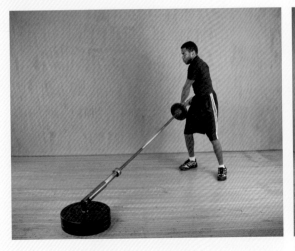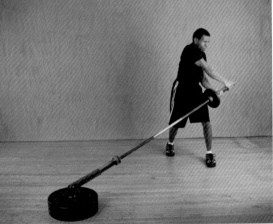

■ **FIGURE 13.60.**

- An Olympic bar is loaded on only one side with the opposite side fixed in a corner acting as a fulcrum for motion. A device that freely allows the bar to rotate (Landmine or Renegade) is recommended.
- Athlete grasps one end of the bar with both arms (one hand over, one under), elbows extended, and at one side.
- While keeping arms straight, the athlete rotates to the opposite side lifting the bar up, extending the bar outward, and across the body to the contralateral side.

- Athlete reverses the action back to the starting position.

⊘ OTHER VARIATIONS AND SIMILAR EXERCISES *Loading medleys with sand bag, DB, or other implements.*

SKIER
Rating: B

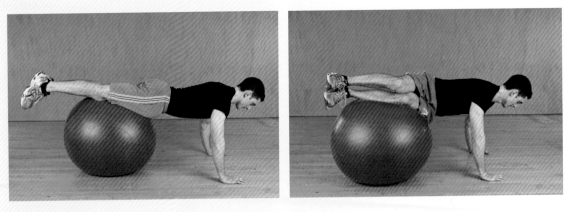

■ **FIGURE 13.61.**

- Athlete begins in a push-up position with shins resting on the SB and knees flexed.
- While maintaining upper-body position, the athlete rotates the trunk quickly to the left (until legs are parallel to the ground) and then back to the right.

⊘ OTHER VARIATIONS *Exercise can be performed with knees extended.*

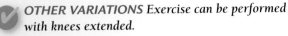

TURKISH GET-UP
Rating: B

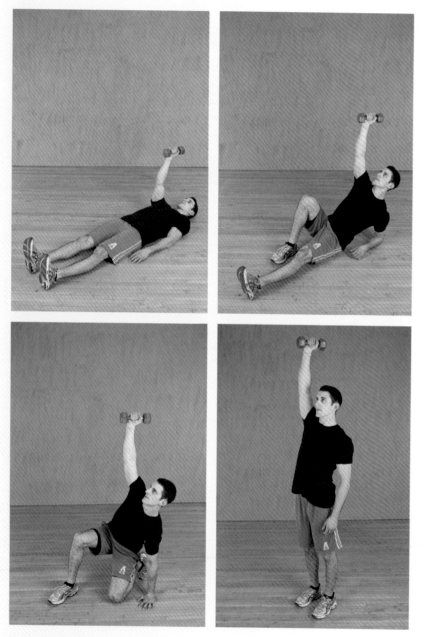

FIGURE 13.62.

- Athlete lies supine on the floor with a KB or DB in one hand with arm perpendicular to the floor. Knee on the same side flexes and foot is flat on the floor while athlete flexes the trunk and supports weight on the opposite elbow.
- While weight is supported by back arm, athlete tucks the opposite leg under the body and begins to rise up to the standing position with KB or DB overhead.

- Athlete returns to the starting position and performs another repetition.

OTHER VARIATIONS *Exercise can be performed with sand bags or core ball.*

GOOD MORNING
Rating: B

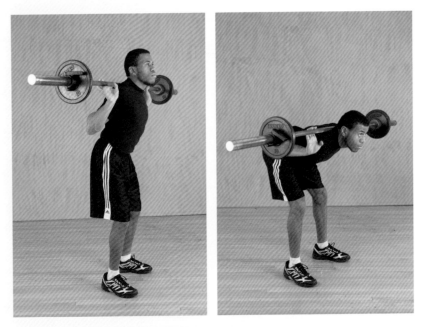

FIGURE 13.63.

- Bar is grasped with a closed, pronated grip slightly wider than the shoulder width while it rests on shoulders (similar to back squat). Feet are shoulder width apart with toes pointed slightly outward. Head is straight or slightly upward with eyes focused on a spot on the wall.
- With chest out, shoulders retracted, and lower back flat (hyperextended), torso and hips are flexed at the waist until almost parallel to the floor. Lower body remains still.
- Athlete returns to the starting position.

OTHER VARIATIONS *Keg/sand bag good morning, DB/KB good morning, good morning on SB/BOSU.*

HYPEREXTENSION
Rating: A

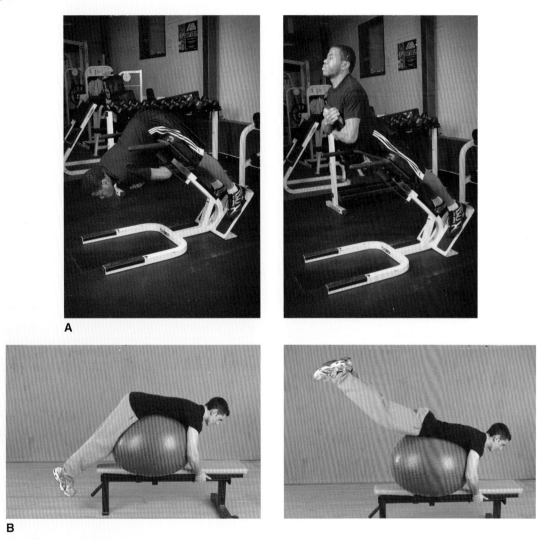

A

B

■ **FIGURE 13.64.** Hyperextension (**left**) and reverse hyperextension (**right**).

- Upper pad of the bench is adjusted so upper thighs lie flat across and there is space for flexion at the waist and knees are not hyperextended. Ankles are positioned under lower pads for support.
- With arms crossed behind head or across chest (holding plate, DB, KB, bar, sand bag), the athlete bends forward at the waist in a full ROM while maintaining a flat back and returns to the starting position in control.
- Hyperextensions and reverse hyperextensions (*image on right*) are excellent exercises working the low-back/glute/hamstring muscles. The extended position on a hyperextension bench can be used as a base for combo exercise building (rotations, press-outs, side raises, and rows).

✔ **OTHER VARIATIONS AND SIMILAR EXERCISES** *Machine back extensions, hyperextensions with straight arms (MB, DB, plate), twisting hyperextensions, rotations (while maintaining the hyperextended back position), single-leg hyperextension, reverse hyperextensions, hypers/reverse hypers on SB, seated BB back extensions, glute-ham raise (BW, BB, DB, KB, MB, sand bag), and press-ups.*

KETTLEBELL SWING
Rating: B

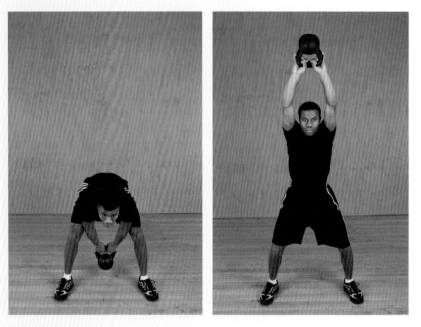

■ **FIGURE 13.65.**

- Athlete begins in a semisquat position with chest out and a slight arch in the lower back. KB is grasped between legs with two hands with arms extended.
- KB is lifted (swung) upward explosively via knee, hip, and back extension to where KB rises above the level of the head.
- KB is returned to the starting position in control.

OTHER VARIATIONS *Exercise can be performed with DB, sand bag, or one arm. A squat can be added at the end (swing squat).*

BACK BRIDGE
Rating: A

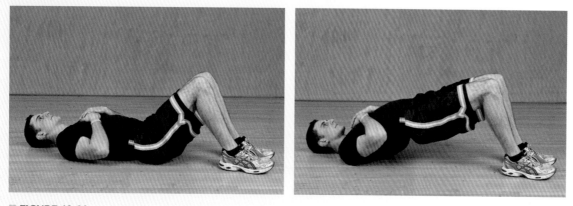

■ **FIGURE 13.66.**

- Athlete lies supine on the floor with arms at side (or across the chest) and knees/hips flexed with feet flat on floor.
- With arms remaining in the starting position, the chest, hips, buttocks, and spine rise (extend) off of the floor to a linear elevated body position (with shoulders supporting upper-body weight) and return back to the starting position.
- ISOM muscle action can be added at the top of the exercise while the body is in a linear position.

> ✔ *OTHER VARIATIONS AND SIMILAR EXERCISES Back bridges on bench, SB/BOSU, single-leg back bridge (floor, MB, SB), straight-leg back bridge, single-leg bridge with opposite leg motion, TRX bridge.*

QUADRUPED
Rating: A

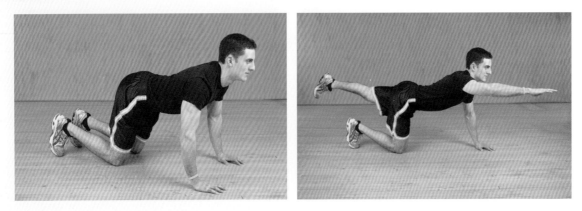

■ **FIGURE 13.67.**

- The athlete assumes a prone position on all fours with hips and knees flexed, arms vertical to the ground, neutral spine, and torso near parallel to the floor.
- Athlete extends the hip (with knee extended) so that it is aligned with the torso. The contralateral arm (shoulder) is flexed so it too is aligned with the torso. A simpler version entails the athlete either lift the leg only or the arm only. To make the exercise more difficult, an ISOM contraction (5–10 s) can be used at the top position.
- This exercise stresses hip and spinal extensors and is performed most often without additional loading.

Athletes should focus on contracting the gluteal muscles tightly.
- The arm and leg are returned to the starting position, and the opposite limbs are trained.

✓ **OTHER VARIATIONS AND SIMILAR EXERCISES** *Quadruped with bent knees, superman (lying prone on the stomach) with both arms and legs extended, superman with ipsilateral arm/leg extension, SB superman.*

KETTLEBELL FIGURE 8S
Rating: A

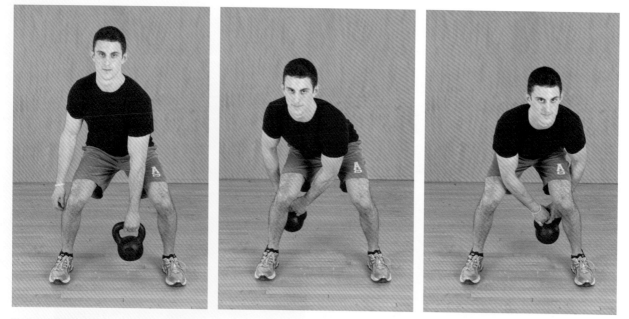

FIGURE 13.68.

- Athlete bends forward with a flat back in a deadlift position and places KB between the legs with one arm extended.
- KB is passed behind right leg in between the legs to left hand.

- KB is passed behind left leg in between the legs to right hand (forming a figure 8).
- Movements are repeated for the required repetition number.

MANUAL RESISTANCE NECK (FOUR-WAY)
Rating: A

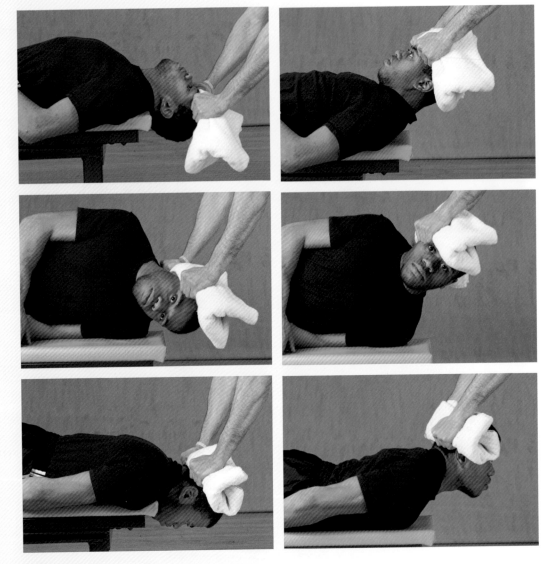

■ **FIGURE 13.69.**

- Athlete begins on all fours or lies on a bench with the neck in the neutral position. A partner applies pressure to the head in four directions.
- Athlete extends the neck against the manual resistance applied by the partner and returns to the starting position. Pressure is applied at multiple points to enable the athlete to laterally flex (right and left) and flex the neck against a resistance.

OTHER VARIATIONS AND SIMILAR EXERCISES *Four-way neck machine, neck flexion/ extension/lateral flexion with head strap, front/back bridges.*

TIRE FLIPPING
Rating: C

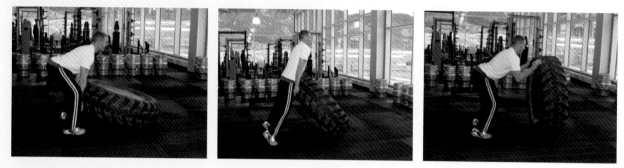

■ **FIGURE 13.70.**

- Athlete begins in a four-point stance with knees and hip flexed using a tire that is at least two times the BW. The height of the tire while it is on the ground should come to approximately knee level.
- Athlete drives the chest into the tire and pushes at approximately 45 degrees. Hips drive forward using a triple extension (of hips, knees, and ankles) lifting the tire up on its side.
- Athlete jumps under the tire on its way up (rather than curling it!) and places the body in a proper

position and extends the arms and continues pushing the tire forward until it flips onto its side. The movement is repeated.

OTHER VARIATIONS AND SIMILAR EXERCISES Tire drags, e.g., pulling or towing a tire during walking/running, backpedaling, or side shuffling. Drags can be performed with sand bags.

FARMER'S WALK
Rating: B

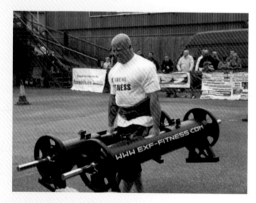

■ **FIGURE 13.71.**

- Athlete uses heavy DB, KB, or a sport-specific farmer's walk device, which enables plate loading of heavy weights.
- Athlete properly bends over, grasps the bar, and lifts the weights into the standing position. Athlete then begins to walk rapidly or run a specified distance while supporting the load in the hands (this exercise is excellent for grip strength training).
- Athlete returns to the staring position and places the weights down on the ground.

COMBINATION EXERCISES

Combination exercises involve combining two exercises into one. Several exercises can be combined into one. Combination exercises increase the complexity and metabolic responses to resistance exercise. Weight is selected based on the weaker of the two (or three) exercises used. The following table lists some common combination exercises used in RT.

- DB push-up with unilateral row (or T rotation)
- Lunge with torso twist (or shoulder press, lateral raise)
- Clean, front squat, and push press
- SB push-up with prone knee-ups
- Step-ups with bicep curl and shoulder press
- BB pullover and press
- Hyperextension with trunk rotation (or shoulder press, lateral raise)
- DB squat with overhead shoulder press

Myths & Misconceptions

Several RT Exercises Should Be Totally Avoided in All Circumstances Because They Cause Injury

Some in the sports and fitness industry have painted with a broad brush in labeling some resistance exercises as inappropriate for everyone regardless of training goals or personal situations. Some common exercises criticized are, *e.g.*, the sit-up, BB squat, behind-the-neck press/pull-down, Olympic lifts, and full ROM bench press. These exercises have been touted as injurious to the lower back, knees, and shoulders. All exercises stress joints to induce adaptations. However, distress to joints is to be avoided, but this concern is multi-factorial. As Dr. Stuart McGill has stated, "there is no such thing as a safe or dangerous exercise — only an ill-prescribed exercise for an individual." Exercises are not injurious provided the athlete has no preexisting condition and performs the exercises properly. Some exercises will not cause injury but could exacerbate an injury if one has a predisposition. Performing a sit-up for someone with low-back pain is contraindicated. However, a healthy individual can benefit from the sit-up. When exercises do pose a risk of injury, many times it is related to improper technique or loading and not the exercise per se. The choice to include or exclude an exercise in an RT program should be made on an individual basis and not because of misinformation.

- Pull-up (or dip) with knee raise or leg scissor
- DB push-up with unilateral row
- T-shoulder raises (lateral to front raise)
- Side plank with lateral raise (or hip abduction)

GRIP STRENGTH TRAINING

Grip strength has long been recognized as an important component of muscular fitness and performance in sports like strength competitions, weightlifting, power-lifting, wrestling, football, and gymnastics. Forearm and hand flexor muscles are the primary muscles involved in gripping whereas the wrist extensors provide stability. Grip strength training involves free weight, machine, and cables/bands wrist flexion/extension exercises, various hand gripping devices, radial/ulnar deviation and circumduction with specific devices, finger flexion/extension, abduction and adduction (pinching) exercises, thick bars, and through performance of pulling exercises without the use of ergogenic aids such as lifting straps.

Gripping Exercises: Power gripping (with ball or gripping devices), ISOM BB, KB, sand bag, or DB grip holds, pinch gripping (with weights), power web finger flexion, machine gripping, lever bar wrist rotations, ISOM bar support, thick bar pulling exercises, climbing board hangs, towel exercises, and push-ups (on finger tips, fists, or back of hands).

OLYMPIC LIFTS AND VARIATIONS

THE CLEAN, SNATCH (FULL, POWER: FROM FLOOR, ABOVE KNEE, BELOW KNEE) ("C" RATING)

The Olympic lifts and variations are total-body lifts that recruit most major muscle groups and are the most complex exercises to perform. They are regarded as the most effective exercises for increasing muscle power, as they require fast force production and Olympic weightlifters generate high degrees of power (14). Critical to performance is the quality of effort per repetition (maximal velocity). The clean and jerk (Fig. 13.72) is a two-staged exercise and can result in greater weights being lifted compared to the single-staged snatch (Fig. 13.73). Both lifts require explosive movements of the lower body and trunk, whereas the arms serve as guides and play a secondary role preparing the body to catch the bar. Variations are partial exercises of the full version that can be used to enhance specific performance aspects of the complete lift or for basic strength and power enhancement. For example, full cleans and snatches require the athlete to squat during the catching of the weight. Power cleans and snatches require the athlete to catch the weight in a more vertical position. The bar needs to be pulled a greater distance because of the higher receiving position. These variations are more commonly used among athletes who are not Olympic weightlifters. Other variations (called **transfer exercises**) are described.

Coaches teach each of these lifts in progressions starting with the clean and later the snatch. Learning the technical aspects of the clean initially assists in the transition to learning the snatch. For example, when teaching the top position of the snatch, a coach may use a sequence such as:

Behind-the-neck press (snatch grip) → overhead squat → drop snatch

The first exercise teaches proper proprioception of the bar in the overhead position. The second exercise builds upon the first by teaching the athlete to descend/ascend (squat) with the bar in the overhead position. The third exercise builds upon the first two by having the athlete drop into the overhead squat position rather than starting

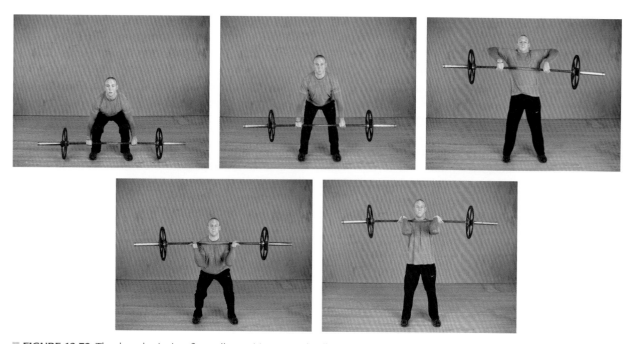

FIGURE 13.72. The clean: beginning, first pull, transition, second pull, and catch positions.

with it. All three exercises build strength and confidence in the athlete to help prepare for further progressions involving snatching, squatting, and catching the bar in the overhead position.

Ideally, these exercises should be performed on a wooden lifting platform with bumper plates that can easily be dropped without causing damage. Although excessive dropping or throwing of weights is not recommended, the athlete is properly taught to drop the

weights when learning the Olympic lifts. This increases safety as there is a greater chance for injury to occur if the bar is not properly dropped on the platform. It is important that the platform remain clear so no ricochet of bar takes place when dropped. If possible, the athlete should attempt to lower his or her center of gravity (COG) as much as possible before releasing the bar. This means the bar will be dropped from a lesser height, which helps preserve equipment as well as ensure safety. The athlete

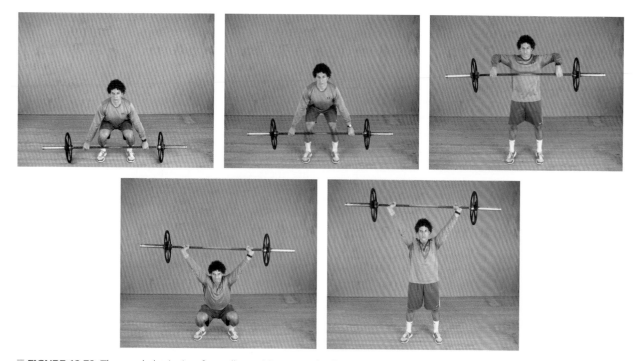

FIGURE 13.73. The snatch: beginning, first pull, transition, second pull, and catch positions.

must keep all body segments behind the falling bar and should use hands (on top of bar) to guide bar downward and minimize rebounding.

For the power clean and snatch, similar phases have been identified. These phases include the starting position, the first pull (BB is pulled from the floor), a transition phase prior to the second pull, the second pull, the catch, and the finish typically performed within 1 second. The duration of the lift and muscle power depends upon the loading, size, and skill level of the athletes (8). Critical here is the displacement of the bar and this is highly related to maximum vertical bar velocity (20). Taller athletes need to move the bar a greater distance with higher velocities. One differentiating factor between skilled and lesser-skilled weightlifters is the timing of the phases especially from the transition to the second pull (8).

The Starting Position

The starting position for each lift will vary in some respects but be similar in others. The feet are placed approximately at hip width (similar to a vertical jump position), toes pointed slightly outward, and the bar is located on the floor near (or touching) the shins. The hips and trunk are flexed forming an angle of 25–50 degrees with the ground, with the hips positioned close to or slightly above the knees (6). The trunk is more upright (larger angle) and hips are higher during the clean because of the narrower grip (using a hook grip) width compared to the snatch. The higher hip position allows heavier loads to be lifted compared to the lower hip position (and less weight) seen with the snatch. Shoulders are positioned directly over or slightly in front of the bar with the body's COG located over the middle of the foot. The low back is kept flat by hyperextending the lumbar spine and retracting the shoulder girdle (sticking the chest out). The head is straight or slightly upward and the arms grasp the bar with elbows extended and out and wrists are flexed. Rotating the elbows outward assists the athlete in maintaining proper bar displacement and keeping the elbow straight throughout pulling. A wide grip width is used for the snatch and a shoulder width grip is used for the clean. For the hang clean or hang snatch, the bar begins either above or below the knee depending on the variation.

First Pull

During the first pull, the bar is pulled toward the body (4–12 cm for the snatch; 3–10 cm for the clean) and is lifted off of the ground to about 31% of the athlete's height for the clean and approximately 35% for the snatch (6). The first pull is produced mostly by knee extension (~35–50 degrees) and plantar flexion (to where shins are vertical) with little change in the trunk angle (remains ~30–32 degrees), and the COG shifts toward the heels.

Trunk angle may slightly increase by the end of this phase and elbows remain extended. Shoulders move in front of the bar. This phase typically begins at a knee angle between 80 and 110 degrees but reaches an angle of 145–155 degrees by conclusion (6). The angle tends to be higher when performing the snatch compared to the clean. In skilled weightlifters observed during competition performing maximal attempts, a rise in force, vertical and horizontal (anterior to posterior) bar velocity, and bar acceleration is seen as the BB is lifted off the floor during this phase (7,14,20). Generally, this phase lasts ~0.50 second and the bar is lifted ~1.5 m·s⁻¹ for the snatch and ~1.2 m·s⁻¹ for the clean (6).

Transition Phase

The transition (or adjustment) phase is characterized by unweighting, or a reduction in force applied to the ground with a negative bar acceleration and slower vertical bar velocity (despite upward movement of the bar) (2,7,14). Approximately 10 degrees or more of knee flexion is seen (*double knee bend*) with a concomitant increase in trunk extension of 35–40 degrees (7). Knees may reach an angle range of 125–135 degrees. The bar reaches the lower third of the thigh for the clean and middle of the thigh for the snatch. Although force applied to the ground and bar acceleration decrease during the transition phase, this phase is critical to optimal lifting technique and performance. Postural realignment occurs, which reduces the back and hip extensor moment arms of resistance; an SSC enhancement is included due to the countermovement; and realignment allows for a second pull with a more vertical torso posture in the strongest area of the ROM, which allows for greater force and power yielding greater bar displacement (7).

Second Pull

The second pull is the most explosive phase and takes ~0.1–0.25 second with the snatch requiring more time than the clean (6). Bar is pulled upward and slightly away from the body by powerful extension of the hip, knee, and ankle joints. A rise in force, bar acceleration, and peak vertical and horizontal bar velocity is seen during the second pull (2,7,14,20). Analyses of Olympic weightlifters show power production is much higher during the second pull than the first pull (13). The second pull poses similar kinetic characteristics to a vertical jump (15). Up to 94% of the work done by a weightlifter is completed by the time the bar reaches peak velocity (13). The bar is pulled slightly away from the athlete and COG shifts toward the toes. Garhammer (14) showed bar velocities during the pull for the snatch compared to the clean tend to be ~10%–20% higher, as the bar is lifted to ~60% of the athlete's stature (2). During competition, bar velocities during the pulling phases are ~1.8–2.1 m·s⁻¹ (14,20). Others have reported second pull bar velocities of 1.65–2.05 m·s^{-1} for the snatch and 1.2–1.6 m·s^{-1} for the clean (6). Force applied to the bar decreases at the top of the second pull as the athlete prepares to pull him/her under the bar for the catch. At no time during the pull are the elbows bent.

The Catch

The next phase entails the athletes positioning themselves under the bar for the catch. The bar is still rising in both lifts when the athlete pulls himself or herself underneath during the catch position. The athlete does not pull to max height and then descend underneath. Rather, they occur almost simultaneously (6). The bar reaches approximately 68%–78% of height for the snatch and 55%–65% of height for the clean. After the second pull, the athlete's feet leave the ground and move laterally into the receiving position. The arms are used to pull the body down under the bar. Optimal bar trajectory entails pulling the bar toward the body during the first pull, moving the bar slightly away from the body during the second pull, and moving the bar closer to the body as the athlete prepares for the catch (resembling an S-shaped pattern of motion) (2,14,20).

The receiving positions for both lifts are critical to optimal performance. For the snatch, after the second pull the feet move out into a squatting position (wider than hip width). The slightly wider stance facilitates stability and brings the hips over the feet. While the feet are moving, the arms pull on the bar thereby accelerating the athlete's ability to descend under the bar (the athlete facilitates descent and does not merely drop under the bar). Elbows are wide, trunk is upright, wrists turn over, and the bar rotates. Throughout the descent the athlete applies force to the bar to support the weight in the full squat position. Lastly, the athlete flexes the shoulders, pushes the head forward, and extends hips into an overhead squat finish.

For the clean, similar lower-body movement is seen (feet move out into a squat position). The athlete pulls himself or herself down forcefully and receives the bar at the shoulder position in a lower position than the snatch because the heavier bar is not lifted as high during the second pull. During foot landing, the wrists rotate around the bar, elbows push forward and upward creating a shelf to catch the weight. The bar is caught on the shoulders and chest and the loading forces the athlete down into a deeper front squat position. Upper arms should be parallel to the ground, knees are over feet, and the athlete completes the lift by performing a front squat.

> ✓ **VARIATIONS AND EXERCISES** *DB or KB snatch (above or below knee, from floor), single-leg DB snatch, one-arm snatch (BB, DB, or KB), pressing snatch balance, drop snatch, DB or KB power clean, squat power clean, hang clean (below or above knee), stop clean and stop snatch, DB or KB hang clean, single-leg DB or KB hang clean, squat hang clean, keg cleans/snatch, keg toss, and log cleans.*

Interpreting Research

Kinematic Analysis of the Snatch

Gourgoulis V, Aggelousis N, Mavromatis G, Garas A. Three-dimensional kinematic analysis of the snatch of elite Greek weightlifters. *J Sport Sci.* 2000;18:643–652.

Gourgoulis et al. (16) performed a kinematic analysis of the snatch in elite Greek Olympic weightlifters and reported the following:

- Knee angles of ~143 degrees (following first pull), ~120 degrees (following transition), and ~156 degrees (following second pull)
- Max ankle and hip extension values of 117 and 177 degrees, respectively
- Knee extension angular velocity (first pull = ~3.86 rad·s^{-1}; second pull = ~6.32 rad·s^{-1})
- Ankle extension angular velocity (first pull = ~1.51 rad·s^{-1}; second pull = ~4.35 rad·s^{-1})
- Hip extension angular velocity (first pull = ~2.81 rad·s^{-1}; second pull = ~8.09 rad·s^{-1})
- Bar displacement (toward lifter = ~6.2 cm; away from lifter = ~3.2 cm)
- Maximal vertical velocity of BB = ~1.67 m·s^{-1}
- Decrease in bar velocity during transition = ~0.05 m·s^{-1}
- Work (first pull = ~612 J; second pull = 413 J)
- Power (first pull = ~1,302 W; second pull = ~2,577 W)
- Phase duration (first pull = ~0.47 s; transition = ~0.15 s; second pull = ~0.16 s; turnover under bar = ~0.23 s)

HOOK GRIP

To optimally perform the Olympic lifting pulling movements, a strong grip is necessary. Isometric grip strength training is important. Most athletes prefer to use the **hook grip**. The hook grip (Fig. 13.74) entails wrapping the thumb around the bar and then wrapping the first three fingers around the thumb and bar. This grip configuration allows for greater support during explosive pulling movements. Because the thumb is relatively weak compared to flexion strength of the fingers as a whole, wrapping the thumb around the bar puts the thumb in a better force-producing position as it can then be supported by the flexion strength of most of the fingers. As flexion strength of the fingers and thumb increase, so does the magnitude of friction between the hand and the bar (static friction force = coefficient of static friction × reactive force). Because of the position of the thumb and the greater static friction observed with the hook grip, pain and discomfort are common in athletes accommodating to the hook grip. Bruising can occur, as well as skin irritations from the knurling of the bar when high levels of pressure are applied. Adaptations take place and eventually the discomfort subsides to where the athlete becomes comfortable. Many athletes release the hook grip (in lieu of a normal grip) when the hands rotate to where the palms are facing up (catch in the pull or preparation for the jerk).

DETERMINING SNATCH GRIP WIDTH

There are two basic ways to estimate proper grip width for the snatch. One method is to have the athlete stand and abduct one arm laterally (parallel to the ground) to the side while making a fist. A tape measure is used to measure the length of the opposite shoulder to the fist. This length is used as the grip width. A second method entails the athlete standing and abducting both arms laterally (parallel to the ground) to the side with elbows flexed. A tape measure is used to determine the length from elbow to elbow as the snatch grip width. Some have recommended using a grip wide enough so that a 49–63 degrees angle is observed between the arms and the bar, or have suggested a position to where the bar comfortably lies in the crease of the hips when trunk/hips are flexed forward with arms fully extended (6). These methods provide a good estimate or at least the starting grip width that can be altered slightly based on technical aspects of the athlete, *e.g.*, shoulder flexibility and strength, elbow joint stability, and pulling mechanics. A good way to assess the grip width is to examine the overhead squat position. The bar should be ~4–6 in. above the head (depending on the comfort level).

Case Study 13.1

Steve is a recent college graduate with a degree in Health and Exercise Science and a concentration in Strength and Conditioning. He was hired by a Division III college and was put in charge of strength and conditioning for the school's football team. As part of his lifting program, Steve required all athletes to perform the power clean because of its utility for power and performance enhancement. However, several incoming freshmen have no experience with Olympic lifting. As a student (and athlete), Steve was properly instructed to teach the power clean in stages (using variations) rather than the complete lift. Thus, Steve grouped these athletes together and began instructional sessions to teach proper technique.

Question for Consideration: If you were Steve, what progressions would you use in order to teach this exercise to this group of athletes?

THE JERK

The jerk is a critical component to Olympic weightlifting (Fig. 13.75). The majority of missed attempts in competition in the clean and jerk result from a missed jerk. The jerk can be described in several phases: the starting position, descent (or half squat or dip), braking, thrust, and split and finish. The athlete starts in the top-front squat position where the hips and shoulders are aligned over the rear segment of the middle of the foot, feet are hip width with toes slightly pointed outward, head slightly back, and arms are relaxed (near parallel to the floor) with elbows in front of the bar as the bar rests in the shelf position. Tensing the arms could result in the athlete

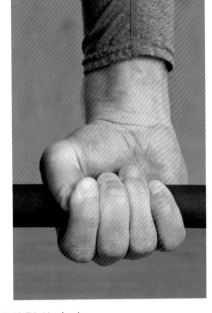
FIGURE 13.74. Hook grip.

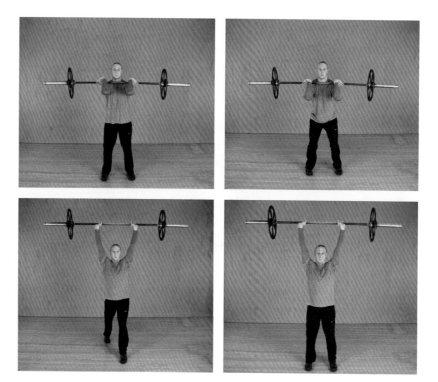

■ FIGURE 13.75. The jerk: beginning, descent, thrust, and finish positions.

pushing the bar forward instead of vertical. The descent or dip provides a countermovement before the explosive thrust of the bar upward. Knee flexion (~114–132 degrees) and ankle dorsiflexion occur in a vertical manner with COG shifting slightly forward (6). Maximum velocities range within 0.8–1.2 m·s^{-1} with peak velocity occurring halfway through the ROM of the dip with a duration of 0.20–0.25 seconds (17). The end of the dip marks the beginning of the braking phase, which takes ~0.12 seconds, and involves further descent equaling a magnitude of one-third of the overall countermovement depth (6). This phase provides a transition between slowing down the countermovement and subsequent beginning of the thrust. The end of this phase is marked by completely stopped downward movement of the bar. Elite weightlifters squat to ~12%–14% of their standing height to knee angles of ~99–110 degrees, spend less time braking toward the bottom of the dip than lesser-skilled individuals, and elite weightlifters tend to show horizontal bar displacements of less than 2 cm compared to lesser-skilled lifters (17).

The thrust encompasses explosive extension of the hips, knees, and ankles driving the bar upward while rising on the toes. Bar velocity ranges between 1.2 and 1.8 m·s^{-1} (6,17). Grabe and Widule (17) showed that the thrust was characterized by peak hip velocities of 4.5–5.0 rad·s^{-1}, peak bar velocities of 1.2–1.4 m·s^{-1}, max knee angles of 145–154 degrees, and performed for 0.22–0.28 seconds. Peak vertical bar velocity allows the bar to reach near its maximal height. The remaining bar elevation is brought about by forceful pushing up on the bar from the arms in order to assist in diving under the bar for the split. Most athletes tend to split when performing the jerk; however, some prefer to use the squat position when diving under the bar. For the split, one hip flexes (front leg) and one extends (back leg) to form a stable base support. The back leg lands before the front leg as the feet leave the ground. The split has been characterized by a duration of 0.20–0.28 seconds and max split velocity of 1.6–2.6 m·s^{-1} (front = 1.6–1.8 m·s^{-1}; rear = 2.2–2.6 m·s^{-1}) (17). The back leg is nearly straight (a little more than 2-ft length posterior from the hip) with a knee angle of ~160 degrees with foot balanced on the toes. The front leg has a knee angle of >90 degrees with shin perpendicular to the floor and is located approximately 1-ft length in front of the hip. The bar is positioned slightly behind the athlete's head on the same vertical plane as the shoulders and hips. Head is forward, and back is hyperextended. Bar trajectory for the jerk is nearly vertical for the decent and vertical with slight backward movement during the thrust and catch. For the finish, weight is transferred to the rear foot as the front leg pushes backward.

OTHER VARIATIONS AND SIMILAR EXERCISES *Power jerk, behind-the-neck jerk (clean and snatch grip), KB jerk.*

Variations of the Olympic Lifts

SNATCH/CLEAN HIGH PULL
Rating: B

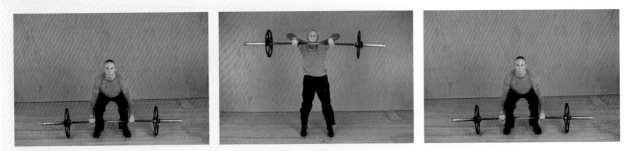

■ **FIGURE 13.76.**

- Starting position is similar to the snatch (wide grip) or clean (narrow grip). Bar rests on the floor or above/below the knees or on the thigh for high pulls from the hang position.
- With torso erect and elbows fully extended, the bar is explosively lifted upward by extending the hip, knee, and ankle joints. Shoulders remain over the bar for as long as possible while keeping the bar close to the body.
- At maximal plantar flexion, the shoulders are elevated and the bar is pulled high.
- Bar is returned to the starting position or safely released to platform.

- This version is less complex as the athlete does not have to descend under the bar and catch the weight. It is an excellent version to teach athletes new to weightlifting. It can be used to train for power as it is performed explosively with less complexity.

> ✔ **OTHER VARIATIONS AND SIMILAR EXERCISES** *DB or KB high pull (from floor or hang position), single-leg DB or KB high pull, snatch pull (to knee), snatch/clean shrugs.*

BEHIND-THE-NECK PRESS (SNATCH AND CLEAN GRIP)
Rating: B

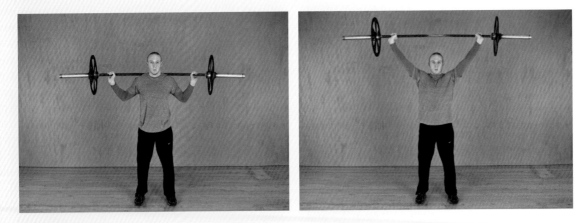

■ **FIGURE 13.77.**

- Athlete assumes a position similar to the back squat with bar resting across the shoulders behind the head. Either a snatch grip or clean grip can be used. Feet are shoulder width or slightly wider apart.
- The bar is pressed upward via shoulder abduction and elbow extension and returned back to the starting

position. Wrists should be hyperextended at top of the movement.
- This exercise helps the athlete learn proper overhead position of the bar.

DROP SNATCH
Rating: C

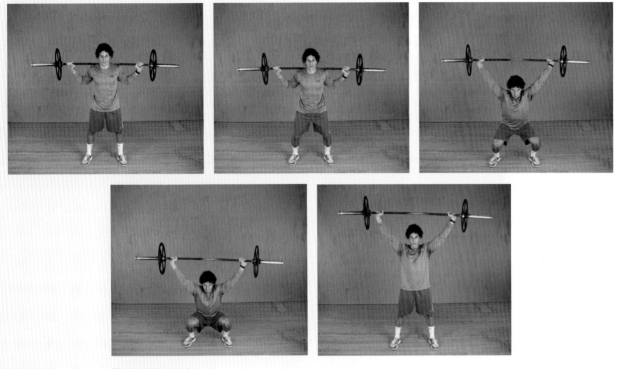

FIGURE 13.78.

- Athlete begins in a back squat position (bar on shoulders) with a snatch grip and feet hip width apart.
- Athlete dips and drives the bar upward, then jumps feet into the normal squat foot width position and drops as quickly as possible into the low receiving snatch position. Athlete should push up on the bar while dropping; the result is to push the body down into position rather than lifting the bar upward.

- The ascent is synonymous with an overhead squat.
- A common mistake is to press first then drop under. The bar moves very little upward when performed correctly.
- Some variations include the pressing drop snatch and the heaving drop snatch.

ROMANIAN DEADLIFT
Rating: B

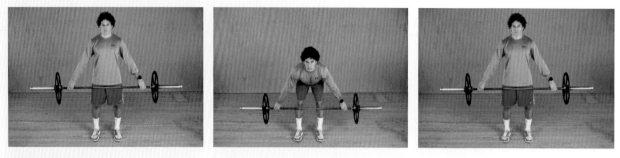

■ **FIGURE 13.79.**

- Athlete starts with a snatch grip or clean grip with the bar at hip level. Knees are slightly bent, elbows are extended, chest is out, and back is hyperextended.
- The bar moves downward close to the thigh to a position below the level of the knees. This is brought about by hip/trunk flexion with slight flexion of the knees.

- The bar is lifted back up to the starting position via hip, trunk, knee, and ankle extension.
- This exercise is useful for learning the proper position during pulling movements.

FRONT SQUAT
Rating: B

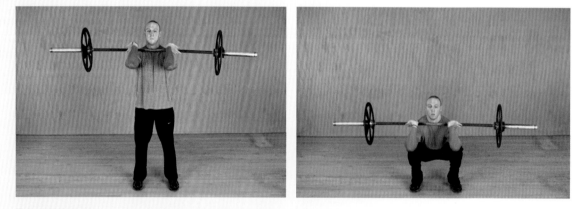

■ **FIGURE 13.80.**

- Athlete unracks the bar in the shelf or rack position with the bar resting comfortably on upper chest and shoulders, elbows up and in, chest out and lower back hyperextended, wrists relaxed and hyperextended, and feet shoulder width apart.
- Athlete descends to the parallel position (or lower) by flexing the hips, knees, and ankles and maintains an erect torso to keep the bar placed in the proper position.

- Athlete ascends by extending the hips, knees, and ankles while keeping the posture erect.
- Excellent for developing strength and balance and serves as a beneficial transfer exercise for the clean. Common mistakes include shifting weight forward, leaning forward excessively, and tightening wrists/ arms to lose rack position.

OVERHEAD SQUAT
Rating: B

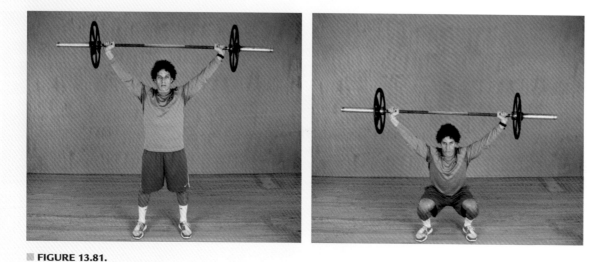

FIGURE 13.81.

- Athlete grasps BB with a snatch width grip behind the neck and presses it into the overhead snatch position. Shoulders are flexed, elbows are fully extended, the chest is out, low back is hyperextended, and the head is forward. Feet are shoulder width or slightly wider.
- Athlete descends to the parallel position (or lower) by flexing the hips, knees, and ankles and maintains an erect torso with the bar maintained in the overhead position.
- Athlete ascends by extending the hips, knees, and ankles while keeping the posture erect. Some common mistakes are heels coming off of the platform (due to not positioning hips properly during descent possibly due to poor shoulder flexibility), forward movement of the bar, bending the elbows, and excessive forward lean.

OTHER VARIATIONS AND SIMILAR EXERCISES *Overhead split squat; can be performed with kegs, DB, KB, and sand bags.*

PUSH PRESS
Rating: B

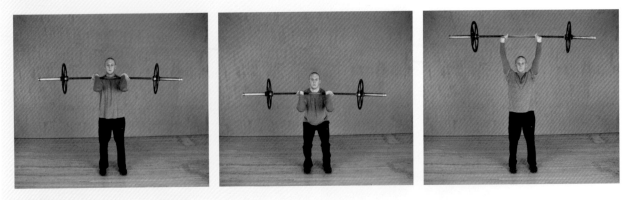

FIGURE 13.82.

- Bar is grasped with a closed, pronated grip slightly wider than or at shoulder width at the level of shoulders. Elbows are out (arm parallel to the ground) and wrists extended. Feet are slightly wider than shoulder width, and hips and knees are slightly flexed.
- A countermovement (dip) is performed followed by an explosive push of the bar upward by extending the knees, hips, and ankles. BW is shifted to the balls of the feet and the foot is plantar flexed. The bar is pushed from shoulder level until elbows are fully extended overhead.

- Bar is lowered to the starting position, and hips and knees are flexed to absorb the weight of bar.

> ✓ **OTHER VARIATIONS AND SIMILAR EXERCISES** DB or KB push press, behind-the-neck push press *(clean and snatch grip)*, keg/sand bag push press, mastiff bar push press.

TIPS FOR SELECTING EXERCISES

Some general tips for selecting/performing exercises include:

1. *Build a base on good technique*—regardless of the exercise; the athlete should have attained good technique prior to progression to heavier weights or more challenging exercises.
2. *Start with basic exercises and progress to more challenging exercises*—the athlete or coach should select some basic exercises to begin and progress to more challenging exercises over time as conditioning improves.
3. *Select exercises that work all major muscle groups*—all major muscle groups should be targeted during RT.

4. *Challenging exercises yield the best results*—in many cases, the exercises that are more difficult and stress several major muscle groups yield better performance results. These core and structural exercises should form the base of the training program. For example, multijoint exercises such as the squat and bench press form the core of many RT programs targeting maximal strength. The Olympic lifts should form the core for power training.
5. *Vary exercises regularly*—exposing the athlete to many exercises can be used as a successful conditioning tool. Over time, coaches can determine which ones work better for certain athletes. Although the coach may have a staple of exercises that form the core of the program, assistance exercises can be varied regularly (every 4–6 weeks).

Summary Points

✔ Proper breathing for most exercises entails inhaling during the negative phase and exhaling during the positive phase. There are exceptions where a Valsalva maneuver is beneficial to increasing IAP for exercises that stress the lower back or are explosive.

✔ Joint motion occurs in sagittal, frontal, and transverse planes. Several exercises are multiplanar where motion takes place in two or three planes.

✔ Resistance exercises may be performed using BW, BBs, DBs, SBs, BOSU balls, MBs, thick bars, KBs, bands/tubing, kegs, sand bags, tires, logs, and other implements.

✔ Any alteration of posture, hand/foot width, and hand/foot position changes muscle activation so each exercise variation is treated as a distinct exercise.

✔ A multitude of lower-body, upper-body, and core resistance exercises can be performed so variation in exercise selection can add new dimensions to RT workouts.

✔ The Olympic lifts and variations are the most complex exercises. Because of their reliance on most major muscle groups, the Olympic lifts are performed at explosive velocities and are excellent for increasing total body strength and power.

Review Questions

1. From the anatomical position, a standing lateral raise (abduction) is performed in:
   a. The sagittal plane
   b. The frontal plane
   c. The transverse plane
   d. No plane

2. When performing the squat exercise, the athlete:
   a. Should lean forward as far as possible during the descent
   b. Should keep his/her head down facing the ground during each phase
   c. Should drive the hips back so the knees and toes are level during the descent
   d. Should hold his/her breath from start to completion of the set

3. The greatest amount of power produced in the power clean and snatch occurs during the:
   a. First pull
   b. Transition phase
   c. Second pull
   d. Catch

4. Which of the following exercises specifically targets the erector spinae muscle group?
   a. Hyperextension
   b. Leg curl
   c. DB fly
   d. Crunch

5. Adding a rotation to a crunch exercise increases the activity of which muscle?
   a. Biceps femoris
   b. Gastrocnemius
   c. Pectoralis major
   d. External oblique

6. The push-up can be made more challenging to shoulder and trunk muscles by performing which exercise?
   a. With one leg abducted and elevated off of the ground
   b. With staggered hands
   c. On an SB
   d. All of the above

7. Using a thick bar during a pulling exercise (deadlift) is a good way to increase grip strength.   T F

8. The conventional deadlift requires the athlete to keep the arms inside the legs while using a wide stance.   T F

9. One method used to determine snatch grip width is to have the athlete stand and abduct one arm laterally and measure the length of the opposite shoulder to the fist with a tape measure.   T F

10. The hyperextension exercise primarily works the quadriceps muscles.   T F

11. Internal/external rotation shoulder exercises are good for athletes involved in throwing sports.   T F

12. The bar velocity for the second pull in the snatch is higher than the clean.   T F

References

1. Barnett C, Kippers V, Turner P. Effects of variations of the bench press exercise on the EMG activity of five shoulder muscles. *J Strength Cond Res*. 1995;9:222–227.

2. Baumann W, Gross V, Quade K, Galbierz P, Schwirtz A. The snatch technique of world class weightlifters at the 1985 world championships. *Int J Sport Biomech*. 1988;4:68–89.

3. Boyle M. *Functional Training for Sports*. Champaign (IL): Human Kinetics; 2004.

4. Cholewicki J, McGill SM, Norman RW. Lumbar spine loads during the lifting of extremely heavy weights. *Med Sci Sports Exerc*. 1991; 23:1179–1186.

5. Cook G. *Athletic Body in Balance*. Champaign (IL): Human Kinetics; 2003.

6. Drechsler A. *The Weightlifting Encyclopedia: A Guide to World Class Performance*. Whitestone (NY): A is A Communications; 1998.

7. Enoka R. The pull in Olympic weightlifting. *Med Sci Sports*. 1979; 11:131–137.

8. Enoka R. Load- and skill-related changes in segmental contributions to a weightlifting movement. *Med Sci Sports Exerc*. 1988; 20:178–187.

9. Escamilla RF, Fleisig GS, Lowry TM, Barrentine SW, Andrews JR. A three-dimensional biomechanical analysis of the squat during varying stance widths. *Med Sci Sports Exerc*. 2001;33:984–998.

10. Escamilla RF, Francisco AC, Fleisig GS, et al. A three-dimensional biomechanical analysis of sumo and conventional style deadlifts. *Med Sci Sports Exerc*. 2000;32:1265–1275.

11. Escamilla RF, Francisco AC, Kayes AV, Speer KP, Moorman CT. An electromyographic analysis of sumo and conventional style deadlifts. *Med Sci Sports Exerc*. 2002;34:682–688.

12. Gallucci JG, Challis JH. Examining the role of the gastrocnemius during the leg curl exercise. *J Appl Biomech*. 2002;18:15–27.

13. Garhammer J. Power production by Olympic weightlifters. *Med Sci Sports Exerc*. 1980;12:54–60.

14. Garhammer J. Biomechanical profiles of Olympic weightlifters. *Int J Sports Biomech*. 1985;1:122–130.

15. Garhammer J, Gregor R. Propulsion forces as a function of intensity for weightlifting and vertical jumping. *J Appl Sports Sci Res*. 1992;6:129–134.

16. Gourgoulis V, Aggelousis N, Mavromatis G, Garas A. Three-dimensional kinematic analysis of the snatch of elite Greek weightlifters. *J Sport Sci*. 2000;18:643–652.

17. Grabe SA, Widule CJ. Comparative biomechanics of the jerk in Olympic weightlifting. *Res Q Exerc Sport*. 1988;59:1–8.

18. Hedrick A. Using uncommon implements in the training program of athletes. *Strength Cond J*. 2003;25:18–22.

19. Hoffman JR, Ratamess NA. *A Practical Guide to Developing Resistance Training Programs*. Monterey (CA): Coaches Choice Books; 2006.

20. Isaka T, Okada J, Funato K. Kinematic analysis of the barbell during the snatch movement of elite Asian weight lifters. *J Appl Biomech*. 1996;12:508–516.

21. Jones B. *The Complete Sandbag Training Course*. Nevada City (CA), Iron Mind Enterprises; 2004.

22. Kubik B. *Dinosaur Training: Lost Secrets of Strength & Development*. Louisville (KY): Brooks D. Kubik, 1996.

23. Santana JC. *The Essence of Program Design*. Boca Raton (FL): IHP; 2004.

24. Schuler L, Mejia M. *The Men's Health Home Workout Bible*. New York (NY): Rodale, Inc.; 2002.

25. Signorile JF, Zink AJ, Szwed SP. A comparative electromyographical investigation of muscle utilization patterns using various hand positions during the lat pull-down. *J Strength Cond Res*. 2002;16:539–546.

26. Simmons L. Bands and chains. *Powerlifting USA*. 1999;22:26–27.

27. Tsatsouline P. *The Russian Kettlebell Challenge: Xtreme Fitness for Hard Living Comrades*. St. Paul (MN): Dragon Door Publications, Inc.; 2001.

28. Urquhart DM, Hodges PW, Allen TJ, Story IH. Abdominal muscle recruitment during a range of voluntary exercises. *Man Ther*. 2005;10:144–153.

29. Vera-Garcia FJ, Elvira JL, Brown SH, McGill SM. Effects of abdominal stabilization maneuvers on the control of spine motion and stability against sudden trunk perturbations. *J Electromyogr Kinesiol*. 2007;17:556–567.

30. Zeller BL, McCrory JL, Kibler WB, Uhl TL. Differences in kinematics and electromyographic activity between men and women during the single-legged squat. *Am J Sports Med*. 2003;31:449–456.

14

Plyometric Training

After completing this chapter, you will be able to:

· Define plyometrics and understand the physiology underlying the ergogenic effects
· Discuss how plyometric training enhances various components of fitness and athletic performance
· Discuss the performance of more than 40 plyometric exercises and variations
· Discuss how to properly manipulate acute program variables when designing plyometric training programs
· Discuss how to integrate plyometric training with other training modalities

The term *plyometrics* has had a few meanings and interpretations over the years depending on whether one is describing pliometrics, classic plyometrics, or modern plyometrics. *Pliometric* exercise translates into "more length" as loaded or explosive eccentric (ECC) muscle actions with no reversible, *e.g.*, concentric (CON), muscle actions are used (63). For example, landing from a jump involves yielding or high ECC loading, where impact forces can exceed the propulsive forces developed during a jump (63). The landing is pliometric where the athlete braces for support (by manipulating the degree of hip, knee, and ankle flexion) but does not follow with a CON or propulsion phase, *e.g.*, performing an exercise called a *depth landing*.

Classic plyometrics (note the different spelling) is the term used to describe the origins of plyometric training where it was originally known as "shock training." Shock training consisted mostly of depth jumps and variations where the intensity was ultrahigh and predominately performed by well-trained to elite strength and power athletes. The term *plyometrics* was first coined in the 1970s by track and field coach Fred Wilt (9) but was based on shock training. European athletes were known to use classic plyometric exercises and were achieving superior athletic performances in sports such as track and field, weightlifting, and gymnastics. One such coach/scientist was Dr. Yuri Verkhoshansky, known by many as the modern-day Father of Plyometrics, published his first study in plyometrics in 1964 (known as the *Shock Method* of training) (59,60). Dr. Verkhoshansky preferred the term *shock training* or *shock method* when describing the classic plyometrics because the high-intensity element distinguished itself from modern plyometrics (60). In fact, Dr. Verkhoshansky has proposed the term

powermetrics to be used in lieu of plyometrics to limit confusion (60). Classic plyometrics were characterized by this ultra-intense system of depth jumping where frequency and volume were kept low to avoid overtraining and rest intervals between repetitions and sets were long.

Modern plyometrics, or simply *plyometrics*, is the term commonly used in the United States which embodies shock training as a segment but also embraces inclusion of exercises that simply consist of *plyometric actions*. *Plyometric actions* refer to the lengthening or prestretching of skeletal muscles under loading that allows a more forceful CON muscle action. Plyometric actions utilize the stretch-shortening cycle (SSC) and are substantially reliant upon loading and the rate of lengthening during the ECC phase. Plyometric actions not only include high-intensity movements such as depth jumps but also include simple activities such as walking, jogging, hopping, and multidirectional movements where the SSC increases mechanical efficiency. By incorporating the premise of plyometric actions into modern plyometric training, many other exercises have been included in athletic training programs. In fact, modern plyometrics consist of a continuum of exercises from low to high intensity whereas classic plyometrics consisted entirely of high-intensity exercises. Although some plyometric drills may be considered low or moderate intensity, they are still performed explosively but consist of less ECC loading than classic plyometrics. Notwithstanding the terminology differences, plyometrics allow an athlete to reach maximal strength and power in the shortest period of time (10). Interest in plyometric training has increased greatly since the 1970s. Coaches and scientists alike began to attribute the performance enhancement to plyometric training since it was a new training modality. The benefits

Myths & Misconceptions

Modern Plyometric Training Consists Entirely of Depth Jumps

Critics of plyometric training have questioned its utility in some populations stating it is too high in intensity. However, the misconception is that plyometrics consist entirely of high-intensity depth jumps. That is, they refer to classic plyometrics as the benchmark but fail to recognize the exercise selection differences in modern plyometric training. Although classic plyometric training consisted mostly of depth jumps, it has evolved into a more comprehensive system of training utilizing diverse explosive exercises of low, moderate, and high intensity. If one accepts the terminology/interpretation that modern plyometrics target plyometric actions, then plyometric training consists of jumps, hops, skips, bounding, and upper-body throws, tosses, and passes in addition to power-specific exercises seen in sports, e.g., throws and swings in baseball and kicks, blocks, and strikes in martial arts. These exercises increase force/power and mechanical efficiency of the athlete. Other modes of exercise also include plyometric actions but are considered separate training modalities, e.g., sprint, agility, and resistance training (RT). Plyometric exercises are based on complexity and intensity and can be modified to train many populations. Thus, many individuals benefit from plyometric training independent of the inclusion of depth jumps.

of plyometric training in enhancing explosive power performance soon were seen by coaches all over the world and became a staple in the training of strength/power athletes into modern day. For example, more than 95% of Major League Baseball (17), 100% of National Basketball Association (55), 100% National Hockey League strength and conditioning (S&C) coaches (16), and ~94% of National Football League S&C coaches (15) incorporate plyometrics in their athletes' workouts.

Plyometric exercises are classified based on the intensity level. *Maximal plyometrics* involve ultrahigh-intense muscular contractions and typically comprise depth jumps and variations (60). *Submaximal plyometrics* involve low- and moderate-intensity drills that comprise most exercises other than depth jumps (60). In addition, plyometric exercises can be impact-oriented (jumps, hops, skips, plyo push-ups) where the reversible action is stimulated by contact with the ground or object, or non-impact-oriented (strikes, thrusts, throws, passes, and tosses without prior catching of the ball) where the drill is an open chain, i.e., the ECC and CON phases are not augmented by direct contact with the ground or object (60). Both types are included in plyometric training programs. For terminology consistency, it is important to note that plyometric training is described in terms of modern plyometric exercises throughout this chapter.

PHYSIOLOGY OF PLYOMETRIC EXERCISE

Plyometric exercise stimulates SSC activity. The countermovement initiates the stretch reflex that leads to an ECC muscle action that precedes a brief ISOM phase and subsequent CON muscle action. The ECC phase (plus prior delay seen between muscle activation via neural action

potentials and muscle contraction [*electromechanical delay*]) is referred to as the *amortization phase*. The length of the isometric (ISOM) phase between ECC and CON actions is referred to as *coupling time*. The subsequent CON muscle action is augmented by the stretch reflex and the release of elastic energy. The muscle-tendon complex acts like a rubber band when it is stretched. It has elastic potential and the ability to rapidly store and release elastic energy. Elastic energy stored primarily within the series elastic component (tendon, actin, myosin, structural proteins) during an ECC muscle action augments muscle force and power during the CON phase when it follows right away. Maximal force and power can be expressed when the ISOM coupling time is minimal. It has been recommended that coupling time be less than 0.15 second, especially in athletes who possess higher percentages of fast-twitch (FT) muscle fibers (60). Thus, minimizing the length of the amortization phase and coupling time is critical for the athlete to develop maximal power. Energy can change forms and elastic energy is wasted as coupling time increases (elastic energy dissipates into heat energy in proportion to the length of the coupling phase). Elastic energy enhances muscular performance whereas heat energy has minimal effects. The use of elastic energy is maximized when the CON phase follows the ECC phase right away. The second major contributor to the SSC is the stretch reflex. Muscle spindles located within skeletal muscle fibers detect the magnitude and rate of length changes. The response is to send action potentials to the central nervous system where the agonist muscle's force production is enhanced while the antagonist muscles relax. In combination, both mechanisms contribute to SSC function although storage/use of elastic energy contributes to a greater extent (by up to 70%). With training, more energy can be stored and utilized as muscle force increases (63). Muscle power and rate of force development increase. This is critical to athletic performance where force must be maximized in short time periods. Plyometric training is designed to train the SSC via neural adaptations, reflex potentiation, and enhanced elastic potential of skeletal muscles. The selective recruitment of FT motor units is advantageous for acute power performance. Lastly, the FT units stay facilitated as activities performed after explosive plyometric exercises are enhanced to a greater extent (37).

PLYOMETRIC TRAINING AND ATHLETIC PERFORMANCE

Plyometric training has increased athletic performance in most studies. Plyometric training can increase jumping height and power (1,12,24,31,33,34,45,61), sprinting ability (11,12,34), agility (14,34), and peak isokinetic strength (30). A meta-analysis of 26 plyometric training studies has shown that plyometric training increases squat jump, countermovement vertical jump, countermovement vertical jump with arm swing, and drop jump performance by 4.7%, 8.7%, 7.5%, and 4.7%, respectively (33). Plyometric training increases muscle strength and hypertrophy, as well as induces fiber-type transitions (type IIX to IIA) similar to RT (45,61). The combination of plyometrics and RT is most effective for increasing vertical jumping ability (1,27,28,47), sprinting speed (14,28,47), agility (14), as well as improving motor performance such as kicking velocity (43). However, not all studies show augmentation of RT and plyometric training (29). Wilson et al. (62) showed that 8 weeks of RT consisting of 6 sets of 6–10 repetitions of squats produced similar increases in vertical jump height to plyometric training consisting of 3–6 sets of 8 repetitions of depth jumps from 20 to 70 cm heights (21% and 18%, respectively). In addition, 6–9 weeks of plyometric training can increase running economy in moderately trained runners and highly trained endurance athletes (53,58), and can improve 3-km race times in runners (56). Plyometric training enhances swimming block start performance (3), lateral reaction time and sprint ability in tennis players (51), throwing velocity in baseball players (8), and kicking speed in soccer players (54).

SIDEBAR   **MECHANICS OF THE VERTICAL JUMP**

The vertical jump consists of five distinct phases: (a) starting position, (b) countermovement, (c) jump or propulsion, (d) flight, and (e) landing. Athletes generate greatest force applied to the ground, power, and jump height from a hip-to-shoulder width stance. The countermovement is characterized by rapid hip and knee flexion, ankle dorsiflexion, and shoulder hyperextension. The jump or propulsion phase consists of explosive hip, trunk, and knee extension, plantar flexion, and shoulder flexion. Take-off velocity during the vertical jump is affected by: knee extension, 56%; plantar flexion, 22%; trunk extension, 10%; arm swing, 10%; and head swing, 2% (32). In the lower body during propulsion the hip, knee, and ankle contribute 40%, 24.2%, and 35.8% to the forces applied to the ground, respectively (50). Studies have documented the importance of the countermovement and arm-swing in maximizing power and height attained during the vertical jump (23). The arm-swing consists of an explosive forward and upward movement of the arms with the thumbs up. The arm-swing helps to keep the torso upright especially as the hips flex. Flight time increases in proportion to the vertical height attained and is dependent upon the power produced by the athlete. The landing style is critical to absorbing shock and minimizing joint stress. Lowering peak ground reaction force and increasing braking (by flexing the knees, hips, and dorsiflexing the ankles for better force distribution and shock absorption) is important. Greater stress is seen during a single-leg landing (greater valgus stress on knee, higher muscle activation, less knee flexion to absorb force) than during a double-leg landing (42). Women show greater valgus stress on the knee and greater relative ground reaction force during double-leg landings compared to men (42). Teaching proper landing mechanics is important to reducing the risk of injuries. Proper breathing consists of inhaling during the countermovement, temporary holding of breath during max propulsion, and exhalation upon elevation off of the ground (46).

DEPTH JUMPS

A staple of plyometric training has been the *depth jump* (or drop jump) since its early introduction in the 1950s into athletic training programs by Dr. Yuri Verkhoshansky (60). One of the most intense types of plyometric exercises, the depth jump has been commonly included in the S&C programs for athletes. The athlete steps off of a box or bench in a relaxed manner, lands (shock), and explosively jumps while spending minimal time on the ground. Biomechanical studies of the depth jump have shown it to be intense, yet effective for maximizing power. Bobbert et al. (4–6) have shown that (in comparison to countermovement jumps) depth jumps result in greater peak forces especially in the knees and ankles whereas the work performed by the hips is lower. The mechanics of the depth jump depend upon individual technique. Peak forces tend to be higher if athletes have minimal flexion of the hips and knees upon landing (a quick rebound) versus athletes who descend lower during the countermovement (4–6). The drop height is another consideration. The higher the drop height, the greater the vertical velocity attained by the athlete during descent, and, coupled with the athlete's mass, the higher drop height results in higher levels of force upon ground contact (63). Intensity increases as drop height increases. Most often, drop heights of 20–100 cm are used. Early literature in athletic training recommended 75–115 cm; however, others have recommended more conservative heights of 20–40 cm (6). Peak propulsion force increases in proportion to drop height (6). Bobbert et al. (6) showed that a depth jump from a 60-cm height produced a higher rate of loading and ground reaction force 1.5 times more than a depth jump performed from a 20-cm height. Greater negative work is performed with increasing drop heights (6). The optimal depth jump height is debatable and individualized as the athlete should demonstrate a smooth transition between ECC and CON phases. Some studies show greater vertical jump heights from higher drop heights (40 cm) up to a certain height whereas some studies show no vertical jump height differences between 20- and 85-cm jump heights (2,6). Similar increases in vertical jump performance following depth jump training at 50- and 100-cm heights were shown (38). Depth jump heights of ~20–40 cm or so may be used initially for athletes beginning depth jump training and gradual progression can take place once the athlete adapts. Because of the intense nature of the exercise, few sets (2–4) of up to 5–8 repetitions with long (2–10 min) rest intervals for 1–3 days per week have been recommended when maximal depth jumps are performed from large heights and/or with external loading (60).

PLYOMETRIC PROGRAM DESIGN

Plyometric training, like other modalities, is a composite of several acute program variables that can be manipulated to achieve a target goal. These variables include exercise selection and order, intensity, volume, frequency, and rest intervals. Designing a plyometric training program for athletes is multifactorial and should include planned progressive overload, specificity, and variation. Many factors need to be considered including the age/training status of the athlete, equipment availability, training surface, and recovery in between workouts, nutrition, and the integration of plyometrics with other training modalities. However, most plyometric training studies are not comparative. A wide variety of programs are effective for increasing performance but few studies compared changes when manipulating program variables. Thus, current plyometric guidelines rely mostly on coaches' practical experience with only some research support. Some other critical factors to plyometric training include the following:

- The quality of training is most critical. Each repetition should be performed with maximal effort, minimal amortization and coupling times, and explosive propulsion.
- Exercise selection should be as specific to the demands of the sport as possible. Sport-specific drills can be

Interpreting Research

The Effects of Resistance, Plyometric, and Combination Training on Power Production

Adams K, O'Shea JP, O'Shea KL, Climstein M. The effect of six weeks of squat, plyometric and squat-plyometric training on power production. *J Appl Sport Sci Res.* 1992;6:36–41.

Adams et al. (1) compared 6 weeks of squat, plyometric, or combined squat and plyometric training on power production. The periodized squat program consisted of a 2-day-per-week frequency where the Tuesday workout was higher in intensity than the Friday workout. Tuesday workouts consisted of 2–4 sets of 2–8 repetitions using 70%–100% of 1 RM whereas Friday workouts consisted of 1–2 sets of 8 repetitions using 50%–70% of 1 RM. The plyometric training program consisted of depth jumps, double-leg hops, and split squats (walking and standing). Depth jumps initiated from a 51-cm height and increased each week reaching 114 cm by week 6 and were performed for 2–3 sets of 6–10 repetitions. The double-leg hops were performed for 2–3 sets of 15 m and the split squats were performed for 1–3 sets of 15 m (walking) and 1–3 sets of 6–10 repetitions (in place). The combination program consisted of both RT and plyometric training programs. The combination of RT and plyometric training produced the most substantial increases in vertical jump (10.67 cm). Individually, RT and plyometric training each produced comparable increases in vertical jump performance (3.3 and 3.81 cm, respectively). These data demonstrated the importance of incorporating plyometric and RT for maximizing lower-body power.

integrated with plyometric exercises to improve skill development along with power. It is critical for the coach to address limb and rotational dominance in athletes (60). Unilateral drills are important for those athletes that, in part, perform explosively with one leg/arm during propulsion and bilateral drills are critical for athletes involved in sports where bilateral limb power is needed. Many sports comprise both, so plyometric training programs in these athletes should include uni- and bilateral drills. For example, a right-handed baseball pitcher needs to explosively push off with the right leg against the rubber on the mound and produce high total-body power during counter-clockwise rotation during the wind-up, delivery, and follow-through phases of pitching. Thus, single-leg push-offs and lateral hops, as well as counterclock-wise MB tosses and throws, can be used to train these actions. Although exercises are included that work the contralateral side or movement to improve muscle balance, emphasis can be given to target these specific movement needs of the athlete's position.

- Gradual progression should be used based on the training level of the athletes. Progression entails increases in intensity via the addition of more complex exercises and perhaps some external loading. Volume can be increased within reasonable limits. Likewise, volume and intensity are inversely related. Low-intensity and moderate-intensity drills should be mastered before progressing to high-intensity drills. It has been suggested that athletes have at least a few years of RT and plyometric training experience prior to performing maximal depth jump training (60). High-intensity workouts require greater recovery time in between workouts so frequency must be decreased accordingly.
- Proper technique should always be coached especially when fatigue manifests. Sufficient rest interval lengths should be used to minimize fatigue when peak power is the goal (and not power endurance).

- Plyometric training should take place in an area where there is sufficient space. For horizontal length-specific drills, at least 30–40 yd is recommended. For vertical drills, ceiling height should be higher than the athletes' maximal reach.

EXERCISE SELECTION

Plyometric exercises consist mostly of jumps-in-place, standing jumps, multiple hops/jumps, bounding, box drills, depth jumps, and throws (10,46). These exercises can be divided into lower-body and upper-body/trunk/core explosive exercises. *Jumps* involve maximizing the vertical and/or horizontal motion component. *Hops* involve maximizing the repeated motion for a given distance or pattern. *Bounds* are exaggerated horizontal movements where an excessive stride length is used. *Box drills* involve jumping on or off boxes of different sizes for varied intensity. *Depth jumps* involve accentuating the ECC component by stepping off of a box of varied height prior to performing an explosive jump. *Tosses* and *passes* involve the upper torso and arms (in addition to lower body and core power) releasing the ball or object below or in front of the head. *Throws* involve the upper torso and arms (in addition to lower body and core power) releasing the ball or object above, over, or across the head. It is important to note that all of these exercises are performed explosively with minimal amortization and coupling phases. Some drills can be combined to form a more complex drill, *i.e.*, adding a sprint or multidirectional hop/jump to a depth jump. In addition, *ballistic exercises* (discussed in Chapter 11) are plyometric due to the release of the load (minimizing deceleration). Exercises such as the jump squat, bench press throw, ballistic leg press, and ballistic shoulder press target the SSC and increase power. It is advantageous to use equipment designed to safely catch the weight via hydraulic braking when released.

Exercises

Lower-Body Plyometric Exercises

TWO-FOOT ANKLE HOP ("POGO")
Intensity: Low

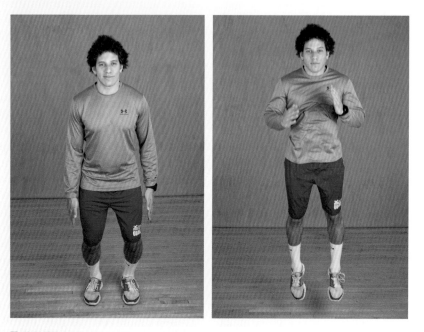

■ **FIGURE 14.1.**

- The athlete begins with arms at the sides and a shoulder width stance.
- After a countermovement, the athlete jumps straight up (with double-arm action), lands, and explosively jumps upright once again. This exercise stresses the plantar flexor muscles to a high degree (Fig. 14.1).

SIDE-TO-SIDE ANKLE HOP
Intensity: Low

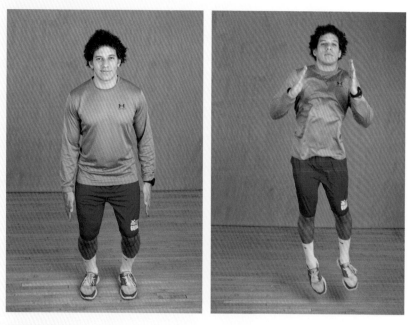

■ **FIGURE 14.2.**

- The athlete begins with arms at the sides and a shoulder width stance.
- After a short countermovement, the athlete jumps with both feet side to side spanning ~2–3 ft. Cones may be used as guide markers.

- This exercise may be performed with one leg where the athlete pushes off on the right leg and lands on the left, and vice versa (Fig. 14.2).

JUMP-AND-REACH
Intensity: Low

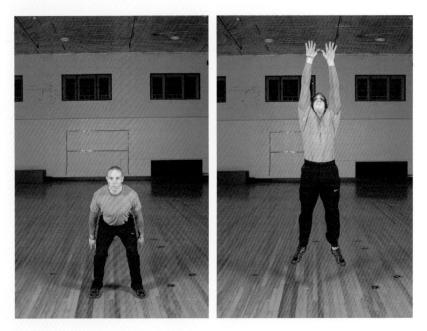

FIGURE 14.3.

- The athlete begins with arms at the sides and a shoulder width stance.
- After a countermovement (and backswing of arms), the athlete jumps straight up and reaches as high as possible simultaneously, lands, and explosively jumps linearly once again. It helps to have a high target for the athlete to strive for to increase jump height, *e.g.*, rim on a basketball court or Vertec (Fig. 14.3).

SQUAT JUMP
Intensity: Low

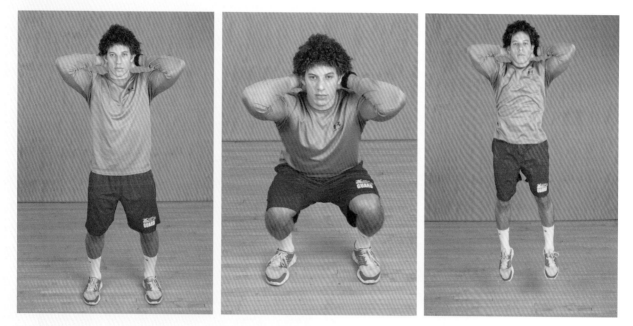

■ **FIGURE 14.4.**

- The athlete begins with the fingers interlocked behind the head and a shoulder width stance. This exercise can be performed with a medicine ball (MB) as well.
- After a countermovement (and backswing of arms), the athlete jumps straight up as high as possible without moving the arms, lands, and explosively jumps for another repetition (Fig. 14.4).

! *CAUTION! Similar to a free-weight squat the athlete should maintain an erect posture during descent and maintain proper knee and toe alignment. The athlete should land softly and the landing directly leads to the countermovement for the next repetition.*

STANDING LONG JUMP
Intensity: Low

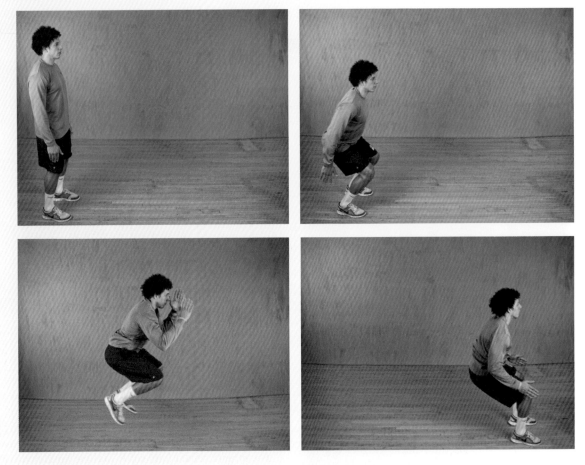

■ **FIGURE 14.5.**

- Athlete begins with arms at the sides and a shoulder width stance with knees slightly bent.
- Following a countermovement (and backswing of arms), the athlete jumps as far forward as possible while using an explosive double-arm action (Fig. 14.5).

! **CAUTION!** *Many times the feet will contact the ground in front of the center of gravity (COG) so balance needs to be maintained during landing.*

VARIATIONS *A variation is to add a multidirectional sprint or sport-specific skill to the end.*

BARRIER JUMPS
Intensity: Low to Moderate

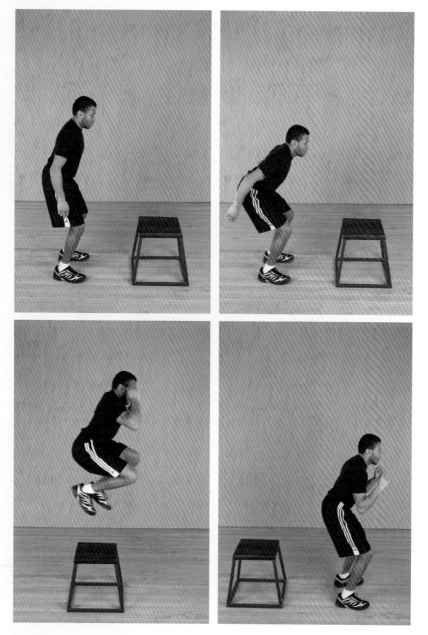

FIGURE 14.6.

- The athlete begins with arms at the sides, shoulder width stance, and knees slightly bent.
- After a quick countermovement and arm backswing, the athlete jumps over a barrier using double-arm action. Some common barriers used are cones, hurdles, and boxes. Increasing the height of the barrier increases the intensity (Fig. 14.6).

CAUTION! *The athlete must focus to ensure clearing the barrier during jumping to avoid tripping, falling, and risking injury.*

VARIATIONS *Variations include lateral, backward, and diagonal barrier jumps or hops. Another variation is to add a multidirectional sprint or sport-specific skill to the end.*

CONE HOPS
Intensity: Low

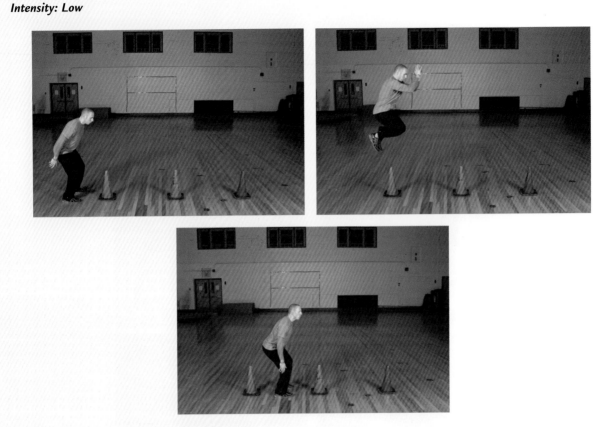

■ FIGURE 14.7.

- The athlete begins with arms at the sides, shoulder width stance, and knees slightly bent.
- Following a quick countermovement and arm backswing, the athlete jumps forward over a cone using double-arm action. A series of cones can be used for multiple repetitions and the spacing in between cones can alter the intensity (Fig. 14.7).

VARIATIONS Variations include lateral cone hops, backward hops, diagonal hops, or adding a 180° rotation to the hop. A multidirectional sprint or sport-specific skill can be added to the end. An advanced variation is to perform hops downhill to accentuate the ECC muscle actions.

TUCK JUMPS
Intensity: Moderate

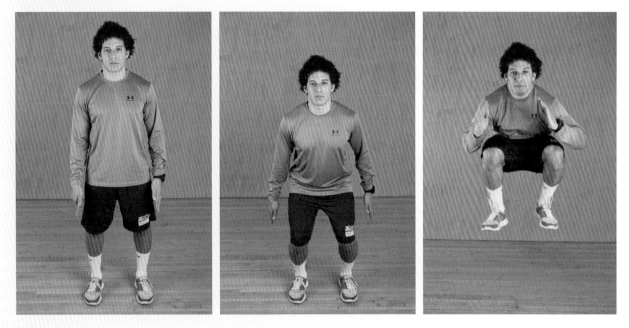

■ **FIGURE 14.8.**

- The athlete begins with arms at the sides, shoulder width stance, and knees slightly bent.
- After a quick countermovement (and backswing of arms), the athlete explosively jumps vertically as high as possible using a double-arm action. While jumping, the athlete raises the knees to the chest and may temporarily hold that position or grasp the knees with both hands.

- The tuck jump is a good exercise to visualize valgus stress (inward bowing) on the knees during landing. This has been successfully used in the evaluation of female athletes who are more likely to sustain anterior cruciate ligament injuries (Fig. 14.8).

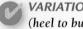 **VARIATIONS** *A variation is to use a heel kick (heel to buttocks) instead of a front tuck.*

SPLIT SQUAT JUMP
Intensity: Moderate

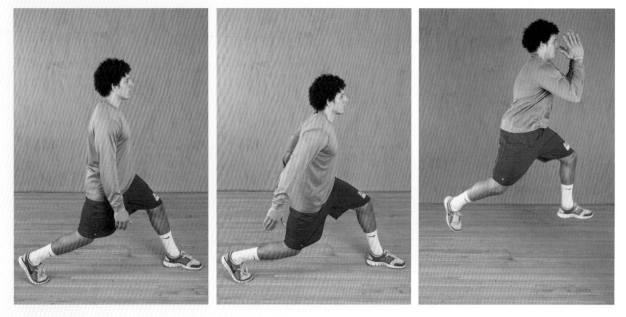

■ **FIGURE 14.9.**

- The athlete begins with arms at the side. One leg is flexed forward while the opposite hip is hyperextended, *e.g.*, resembling a front lunge position. Front knee is flexed ~45–90° whereas back knee is slightly flexed.
- After a short countermovement, the athlete explosively jumps vertically while extending the arms upward.

- The athlete lands in the same position held prior to initiating the jump (Fig. 14.9).

> ✔ **VARIATIONS** *A variation is to cycle the legs during flight, i.e., switch forward/back legs in midair and land in the opposite position (a scissor jump).*

PIKE JUMP
Intensity: Moderate to High

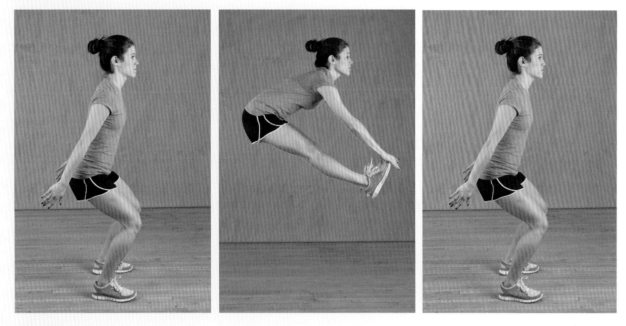

▌FIGURE 14.10.

- Athlete begins with the arms at the sides, shoulder width stance, and knees slightly bent.
- After a countermovement, the athlete explosively jumps upward. While jumping, the athlete lifts both legs upward while keeping the knees only slightly bent and flexes the shoulders to try to touch the toes during flight. The athlete lands and repeats the jump (Fig. 14.10).

VARIATIONS *Variations include widening the legs (abduct the hips) during flight or lifting the legs laterally during flight.*

SINGLE-LEG VERTICAL JUMP
Intensity: High

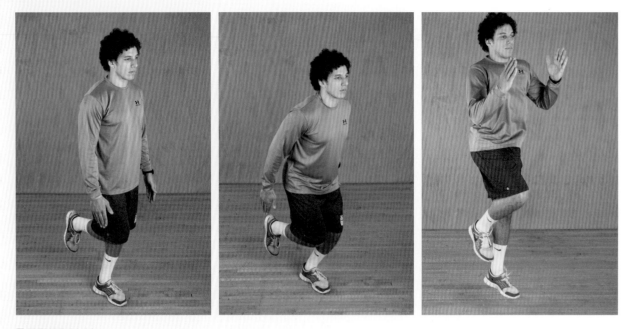

■ **FIGURE 14.11.**

- The athlete begins with arms at the side. Body weight is placed on one leg while other nonjumping leg is flexed off of the ground. The front knee is slightly flexed while supporting body weight.
- After a countermovement, the athlete explosively jumps vertically off of the front leg using a double-arm action. The athlete lands and explosively performs another jump with the same leg. Some recovery time may be needed in between jumps to maintain balance prior to the next repetition (Fig. 14.11).

> **VARIATIONS** *Variations include the single-leg jump and reach and the single-leg tuck jump. The athlete can land and jump off of the opposite leg (cycle legs between repetitions).*

DOUBLE-LEG HOPS
Intensity: Moderate

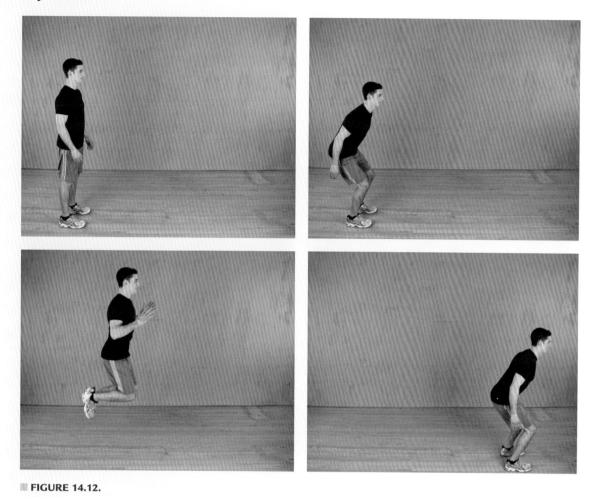

FIGURE 14.12.

- Athlete begins with arms at the sides, shoulder width stance, and knees slightly flexed.
- Following a countermovement (and arm backswing), the athlete jumps forward explosively, lands, and repeatedly hops for a specific distance.
- Barriers such as cones, boxes, mini hurdles, and bags can be used as guides (Fig. 14.12).

VARIATIONS *Variations include lateral hops, backward hops, and diagonal or zigzag hops. The coach can prescribe specific patterns of hopping to the sport (in shapes of triangle, rectangle, hexagon, a "T, M, W", etc.). Another variation is to perform the hops up stadium steps. A multidirectional sprint or sport-specific skill can be added to the end of the hop sequence.*

SINGLE-LEG HOPS
Intensity: Moderate to High

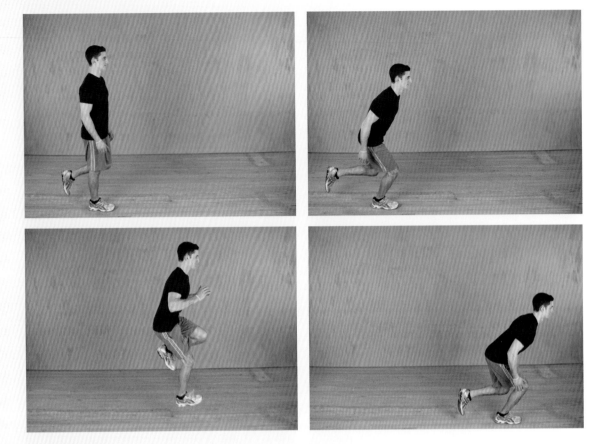

■ **FIGURE 14.13.**

- Athlete begins with arms at the sides. The jumping leg is slightly flexed while supporting the weight of the body whereas the nonjumping leg is flexed at the knee ~60°–90°.
- After a countermovement (and arm backswing), the athlete jumps forward explosively, lands, and repeatedly hops for a specific distance (Fig.14.13).

VARIATIONS *Variations include lateral hops, backward hops, and diagonal or zigzag hops. The coach can prescribe specific patterns of hopping to the sport. A multidirectional sprint or sport-specific skill can be added to the end of the hop sequence. Intensity can be increased by performing single-leg hops uphill or up stadium steps.*

STANDING TRIPLE JUMP
Intensity: Moderate to High

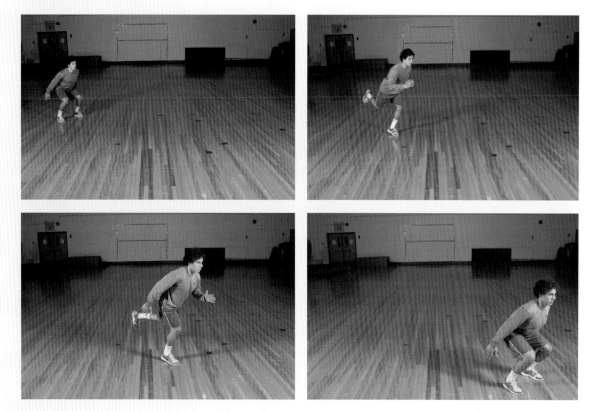

■ **FIGURE 14.14.**

- The athlete begins with arms at the sides, shoulder width stance, and knees slightly bent.
- Following a countermovement, the athlete jumps forward explosively and lands on one foot. The athlete explosively jumps off of the landing leg and lands on the opposite leg. The athlete explosively jumps off this leg and lands on both feet.

- It helps if the athlete lands on a softer surface such as a landing pit (Fig. 14.14).

> ✔ **VARIATIONS** *A variation is to begin with a running start instead of standing. Barriers can be used as jump guides.*

SINGLE-LEG BOX JUMP
Intensity: Moderate to High

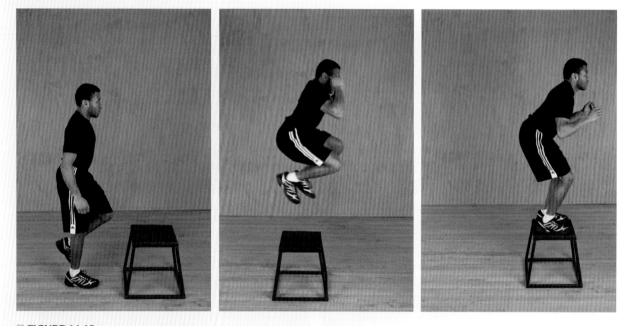

■ **FIGURE 14.15.**

- The athlete begins with arms at the sides, support leg on the ground with knee slightly flexed, and nonsupport leg flexed close to or near 90° (Fig. 14.15).
- A box 15–115 cm high is placed in front of the athlete.
- After a countermovement (and arm backswing), the athlete jumps vertically (with double-arm action) and lands on top of the box.
- Another single-leg box exercise is the *single-leg push-off*. Here, the athlete begins with arms at the sides, front foot on the box, and rear leg in contact with the ground. A box 15–46 cm high should be used (appropriate height should yield jump leg close to parallel to the ground [or hip and knee flexed close to ~90°]). The higher the box the higher the intensity. The athlete explosively jumps vertically (with double-arm action), reaches as high as possible, and lands with the same leg atop the box.

> **! CAUTION!** *For all box jumps caution must be used to ensure proper landing on the box. The athlete should land with both feet toward the center of the box while maintaining equilibrium.*

> **✓ VARIATIONS OF THE SINGLE-LEG PUSH-OFF**
> *Variations include alternating legs (landing on the opposite leg while legs cycle in the air), a lateral push-off (where the athlete lands on the same leg), and a lateral push-off where the athlete jumps over the box and lands on the opposite leg.*

BOX JUMP
Intensity: Low to Moderate

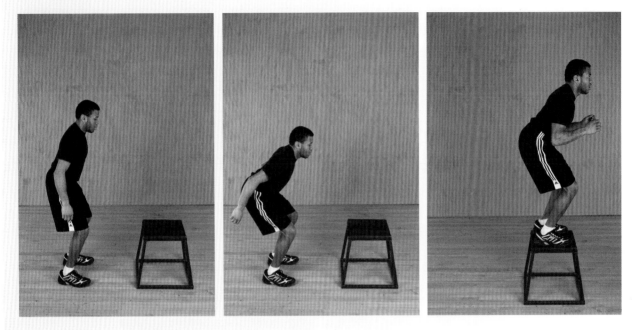

■ FIGURE 14.16.

- Athlete begins with arms at the sides, shoulder width stance, and knees slightly bent.
- A box 15–115 cm high is placed in front of the athlete.
- The athlete jumps explosively up and forward (with double-arm action) on top of the box. The athlete steps off of the box and performs another repetition (Fig. 14.16).

> **VARIATIONS** *Variations of this exercise include a lateral box jump, diagonal box jump, and a squat box jump (with fingers clasped behind the head and no arm action). A multidirectional sprint or sport-specific skill can be added to the end of the drill.*

MULTIPLE BOX JUMPS
Intensity: Moderate to High

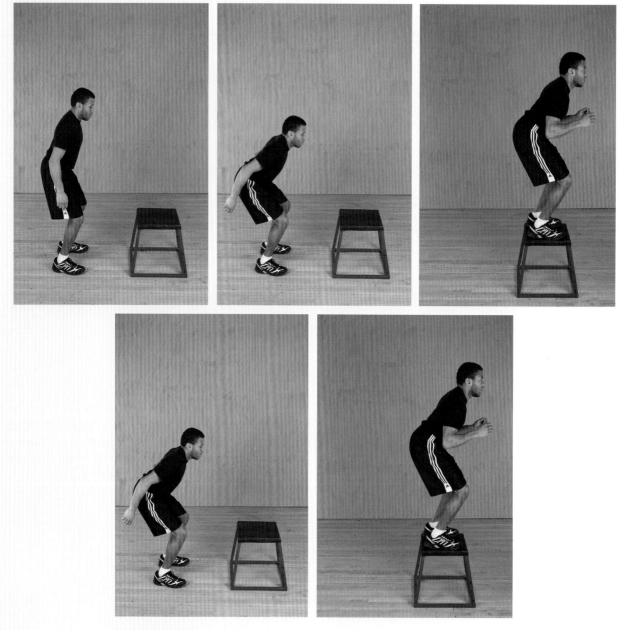

■ **FIGURE 14.17.**

- This exercise is similar to the box jump. Multiple boxes are used in succession. Typically, three to five boxes of similar height are used.
- The athlete jumps onto the first box, off onto the floor, and then onto the second box, and repeats until the set is complete (Fig. 14.17).

> **VARIATIONS** Variations to this exercise include lateral box jumps and single-leg landings. Box heights that increase in succession to increase the intensity can be used.

Another variation is to have the athlete jump from a box to stress the element of the landing. This drill stresses the yielding component and works to develop ECC strength.

Another variation (box double leap) entails the athlete jump on top of the box, then explosively jumps off of the box (with double-arm action) in one motion for height and distance, and sticks the landing. This drill also targets yielding or ECC strength once the athlete jumps on top of the box. Having a soft landing area is recommended.

A multidirectional sprint or sport-specific skill can be added to the end of the drill.

SKIPPING
Intensity: Low

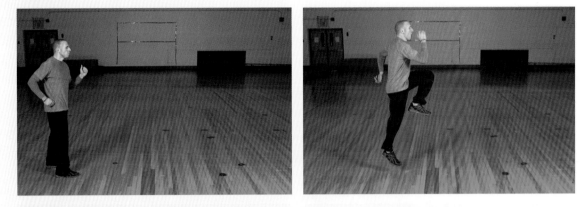

FIGURE 14.18.

- Athlete begins with arms at the sides, shoulder width stance, and knees slightly bent.
- After a quick countermovement, the athlete explosively raises one leg (to a 90° knee angle) and the opposite arm (to a 90° elbow angle). Upon return, the opposite limbs are raised and the cycle is repeated until the targeted number of repetitions has been completed (Fig. 14.18).

VARIATIONS Variations include backward skipping and skipping with double-arm action (as opposed to one).

ALTERNATE BOUNDING
Intensity: Moderate to High

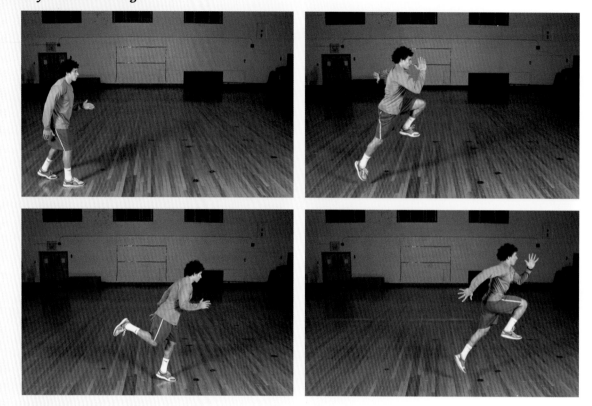

FIGURE 14.19.

- The athlete begins with arms at the sides, shoulder width stance, and knees slightly bent.
- After a quick countermovement (preferably from a jog), the athlete pushes off explosively with one leg. The opposite leg will flex forward in an exaggerated manner with the leg parallel to the ground. The athlete reaches forward with the opposite arm. The goal is to cover as much ground as possible during each exaggerated stride.

- Upon landing, the athlete explosively pushes off of the landing foot and repeats (Fig. 14.19).

VARIATIONS *Variations to this exercise include double-arm bounding. A multidirectional sprint or sport-specific skill can be added to the end of the drill.*

SINGLE-LEG BOUNDING
Intensity: Moderate to High

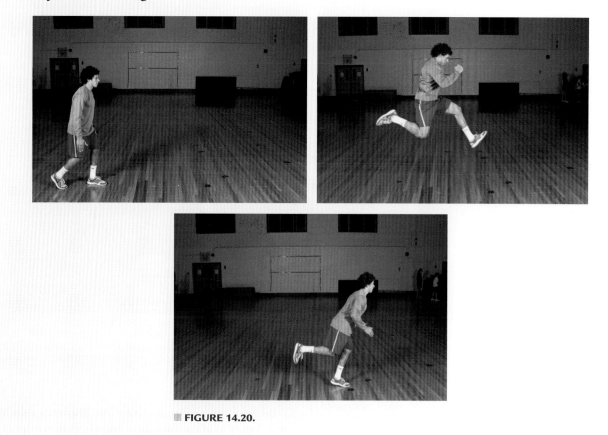

FIGURE 14.20.

- The athlete begins with arms at the sides, shoulder width stance, and knees slightly bent.
- After a quick countermovement (preferably from a jog), the athlete pushes off explosively with one leg. The opposite leg will flex forward in an exaggerated manner with the leg parallel to the ground. The athlete reaches forward with the opposite arm.

- The athlete pushes off and lands on the same foot (different from alternate bounding). The opposite side is drilled following completion of the first side.
- A multidirectional sprint or sport-specific skill can be added to the end of the drill (Fig. 14.20).

DEPTH JUMP (DROP JUMP)
Intensity: Very High (Depending on Box Height)

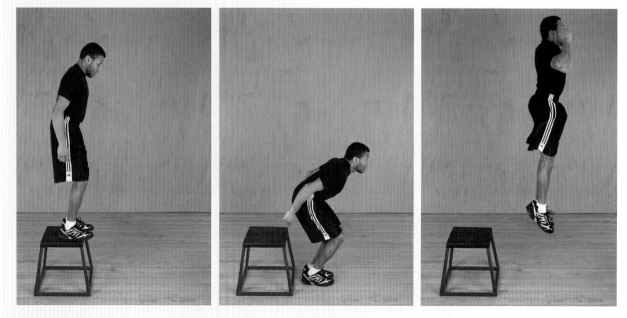

■ **FIGURE 14.21.**

- The athlete begins with arms at the sides, shoulder width stance, and knees slightly bent on top of a box (with toes near or hanging over the edge of the box). Box heights vary between 20 and 115 cm. Intensity increases as box height increases.
- The athlete steps off of the box, lands on the ground, and explosively jumps vertically (with double-arm action) as high as possible upon landing (Fig. 14.21).

! **CAUTION!** *Athletes must be able to have a smooth transition between ECC and CON phases. If the athlete hesitates to regain stability then the box height should be reduced. The athlete should not break the exercise into a distinct landing and subsequent jump. Rather, it should be one continuous motion. This is an intense exercise, so volume and frequency should be adapted to allow adequate recovery in between workouts. Because of the intense nature of this exercise, it is recommended that only experienced (at least 1–2 years) athletes perform this drill.*

✔ **VARIATIONS** *Many variations can be performed. Several of the jumps discussed in this chapter can be performed once the athlete steps off from the box (jump and reach, squat jump, tuck jump, long jump, pike jump, etc.). A multidirectional sprint or sport-specific skill can be added to the end of the jump.*

DEPTH JUMP (DROP JUMP) TO ANOTHER BOX OR BENCH
Intensity: Very High

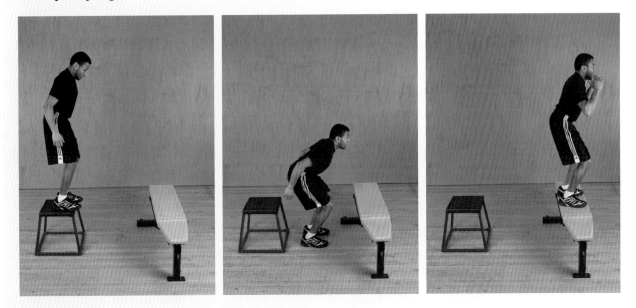

■ **FIGURE 14.22.**

- Athlete begins with arms at the sides, shoulder width stance, and knees slightly bent on top of a box (with toes near or hanging over the edge of the box). Box heights vary between 20 and 115 cm. Intensity increases as box height increases.
- The athlete steps off of the box, lands on the ground, and explosively jumps vertically (with double-arm action) as high as possible upon landing.
- The athlete jumps and lands on to a second box or bench. The distance between boxes and height of the boxes can vary based on goals of the exercise. A smaller box with a greater distance from the start box can

be used to stress the long jump whereas a taller box located close to the start box can be used to train the vertical jump. Some have suggested a length of 24 in. in between boxes to start with (10,44) (Fig. 14.22).

VARIATIONS *A variation of this exercise is to use one box. The athlete begins on top of the box facing backward (toward the box as opposed to away from the box). The athlete drops off of the box, lands on the ground, and explosively jumps back on to the top of the box as quickly as possible.*

SINGLE-LEG DEPTH JUMP
Intensity: Very High

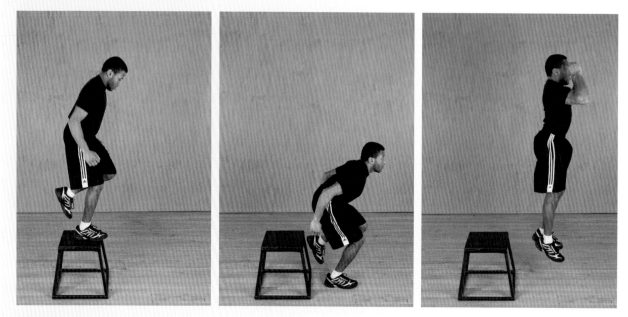

■ **FIGURE 14.23.**

• Similar to the depth jump with the exception, the athlete lands on one foot and explosively jumps off the landing foot (Fig. 14.23).

✔ VARIATIONS *This variation is very intense and requires a shorter box in comparison to the double-leg depth jump. It is reserved for trained to highly trained athletes.*

Upper-Body and Core Plyometric Exercises

MEDICINE BALL CHEST PASS
Intensity: Low

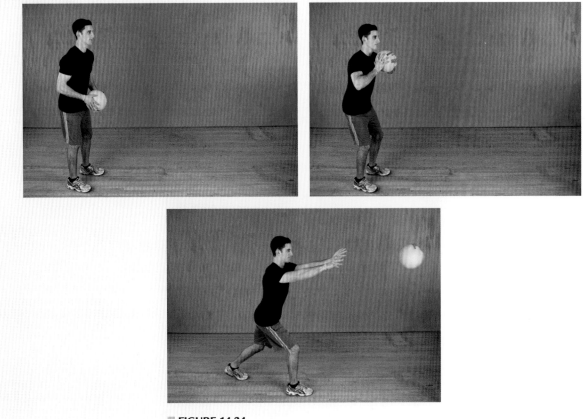

■ **FIGURE 14.24.**

- Athlete begins with a shoulder width stance with knees slightly bent and grasps an MB or core ball (2–15 lb or more) at chest height with shoulders flexed and abducted with elbows pointing outward.
- After a countermovement, the athlete explosively puts or throws the ball forward. The athlete may maintain his/her stance during the pass or take a step forward to generate momentum.
- The athlete may use a partner, wall, open space, or rebounder when performing this exercise. A partner or rebounder is advantageous because the ball is returned to the athlete after release. This forces the athlete to catch the ball prior to performing the next repetition. Catching the ball and explosively performing another pass stress the SSC to a greater extent (via loaded ECC action). A rebounder is an angled trampoline-like device which forcefully returns the ball back to the athlete upon contact (Fig. 14.24).

CAUTION! *The athlete must focus on catching the MB if a partner or rebounder is used. Failure to properly catch the ball could lead to injury and disrupted technique.*

VARIATIONS *Variations of this exercise include performing the chest pass from a running start and seated or kneeling position. This exercise can also be performed simultaneously with a sit-up where the MB is passed to a partner. A rotation can be added to the chest pass.*

This exercise may be preceded by a lower-body plyometric exercise.

OVERHEAD MEDICINE BALL THROW
Intensity: Low

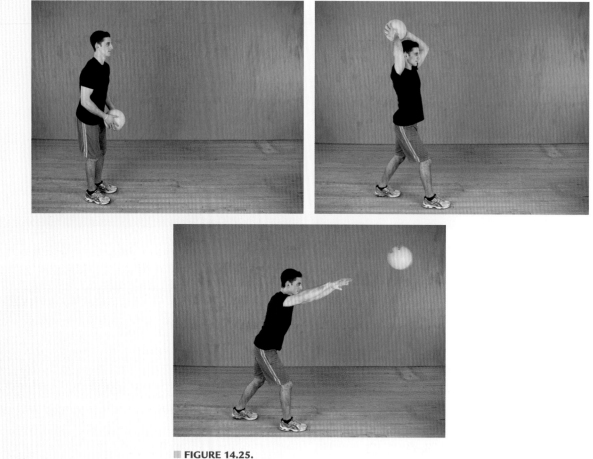

FIGURE 14.25.

- Athlete begins with a shoulder width stance with knees slightly bent, and grasps an MB or core ball at chest height.
- The athlete lifts the MB to an overhead position, steps forward with one foot, and explosively throws the ball.
- The athlete may use a partner, wall, open space, or rebounder when performing the exercise (Fig. 14.25).

VARIATIONS *Variations of this exercise include performing the overhead MB throw from a staggered stance, running start, and seated or kneeling position. This exercise can be performed with one arm using a lighter MB. This version is used to mimic the demands of throwing a ball and is an excellent exercise for baseball and softball players, quarterbacks, etc. The single-arm overhead throw with a small MB can be performed from a shoulder width stance, staggered stance, running start, or kneeling position. The direction of the throw can vary (athlete can throw the ball to a partner, off of a wall, for distance, or throw the ball off of the ground).*

MEDICINE BALL BACK THROW
Intensity: Low

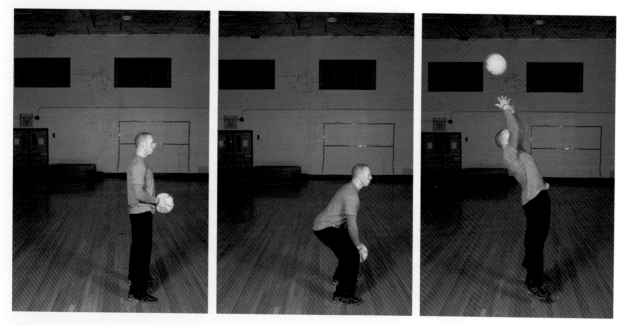

FIGURE 14.26.

- The athlete begins with a slightly past shoulder width stance, knees bent, and arms extended in front of the body grasping an MB or core ball.
- A countermovement is performed where the athlete flexes at the hip and knees, and then explosively extends and hyperextends the hips and back, flexes the shoulders, and throws the ball backward as far as possible (Fig. 14.26).

 VARIATIONS *A variation of this exercise is to perform it seated.*

SINGLE-ARM VERTICAL CORE BALL THROW
Intensity: Low to Moderate

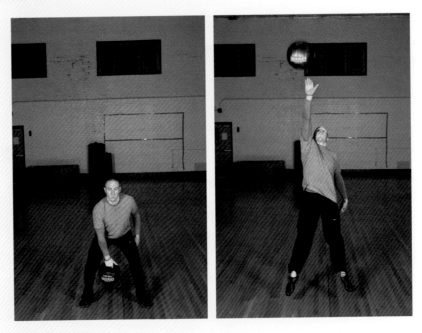

■ **FIGURE 14.27.**

- The athlete begins with a slightly past shoulder width stance, knees bent, and throwing arm extended in front of the body between the legs grasping a core ball.
- A countermovement is performed where the athlete flexes at the hip and knees, and then explosively extends and hyperextends the hips and back, flexes the shoulders, and throws the core ball vertically up as high as possible. This technique is similar to performing a single-arm dumbbell snatch with the exception the core ball is released vertically (Fig. 14.27).

OVERHEAD MEDICINE BALL SLAMS
Intensity: Low

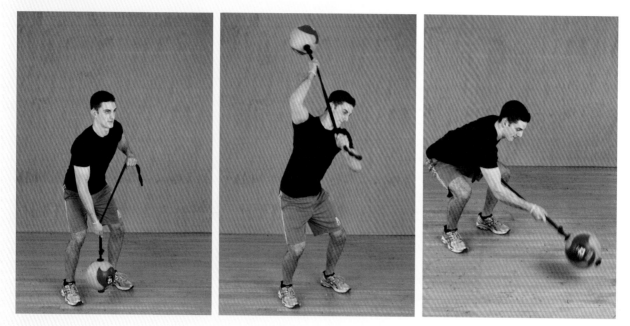

FIGURE 14.28.

- The athlete begins with a slightly wider than shoulder width stance, knees bent, and an MB held at arm's length in front of the body.
- The countermovement entails the athlete extends the hips back and raises the MB to the overhead position.

- Athlete explosively flexes the waist and hips and throws the MB forcefully off of the ground.
- This exercise may be performed with a core ball, slam ball (Fig. 14.28), or keg. If a slam ball is used, the athlete can slam it off of the floor or wall in front of the body.

MEDICINE BALL UNDERHAND TOSS
Intensity: Low

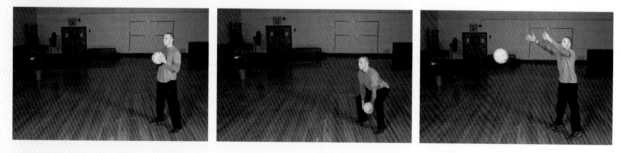

FIGURE 14.29.

- The athlete begins with a slightly wider than shoulder width stance, knees bent, and an MB held at arm's length in front of the body.
- A countermovement is performed where the athlete flexes at the hip and knees, and then explosively extends and hyperextends the hips and back, flexes the shoulders, and tosses the ball forward.
- The athlete may use a partner, wall, open space, or rebounder when performing the exercise. A partner or rebounder is advantageous because the ball is returned to the athlete after release (Fig. 14.29).

VARIATIONS A variation is to perform the exercise from the side. Athlete will begin the throw from a side position (where the MB is located lateral to the knee), rotate, and explosively toss the MB underhand for distance and/or speed. Another variation is to perform exercise from a kneeling position. The exercise may also be performed while doing a back hyperextension in the weight room.

PULLOVER PASS
Intensity: Low

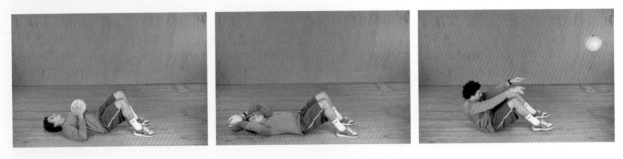

■ **FIGURE 14.30.**

- The athlete lies on the ground or stability ball with knees flexed and feet flat on the floor.
- Athlete lifts the MB or core ball overhead and passes the ball to a partner with straight arms (Fig. 14.30).

✓ **VARIATIONS** *A variation is to incorporate a sit-up or torso rotation while throwing the ball.*

MEDICINE BALL SIDE TOSS
Intensity: Low

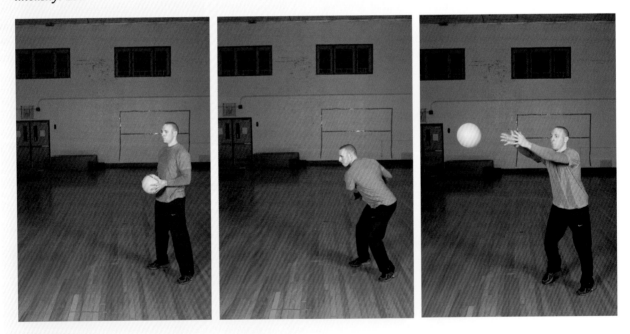

■ **FIGURE 14.31.**

- The athlete begins with a slightly wider than shoulder width stance, knees slightly bent, and arms extended to one side of the body grasping an MB or core ball.
- The countermovement entails the athlete rotate to the side of the MB and explosively tosses the ball in the opposite direction across the body (rotating the opposite side to toss the ball).

- The athlete may use a partner, wall, open space, or rebounder when performing the exercise. This exercise may be performed kneeling, seated, or with a slam ball (against the wall).
- Throws are then performed to the opposite side (Fig. 14.31).

MEDICINE BALL FRONT ROTATION THROW
Intensity: Low

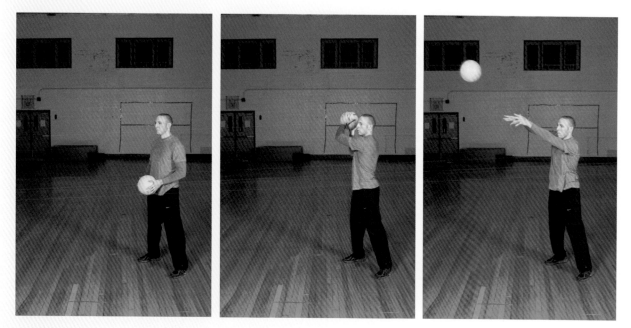

FIGURE 14.32.

- The athlete begins with a shoulder width stance, knees slightly flexed, and elbows flexed in front of the body with hands grasping an MB or core ball.
- The countermovement entails the athlete raise the MB over the shoulder and rotates toward the side of the ball.

- The athlete explosively throws the ball semi-cross body forward. The athlete may use a partner, wall, open space, or rebounder when performing this exercise.
- This exercise can be performed kneeling, seated, from running start, and with one arm using a smaller ball (Fig. 14.32).

MEDICINE BALL POWER DROP
Intensity: High

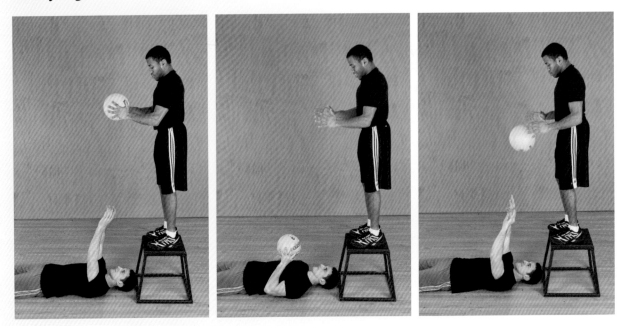

■ **FIGURE 14.33.**

- A partner is needed for this exercise. The partner stands on a plyo box or bench 20–115-cm high holding an MB at arm's length with arms parallel to the ground.
- The athlete begins lying on the ground with arms extended upward and (perpendicular to the floor) with the head near the base of the plyo box or bench. The athlete's arm should be located directly under the MB held by the partner.

- The partner drops the ball and the athlete catches and lowers the ball to chest level (accentuated ECC countermovement). The athlete then explosively passes (chest presses) the ball back up to the partner (Fig. 14.33).

⚠ *CAUTION! Caution needs to be used because failure to catch the ball (by either the athlete or partner) could result in injury.*

PLYOMETRIC PUSH-UP
Intensity: Moderate

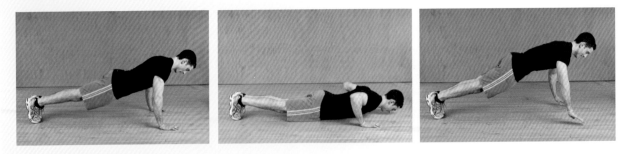

■ **FIGURE 14.34.**

- The athlete begins the exercise in a standard push-up position.
- The athlete descends and explosively performs a push-up where the athlete's hands temporarily leave the ground. Some athletes will clap their hands at this point.
- The athlete lands, descends, and continues to perform another repetition (Fig. 14.34).

DEPTH PUSH-UP
Intensity: High

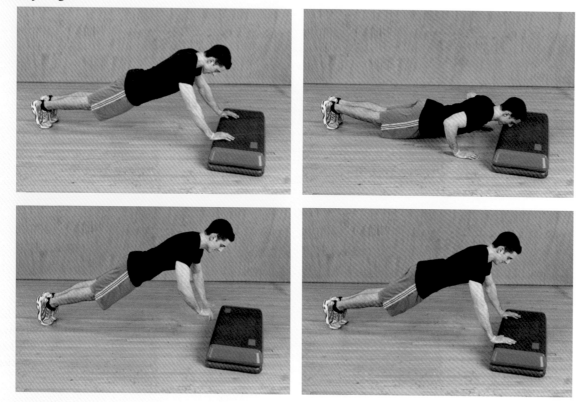

FIGURE 14.35.

- This exercise is similar to the plyometric push-up except the athlete begins the exercise from an elevated position. MBs, steps, or small boxes can be used for elevation.
- The athlete drops from the elevated height, performs a plyo push-up, and completes the repetition by maintaining the starting position elevated from the

ball or box. The athlete needs to explode high enough to ensure he or she can transition to the elevated starting position (Fig. 14.35). Using two boxes or steps laterally placed at the level of each arm is recommended when large elevations are used as it provides a clear path for the head during discent.

BAG THRUSTS
Intensity: Low

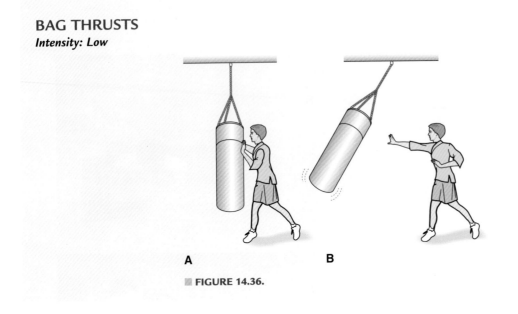

A   B

■ **FIGURE 14.36.**

- A heavy bag or floor bag (Wavemaster) is needed for this exercise.
- The athlete begins with shoulder width stance with feet staggered. The athlete then explosively thrusts hand into the bag (using the limb on the same side of the back leg) (Fig. 14.36).

VARIATIONS Variations of this exercise include a two-handed thrust. The athlete may also use the heavy bag for boxing or martial art strikes. These include various forms of punches, blocks, and kicks.

PENDULUM EXERCISES
Intensity: Low to Moderate

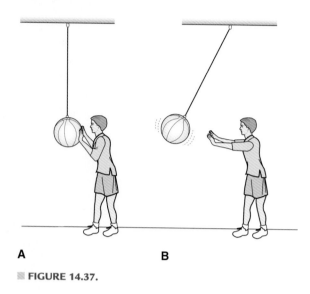

A   **B**

FIGURE 14.37.

- An MB suspended from a rope hanging from a tall structure is needed for these drills.
- The athlete can perform multiple throws using an MB as a pendulum.
- Variations include one- and two-arm overhead throws and chest pass. These can be performed from a standing or kneeling position.
- Catching the ball is required for these drills, which increases the difficulty (Fig. 14.37).

> ✔ *VARIATIONS A lower-body variation can be performed. The athlete uses a swing-type apparatus suspended from a high support mechanism in close proximity to a wall. Upon swinging, the athlete will contact the wall and explosively push off leading to a subsequent oscillation. The swing can be made heavier to increasing loading during the ECC component to target the yielding phase (60,63). In addition, sturdy uprights can be placed before the swing (in the swings path) to modify the exercise to target the upper body (60). For both variations, the height of the backswing (in addition to loading) affects intensity, e.g., greater backswing yields greater impact force. This variation is a high-intensity drill.*

Case Study 14.1

Kevin is a high school soccer player who wants to begin a plyometric training program. He comes to you for a consultation and wants to know which plyometric exercises would be appropriate for him and specific for the skills needed by a soccer player.

Question for Consideration: What plyometric exercises would you recommend for Kevin based on his training level?

INTENSITY

The intensity of plyometric exercises depends on several factors including the exercise complexity, loading, speed, and the size and length of boxes or barriers used. The complexity relates to the type of drill used. Jumps-in-place are lowest in intensity, followed by standing jumps, multiple hops and jumps, bounding, and box drills (9,10). Depth jumps are the most intense type of plyometric exercise. Higher loading during landing increases the intensity of the plyometric drill. Loading increases when the mass of the athlete increases (from external loading with weighted vests or weights) and when the velocity of impact increases (from higher jump heights). Single-leg jumps are more intense than comparable double-leg jumps. Each exercise presented in this chapter is categorized as low, moderate, or high intensity as a guide for exercise selection. The intensity of plyometric training can be increased by adding a low to moderate amount of external loading. For example, using a weighted vest, MB, dumbbells, or other loading device can increase the intensity of plyometric training. Also, the athlete's body weight plays a role as one plyometric drill may be more intense in an athlete of greater size than a smaller athlete. Intensity is increased by using larger barriers or boxes, or by setting cones/barriers further apart. This requires the athlete to jump higher or further per repetition. Plyometric training programs begin with low- and moderate-intensity exercises and progresses to higher intensity exercises over time. Thus, plyometric exercise prescription is a common means of altering training intensity. Table 14.1 illustrates a continuum of plyometric exercises based on intensity. Low-, moderate-, and high-intensity classifications are used. It is important to note that any exercise listed (including low-intensity drills) can be made more intense via methods previously described.

EXERCISE ORDER

Plyometric exercises can be sequenced in numerous ways. As opposed to RT, there are essentially no sequencing recommendations for plyometric training. Most sequencing patterns can be beneficial provided adequate recovery is given in between sets and exercises. Low-intensity drills can be included anywhere in sequence. Many coaches prefer to include one or two at the beginning of

TABLE 14.1 PLYOMETRIC EXERCISE INTENSITY CONTINUUM

LOW INTENSITY	MODERATE INTENSITY	HIGH INTENSITY
Pogos	Barrier jumps	Pike jump
Side-to-side ankle hop	Tuck jumps	Single-leg vertical jump
Jump and reach	Split squat jump	Single-leg hops
Squat jump	Double leg hops	Depth plyo push-up
Standing long jump	Box jumps	MB power drop
Cone hops	Alternate bounding	Single-leg bounding
Single-leg box jump	Single-arm vertical CB throw	Depth jump and variations
Skipping	Plyo push-up	
MB chest pass	Triple jump	
Overhead MB throw	Multiple box jumps	
MB back throw		
Overhead MB slam		
MB underhand throw		
Pullover pass		
MB side throw		
MB front rotation throw		
Bag thrusts		

a workout to help the athlete better warm up or become more prepared for subsequent high-intensity drills. Low-intensity drills can be performed later in the workout after other key moderate- and high-intensity drills are performed. Moderate- and high-intensity drills are typically performed near the beginning (following appropriate warm-up and low-intensity drills) while fatigue is minimal and energy levels are high. Because the intensity level is greater, it is most beneficial to the athlete to perform these drills early to maximize SSC activity. When upper-body plyometric drills are included, the athlete may choose to alternate between lower- and upper-body drills (similar to RT). The rationale is to provide greater recovery in between exercises. Upper-body plyometric exercises can be staggered in between lower-body drills to maximize workout efficiency without compromising SSC performance. Lastly, plyometric exercises may be incorporated into an RT workout (known as **complex training**) (9,10). A technically similar plyometric exercise can be performed in between sets of a similar resistance exercise. Some sample pairings may include performing squat jumps in between the sets of barbell back squats, tuck jumps in between sets of front squats, box jumps in between sets of hang cleans, an MB chest pass in between sets of the bench press, and bag thrusts (or striking a heavy bag) in between sets of ISOM wall pushes or the close-grip bench press. Postactivation potentiation occurs during the performance of plyometric drills after resistance exercises. Acute power enhancement may be augmented when using complex training. Although research shows that complex training acutely enhances athletic power (52), short-term training studies

have not shown complex training to be more effective for enhancing power or vertical jump performance to a greater degree than performing plyometric and RT separately (41). Thus, integrating plyometric exercises into an RT workout appears equally as effective for enhancing power as separate workouts.

VOLUME

Volume represents the total number of sets and repetitions performed during a plyometric workout and depends on training intensity and frequency as well as the impact of other training modalities. For lower-body plyometrics, the number of foot contacts or distance covered denotes training volume. For upper-body or core plyometrics, the number of repetitions (throws, passes, or tosses) represents training volume. Similar to other modalities of exercise, plyometric volume and intensity are inversely related. Few guidelines regarding plyometric training volume are available. Chu (10) has recommended some guidelines for plyometric training that are listed in Table 14.2.

FREQUENCY

Frequency refers to the number of training sessions per week. Plyometric training typically takes place 1–4 days per week. Training frequency will depend on other variables such as intensity and volume, as well as the inclusion of other training modalities. High-intensity training may necessitate a lower frequency especially when depth

TABLE 14.2 PLYOMETRIC TRAINING VOLUMES BASED ON EXPERIENCE[a]

STATUS	OFF-SEASON	PRESEASON	IN-SEASON
Beginner	60–100	100–250	Depends on Sport
Intermediate	100–150	150–300	Depends on Sport
Advanced	120–200	150–450	Depends on Sport

[a]Numbers represent foot contacts per workout. Warm-up exercises are not included. The wide range of values during preseason indicates variations in intensity. That is, high-intensity drills yield lower volumes whereas low- and moderate-intensity drills yield higher volumes. In-season volume depends on the sport as volume will be low in sports that are highly plyometric in nature. Adapted with permission from Chu DA. *Jumping into Plyometrics.* 2nd ed. Champaign (IL): Human Kinetics; 1998. pp. 1–138.

jumps are performed, and frequency may be lower when other modalities are included. In-season training of athletes necessitates a low training frequency. Sport practices and competitions include plyometric actions so training must be developed around the intensity/volume of plyometric actions seen in the sport. Thus, maintenance plyometric training of 1–2 days per week may suffice which could offset any potential detraining effects. Because of the intense nature of plyometric training, ~48–72 hours of recovery in between training sessions is recommended (10,44). Few frequency-comparative studies have been conducted. de Villarreal et al. (12) showed that 1 day per week and 2 days per week (with double the number of drop jumps) frequencies produced greater improvements in vertical jump and sprinting speed than high-frequency (4 days per week with quadruple the number of drop jumps) training. Thus, coaches must use their best judgment in prescribing plyometric training frequencies. Similar to RT, it is the intensity and volume that may be the key variables provided that the frequency selected allows adequate recovery time between workouts.

REST INTERVALS

Rest intervals between sets, repetitions, and plyometric exercises is critical for training adaptations. Adequate rest intervals are needed when maximizing power is the goal. For noncontinuous or single-repetition jumps (depth jump) or throws, intraset rest intervals are useful for maximizing power. For example, 5–10 seconds of rest in between submaximal depth jumps is recommended with 2–3 minutes of rest in between sets (44). However, maximal depth jumps require longer intraset (up to 2–4 min) and interset (>5–10 min) rest intervals (60). Rest interval lengths are exercise-specific and depend on the intensity. More recovery may be needed in between sets for high-intensity drills than low- or moderate-intensity drills. For example, a 30-second rest interval between sets of ankle hops is sufficient but maybe not sufficient when performing sets of box jumps. Work-to-rest ratios of 1:5–1:10 are recommended (10,44). Using a 1:10 ratio, an athlete would rest ~100 seconds if the total set length was 10 seconds. Thus, 1:5 ratio may be applied to low- and moderate-intensity drills and 1:10 ratio to

higher-intensity drills. Shorter rest interval lengths minimize recovery and train power endurance in the athlete. This could be a goal of the coach during anaerobic conditioning phases but rest interval prescription for plyometric training targeting maximal power should allow adequate recovery and will be longer in length.

OTHER CONSIDERATIONS IN PLYOMETRIC TRAINING PROGRAM DESIGN

Designing plyometric training programs depends on additional factors. These include the warm-up, age, training status, surface, and equipment availability.

WARM-UP

All plyometric training programs must begin with a proper warm-up. A general warm-up may be used initially (5–10 min of jogging) followed by a specific warm-up. The specific warm-up exercises selected are used to physiologically prepare the athlete for the workout. They are used to develop fundamental movement skills and coordination transferable to plyometric training. Drills are low in intensity. Some examples of good plyometric training warm-up drills include marching, high-knees, butt kicks, skipping, lunges, back pedaling, side shuffles, cariocas, and progressive form running. These drills are commonly used in preparation for sprint and agility training. The warm-up can consist of 10–20-m length drills where the athlete performs the set up, rests, and returns back for a second set, or performs a set up and walks back to increase recovery in between sets. If a group of athletes are warming-up together, each athlete can rest a few seconds more while another squad is performing the drill. At least 10 total sets are performed (1–3 sets per drill).

AGE

The majority of scientific and practical information regarding plyometric training has focused on young adults and adults typically in their 20s and 30s. However, the use of plyometric training in children, adolescents, and middle-aged to older adults has received some attention, and in some cases scrutiny. Part of the issue dealing with plyometric training in these populations has been the diverse terminology in defining plyometrics. Some view plyometrics in classic terms as predominantly depth jumping at high levels of intensity. In contrast, many view plyometrics in modern terms as exercises that stress the SSC which vary greatly in intensity. A proponent of modern plyometrics may propose that plyometrics can be beneficial for most individuals regardless of age. Throughout this chapter numerous plyometric exercises were illustrated and explained. These exercises vary in intensity and many low-intensity drills are appropriate for many populations. Plyometric training can be safe and effective for individuals regardless of age when properly administered and supervised.

Plyometric exercises can benefit middle-age and older adults. Muscular power deteriorates at a faster rate than strength with aging and attempts to maintain or improve power can be beneficial to improving fitness. Part of the perception in society is that plyometric exercises are more reserved for young adults. However, plyometric actions are commonly performed in middle-age and older adults who frequently play pick-up games of basketball or racquetball for example. Masters athletes benefit greatly from plyometric training. Precaution must be used regarding potential orthopedic limitations and plyometrics may be contraindicated for some. Plyometric training guidelines for adults may be used for masters athletes with the exception that volume may be lower and low- to moderate-intensity drills are preferred (44).

TRAINING STATUS

Plyometric training program design depends on the training status of the athlete. Novice athletes should begin with a basic program comprised of low-intensity drills and progress to high-intensity drills gradually over time as conditioning and coordination improve. Trained athletes have greater tolerance and can perform higher-intensity drills and a higher volume of exercise. In the past, the strength level of the athlete was considered within the training status domain. Early European coaches recommended that athletes needed to have great strength, *e.g.*, able to squat at least 1.5–2.5 times their body weight and have high levels of ECC and explosive ISOM strength, before beginning plyometric training (60). These guidelines were never intended to apply to submaximal plyometric drills. If this were the case, few athletes would qualify and this suggestion no longer is relevant for several plyometric exercises. These early suggestions were

Myths & Misconceptions

Plyometric Training is Harmful for Children and Adolescents

Children and adolescents benefit from plyometric training, and plyometric training can help children and adolescents become physically fit and adequately prepared for various youth sports. Many activities and games (hopscotch) children play are plyometric in nature (activate the SSC) so the thought of plyometric training in youth is not novel. Plyometric training in children and adolescents has been embraced by prominent S&C organizations (20). Some misconceptions concerning plyometric training in youth is that it is unsafe (causes growth plate injuries) and children lack the necessary strength needed to engage in a training program. However, research does not support the contention that plyometrics are dangerous or that a minimal level of strength is needed to perform low- to moderate-intensity plyometric actions (20). Studies investigating youth plyometric training have shown it to be safe and effective for performance improvements (13,20). Youth plyometric training improves jumping ability, running time, push-up performance, and speed (13,20,26), and these augmentations have occurred beyond the changes that are associated with typical activity experienced in physical education classes (26). MB training is effective in children and adolescents (18-20,40). Marginson et al. (35) showed that a plyometric workout resulted in mild postexercise soreness (compared to adult men) but repeated exposure limited muscle damage and dysfunction in children. Children and adolescents respond more favorably than adults to plyometric training when it comes to soreness responses after exercise. However, it may not be prudent for youths to perform high-intensity drills such as depth jumps but these exercises represent only a myriad of the number of plyometric exercises young athletes can perform. Youth plyometric training programs should begin with low-intensity drills where proper form and technique are stressed. A gradual progression to moderate-intensity drills should be used where the major goals are to increase youth fitness, balance and coordination, and performance. Research has not determined an appropriate minimal age for initiating a plyometric training program but some S&C professionals have had success training children 7-8 years of age provided they have the emotional maturity to listen to instructions and perform the exercises properly (44). The decision to allow a child/adolescent to perform plyometric training is up to a parent or coach as it is safe and effective when properly supervised.

made due to the fact that depth jumping comprised classic plyometrics and impact forces could exceed six times the athlete's body weight (60). It would not be logical to force an athlete to have high levels of strength in order to begin a program consisting of basic vertical jumps or pogos. Others have recommended that athletes be able to squat 1.5 times their body weight, bench press their body weight (for heavy athletes) or 1.5 times their body weight (for athletes who weigh less than 220 lb), perform five plyo push-ups in a row, and be able to perform speed squats and bench presses (5 repetitions in less than 5 s with 60% of body weight) (44). These standards are applied mostly to high-intensity drills. Some coaches have used balance/stability assessments prior to engaging in plyometric training. A coach may use periodic evaluation of their athletes to determine if that athlete is ready to proceed to more intense training. Although it may be helpful for an athlete to have a solid strength foundation (especially adequate ECC strength), other fitness components are critical including balance, coordination, power, speed, and agility. Because plyometric training helps improve all of these fitness components, an athlete of lesser conditioning and strength can greatly benefit from plyometric training but mostly via low- to moderate-intensity drills.

TRAINING SURFACE

Plyometric training can be performed in a variety of places. The surface selected should be yielding and provide some give to reduce the overall joint stress to the body. However, the surface should not be too yielding. Impellizzeri et al. (25) reported 4 weeks of plyometric training on grass and sand increased jumping and sprint performance. However, grass produced superior results while less soreness was shown after plyometric training in the sand. Grass is a popular choice for plyometric training as open fields have the benefit of enabling longer-distance drills to be performed. Matted floors and gymnastics floors are acceptable training surfaces. The mats cannot be too thick as this can excessively increase the amortization phase (44) and not maximize the SSC. Concrete and hardwood floors lack the shock-absorbing ability and may cause undue strain to the athlete. A few studies have examined the potential of aquatic plyometric training. Training in the water has the advantage of increasing resistance during jumping (based on the depth of the water) but the disadvantage of minimizing ECC loading due to the buoyancy of the water. Stemm and Jacobson (57) and Martel (36) showed that aquatic plyometric training increased vertical jump. Thus, aquatic plyometric training can be effective especially for single-leg exercises (60). Lastly, the level of inclination or declination in the surface is important. Many times plyometric training will take place on a relatively even surface. However, surface angular alterations can pose a new stimulus for training.

Plyometric training uphill increases the metabolic demand and force requirement whereas plyometric training downhill increases the ECC component, intensity, and results in greater postexercise muscle soreness.

PLYOMETRIC TRAINING EQUIPMENT

Plyometric training can be performed without any specialized equipment. However, some pieces of equipment may be needed in order to perform some drills. Some common pieces of equipment include cones, boxes, jump ropes, mini hurdles, bands, bags, weighted vests, MBs, slam balls, and core balls. Cones can be used as barriers or guides, or can be used as obstacles for various hops and jumps. Cones usually range in size from small (4.5 in.) to large (18 in.). Boxes are used for box jumps, depth jumps, and variations. Plyo boxes come in various sizes but must be sturdy to offset the explosive nature of plyometric exercises. Many boxes will be made of wood or tubular steel capable of withstanding large levels of force. Boxes come in various sizes from small (~6 in.) to large (~42 in. or greater). Smaller boxes are used for hops with larger boxes used for box jumps and depth jumps. Important to box selection is the upper surface. The box top surface should be made of nonskid rubber for greater friction and stability upon landing. The surface dimensions may range from 14 × 14 in. for smaller boxes to 20 × 20 in. for larger boxes. Some smaller boxes have added utilities. There are angled boxes with multiple surfaces that allow for lateral plyometric exercises. Jump ropes come in various forms and sizes with some designed more for speed and some to provide some resistance. Hurdles serve as barriers/obstacles for hops and jumps. Hurdles typically range in size from 6 to 12 in. up to 42 in. or higher. Some hurdles are adjustable which can be used for multiple exercises.

Bands provide resistance to jumping. Several styles are currently on the market. One particular resisted jump training device is the Vertimax (Fig 14.38). The Vertimax consists of a matted platform with resistance bands attached to a waist harness that gives the athlete resistance during several types of jumps. The loading from the bands creates greater ECC loading upon landing which serves as a potent stimulus for plyometric training. Several studies have examined jump training with the Vertimax. Rhea et al. (48,49) reported that 12 weeks of training with the Vertimax produced superior increases in vertical jump height and power in athletes than unloaded plyometric training. However, McClenton et al. (39) showed that 6 weeks of depth jump training versus jump training on the Vertimax produced similar increases in performance, and Carlson et al. (7) showed that 6 weeks of jump training on the Vertimax was no more effective than RT or plyometric training for increasing jump performance. Nevertheless, jump training on the Vertimax is effective for enhancing jump performance. Weighted vests can be

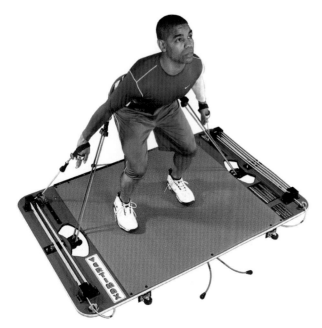

FIGURE 14.38. The Vertimax. (Courtesy of Perform Better, Cranston, RI.)

used for additional resistance during plyometric drills. Various vests are available but typically allow external loading of up to 30 lb or more but caution must be used as external loading may be most appropriate for low- and moderate-intensity drills. Bags (boxing, football) can be used as obstacles for jumping over. Medicine, core, and slam balls come in various sizes and are used for upper- and lower-body plyometrics.

PLYOMETRICS AND SAFETY CONSIDERATIONS

Plyometric training is safe for athletes of all ages provided that common sense is used in the program design and it is properly supervised. The most common reasons for injuries during plyometric training are: (a) violation of training guidelines, (b) inadequate warm-up, (c) too high a rate of progression, (d) lack of skill, (e) poor surface selection, (f) improper volume or intensity, and (g) undisclosed predisposition (44). Violations of training guidelines, coupled with high volume with too high intensity (or progressing too much too soon), could result in overreaching and subsequent overtraining of the athlete. Overtrained athletes are more susceptible to injury. For plyometric training it is the quality of the workout that is important and not quantity per se especially when depth jumps are performed. Volume and frequency need to be carefully prescribed based on the training phase. Inadequate warm-ups force the athlete to embark upon intense, explosive muscular contractions without proper physiologic preparation thereby increasing the risk of injury.

Lack of skill is a particular problem for coaches and athletes. Poor technique among athletes may limit

exercise selection. Sufficient coordination, balance, and strength are needed for performance of several plyometric exercises including those moderate to high in intensity. Coaches need to stress proper jumping mechanics with athletes at all phases of training. Critical to proper jump technique is the landing where large levels of force are absorbed by the athlete's body. Peak impact forces during jumping can be greater than the peak propulsion forces. Improper landing can place the athlete at greater risk of injury. Exercise selection can accommodate athletes with subpar skill development. Plyometric drills range in complexity. Beginning exercises may comprise the entire workout for poorly conditioned athletes. The athletes need to demonstrate improvement in technique plus increases in neuromuscular conditioning before progressing to more challenging exercises. Particular caution must be used with larger athletes. Large athletes place greater loading to musculoskeletal system thereby increasing the risk of injury if not careful. The volume of plyometric training should be lower for large athletes and the intensity must closely be monitored (44). It has been suggested that large athletes not perform depth jumps off of boxes greater than 18 in. (44). Plyometric training is safe when athletes are not previously injured. A prior injury or predisposition to injury can place the athlete at greater risk. Careful monitoring of the athletes is necessary. An injury may necessitate altering or temporarily discontinuing plyometric training until medical clearance has been attained. Lastly, proper breathing during plyometrics is important. Similar to high-intensity RT, a Valsalva maneuver is typically used during the ECC and early CON phases of the drill to ensure proper stability, shock absorption, and force and power production during propulsion. Exhalation ensures shortly afterward during the latter stages of the CON action.

INTEGRATING PLYOMETRIC WITH OTHER TRAINING MODALITIES

Plyometric training is a modality that is commonly performed with other modalities during a training cycle to optimize athletic performance. A program consisting of plyometric and RT can be employed simultaneously. For example, plyometric training 2 days per week can easily be incorporated into an RT program. Plyometric training can be performed on off-lifting days or on the same day. If performed on the same day, plyometric training may be given priority and performed first. Resistance training can be performed after or later in the day. The muscle groups trained for each workout is important. If only the upper body is resistance trained that day, then lower-body plyometrics can be performed uninhibited and the sequence can vary. It is not recommended that high-intensity lower-body RT and lower-body plyometric training be performed on the same day as the modality-trained second would do so in a

TABLE 14.3 INTEGRATING PLYOMETRIC AND RESISTANCE TRAINING (UPPER/LOWER-BODY SPLIT)

	DAY	RESISTANCE TRAINING	PLYOMETRIC TRAINING
Upper/lower-body split workout	Monday	Upper body	Off
	Tuesday	Lower body	Off
	Wednesday	Off	Total body
	Thursday	Upper body	Off
	Friday	Lower body	Off
	Saturday	Off	Total body
	Sunday	Off	Off
Total-body workout	Monday	Total body	Off
	Tuesday	Off	Upper body
	Wednesday	Total body	Off
	Thursday	Off	Off
	Friday	Total body	Off
	Saturday	Off	Lower body
	Sunday	Off	Off
Advanced upper/lower-body split	Monday	Upper body	Lower body
	Tuesday	Lower body	Upper body
	Wednesday	Off	Off
	Thursday	Upper body	Lower body
	Friday	Lower body	Upper body
	Saturday	Off	Total body
	Sunday	Off	Off

semifatigued state. Plyometric drills can also be incorporated into a weight training workout, *e.g.*, complex training.

Plyometric training coincides with sprint and agility training so effective combination programs can be developed. These modalities train similar physiological mechanisms and work in tandem to optimize neuromuscular performance so integration of these modalities into a workout is common. Plyometric, sprint, and agility drills can be alternated within a workout or trained in sequence. In some sports, athletes need a good aerobic base, and aerobic training may be performed along with plyometric training. It is important to point out that an incompatibility does exist between high-intensity anaerobic and aerobic training modalities. However, low to moderate levels of aerobic training (low frequency) may be performed without compromising performance. If this is the case, it is recommended that

plyometric training be performed first followed by aerobic exercise. It is better to perform the two during a workout as aerobic training in between anaerobic training sessions can impede recovery. Flexibility training should be incorporated at the conclusion of a plyometric workout and not before. Table 14.3 depicts some examples of integrating RT and plyometric training. The first two samples are intermediate programs where upper/lower-body split or total-body workouts are performed. The third sample is more advanced as it incorporates a higher frequency of plyometric training. Table 14.4 depicts a sample of combined plyometric and sprint training workout using an alternate integration model.

In-season plyometric training necessitates a lower training volume and frequency. The athletes' sport takes presentence so the frequency and volume of plyometric and resistance training decrease accordingly. Coaches

TABLE 14.4 SAMPLE COMBINED PLYOMETRIC AND SPRINT TRAINING WORKOUT[a]

GENERAL WARM-UP	3–5 MIN OF SLOW JOGGING
Dynamic range of motion drills	1 × 5 drills
High knees	2 × 20 yd
Butt kickers	2 × 20 yd
Lunge walks	2 × 20 yd
Truck jumps	3 × 10
Gears (10-yd intervals)	3–5 × 40 yd
Double-leg hops with lateral sprints	3 × 30 yd with 20-yd sprints
Box jumps	3 × 8
Sprints	3 × 40 yd
Cool-down	

[a]Specific sprint drills are discussed in Chapter 15.

TABLE 14.5 SAMPLE OFF-SEASON TOTAL-BODY PLYOMETRIC TRAINING PROGRAMS[a]

INTERMEDIATE WRESTLING PROGRAM (2×/WEEK)	INTERMEDIATE BASEBALL PROGRAM (2×/WEEK)
Squat jumps — 3 × 10	Tuck jumps — 3 × 10
MB side throw — 3 × 8 (each side)	MB overhead throw — 3 × 8
Split squat jump with cycle — 3 × 10	Barrier jumps — 5 × 5
MB back throw — 3 × 5	MB kneeling side throw — 3 × 8 (each side)
Single-leg push-off — 3 × 6 (each leg)	Lateral step-ups — 3 × 10
Plyo push-up — 3 × 10	Alternate-leg bounding — 3 × 25 yd
Box jumps — 3 × 8	
Low- to moderate-intensity drills	
Foot contacts = 120	Foot contacts = 103
Upper-body repetitions = 93	Upper-body repetitions = 72
Alternate exercises	
Single-leg hops	Standing long jump with lateral sprint
Bag/sandbag side throw	Lateral cone hops
Core ball overhead slams	Box jumps
Stadium hops	Slam ball rotations
MB chest pass	MB front rotation throw
Slam ball side rotation slams	

[a]All workouts are to be preceded by a warm-up and finished with a cool-down consisting of stretching. Jump lengths, box heights, barrier heights, etc. are based upon the conditioning of the athlete.

must closely monitor athletic performance in examination of potential overreaching/overtraining, and training volume can be adjusted accordingly. All sports consist of plyometric actions so practice and competition can be viewed as a training stimulus. Anaerobic sports that require high levels of power and strength necessitate the athlete train intensely during the season to maintain performance. Thus, too much plyometric training can be excessive or counterproductive when the demands of the sport are considered, especially when depth jumps are performed.

TABLE 14.6 SAMPLE OFF-SEASON TOTAL-BODY PLYOMETRIC TRAINING PROGRAMS[a]

ADVANCED BASKETBALL PROGRAM (2×/WEEK)	ADVANCED WEIGHTLIFTING PROGRAM (2×/WEEK)
Jump and reach — 4 × 10	Tuck jumps — 4 × 10
MB chest pass — 3 × 8	Split squat jump (cycle) — 4 × 10
Box jumps — 5 × 5	MB back throw — 3 × 8
MB overhead throw — 3 × 8	Depth jumps to box — 5 × 3
Depth jumps to box — 5 × 3	Multiple box jumps — 5 × 3
Power drop — 3 × 6	
Single-leg push-off — 4 × 8 (each leg)	
Low- to high-intensity drills	
Foot contacts = 144	Foot contacts = 125
Upper-body repetitions = 66	Upper-body repetitions = 24
Alternate exercises	
Single-leg hops	Squat jumps
Alternate-leg bounding	Double leg hops
Barrier jumps	Single-arm vertical core ball throw
Single-leg depth jumps	Single-leg depth jumps
MB front rotation throw	Depth push-ups

[a]All workouts are to be preceded by a warm-up and finished with a cool-down consisting of stretching. Jump lengths, box heights, barrier heights, etc. are based upon the conditioning of the athlete.

PUTTING IT ALL TOGETHER

The program designed should incorporate all of the factors discussed in this chapter. Numerous effective programs can be developed provided that the progressive overload, specificity, and variation are used appropriately and the program is well supervised. Tables 14.5 and 14.6 depict sample plyometric training programs. The key elements are selecting sport-specific exercises and prescribing appropriate levels of intensity and volume. Each repetition should be performed explosively and coaches should constantly monitor technique and stress proper mechanics to their athletes.

Summary Points

✔ Modern plyometrics are explosive exercises that utilize the SSC and target power, speed, and strength development.
✔ Plyometric training increases jumping height and power, sprinting speed, agility, muscle strength, hypertrophy, running economy and race times, swimming block start performance, reaction time, throwing velocity, and kicking speed.
✔ Plyometric exercises consist of hops, jumps, bounding, box jumps, depth jumps, and throws, and the intensity is based on complexity, use of external loading, uphill/downhill, height/distance of jump/throw, height of box, and unilateral versus bilateral exercises.
✔ Plyometric exercise volume is based upon the number of foot contacts or throws/repetitions. Volume depends on the athlete's training status and whether the athlete is in the off-season, preseason, or in-season training period.
✔ Plyometric exercises can be performed with just body weight and various pieces of equipment including cones, boxes, jump ropes, mini hurdles, bands, bags, weighted vests, MBs, slam balls, and core balls.

Review Questions

1. The time between the end of the ECC action and beginning of the CON muscle action is known as the:
   a. SSC
   b. Coupling time
   c. Isokinetic phase
   d. Relaxation time

2. Which of the following exercises is considered to be the most intense?
   a. Ankle hops
   b. Lateral cone hops
   c. Tuck jumps
   d. Depth jumps

3. An appropriate number of foot contacts of lower-body plyometric drills for a beginner during an off-season program is:
   a. 30
   b. 75
   c. 150
   d. 250

4. A plyometric drill involving exaggerated horizontal movements where an excessive stride length is targeted is known as:
   a. Bounding
   b. A hop
   c. A box jump
   d. A throw

5. Which of the following would be the most appropriate surface for plyometric training?
   a. Hardwood floor
   b. Concrete
   c. Grass
   d. Sand

6. Greatest CON power output is seen during the _____ phase of the vertical jump.
   a. Starting position
   b. Countermovement
   c. Propulsion
   d. Flight

7. Performing a plyometric exercise in between sets of a similar resistance exercise during a workout is known as complex training.   T F

8. Plyometric training leads to fiber-type transitions (type IIX to IIA) similar to resistance training.   T F

9. Double-leg jumps are more intense than single-leg jumps.   T F

10. A low-intensity plyometric exercise simply means that it should not be performed explosively.   T F

11. A 1:1 work/relief ratio is recommended for most plyometric training programs.   T F

12. Plyometric training frequency depends on intensity, volume, and the inclusion of other training modalities.   T F

References

1. Adams K, O'Shea JP, O'Shea KL, Climstein M. The effect of six weeks of squat, plyometric and squat-plyometric training on power production. *J Appl Sport Sci Res*. 1992;6:36–41.

2. Bedi JF, Cresswell AG, Engel TJ, Nicol SM. Increase in jumping height associated with maximal effort vertical depth jumps. *Res Quart*. 1987;58:11–15.

3. Bishop DC, Smith RJ, Smith MF, Rigby HE. Effect of plyometric training on swimming block start performance in adolescents. *J Strength Cond Res*. 2009;23:2137–2143.

4. Bobbert MF, Mackay M, Schinkelshoek D, Huijing PA, van Ingen Schenau GJ. Biomechanical analysis of drop and countermovement jumps. *Eur J Appl Physiol*. 1986;54:566–573.

5. Bobbert MF, Huijing PA, van Ingen Schenau GJ. Drop jumping I. The influence of jumping technique on the biomechanics of jumping. *Med Sci Sports Exerc*. 1987;19:332–338.

6. Bobbert MF, Huijing PA, van Ingen Schenau GJ. Drop jumping II. The influence of dropping height on the biomechanics of drop jumping. *Med Sci Sports Exerc*. 1987;19:339–346.

7. Carlson K, Magnusen M, Walters P. Effect of various training modalities on vertical jump. *Res Sports Med*. 2009;17:84–94.

8. Carter AB, Kaminski TW, Douex AT, Knight CA, Richards JG. Effects of high volume upper extremity plyometric training on throwing velocity and functional strength ratios of the shoulder rotators in collegiate baseball players. *J Strength Cond Res*. 2007;21:208–215.

9. Chu DA. *Explosive Power and Strength*. Champaign (IL): Human Kinetics; 1996. pp. 153–165.

10. Chu DA. *Jumping Into Plyometrics*. 2nd ed. Champaign (IL): Human Kinetics; 1998. pp. 1–138.

11. Delecluse C. Influence of strength training on sprint running performance: current findings and implications for training. *Sports Med*. 1997;24:147–156.

12. De Villarreal ES, Gonzalez-Badillo JJ, Izquierdo M. Low and moderate plyometric training frequency produces greater jumping and sprinting gains compared with high frequency. *J Strength Cond Res*. 2008;22:715–725.

13. Diallo O, Dore E, Duche P, Van Praagh E. Effects of plyometric training followed by a reduced training programme on physical performance in prepubescent soccer players. *J Sports Med Phys Fitness*. 2001;41:342–348.

14. Dodd DJ, Alvar BA. Analysis of acute explosive training modalities to improve lower-body power in baseball players. *J Strength Cond Res*. 2007;21:1177–1182.

15. Ebben WP, Blackard DO. Strength and conditioning practices of National Football League strength and conditioning coaches. *J Strength Cond Res*. 2001;15:48–58.

16. Ebben WP, Carroll RM, Simenz CJ. Strength and conditioning practices of National Hockey League strength and conditioning coaches. *J Strength Cond Res*. 2004;18:889–897.

17. Ebben WP, Hintz MJ, Simenz CJ. Strength and conditioning practices of Major League Baseball strength and conditioning coaches. *J Strength Cond Res*. 2005;19:538–546.

18. Faigenbaum AD, McFarland J, Keiper F, et al. Effects of short-term plyometric and resistance training program on fitness performance in boys age 12 to 15 years. *J Sport Sci Med*. 2007;6:519–525.

19. Faigenbaum AD, Farrell A, Radler T. "Plyo Play": A novel program of short bouts of moderate and high intensity exercise improves physical fitness in elementary school children. *Phys Educ*. 2009; 66:37–44.

20. Faigenbaum AD, Kraemer WJ, Blimkie CJ, et al. Youth resistance training: updated position statement paper from the National Strength and Conditioning Association. *J Strength Cond Res*. 2009; 23(suppl):S60–S79.

21. Fleck SJ, Kraemer WJ. *Designing Resistance Training Programs*. 3rd ed. Champaign (IL): Human Kinetics; 2004. pp. 230–236.

22. Gambetta V, Odgers S. *The Complete Guide to Medicine Ball Training*. Sarasota (FL): Optimum Sports Training; 1991. pp. 18–52.

23. Harman EA, Rosenstein MT, Frykman PN, Rosenstein RM. The effects of arms and countermovement on vertical jumping. *Med Sci Sports Exerc*. 1990;22:825–833.

24. Holcomb WR, Lander JE, Rutland RM, Wilson GD. The effectiveness of a modified plyometric program on power and the vertical jump. *J Strength Cond Res*. 1996;10:89–92.

25. Impellizzeri FM, Rampinini E, Castagna C, et al. Effect of plyometric training on sand versus grass on muscle soreness and jumping and sprinting ability in soccer players. *Br J Sports Med*. 2008; 42:42–46.

26. Kotsamidis C. Effect of plyometric training on running performance and vertical jumping in prepubertal boys. *J Strength Cond Res*. 2006;20:441–445.

27. Kraemer WJ, Newton RU. Training for improved vertical jump. *Gatorade Sport Science Exchange*. 1994;7:53.

28. Kraemer WJ, Ratamess NA, Volek JS, Mazzetti SA, Gomez AL. The effect of the Meridian shoe on vertical jump and sprint performances following short-term combined plyometric/sprint and resistance training. *J Strength Cond Res*. 2000;14:228–238.

29. Kramer JF, Morrow A, Leger A. Changes in rowing ergometer, weight lifting, vertical jump and isokinetic performance in response to standard and standard plus plyometric training programs. *Int J Sports Med*. 1983;14:449–454.

30. Lephart SM, Abt JP, Ferris CM, et al. Neuromuscular and biomechanical characteristic changes in high school athletes: a plyometric versus basic resistance program. *Br J Sports Med*. 2005; 39:932–938.

31. Luebbers PE, Potteiger JA, Hulver MW, et al. Effects of plyometric training and recovery on vertical jump performance and anaerobic power. *J Strength Cond Res*. 2003;17:704–709.

32. Luhtanen P, Komi RV. Segmental contribution to forces in vertical jump. *Eur J Appl Physiol Occup Physiol*. 1978;38:181–188.

33. Marcovic G. Does plyometric training improve vertical jump height? A meta-analytical review. *Br J Sports Med*. 2007;41: 349–355.

34. Marcovic G, Jukic I, Milanovic D, Metikos D. Effects of sprint and plyometric training on muscle function and athletic performance. *J Strength Cond Res*. 2007;21:543–549.

35. Marginson V, Rowlands AV, Gleeson NP, Eston RG. Comparison of the symptoms of exercise-induced muscle damage after an initial and repeated bout of plyometric exercise in men and boys. *J Appl Physiol*. 2005;99:1174–1181.

36. Martel GF, Harmer ML, Logan JM, Parker CB. Aquatic plyometric training increases vertical jump in female volleyball players. *Med Sci Sports Exerc*. 2005;37:1814–1819.

37. Masamoto N, Larson R, Gates T, Faigenbaum A. Acute effects of plyometric exercise on maximum squat performance in male athletes. *J Strength Cond Res*. 2003;17:68–71.

38. Matavulj D, Kukolj M, Ugarkovic D, Tihanyi J, Jaric S. Effects of plyometric training on jumping performance in junior basketball players. *J Sports Med Phys Fitness*. 2001;41:159–164.

39. McClenton LS, Brown LE, Coburn JW, Kersey RD. The effect of short-term VertiMax vs. depth jump training on vertical jump performance. *J Strength Cond Res*. 2008;22:321–325.

40. Mediate P, Faigenbaum A. *Medicine Ball for All Kids: Medicine Ball Training Concepts and Program-Design Considerations for School-Age Youth*. Monterey (CA): Coaches Choice; 2007.

41. Mihalik JP, Libby JJ, Battaglini CL, McMurray RG. Comparing short-term complex and compound training programs on vertical jump height and power output. *J Strength Cond Res*. 2008;22: 47–53.

42. Pappas E, Hagins M, Sheikhzadeh A, Nordin M, Rose D. Biomechanical differences between unilateral and bilateral landings from a jump: gender differences. *Clin J Sports Med.* 2007; 17:263–268.

43. Perez-Gomez J, Olmedillas H, Delgado-Guerra S, et al. Effects of weight lifting training combined with plyometric exercises on physical fitness, body composition, and knee extension velocity during kicking in football. *Appl Physiol Nutr Metab.* 2008;33: 501–510.

44. Potach DH, Chu DA. Plyometric training. In: Baechle TR, Earle RW, editors. *Essentials of Strength Training and Conditioning.* 3rd ed. Champaign (IL): Human Kinetics; 2008. pp. 413–456.

45. Potteiger JA, Lockwood RH, Haub MD, et al. Muscle power and fiber characteristics following 8 weeks of plyometric training. *J Strength Cond Res.* 1999;13:275–279.

46. Radcliffe JC, Farentinos RC. *High-Powered Plyometrics.* Champaign (IL): Human Kinetics; 1999. pp. 23–115.

47. Ratamess NA, Kraemer WJ, Volek JS, et al. The effects of ten weeks of resistance and combined plyometric/sprint training with the Meridian Elyte athletic shoe on muscular performance in women. *J Strength Cond Res.* 2007;21:882–887.

48. Rhea MR, Peterson MD, Oliverson JR, Ayllon FN, Potenziano BJ. An examination of training on the VertiMax resisted jumping device for improvements in lower body power in highly trained college athletes. *J Strength Cond Res.* 2008;22:735–740.

49. Rhea MR, Peterson MD, Lunt KT, Ayllon FN. The effectiveness of resisted jump training on the VertiMax in high school athletes. *J Strength Cond Res.* 2008;22:731–734.

50. Robertson DG, Fleming D. Kinetics of standing broad and vertical jumping. *Can J Sport Sci.* 1987;12:19–23.

51. Salonikidis K, Zafeiridis A. The effects of plyometric, tennis-drills, and combined training on reaction, lateral and linear speed, power, and strength in novice tennis players. *J Strength Cond Res.* 2008;22:182–191.

52. Santos EJ, Janeira MA. Effects of complex training on explosive strength in adolescent male basketball players. *J Strength Cond Res.* 2008;22:903–909.

53. Saunders PU, Telford RD, Pyne DB, et al. Short-term plyometric training improves running economy in highly trained middle and long distance runners. *J Strength Cond Res.* 2006;20:947–954.

54. Sedano Campo S, Vaeyens R, Phillippaerts RM, et al. Effects of lower-limb plyometric training on body composition, explosive strength, and kicking speed in female soccer players. *J Strength Cond Res.* 2009;23:1714–1722.

55. Simenz CJ, Dugan CA, Ebben WP. Strength and conditioning practices of National Basketball Association strength and conditioning coaches. *J Strength Cond Res.* 2005;19:495–504.

56. Spurrs RW, Murphy AJ, Watsford ML. The effect of plyometric training on distance running performance. *Eur J Appl Physiol.* 2003; 89:1–7.

57. Stemm JD, Jacobson BH. Comparison of land- and aquatic-based plyometric training on vertical jump performance. *J Strength Cond Res.* 2007;21:568–571.

58. Turner AM, Owings M, Schwane JA. Improvement in running economy after 6 weeks of plyometric training. *J Strength Cond Res.* 2003;17:60–67.

59. Verkhoshansky Y. Are depth jumps useful? *Yessis Rev Soviet Phys Ed Sports.* 1968;3:75–78.

60. Verkhoshansky Y, Siff M. *Supertraining.* 6th ed. Ultimate Athlete Concepts; 2009. pp. 267–284.

61. Vissing K, Brink M, Lonbro S, et al. Muscle adaptations to plyometric vs. resistance training in untrained young men. *J Strength Cond Res.* 2008;22:1799–1810.

62. Wilson GJ, Murphy AJ, Giorgi A. Weight and plyometric training: effects on eccentric and concentric force production. *Can J Appl Physiol.* 1996;21:301–315.

63. Zatsiorsky V, Kraemer WJ. *Science and Practice of Strength Training.* 2nd ed. Champaign (IL): Human Kinetics; 2006. pp. 1–35.

CHAPTER 15

Sprint and Agility Training

After completing this chapter, you will be able to:

- Define speed, agility, quickness, reaction ability, and speed endurance
- Discuss the roles stride length and stride rate have on speed development
- Discuss the mechanics of proper sprint technique relative to the phases of sprinting
- Discuss the importance of overspeed and resisted sprint training on speed development
- Identify several drills which can improve an athlete's technique, speed, quickness, agility, and reactive ability
- Discuss relevant elements to agility and ways to specifically train each to enhance performance
- Discuss the elements of sprint and agility program design
- Discuss methods of improving speed endurance

Speed and agility are critical components to several sports. Many have heard coaches say that "speed kills" meaning it is a differentiating factor between teams and athletes in competition. Speed is the change in distance over time and maximal speed is a critical component to anaerobic sport performance. This is especially important for track and field athletes such sprinters. However, maximal speed may not be attained until the athlete has run at least 20–40 m in a linear path. In many cases, the athlete may not have the option of running optimally (or unimpeded) for 20–40 m but may have to move rapidly for shorter distances covering multiple directions. Thus, acceleration ability becomes a critical training component. **Acceleration** is the rate of change of velocity over time. In athletic terms, it entails the athlete's ability to reach high velocities in a short period of time following a change of direction, deceleration, or from a static position. Athletes with explosive acceleration ability have a major advantage in sports such as football, basketball, and baseball. Highest rates of acceleration are seen within the first 8–10 strides where the athlete may reach ~75% of his/her max velocity within the first 10 yd (26). Training to increase acceleration is critical to athletic success. Acceleration ability is highly related to reaction time. *Reaction time* refers to the athlete's ability to react to a stimulus. Fast reaction times increase the likelihood of athletic success. For example, the quicker a sprinter reacts to the gun, the better the race time. Goalies in hockey or a baseball player getting ready to hit a 90-mph-fast ball may have less than 0.40 second to react. The quicker the first response, the more likely an athlete will be able to accelerate into a successful position.

Sprints of sufficient duration will force the athlete to reach maximal speed and maintain it for as long as possible so **speed endurance** is critical to many sports. Speed endurance also refers to the ability to maintain maximal speed over several repetitions. Reducing fatigue-induced deceleration is a critical conditioning component. For example, an athlete with the ability to have the same burst of speed in the second half of a game as he/she did in the first half will have good speed endurance. In a linear sprint of sufficient duration (100 m), three distinct phases can be seen: (a) acceleration, (b) maximum speed maintenance, and (c) speed endurance or deceleration.

The ability to move rapidly while changing direction in response to a stimulus is agility. Agility is quite complex and requires the optimal integration of several physiological systems and components of fitness (Fig. 15.1). Although an athlete may have sufficient linear speed, this does not mean he/she will be very agile and coordinated. There is some evidence that linear sprinting ability has only limited transferability to various agility drills (40). For example, the ability to backpedal is an independent skill. Maximal backward running velocities range from 60% to 80% of one's sprint speed (40). Backpedalling produces shorter stride lengths, greater stride rates, longer support time, lower peak ground reaction force and time to produce it, and smaller range of motion (ROM) of the hip, knee, and ankle compared to forward sprinting (40). Thus, components of agility must be trained independently in order to maximize athletic performance.

Agility requires the athlete to coordinate several activities including the ability to react and start quickly,

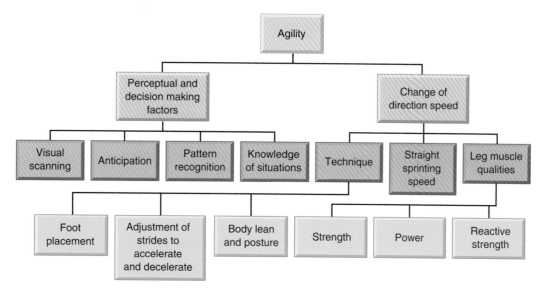

FIGURE 15.1. Components of agility. (Reprinted with permission from Young WB, Farrow D. A review of agility: practical applications for strength and conditioning. *Strength Cond J.* 2006;28:24–29.)

accelerate, decelerate, move in the proper direction, and maintain the ability to change direction as rapidly as possible while maintaining balance and postural control. The athlete must adapt to the environment, react quickly, adjust bodily position accordingly, and transition from one skill to another as efficiently as possible. Agility will allow the athlete to reduce the risk of injury, evade other athletes on the field or court, maintain the proper position to catch, strike, and kick a ball, and maintain the proper position to block or tackle an opponent. Often the athlete may have a small window within which to accelerate or decelerate before a change of direction takes place. This complexity provides a challenge to the athlete when training for optimal bodily control. The rapid change of direction may take place from a variety of stable or unstable bodily positions, *e.g.*, standing (unilateral or bilateral), lying (prone or supine), seated on the ground, and/or kneeling positions forcing the athlete to react to a number of situations. The athlete who can change position fluently and rapidly will be more likely to experience success in his/her respective sport. Although the actual practice/competition for the sport increases agility, many strength and conditioning (S&C) coaches see the value of off-season and preseason sport-specific agility training to increase athleticism beyond the improvements seen from just participating in the sport. Training each fitness component throughout the year is important for the athlete just to stay competitive with other athletes.

INCREASING SPRINT SPEED

Sprint speed is the product of stride length and frequency (rate) and faster athletes display higher stride rates and greater stride lengths than slower runners (48). **Stride length** is the length of each stride (from toe-off to heel strike on the same side) during sprinting and is determined by leg length, leg strength and power, and sprinting mechanics. Stride length is improved by increasing the athlete's ability to develop explosive forces applied to the ground (48). This should be a natural occurrence because stride length can be intentionally increased forcibly, a common sprinting error known as overstriding. Overstriding creates equilibrium problems and slows the athlete down. **Stride rate** or *frequency* refers to the number of foot contacts per period of time. Rapid turnover of the feet during the sprint cycle is seen at higher speeds and is a goal of maximal sprint training. Sprint, agility, plyometric, and ballistic training are the most effective ways to increase stride rate. Forcing a greater stride rate can decrease stride length and vice versa. *Maximal sprint speed occurs only when the optimal proportion or combination of stride length and rate are utilized by the athlete.* These are athlete-dependent and it is paramount that the coach closely monitors the technique to prevent flaws, *e.g.*, overstriding, which can slow the athlete down.

Training programs designed to increase maximal speed are multifactorial. An integrated approach is most effective where a combination of plyometric, sprint (nonresisted, overspeed, resisted [chutes, sleds, weighted vests]), and resistance training (RT) (13) is used in the training of athletes. Nonresisted (54), uphill/downhill (39), and resisted sprint training programs (23,45,54) increase acceleration and sprint speed. The combination of sprint and RT is effective for enhancing maximal speed, speed endurance, power, and strength of the lower body (24,41). Resistance training increases muscular strength and power, and in combination with sprint training, enables the athlete to exert greater force with each foot contact leading to an increase in running acceleration and velocity. Maximal strength for sport-specific exercises like the half-squat and hang clean correlate highly to sprint performance (12,50). Young et al. (53) showed correlations between peak force application and starting ability, acceleration out of the block, and maximum sprinting speed.

TABLE 15.1 WAYS TO INCREASE COMPONENTS OF SPRINTING

SPRINT COMPONENT	TRAINING MODALITIES
Reaction time and start ability	Overspeed training Reactive drills Power training
Acceleration	Resistance and ballistic training Acceleration training Resisted and overspeed training Basic sprint drills and plyometrics
Stride length	Resistance and ballistic training Acceleration training Resisted and overspeed training Basic sprint, stick/line drills and plyometrics Flexibility training
Stride frequency	Resistance and ballistic training Resisted and overspeed training Basic sprint drills and plyometrics Quick feet drills
Max speed and power	Resistance and ballistic training Acceleration training Resisted and overspeed training Basic sprint drills and plyometrics Power training and quickness drills

Adapted with permission from Dintiman G, Ward B, Tellez T. *Sports Speed*. 2nd ed. Champaign, IL: Human Kinetics; 1998. pp. 191–220.

Thus, a comprehensive sprint enhancement program consists of sprint-specific drills in addition to plyometric, flexibility, and RT (Table 15.1).

SPRINT TRAINING

MECHANICS OF SPRINT RUNNING

The phases of sprinting begin with the starting position, acceleration, and maximum speed. The starting position is essential for attaining optimal stability allowing maximal propulsive forces for acceleration. Acceleration is marked by an increase in velocity. Once the athlete begins to accelerate and reaches peak speed or velocity, several phases can be identified that assist the coach in stressing proper technique (Fig. 15.2). Sprinting can be characterized by two major phases: (a) **flight phase** and (b) the **support phase**. The flight phase describes motion of the leg that is not in contact with the ground. It can further be broken into the early, middle, and late flight phases. The early flight phase describes recovery motion of the back leg from the time it leaves the ground

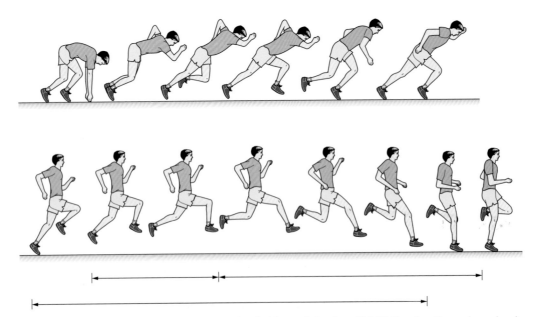

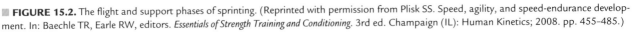

■ **FIGURE 15.2.** The flight and support phases of sprinting. (Reprinted with permission from Plisk SS. Speed, agility, and speed-endurance development. In: Baechle TR, Earle RW, editors. *Essentials of Strength Training and Conditioning*. 3rd ed. Champaign (IL): Human Kinetics; 2008. pp. 455–485.)

until there is moderate knee flexion and further hip hyperextension. The hip and knee musculature decelerates backward rotation of the thigh and lower leg/foot. The midflight phase describes motion of the back leg as knee flexion increases and hip flexion positions the thigh in alignment with the torso. The late flight phase describes motion for preparation of ground contact. The hip flexes forward and the knee extends to attain an optimal unilateral landing position and signifies the beginning of the support phase. The support phase describes motion of the leg that is in contact with the ground. It can further be broken into the early and late support phases. The early support phase describes motion of the leg as it contacts the ground. Braking and shock absorption take place as the hip extends, knee slightly flexes, and the ankle dorsiflexes. The late support phase describes triple extension of the leg to maximize propulsive forces during push-off thereby continuing the motion of the center of gravity (COG) forward. Triple extension involves hip and knee extension and ankle plantar flexion. The final segment of the late support phase concludes with the propulsion leg leaving the ground indicating the beginning of the early flight phase. The cycle repeats for the duration of the sprint.

Starting Position

The proper starting position entails the athlete maintain a three-point (one hand touching the ground) or four-point (two hands touching the ground) stance with the legs in a staggered stance (with the stronger or dominant leg forward [left leg for a right-handed athlete]). Body weight is evenly distributed with a front knee angle of ~90°, rear knee angle of ~110°–135°, front hip angle of ~40°–50°, a rear hip angle of 80°–90°, and a torso angle of ~42°–45° from the horizontal (40). The height of the COG may range from 0.61 to 0.66 m vertically and is located ~0.16–0.19 m from the starting line horizontally (35). Athletes with stronger arms can maintain a position where the COG is closer to the starting line (35) although weight should be balanced, or the athlete may lose force applied to the ground during propulsion and lose balance forward during initial acceleration. Upon initial motion, both legs explosively push off where the front leg completes its extension as the rear leg swings forward. Knee and hip angles increase while ankle angles decrease. The rear leg produces greater initial force while pushing backward and downward and lifts off first whereas the front leg plays a vital role in starting velocity and will exert force for a longer period of time (40). In elite sprinters the front leg applies force for ≤0.37 second and the rear leg produces force for ≤0.18 second (twice as much time for the front leg) (40). Force production is greater in elite sprinters than lesser-trained athletes (35). Simultaneously, the opposite arm swings forward and up as the rear foot lifts up to increase momentum and reduce inertia. Backward arm countermovement helps forward flexion of the leg. Forward lean of trunk helps overcome inertia while accelerating from the starting position.

Acceleration

Acceleration phase consists of the ability to rapidly increase velocity from the starting position. The back leg drives forward while the shin is ~45° to the ground. The angle of the shin decreases ~6°–7° with each stride over the first 10 m as the torso gradually reaches an upright position during the first 8–10 strides. Arms are swung back and forth (at a 90° elbow angle) in a sagittal plane while shoulders remain as relaxed as possible. Wrists remain neutral and fingers are extended. The arms work in opposition to the legs with right arm and left leg moving forward and vice versa. The face, shoulders, hands, and neck muscles remain relaxed. The head begins down in front of the body's COG during acceleration but will eventually extend and form a vertical line with the body when maximal speed is attained. Legs are cycled back and forth in a sagittal plane with high knee action when driving forward and a pawing type of action is used when the ball of the foot strikes the ground. It is important that force be developed through the ball of the foot and not the toes to maximize force applied to the ground (15). The ankles remain dorsiflexed (toes up) for most of the sprint cycle except when the feet come in contact with the ground. Both stride length and frequency increase as speed increases (Fig. 15.3) and the acceleration phase length ranges from 30 to 50 m (35). The athlete's height and/or leg length correlate to stride length, and gender differences in height is a critical factor in viewing differences in max speed, *e.g.*, men typically have longer limbs

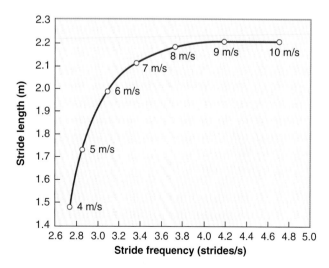

■ FIGURE 15.3. Stride length and rate relationship to sprint speed. (Reprinted with permission from Plisk SS. Speed, agility, and speed-endurance development. In: Baechle TR, Earle RW, editors. *Essentials of Strength Training and Conditioning*. 3rd ed. Champaign (IL): Human Kinetics; 2008. pp. 455–485.)

and faster running speeds (35). At higher speeds there is a small increase in stride length and a greater increase in stride rate (48). In elite sprinters, support (early and late) phases are ≤0.20 and 0.18 second, respectively, and flight phases (early-to-mid, mid-to-late) are ≤0.70 and 0.90 second, respectively, stride length increases for the first 45 m, stride frequency increases for the first 25 m, forward body lean decreases from ~45° to ~5° within ~20 m, and peak acceleration rate can reach ~11.8 m · s^{-2} (40). Impact forces increase and ground contact time decreases as speed increases (48). The force applied to the ground increases as speed increases; however, impulse reaches a peak and declines slightly due to shorter foot contact times with the ground (48). Lower-extremity muscle activity increases as velocity increases and muscle activation during acceleration is ~5% higher than the max speed phase (35). Positive relationships exist between propulsive forces and running velocity during acceleration (35).

Maximum Speed

Stride rate and length are maximized when the athlete reaches peak speed. Stride length at maximal speed is typically around 2.3–2.5 times the athlete's leg length (26). Stride rate plays a more substantial role as the athlete reaches the maximum speed phase (35). Flight phase duration is typically ~0.12–0.14 second whereas support phase duration is ~0.08–0.10 second in sprinters (35,40). During the support phase, the torso remains erect (<5° forward lean), weight is balanced as only the ball of foot contacts the ground, and horizontal braking forces and vertical displacement are minimized (40). Vertical displacement of the COG decreases as speed increases and elite sprinters with greater speed demonstrate lower vertical displacement values than lesser-skilled athletes (35). The push-off angle of the rear foot during propulsion is ~50°–55° and peak forces applied to the ground are generated rapidly (<0.04 second in elite sprinters) (40). Weyand et al. (48) have shown that applying greater force to the ground is vital for maximizing sprint speed more so than the movement velocity of the legs during the swing phase. Ground reaction forces during maximal sprints may range from 2.5 to 5 times an individual's body weight (48,49). Leg drive is enhanced by powerful arm action. Elbows are flexed to ~90° and arms are kept close to body to minimize wind resistance. Flexing the hips (close to 90°) and knees (thigh nearly parallel to the ground during late flight and "heel-to-butt" during midflight) is vital to maximizing hip angular velocity by lowering the hip's moment of inertia during flight. The athlete keeps torso, head/neck, and upper extremity muscles as relaxed as possible. The phase of maximal sprinting affects performance. Athletes transiently slow down during the impact (by ~5%) or braking phase but compensate by increasing velocity during

propulsion (33,35). The deceleration during braking is thought to limit maximal speed in addition to the short contact period of propulsion and potential air resistance (6). Muscle activation is greater during impact than in the propulsion phase presumably due to the effects of the stretch-shortening cycle (SSC) (35). Interestingly, preactivation of lower-body musculature occurs where lower body muscles increase activity up to ~50%–70% of their maximum during preactivation (the period of time directly prior to impact with the ground) to increase stiffness and prepare for shock absorption (34).

COMMON ERRORS IN SPRINTING

Sprinting occurs primarily in the sagittal plane. Thus, movements should be confined to the sagittal plane as much as possible. Proper sprint technique focuses on maintaining correct posture, arm, and leg action. Sprint training entails technique training in addition to conditioning drills as minor improvements in technique can lead to increases in sprint speed. Deviations lead to unnecessary movements that lower efficiency and reduce speed. Some common errors include:

1. improper stance (hands too far apart, hips too high or low)—can be corrected by narrowing hands and coaching proper hip position
2. pushing off too high during acceleration—can be corrected by coaching athlete to push downward
3. rising too quickly during acceleration from the start—can be corrected by coaching athlete to stay low and gradually rise as a *power line* should be formed through the head, spine, and rear leg while maintaining a ~45° torso angle to the ground
4. excessive head movement—can be corrected by coaching athlete to focus eyes on a target straight ahead
5. not explosively using the arms to accelerate (movement of the arms counteracts rotational motion initiated by the lower body to help keep the body in proper alignment)—can be corrected by form drills such as arm swings and marches
6. arm movements occurring out of the sagittal plane (across the body) and not close to the body—can be corrected by coaching front-to-back motion and including form drills such as arm swings, skips, and marches
7. failing to keep muscles (especially shoulders) as relaxed as possible (fluid, rhythmic motion is important)—can be corrected by coaching athletes to relax and enforcing relaxation during sprints and form drills such as arm swings
8. excessive bending (flexion/extension) of elbows—can be corrected by coaching the athlete to keep elbow angle close to 90° and including form drills such as arm swings and marches
9. not fully extending the legs during propulsion (lowers force applied to the ground and could result from

weak posterior muscles and tight hip flexors and ankle muscles)—can be corrected by RT, plyometric and sprint drills, and flexibility training

10. limited hip and knee ROM during lower-body motion—can be corrected by coaching "driving the legs" and through flexibility training, RT, and form drills such as high knees, marching, TRX mountain climbers, and resisted hip flexion

11. not dorsiflexing the foot during flight—can be corrected by coaching proper foot position (dorsiflexion) and with form drills (skips), flexibility training, and resisted dorsiflexion exercises

12. failing to maintain upright position during maximal speed—can be corrected by coaching proper body position and core RT and sprint training drills

13. too much vertical bouncing—can be corrected by coaching the athlete to push off horizontally and minimize vertical motion

BASIC SPRINT TRAINING DRILLS

The most specific way to increase sprint speed is by sprinting. However, drills can be used which improve athletic conditioning and technique simultaneously. These drills are used at the beginning of a workout following a general warm-up and dynamic ROM exercises to help prepare the body for more intense sprints and/or plyometric exercises performed later in the workout. Figures 15.4–15.17 depict common basic sprint training/technique drills. Drills shown in this chapter were not previously discussed. It is important to note that some linear plyometric drills can be effectively used to enhance sprint speed. For example, drills such as multiple forms of bounding and skipping have high transfer ability to sprinting mechanics.

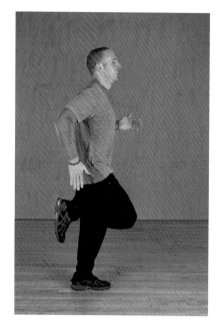

■ **FIGURE 15.5.** "Butt kickers." The athlete begins by jogging and pulls the heel of the foot until it bounces off the buttocks. A variation is a drill known as the "wall slide," which is very similar except during recovery the athlete's heels never move behind the athlete's body.

OVERSPEED AND RESISTED SPRINT TRAINING

Overspeed Sprint Training

Overspeed training allows the athlete to attain supramaximal speed, or an assisted speed that is greater than the athlete's maximal effort. The objective is to provide assistance to the athlete without altering sprinting mechanics and to improve the quality of effort (40). Overspeed training increases stride

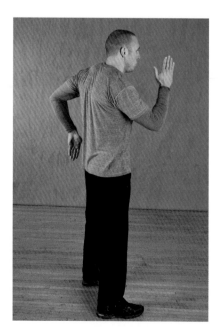

■ **FIGURE 15.4.** Standing arm swings. The athlete stands with feet together and swings arms in a sagittal plane with elbows flexed at 90°.

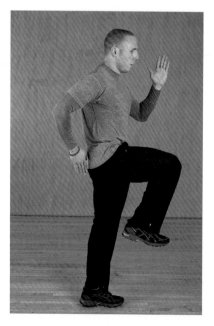

■ **FIGURE 15.6.** "High knees." The athlete drives the knees upward with each step trying to maximize ROM with each movement.

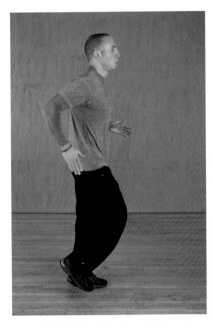

■ **FIGURE 15.7.** Ankling. The athlete jogs with very short steps and emphasizes plantar flexion during ground contact.

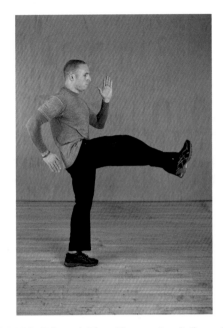

■ **FIGURE 15.9.** "B" march. The athlete marches similar to the "A" march (seen in Fig. 15.8) except the recovery leg extends in front of the body.

length and rate as it poses an intense neuromuscular stimulus and maximizes motor unit recruitment. Supramaximal speed can be achieved with a tail wind, downhill running (~1°–7°), high-speed towing, and high-speed treadmill running (35). The supramaximal velocity attained should not exceed a value >10% or greater than the athlete's own ability, or technical breakdowns could occur such as overstriding and leaning back to augment braking (40). Mero

et al. (35) showed supramaximal sprinting increases stride rate by ~6.9% and stride length by ~1.5%. It is important that the athletes are properly warmed up prior to overspeed training. Overspeed training is most effective when performed early in the workout where the athlete's energy levels are high and fatigue is minimal (15). The intensity is high and can result in greater muscle soreness so adequate recovery in between workouts is essential.

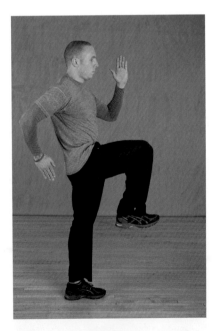

■ **FIGURE 15.8.** "A" march. The athlete marches with proper posture and arm action as the knee is fully flexed and the ground foot is plantar flexed when recovery knee is at the highest point. A skip can be used in lieu of marching.

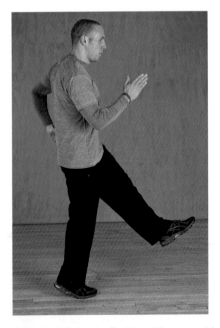

■ **FIGURE 15.10.** Straight leg shuffle. The athlete runs with the legs straight and foot dorsiflexed.

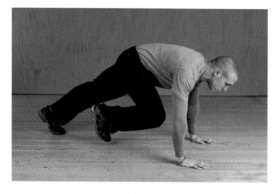

FIGURE 15.11. Mountain climbers. The athlete begins in a push-up position and drives legs forward.

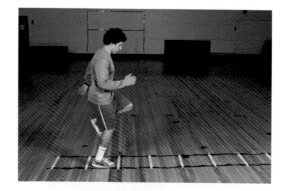

FIGURE 15.12. Ladder runs. To increase foot speed (stride frequency), the athlete runs through an agility ladder as fast as possible while touching one foot down between each rung. Stride length can be emphasized by increasing the slat length or by touching down every second or third run. Sticks can be used in lieu of a ladder.

Sprinting with a tailwind is dependent upon environmental conditions. On a gusty day, the athlete could time his/her sprints with the wind and in the same direction. Maximal effort is given and the tailwind propels the athlete forward at a slightly greater speed (increase in speed is related to wind velocity). It is difficult to predict weather patterns so other forms of supramaximal sprinting are more reliable.

Downhill sprinting is a safe form of overspeed training that is practical provided the athlete has access to a training area with a downward slope of at least 50 m. The higher speed attained during downhill sprinting is due mostly to greater force applied to the ground compared to sprinting on a level surface (48). The level of decline need not be high, e.g., at least 1° but up to ~7° (15,40). The steeper the decline, the greater the chance of falling and can produce some technical flaws including overstriding, landing on one's heels, and forcing the athlete to contact the ground beyond the COG (15). Ebben et al. (16) studied downhill sprinting on slopes ranging from 2.1° to 6.9° and showed optimal sprinting kinematics was seen at a decline of 5.8°.

At this 5.8° slope, the athletes' maximal speed increased by ~7.1% and acceleration increased by ~6.5% (16). It could be advantageous if a flat or uphill surface is located near the declined surface which can allow some contrasts in maximal sprinting sets. Paradisis and Cooke (39) showed 6 weeks of downhill sprinting increased sprint speed and stride frequency by 1.1% and 2.4%, respectively. However, a group which combined uphill and downhill sprinting experienced greater improvements in sprint speeds and stride frequency (3.5% and 3.4%, respectively). Downhill sprinting is less metabolically demanding (2) and increases the eccentric (ECC) component. Thus, muscle damage and delayed onset muscle soreness may ensue and coaches and athletes must be aware of overuse injuries if the volume and/or frequency of downhill sprinting are too high. Peak impact ground reaction forces may be up to 54% higher (at a 9° decline) during downhill running than running uphill (18).

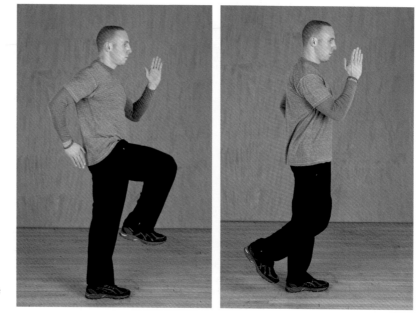

FIGURE 15.13. Pawing. The athlete walks or skips with front leg pulling through and pawing the ground in an exaggerated manner.

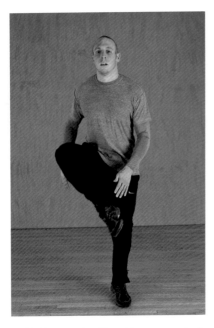

FIGURE 15.14. Drum major. The athlete rotates the forward leg inward and touches the heel to the hand while running forward. The opposite may also be performed to the rear leg (heel to toe) where the athlete touches the foot externally.

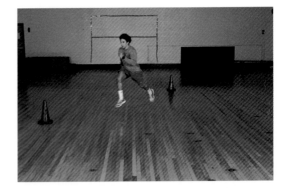

FIGURE 15.15. Gears. Numerous variations of this drill exist of which three are described here. In the first variation, cones (usually five) are placed ~15–20 yd apart. The athlete runs from cone to cone, increasing speed at each cone. This drill is useful for teaching the athlete acceleration and transitioning between speeds. This drill can be varied by altering the pattern of acceleration and decelerations, *e.g.,* accelerate, decelerate, accelerate, decelerate, or accelerate, accelerate, decelerate, accelerate, accelerate. The second variation is known as *ins and outs* (different from the agility ladder drill) where the athlete accelerates, cruises, sprints, cruises, sprints, and decelerates at 10- to 20-yd intervals. The third variation is to use a partner for in-line rolling sprints. The partner stands 10 yd in front of the athlete and begins running. The trailing athlete accelerates and passes the lead athlete and then decelerates. The new trailing athlete accelerates and passes the athlete, and so on. Place exchanges ("changing gears") take place until cessation of the drill. Multiple (>2) athletes can be used.

Towing is a popular mode of overspeed training (Fig. 15.17). The athlete is towed or assisted to attain a supramaximal sprint speed. Athletes have used towing to increase their sprint speed since the 1950s (15) although methods used currently are much more efficient, safer, and the popularity of towing has increased. Towing can acutely produce a higher stride length, rate, decreased foot contact times, and sprinting speed and is a potent stimulus to the neuromuscular system (8,10). The magnitude of the towing force is critical to sprint mechanics and the overall training effect. Clark et al. (8) showed that a towing force of greater than 3.8% of the athlete's body weight had negative impacts on sprint training. A small-to-moderate amount of force is all that is needed.

The athlete may be towed in different ways. Elastic tubing can be used and attached around the waist.

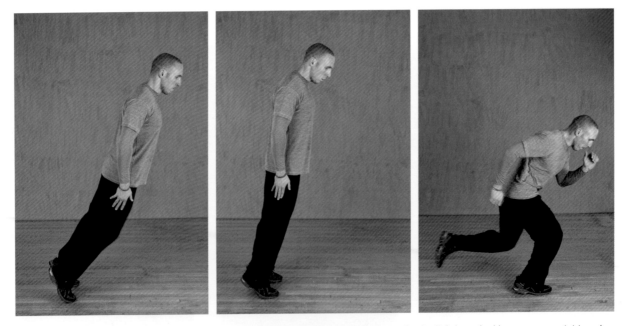

FIGURE 15.16. Falling starts. From a standing position, the athlete either leans/falls forward or is slightly pushed by a partner to initiate the sprint. Upon catching himself/herself (self-imposed reaction) the athlete sprints forward to train his/her acceleration ability.

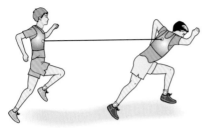

FIGURE 15.17. Overspeed training: towing.

The opposite end can be attached to another athlete or a stationary object. If a stationary object is used, the athlete will connect the tube in front, back up several yards (at least 20–25 yd depending on the strength and length of tubing used), and begin running while being towed by the elastic tubing. The farther the athlete backs up, the greater the stretching and elastic response of the tubing as more force will be applied to the athlete. Thus, sprinting speed increases during towing. The athlete may connect the other end of the tubing to another athlete. The athlete will attach the tubing to the front while the athlete doing the towing will have the other end of the tubing attached to his/her rear. The lead athlete begins sprinting thereby increasing the tension applied to the tubing. As a result, the rear athlete is towed forward and stride length and frequency increase. The lead athlete finishes the sprint first and propels the trailing athlete forward for the specified distance. Another way is to ensure that the lead athlete is faster than the trailing athlete. The lead athlete can tow the trailing athlete. At the same time the lead athlete can use the trailing athlete as resistance (for resisted sprint training).

Current overspeed trainers sold on the market come in various forms. Bungee cords are used. Latex tubing provides the athlete with a steady force transition during stretching that prevents abrupt motion changes. The tubing may be sheathed in nylon which helps prevent cuts and backlash that could occur if the tubing rips. Tubing comes with a belt (or harness although a belt is preferred for overspeed towing) for attachment, vary depending on the size of the athlete (above or below 140 lb), may provide various degrees of tension (light, medium, or heavy),

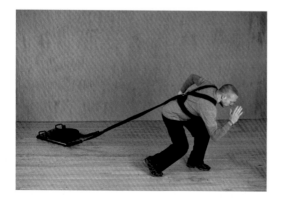

FIGURE 15.18. Sled towing.

and may stretch up to 40 yd or usually three times the original length. Precautions need to be taken with tubing as it can break perhaps leading to an injury for the athlete or it can become loose and disconnected from the belt if not carefully fastened. If any nicks or damage to the tubing is observed, the tubing should be replaced immediately. The athlete should avoid standing too long with the tubing in a stretched position. The athlete should begin sprinting as soon as the desired position is reached. Standing with the tubing stretched for prolonged periods of time can loosen the tubing. In past, it was common for the trailing athlete to be towed by an individual in front riding a bicycle, moped, or other slow-moving vehicle. The use of elastic tubing attached to a stationary object or another athlete is preferred and is safer. Towing is recommended to take place on a grassy surface to lessen the shock on the athlete. The elastic tubing can easily be used on fields and train multiple athletes at a time. Lastly, towing can be used for other drills such as backpedalling and side-to-side movements.

Overspeed training can be performed on an advanced model treadmill. Treadmills that exceed the athlete's max sprint speed can be used to force the athlete to increase stride rate and length. Treadmills that reach high speeds in short periods of time are preferred as a slow increase in belt speed could excessively fatigue the athlete. As with treadmills in general, there are inherent risks and concerns. It is recommended that a spotter be used and a safety harness (in addition to the support rails) supports the athlete to reduce injury risk. The coach should control the treadmill speed so the athlete can maintain proper form without any additional responsibilities especially during deceleration. The treadmill used should slow belt speed rapidly. It is critical to note that with treadmill sprinting, there is slight deceleration or braking due to belt mechanics with each step. This becomes more pronounced with larger athletes and those sprinting at high speeds (14,15). Some of the braking can be reduced with familiarization.

Resisted Sprint Training

Sprint speed is enhanced through resisted sprint training. The athlete sprints maximally against a resistance. Resistance may come in the form of:

- *Wind*—a headwind provides resistance to the athlete. The wind is inconsistent so using a headwind can only occur at sporadic periods of time.
- *Sleds*—a sled or other object that can be dragged posteriorly on the ground (pulling a tire) is a popular means of resisted sprinting (Fig. 15.18). Sleds are made of steel, have a handle and/or harness attachment, and have a post(s) which hold Olympic plates. Some sleds can be loaded with heavy weights and can sustain more than 540 lb. However, weight selection will depend on goals. For sprint training, low-to-moderate loading

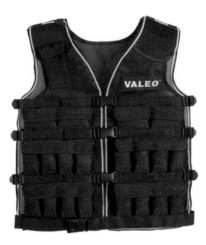

■ **FIGURE 15.19.** Weighted vest sprint.

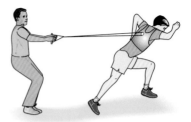

■ **FIGURE 15.20.** Towing sprint with resistance.

(up to 10% of body mass) should be used which allows the athlete to maintain proper form, to be explosive, and to reach a speed at least 85%–90% of his/her max speed. The athlete begins in a three- or four-point stance, with the sled strap elongated, and maximally accelerates to peak speed as quickly as possible as if he/she were running an unloaded sprint. Sleds can be used for sport-specific power development. For example, the Monster Sled has a waist-high attachment arm which enables the athlete to push the sled forward at hip level while leaning forward rather than pulling the sled for speed using a shoulder or belt harness. This motion mimics movements seen in sports such as football and wrestling. Sleds have attachments on the base which forces the athlete to bend over farther prior to pushing the sled. Thus, heavier-loaded sleds could be useful for enhancing sport-specific running power and forces the athlete to maintain a low COG. A shoulder harness makes it more difficult to overcome inertia forcing the athlete to lower the COG. This teaches athletes to develop power and stay low. A belt harness is excellent for speed training to maximize sprint speed. Sprints of 10–50 yd with a sled are commonly used. In some cases, an athlete may use a tire in lieu of a sled for resistance. Tires and sleds can also be used for other drills such as backward, side shuffle, and carioca sprints.

- *Parachutes*—*speed chutes* are another popular source of resistance for sprinting. The chute opens as the athlete accelerates and increases resistance as it opens and ascends upward. Chutes come in different sizes and provide different levels of resistance especially at higher speeds of motion. Some newly designed chutes provide variable resistance. For example, they have an adjustable cord-lock on the lines which can change the shape and diameter of the chute and alter the resistance (more resistance with wide expansion, less resistance with narrow expansion). Some chutes contain a velcro belt which allows for mid-stride release thereby

enabling the athlete to continue sprinting unimpeded. This type of loaded/unloaded sprint cycling of training has been called *sensation training* (44), or contrast training.
- *Sand*—sand is a highly compliant surface which increases resistance with each stride. Running in sand increases energy expenditure 1.6 times more than running on a hard surface (25) and can pose a novel stimulus for sprint and speed endurance training. The instability of the sand alters muscular activation of the lower limbs. The greater metabolic demand is due, in part, to decreased mechanical efficiency and SSC activity (25).
- *Weighted Vests*—weighted vests and/or other weighted body wear (pants, suits, shoes, and strength shoes) can be used for resisted sprint training (Fig. 15.19). Weighted vests are light, durable, and have the capacity to add or exchange weights. The vest may come with pockets that can hold small amounts of weights (½–2 lb) totaling perhaps 10–20 lbs or more depending on the vest. External loading should not be excessive to impede technique and explosive acceleration. Weighted vests are multipurpose and can be used for plyometric, agility, calisthenics, body weight, and sport-specific exercises.
- *Harness*—harnesses have multiple purposes. A harness can be used between two athletes (Fig. 15.20). For example, the trailing athlete can provide resistance to the lead athlete. The trailing athlete should supply enough resistance to allow the lead athlete to sprint to at least 85%–90% of their max. Some harnesses will have a quick release mechanism which allows the

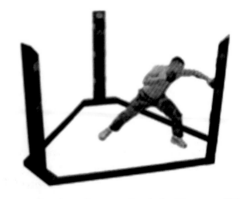

■ **FIGURE 15.21.** The Makoto reaction device (Courtesy of Makoto USA, Centennial, Co).

harness cord to disengage, enabling the lead athlete to continue sprinting unimpeded. Some heavy-duty harnesses can be attached to heavy objects. For example, athletes have been known to pull cars or trucks. Although this type of training is more oriented toward developing total-body power, speed and acceleration are enhanced. Some harnesses have multiple resistance bands that can attach to the ankles, waist, shoulders, and/or arms. These can be used for other modalities besides linear sprinting, *e.g.*, backpedalling, lateral movements, etc.

- *Uphill and/or stairs*—sprinting uphill or up stadium stairs provides other sources of resistance. The athlete is forced to contract his/her muscles at a higher magnitude to accelerate his/her COG against the force of gravity. Sprinting uphill provides a great metabolic challenge to the athlete and is a good way to increase muscle or speed endurance. Because of the added force requirement, uphill sprinting increases acceleration ability. Dintiman et al. (15) have recommended steep inclines (8° or higher) for 10–30 yd for increasing acceleration and start ability, and angles ranging from 1° to 3° for starts and speed endurance for distances greater than 20 yd. Sensation training can be performed if the hill flattens to a plateau. The athlete sprints uphill (to maximize muscle fiber recruitment) and continues to sprint on the flat surface (creating a sense of overspeed training by making the athlete feel like he/she is running faster).

- *Partner*—a partner can physically provide resistance to the athlete to improve acceleration by either holding on to the belt/cord, towel, or by placing hands around the athlete's waist. The utility is that the partner supplies resistance for all or only part of the drill. The partner supplies some resistance for 8–10 strides to improve the athlete's starting acceleration. However, the partner may let go and release the athlete (for sensation training) to allow the athlete to sprint maximally for a specified distance without resistance in a variation known as the *partner-assisted release*. This is a version of a *quick release mechanism* thought to enhance speed and power due to the high-intensity contraction preceding the release. Quick release techniques have been used in ballistic, resistance, and plyometric training. Because of the need for a high rate of force development (RFD), inadequate time is provided by most explosive exercises less than 1 second in duration. The resultant force output is lower than what is seen during a slower high-intensity contraction (based on the *force-velocity relationship*). Quick release techniques are used to maximize the force-velocity relationship where a loaded dynamic or maximum isometric (ISOM) contraction (locked against a resistance) is performed for 1–3 seconds (to increase force and motor unit recruitment) and quickly released to allow unresisted motion the rest

of the way (55). Upon release, these motor units are still facilitated, force is higher, and the athlete is thought to generate greater speed and power. Thus, it is a technique designed to maximize performance by creating a more favorable force-velocity environment. Sufficient resistance should be applied by the partner before the release.

Acute sprint speed and technique are altered by the presence of external loading. As loading increases, sprint speed decreases in proportion. Cronin et al. (11) compared sled towing and weighted vest training (with 15% and 20% of body mass) with nonresisted sprints and showed increased sprint times (by 7.5%–19.8%) in both resisted conditions with a concomitant decrease in stride length (–5.2% to –16.5%) and stride frequency (–2.7% to –6.1%). Sled towing and weighted vests increased stance phase duration and decreased swing phase duration whereas sled towing increased trunk and knee angles and weighted vests decreased trunk angle. Lockie et al. (27) showed that sled towing with 12%–32% of body mass decreased stride length (10%–24% depending on the magnitude of loading) and stride frequency, and increased ground contact time, trunk lean, and hip flexion. Of concern to resisted sprint training is the loading used. The use of too heavy a load negatively affects sprinting. Sprint start technique and kinematics are not affected by pulling a load of up to 10% of body mass while using a sled (31). However, using a load of 20% of body mass increased time spent in the blocks, decreased stride length during initial steps, and produced more horizontal position during propulsion. Reductions in stride length and acute sprint velocity were shown as expected but technique was not altered.

Resisted sprinting can enhance sprint performance (23). Alcaraz et al. (1) showed resisted sprint training with a sled, chute, or weighted belt was effective for training the maximum speed phase of sprinting. Myer et al. (37) compared inclined treadmill training to partner-resisted sprint training for 6 weeks and showed that both groups increased sprint speed and stride frequency but not stride length with no differences between groups. However, the ability of resisted sprint training to augment sprint performance more than traditional nonresisted sprint and plyometric training is less clear. Clark et al. (9) showed that resisted sprint training with weighted vests or sleds (18% and 10% of body mass) did not augment speed development more than nonresisted sprint training over 7 weeks of training. Spinks et al. (45) showed that resisted and nonresisted sprint training produced similar increases in acceleration over 8 weeks of training. Zafeiridis et al. (54) found nonresisted sprint training more effective for enhancing the maximum speed phase whereas resisted sprint training was more effective for increasing acceleration.

Interpreting Research

Resisted Treadmill Sprinting and Ground-Based Sprint Performance

Ross RE, Ratamess NA, Hoffman JR, Faigenbaum AD, Kang J, Chilakos A. The effects of treadmill sprint training and resistance training on maximal running velocity and power. *J Strength Cond Res.* 2009;23:385–394.

Ross et al. (42) investigated the effects of combined resisted/nonresisted sprint training alone or in combination with RT on sprint kinematics. Unique to this investigation was the type of treadmill used for sprint training. A newly designed treadmill (Woodway Force 3.0, Woodway, Inc.) which consisted of a belt that was user-driven (moved in proportion to sprint speed) and contained an electromagnetic braking system, which provided up to 68.2 kg of resistance to the treadmill belt, was studied. The resistance applied occurred within the belt as opposed to the waist, trunk, or limbs which is characteristic of other resisted sprint training devices. The treadmill training program was performed 2 days per week and consisted of 8–12 sets of maximal sprints for 40–60 m at 0%–25% of each athlete's body mass with rest intervals of 2–3 minutes. The program rotated between loaded and unloaded sprint sets. 30-m sprint times and treadmill sprint velocity improved in both groups. Only the combination sprint/RT group increased treadmill sprint peak power. Interestingly, sprint training also increased 1 RM squat strength. This study showed that treadmill sprint training enhanced land-based sprint performance.

AGILITY TRAINING

Agility training involves an integrated approach. Agility requires mobility, coordination, balance, power, optimal SSC efficiency, stabilization, proper technique, strength (in the development of forces applied to the ground for impact and propulsion), flexibility, body control, footwork, and a rapid ability to accelerate and decelerate (19,47). There is a cognitive component to agility such as visual scanning, scanning speed, and anticipation (43). All of these factors work together in improving agility. As a result, some studies have shown low correlations between specific components of fitness and agility. Young et al. (52) found a positive relationship between reactive strength and agility but leg concentric power (during an isokinetic squat) was poorly correlated to agility. Marcovic (28) and Marcovic et al. (30) have shown that leg extensor strength and power were poor predictors of agility. These results demonstrate the complex nature of agility. Sufficient ECC muscle strength and reactive ability are needed to maximize acceleration. Although strength and power are critical to agility performance, individually they may not correlate highly to agility owing to the fact that it is the interaction of these components rather than the independent effects of just a few. Thus, agility training includes multiple modalities including strength and power, sprint, specific agility, balance and coordination, and flexibility training.

TECHNICAL ASPECTS OF AGILITY TRAINING

Exercise has the ability to improve agility. Some modalities are more effective than others. Plyometric, RT, and flexibility training may positively enhance agility.

Although RT by itself may not improve agility per se (17,21), the increase in strength and power may augment other modalities of training used to increase agility. Plyometric and sprint training are critical to agility enhancement (36). Most often, an integrated workout will take place where plyometrics, sprint, and agility drills will be included to comprehensively train agility.

Although many drills can be used to enhance agility, these drills share some common fundamental movements which are critical to rapidly changing direction, accelerating, and decelerating. The following list displays some common targets of sport-specific agility drills:

- *Balance*—the ability to maintain equilibrium is critical to agility training. Balance is maintained via input from the visual, vestibular, and proprioceptive systems. The vestibular center lies in the inner ear and responds to head movement and bodily motion by fluid movement. Selected proprioceptive systems (muscle spindles, Golgi tendon organs) and other joint receptors provide feedback to the central nervous system (CNS) to help control equilibrium and kinesthetic awareness. Motion is detected and an appropriate muscular response ensues. Controlling the COG is an underlying component to all agility drills. Balance and stability are greatest when the COG is lowered, the base support is larger, and the line of gravity is centered within the base support. Controlling the COG and base support are critical during agility drills to place the body in a more stable position. Force production is highest in stable positions. A stable athlete can develop greater forces applied to the ground and this, in turn, can increase agility. The ability to maintain equilibrium is vital to agility training. Static balance training includes drills that improve the athlete's ability to stand in place, whereas dynamic balance training drills improve the athlete's ability to maintain equilibrium during motion. Although many exercises may be included, some exercises are designed to target balance improvements more than others. Performing an exercise unilaterally instead of bilaterally, narrowing the base support, and performing an exercise in a nonstable environment (stability ball, BOSU ball) or with one's eyes closed, performing a combination exercise, or performing an exercise from an unstable position (performing a shoulder press from a lunge position) are all specific ways to improve balance during RT. Plyometric and sprint drills require the athlete to maintain dynamic balance. Agility drills require high levels of balance and are performed on varying surfaces where rapid movement is crucial. As Verstegen and Marcello (47) have pointed out, a "solid base support creates the foundation on which the athlete can apply positive angles." *Positive angles* refer to the correct position of the hips, knees, and ankles relative to the trunk, which allow the athlete to optimally produce force applied to the ground to accelerate, decelerate, and change directions. Proper control of balance allows the athlete to maintain a position where agility can be maximized.

- *Posture*—proper posture is essential to agility training. Preventing excessive amounts of forward lean during acceleration and decreasing forward lean as deceleration increases are critical to properly performing the agility drill. The head should remain in a neutral position and eyes should be focused directly ahead. The athlete should try as best as possible to maintain the power line position during propulsion. Posture is enhanced by strong core stability so core training is essential.
- *Foot contact*—foot contact with the ground is critical to agility. The athlete should maintain a dorsiflexed (toes up) ankle position upon contact with the ground. The dorsiflexed ankle position allows the athlete to quickly explode off of the ground. The athlete lands on the ball of the foot (not the toes) to optimize force applied to the ground. Upon acceleration, the feet rise only slightly off the ground as this reduces time for the next cycles of foot contact. A distinct sound will be heard when the athlete is landing properly and pushing off. The lack of a crisp sound may indicate landing on the toes.
- *Arm action*—similar to sprinting, explosive arm action facilitates leg drive and enhances agility performance during acceleration.
- *Reaction*—the ability of the athlete to react to the stimulus is critical to optimal agility training. Reaction ability comprises vision, hearing, and anticipation, in addition to the appropriate neuromuscular response, which can be enhanced through proper practice over time (47).

- *Quickness*—foot speed and the ability of the athlete to possess a quick first step is critical to agility training. Quickness is dependent upon stance, posture, reactive ability, and knowledge of on which direction movement will initiate.
- *Acceleration/deceleration*—the ability to accelerate and decelerate forms the core of agility training. Each drill targets the athlete's ability to accelerate and decelerate.
- *Targeted movements*—agility drills involve multiple movements including linear sprints, backpedalling, side shuffling, drop stepping, cutting, pivoting, and crossovers. Jumps may be integrated with agility drills.

AGILITY EQUIPMENT

Agility training can be performed with no equipment. A football field with marked lines can be used for many drills. However, some pieces of equipment expand the types of drills that can be used. *Cones* come in various sizes and are used as markers that guide the movements and change of direction. Smaller cones force the athletes to reach further when performing drills where the cone needs to be touched upon directional change. *Agility ladders* enable performance of a multitude of quickness drills that are excellent for developing foot speed, balance, and coordination. *Rings* and *agility dots* can be used for a multitude of single- and double-leg movements. *Reaction balls* contain ridges that force the ball to bounce in different directions while the athlete tries to catch it. Use of a reaction ball can help the athlete improve hand-eye coordination, reaction ability, and first-step quickness. *Agility bags* provide obstacles for athletes to perform several multidirectional drills especially front sprints, side shuffling, and backpedalling. *Tires* have been used especially by football players to increase foot speed and agility. *Agility poles* can be set up at various distances and configurations to create an obstacle course for athletes during agility training. *Mini-hurdles* and *boxes* may also be used as obstacles in addition to their regular use for hopping and jump drills. *Reaction belts* are excellent for athletes to use during shadow drills. *Jump ropes* are excellent for increasing foot speed. Lastly, the Makoto tester (Makoto USA) can be useful (22). It measures and trains reaction ability and agility (Fig. 15.21). The athlete stands in the middle of the triangle and reacts to visual and auditory stimuli. Random lighting forces the athlete to strike that area to fine-tune hand-eye coordination, anticipation, and reaction time, and a score is given once the trial time has been completed.

AGILITY TRAINING DRILLS

It is essential to minimize the loss of speed during deceleration when training for agility. Drills that require changes of direction of the COG forward, backward, vertically, and laterally train the athlete to optimally move in

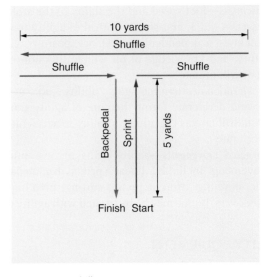

■ **FIGURE 15.22.** T-drill.

response to a stimulus. Agility training drills can be classified into three general types: (a) programmed, (b) reactive, and (c) quickness. *Programmed drills* are those that are preplanned (sometimes referred to as *closed skills*). The athlete is aware of the movements prior to beginning the drill. For example, during the T-drill the athlete knows he/she has to sprint forward, side shuffle right, side shuffle left, and back pedal to the finish.

Reactive drills are continued based on the information from a coach, other athlete, or object such as a ball. They are not preplanned (sometimes referred to as *open skills*). Athletes from many sports participate in reactive drills as part of their athletic practices. Direct competition forces athletes to react to game situations but reactive drills are used in training as well. For example, from a box jump the athlete may sprint forward 10 yd. At the yard marker a coach may be located and will point in a direction for the athlete to continue. If the coach points right then the athlete may pivot and sprint to the right or side shuffle to the right. Partner drills may be reactive. Shadow or mirror drills involve two athletes attached by a reaction belt (which may have velcro straps to disengage) or not attached. One athlete assumes the lead and the other athlete shadows the athlete's every move. This entire drill is based on reaction. Another example is slap or tag drills. One athlete must tag or touch a partner. A game of *tag* forces one athlete to be evasive and the other to react and apply a tag. Modifications of tag drills can be used from standing positions but sport-specific positions. For example, the *push-up slap* drill involves two athletes facing each other (head-to-head) in a starting push-up position. While maintaining their posture, each athlete tries to slap the hand of the other athlete and the other athlete tries to evade the slap by moving the hand. This not only trains reactive ability but also core strength as the athlete is forced to support his/her prone body weight with one arm for some periods of time. Wrestlers incorporate many

reactive drills in their training (as wrestling is a reactive sport) where one athlete may try to slap the partner's foot while the other tries to evade the slap during takedown simulations. Another drill is to place flags/strings around the wrestlers' waist during shooting drills for takedowns. The athlete who first grabs the other's flag wins the drill. Some reactive drills involve ball tosses and catch which force the athlete to react quickly. For example, the *blind partner toss* involves an athlete standing behind another athlete, throwing a ball against a wall, and the primary athlete reacts by catching the ball wherever it bounces. Medicine balls can be used, thrown against a wall at short distances, and the athlete reacts quickly to catch the ball.

Quickness drills are designed to produce fast movements and quick feet. Many agility ladder drills are designed to have rapid movement of the feet. Some quickness drills may involve minimal locomotion but very fast foot movements in a specified area. Some common quickness drills necessitate starting on the ground and quickly popping up to one's feet as fast as possible. Other drills include beginning on the feet, falling to the ground (sprawl in wrestling), and then rapidly getting up. The *resisted let-go* is a useful drill for increasing quickness. One athlete holds or provides resistance to another athlete from the rear (although other angles can be used). The resisted athlete begins to sprint forward or begin a specific agility drill. Resistance is applied at the beginning of the drill. The other athlete then abruptly releases the athlete, eliciting a quick response. In any instance, a drill which forces the athlete to move the body rapidly in any direction can improve quickness.

Programmed drills invoke a more varied response than reactive drills during cutting maneuvers especially in the knee. Besier et al. (5) showed greater stabilization of the knee (via selective activation of medial/lateral, internal/external rotator muscles, and cocontraction of the flexors/extensors) in a programmed cutting maneuver versus generalized cocontraction in reactive cutting. The reactive maneuvers resulted in greater valgus and varus moments on the knee. Programmed drills allow for postural adjustments while reactive cutting drills increased stress on the knee (3). Stress on the knee is greater during side stepping and crossover steps than linear running (4). These data demonstrate that neuromuscular mechanisms help limit joint distress when the moves are anticipated.

Agility drills come in many forms and it is beyond the scope of this chapter to depict several hundreds of potential drills. Basic agility drills can be used without special equipment or markings. These focus on specific movements and may come in the form of calisthenics such as cartwheels, jumping jacks, forward/backward rolls, shoulder rolls, and other more sport-specific drills such as get-up-and-gos (common in football), sprawl drill (seen in wrestling), pitter-patter (wrestling and football), duck unders (used by boxers), base running drills (baseball and softball), and specific footwork drills (for multiple sports).

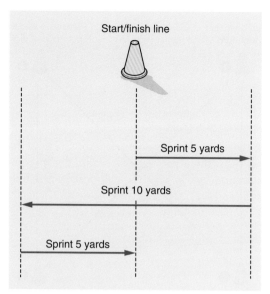

■ FIGURE 15.23. 20-yd shuttle (pro agility drill).

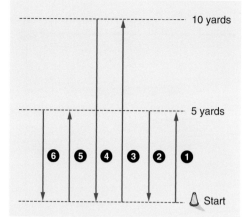

■ FIGURE 15.25. 40-yd sprint. Variations: backpedalling or side shuffling. Can change the length of the drill and mix linear sprints with backpedalling and side shuffling.

Several agility drills consist of basic movements such as forward sprints, backpedalling, side shuffling, drop-steps, crossover steps, diagonal steps, and cutting and pivoting. One popular agility drill commonly used in warm-ups and training is the *carioca*. The carioca involves lateral motion where the right leg steps over the left with one step, right leg steps behind the left with the second step, and the cycle repeats with proper hip motion. This drill is performed quickly once proper technique is learned.

Many agility drills are composed of the aforementioned movements but for different patterns. That is, many agility drills are marked by different courses or patterns of movement. The following drills are some examples of agility exercises commonly performed by athletes (Figs. 15.22–15.44). It is important to note that there are numerous drills that can be designed. The coach should choose drills that are similar to motions encountered in the sport and can design patterns that replicate actual movement, *e.g.*, setting cones to replicate a crossing pattern for a football-wide receiver. At the end of the drill, a pass may be thrown to the athlete to increase the level of sport specificity. Drills should encompass the basic movements of linear sprints, accelerations/decelerations, backpedalling, side and diagonal shuffling, cariocas, cutting, and pivoting. Coaches should constantly monitor technique and be especially instructional to athletes as they touch or run around the cones. Body control is needed to ensure athletes stay close to the cones and do not drift too far away. Correct foot placement, lowering of the COG, deceleration and acceleration, posture, and approach angles are critical when encountering the cones as these can be areas where athletes may lose critical time due to technical flaws. On the field this may result in a negative play as any additional time taken could mean the difference between making the play and allowing the opponent a major competitive advantage. Cone lengths (and the number of cones) modulate the level of changing direction and pattern of acceleration/

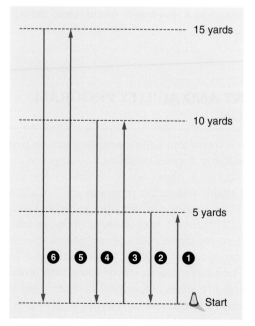

■ FIGURE 15.24. 60-yd shuttle run.

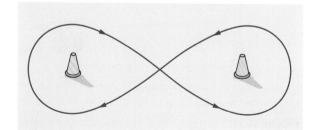

■ FIGURE 15.26. Figure 8 drill.

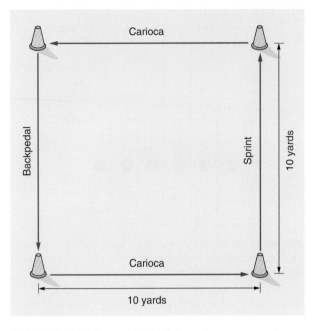

■ **FIGURE 15.27.** Square drills. Variations: change cone spacing. A cone can be placed in the middle to add further movements (in the shape of a "*star*").

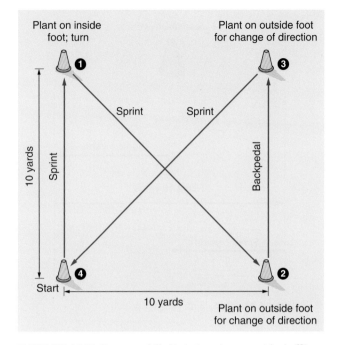

■ **FIGURE 15.29.** X-pattern drills. Variations: integrate side shuffling, backpedalling.

deceleration. Close distances force the athlete to change direction quickly without large windows of acceleration whereas large distances enable the athlete to accelerate over greater lengths which also creates an opportunity for deceleration management upon changing direction. Drills may be integrated to increase the complexity.

Case Study 15.1

Jim is a baseball player who wants to improve his agility over the off-season. He approaches you and wants you to prescribe him some good agility drills he can use to improve his baseball performance. Based on your knowledge of the movement demands of baseball (Jim plays right field), prescribe or design 10 drills which have high baseball specificity. For each one, give an example of how the drill relates to a movement encountered during a baseball game.

SPRINT AND AGILITY PROGRAM DESIGN

Although sprint and agility workouts can be performed independently, for most athletes an integrated approach works very well. There has been little study comparing various sprint and agility programs for efficacy. Most of the available training information is derived from practitioners so there is a wide latitude of design and implementation strategies. Similar to plyometric training, beginning sprint and agility programs should focus on proper technique and footwork using basic drills. Basic drills have low levels of footwork complexity and change of directions. Mastery of early drills leads to progression to more challenging drills. Intensity of drills increases with greater complexity. For sprint training, overspeed

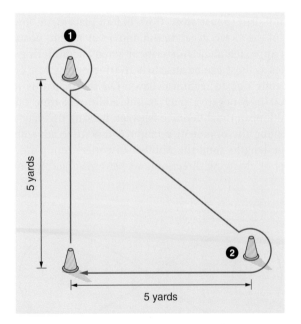

■ **FIGURE 15.28.** Right triangle drills. Variations: change the distance between cones, place the second cone on the opposite side, and alter turns at each cone.

Myths & Misconceptions

Sprint Speed and Agility are Entirely Genetically Determined

This statement is partially true in that genetics do play a role in sprint speed and agility. For example, muscular (fiber types, architecture, protein expression), neural (recruitment, rate, synchronization, coactivation/activation strategies), and skeletal (limb lengths) factors contribute greatly to maximal sprint speed and all these have a genetic component to them. Elite athletes may have some performance-enhancing gene polymorphisms that enable higher levels of performance (38). Genetic expression of proteins involved in muscle contraction appear to be upregulated more in athletes gifted with high sprinting capacity and ability to rapidly accelerate and decelerate. Some of these do not change once the athlete is fully mature, *e.g.*, tendon insertions, limb lengths. However, other factors are trainable and every athlete can improve upon their maximal speed and agility via specific training. Some evidence shows that skill acquisition involved in sprint and agility training may be most trainable during the preadolescent years (40). Proper coaching and/or physical education instruction emphasizing motor development and learning early in life are very beneficial for athleticism later in life. Although genetics may separate the great sprinters from the average sprinters or great athletes from average athletes, every athlete has the ability to improve his/her sprint speed and agility by proper training, diet, and recovery in between workouts.

and resisted sprint drills are more intense and may be introduced once basic sprint technique is mastered and the athlete has improved sprinting ability (developed a base). When used, these drills are typically performed earlier in the workout when energy is high and fatigue is minimal to facilitate skill acquisition. For agility training, basic drills with few turns should be mastered first. These tend to be more one-dimensional in that they consist of only one or two major footwork components. This is true for ladder drills where basic drills (hopscotch drill, multiple hops) should be mastered first and progress later to more complex drills that involve a large number of foot contacts and motions. Higher intensity agility drills include those with complex movement patterns, multiple directions, involve high rates of acceleration/deceleration, are reactive, and may incorporate some moderate-to-high plyometric drills in addition to basic agility movements.

Drill progression (upon mastery) is unique. With RT the athlete can keep increasing load over time. However, with sprint and agility training there is finite loading (unless external loading is used) so progression entails

improving drill times while maintaining optimal technique and mastering more complex drills. Drills can be made more complex by adding other movements, changing the lengths/position of cones or other agility markers, or adding a reactive sport-specific skill to the drill. Thus, agility training progression may be viewed similarly to a martial artist in training. Martial arts progression is based upon a system of belts. Each belt signifies the athlete has mastered certain skills from a beginning level (white or yellow belt) to advanced levels (black belt and associated ranks). Progression in agility training can be viewed similarly where the athlete masters basic drills, improves his/her times in these drills, and progresses to more complex drills. Upon progression, basic drills can still be used as part of the program to maintain the athlete's performance level of these drills.

There is little consensus as to specific guidelines for sprint and agility training. Examination of training programs of the some of the world's greatest athletes and practices of elite coaches reflect that there are many ways to train speed, quickness, and agility. However, there are

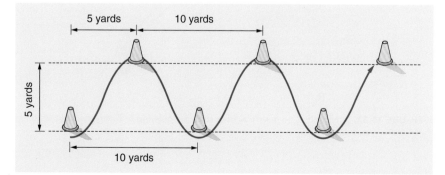

■ **FIGURE 15.30.** Z-pattern drills. Variation: change cone spacing.

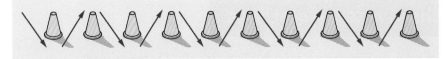

■ **FIGURE 15.31.** Zig-zag drills. Variations: can use agility poles, integrate backpedalling or side shuffling. Cones can be spaced farther apart (with fewer cones, *e.g.,* four) to form the "S" shape.

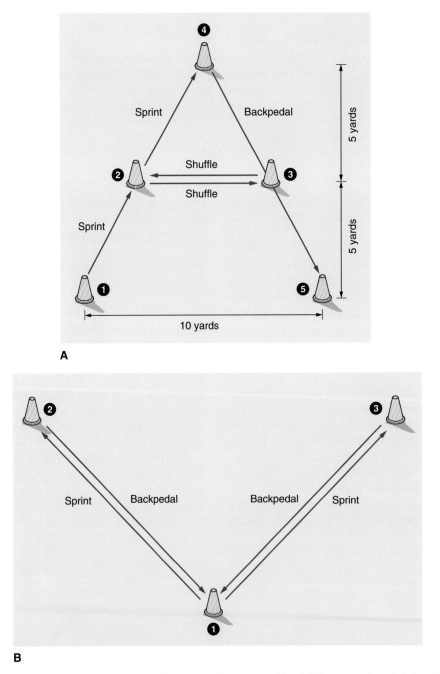

■ **FIGURE 15.32.** Letter drills. Cones are placed at strategic locations to form letters of the alphabet, *e.g.,* A (see **A**), V (see **B**), and N. Sprints, backpedalling, and side shuffling are used during each drill.

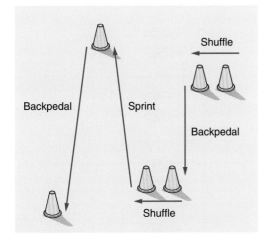

FIGURE 15.33. EKG drill.

certain recommendations/suggestions that can be used in the design of sprint and agility programs. Manipulation of acute program variables targets specific aspects of speed, quickness, and agility. Similar to other modalities of training, the variation of volume and intensity of sprint and agility is more conducive to progression rather than just increasing each over time as overtraining may occur. The following general guidelines can be helpful in program design:

- **Structure and Sequencing**: the structure of the program needs to be determined right away. That is, whether or not speed and agility workouts will be independent or integrated. The following are structure and sequencing recommendations for both types:
  - Sprint training only: general warm-up → dynamic ROM exercises → sprint technique → overspeed/resisted sprint drills → basic speed → cool-down

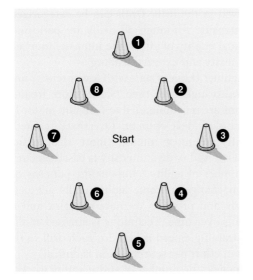

FIGURE 15.34. Diamond reaction drill. A coach is located in the middle to indicate left or right direction to the athlete.

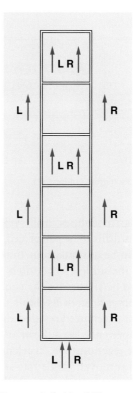

FIGURE 15.35. Hopscotch (ladder drill).

- Agility training only: general warm-up → dynamic ROM exercises → agility drills (most complex to least complex) → cool-down
- Integrated sprint/agility training: general warm-up → dynamic ROM exercises → sprint technique → agility drills (most complex to least complex) → basic speed → cool-down
- Sprint and agility take presentence in sequence if RT is performed the same day.
- **Exercise Selection**: the types of drills and exercises included are critical to program design. Many drills have been discussed in this chapter and numerous others exist as well. Drill selection should be based on a continuum from basic to complex. The following recommendations categorize drills which should be used in successful speed and agility programs.

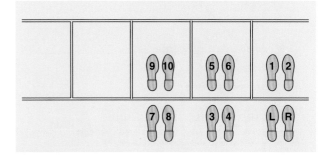

FIGURE 15.36. Ins and outs (ladder drill). Variation: to exit the ladder on the opposite side.

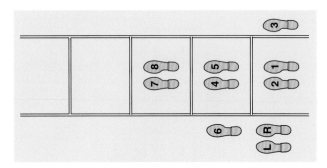

■ **FIGURE 15.37.** Icky shuffle (ladder drill).

Similar to other modalities, drill cycling (periodizing many exercises/drills to be performed at certain points in training) can be advantageous to the athlete as the more stimuli the athlete encounters in training, the better prepared he/she are for the competition.

- Sprint training: form drills, basic speed drills (varied lengths), overspeed/resisted drills (with some training experience as a form of progression)—drills target reaction time, acceleration, and maximum speed turnover (stride rate and length).
- Agility training: sport-specific drills stressing body movement and control, balance exercises, reactive drills, basic movement agility drills—patterns and components are simple and progress to more

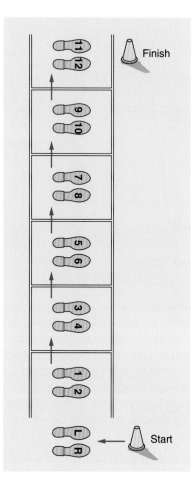

■ **FIGURE 15.39.** Left-right shuffle (ladder drill).

complex as technique mastery is observed and performance improves.

- Warm-up drills: performed after a general warm-up. Some are also form drills (Table 15.2).
- **Intensity**: refers to the complexity and loading involved in the drill. Drills can be categorized based on intensity. Although all drills are performed with maximal quality of effort, the intensity increases with complexity and external loading.
- Beginner trainees start with low intensity and progress to high over time. Short, more frequent sessions are recommended to facilitate motor learning and skill development. Overspeed/resisted sprint drills are most intense (more than basic speed drills). Agility drill intensity is based on complexity (number of agility components, patterns of direction change). Simple agility drills are performed early and progress to more complex and reactive drills over time. Technique is stressed at all phases of training. Speed is high for each drill so the quality of effort per set/repetition is critical.
- **Frequency**: the number of sprint/agility workouts per week. Frequency depends on many factors including practice/competition schedule, other modalities of

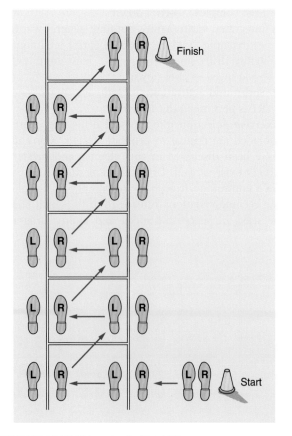

■ **FIGURE 15.38.** Side rocker (ladder drill).

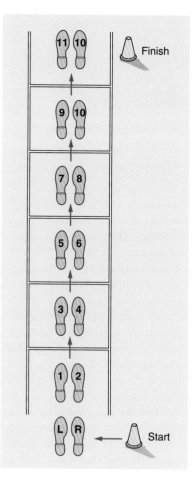

FIGURE 15.40. Two-feet forward (ladder drill).

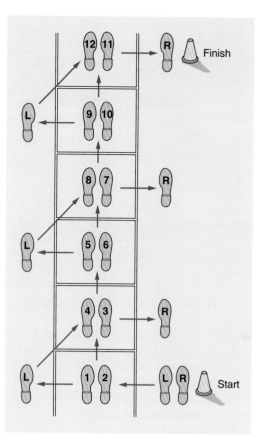

FIGURE 15.41. Two-in lateral shuffle (ladder drill).

training (resistance, plyometric), diet, and recovery practices.

- 1–3 days per week is typically recommended. Higher frequency can be used with caution in advanced athletes. Undulating variations in intensity and volume can accommodate higher training frequencies.
- **Volume**: the total number of repetitions and work performed. Volume load can be used as the measure which is the product of drill distances and intensity (speed or loading). Volume load is quite variable and depends upon several factors including intensity, frequency, diet, recovery, and training status. Advanced athletes can tolerate higher training volumes but caution still needs to be used.
- 1–3 sets for form drills and dynamic exercises; 3–5 sets for sprint and agility workload sets. Volume of overspeed drills should be max 10% of volume. The length/duration of each drill contributes to total volume. For maximal speed and agility training, most drills will be somewhat short in duration to maximize ATP-PC metabolism. Drills longer in length and/or duration (>10–15 s) begin to stress speed or agility endurance (*anaerobic conditioning*)

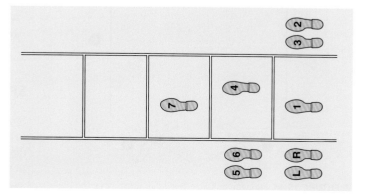

FIGURE 15.42. Zig-zag cross-over shuffle (ladder drill).

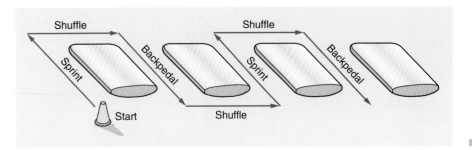

■ **FIGURE 15.43.** Bag weaves.

in proportion. Thus, short, quick, explosive drills are recommended for pure speed and agility development. The United States Track and Field Association has recommended acceleration and maximum speed drills be 20–80 yd in length and that the volume per workout range for 300–500 yd (acceleration) and 300–800 yd (maximum speed) in collegiate athletes (7).

- **Rest Intervals**: rest in between sets and exercises. Speed and agility training requires adequate recovery in between sets and exercises. A fatigued athlete cannot develop the speed and/or agility needed to optimally train the neuromuscular system. A constant rest interval or work:relief ratio can be used.
  - 1–3 minutes of rest between sets depending on the intensity. Work-relief intervals of 1:10 and beyond can be used to target the ATP-PC system and to allow adequate recovery. Less rest is needed between sets of form drills.

PUTTING IT ALL TOGETHER

The program designed can be implemented and periodically assessed. Sprint and agility programs must accommodate other modalities of training such as RT and depends on whether the athlete is in the off-, pre-, or in-season periods. Table 15.3 depicts a sample basic

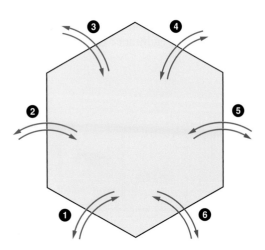

■ **FIGURE 15.44.** Hexagon drill.

3-day sprint and agility training program. Day 1 focuses on sprint training, day 2 agility training, and day 3 is an integrated workout. The structure is based upon performing a general warm-up initially followed by dynamic ROM drills. The athlete can select five drills and perform 1 set of each one. Drills may be rotated for each workout. For sprint or integrated workouts, form drills follow. In this example, each drill is performed for 20 yd for 2 sets, *i.e.*, 20 yd up and 20 yd back with little rest in between sets (30 s–1 min). For agility workouts, basic structural movements replace sprint form drills. Structural movements and form drills are used during integrated sprint/agility workouts. The primary drills are performed next. The cool-down follows if no speed or agility endurance work will be performed. If speed/agility endurance training takes place, it should take place at the end of the workout prior to the cool-down as to not interfere with the maximal speed and agility drills. Progression may take place by incorporating more challenging agility drills and by introducing overspeed and resisted sprint drills.

Case Study 15.2

Power training for anaerobic athletes requires an integrated approach consisting of RT, plyometric, sprint, and agility training. Balance between all modalities is imperative to developing effective power training programs.

Questions for Consideration: **Consider a training phase where all modalities are included. How might an athlete or coach design a program to include all of these modalities into a weekly workout schedule? Be sure to discuss training frequency, workout structures, general exercise selection, and sequencing.**

SPEED ENDURANCE TRAINING

Speed endurance is the maintenance of maximal speed over an extended period of time. Although speed is discussed here, the ability to maintain other components such as agility and power are critical to athletic success. Collectively, these are measures of anaerobic

TABLE 15.2 SELECTED SPRINT AND AGILITY TRAINING WARM-UP DRILLS

DYNAMIC ROM	SPRINT	AGILITY
Toe walks	High knees	Ankle hops
Knee circles	Butt kickers	Accelerations
Scorpion	Lunge walks	Side shuffles
Straddled hip circles	Skips	Backpedalling
Lunge with torso rotation	Mountain climbers	Cariocas
BW squat	A and B marches	Side lunges
Press-ups	Ankling	Resisted walks—4 directions (bands)
Lying hip adduction/abduction	Pawing	
	Resisted knee-ups (bands)	
	Arm swings	

conditioning, or the ability to maintain high anaerobic exercise performance over time. Athletes with high levels of speed endurance do not experience the same level of fatigue over time as a lesser-conditioned athlete. They may not demonstrate as substantial a deceleration phase during a long sprint or, during multiple bouts of explosive activities, and they will not experience the same level of fatigue as the game, practice, or workout continues. The basketball player will still have the burst of power late in the second half when the game is on the line. The football player will still have the speed, agility, and power needed to make a critical play in the fourth quarter. Speed endurance training leads to favorable muscle fiber-type transitions, increased buffering capacity and ability to tolerate higher levels of blood lactate, and increased glycolytic enzyme activity all of which enable the athlete to maintain higher speeds for an extended period of time.

Speed endurance training is characterized by longer sprint distances and reduced rest intervals in between sets and repetitions. Drill lengths may range from 30 yd to more than 300 yd and are run at intensities ranging between 75% and 100% of maximal speed (7). Unlike maximal speed and agility training, fatigue is not avoided here but becomes an important stimulus. Drills consist of repeated sprints (sprints with short rest intervals such as *wind sprints*), interval sprints (where the athlete sprints part of the course and jogs part of the course at regular fixed intervals), repetitive flying sprints, rolling sprints (with groups of athletes where the last athlete sprints to the front upon indication from a coach), or repetitive relays (20). *Pick-up sprints* are effectively used where groups of athletes run on a track as four intervals are used: (a) jog for 25 m, (b) stride for 25 m, (c) sprint for 25 m, and (d) walk for 25 m (15). Partial recovery is seen during the jogging and walking phases. Agility runs such as shuttle runs can be used, so change of direction ability is challenged by the fatiguing stimulus. The work:relief ratio is lower (1:5 or lower). Less rest is taken in between to limit recovery thereby requiring the athlete to sprint maximally in a fatigued state. Speed endurance

TABLE 15.3 SAMPLE 3-DAY SPRINT AND AGILITY PROGRAM

MONDAY	WEDNESDAY	FRIDAY
General warm-up 3–5-min jog	General warm-up 3–5-min jog	General warm-up 3–5-min jog
Dynamic ROM drills 1 × 5 drills	Dynamic ROM drills 1 × 5 drills	Dynamic ROM drills 1 × 5 drills
High knees 2 × 20 yd	Ankle hops 2 × 10	Mountain climbers 2 × 20 s
Butt kickers 2 × 20 yd	Runs (50% of max) 2 × 20 yd	"B" marches 2 × 20 yd
Lunge walks 2 × 20 yd	Backpedals 2 × 20 yd	Backpedals 2 × 20 yd
"A" march 2 × 20 yd	Side shuffles 2 × 20 yd	Cariocas 2 × 20 yd
Gears (10-yd int) 3–5 × 40 yd	Ladder hopscotch 3×	T-drill 3×
Sprints 5 × 20 yd	Ladder ins and outs 3×	Sprints 6 × 40 yd
Flying sprints 3 × 40 yd	20-yd shuttle 3×	Zig-zag drill 3×
Cool-down	Square drill 3×	60-yd shuttle run 3×
	"V" drill 3×	Cool-down
		Cool-down

workouts are challenging, require greater recovery times, and drills are performed at the end of the workouts. Total volume of speed endurance training depends upon the sport. Advanced athletes can tolerate greater volume than novice athletes. For speed endurance training involving low-to-moderate intensity drills for moderate distances, 8–20 repetitions have been recommended for advanced athletes and 5–12 for novice athletes (40). For speed endurance training involving high-intensity drills for short-to-moderate distances, 4–12 repetitions have been recommended for advanced athletes and 4–8 for novice athletes (40). It is important to break down the sport by analyzing the typical lengths the athlete may sprint, the number of plays or explosive activities seen during a typical game, and the amount of rest seen in between plays. For example, in football some data show that on offense a team may have ~12–15 series per game, average ~4.5–5.6 plays per series, with each play lasting ~5.0–5.5 seconds (up to ~13 s for a long play), and have ~25–36 seconds of rest in between plays yielding a work:relief ratio of 1:5 (20). These data provide a valuable framework for S&C coaches to develop a speed endurance training program.

Speed endurance training programs are easy to administer. The major components to training progression are the distance sprinted, the number of sprints, and the rest intervals in between sprints. The distance sprinted and the number of sprints can increase, and/or the rest intervals may decrease during speed endurance training progression. The following example depicts basic progression concept applied to an 8-week program. The numbers are based on two workouts per week so 20 × 50 yd indicates 10 repetitions per workout at 50 yd each. When possible, the coach should time each repetition to ensure maximal effort and to use the times to evaluate training especially those last few repetitions at the end of the workout. Comparisons can be made to those repetitions with similar lengths and rest intervals. Athletes should see improvements in times as training progresses.

- Week 1: 20 × 50 yd with 2-minute rest intervals
- Week 2: 20 × 50 yd with 1.5-minute rest intervals
- Week 3: 22 × 60 yd with 2-minute rest intervals
- Week 4: 22 × 60 yd with 1.5-minute rest intervals
- Week 5: 24 × 70 yd with 2-minute rest intervals
- Week 6: 24 × 70 yd with 1.5-minute rest intervals
- Week 7: 26 × 80 yd with 2-minute rest intervals
- Week 8: 26 × 80 yd with 1.5-minute rest intervals

Summary Points

✔ Speed, agility, acceleration ability, reaction time, and quickness are essential elements to improving athleticism. An athlete with sufficient linear speed does not mean that he/she will have sufficient agility, reaction time, and quickness. Each component needs to be specifically trained in order to maximize athletic performance.

✔ Maximal sprint speed is the product of stride rate and length. Increasing stride length and rate through training creates faster athletes.

✔ Sprinting speed is a skill which can be improved by technical training and conditioning. Coaches need to monitor and institute correct sprinting technique to maximize benefits.

✔ Sprint training is characterized by the use of form drills, sprints of specific lengths (to mimic athletic demands and target correct metabolic systems), over-speed, and resisted sprint training drills. Technique mastery should be used as a guide before progressing to more intense and complex drills.

✔ Training for improved agility is multifactorial and requires mobility, coordination, balance, power, optimal SSC efficiency, stabilization, proper technique, strength, flexibility, a rapid ability to accelerate and decelerate, visual scanning, scanning speed, and anticipation.

✔ Training for speed, agility, and quickness requires an integrated approach consisting of resistance, ballistic, flexibility, balance, and plyometric training in addition to specific sprint and agility training.

✔ Agility drills may be programmed or reactive. Quickness is best improved by incorporating explosive drills that maximize body movement speed and locomotion.

✔ Speed endurance is needed by those athletes involved in anaerobic sports where prolonged explosive movements are used with short recovery intervals. Speed endurance training takes place at the end of workouts and can be increased by increasing drill length, drill repetition number, and/or decreasing rest intervals between repetitions.

Review Questions

1. The rate of change of velocity over time is:
   a. Speed
   b. Acceleration
   c. Reaction time
   d. Speed endurance

2. A common technical error seen during sprinting is:
   a. Relaxed facial, neck, and shoulder muscles
   b. Explosive arm actions with elbows ~90° angles
   c. Limited knee and hip ROM
   d. Upright torso position during the maximum speed phase

3. Which of the following is the best sequence of drills/exercises for sprint and/or agility training?
   a. General warm-up, dynamic ROM exercises, form drills, overspeed drills, and basic sprinting drills
   b. General warm-up, basic sprint drills, dynamic ROM exercises, overspeed drills, and form drills
   c. Resisted sprint drills, form drills, basic sprint drills, dynamic ROM exercises, and general warm-up
   d. General warm-up, basic agility drills, dynamic ROM exercises, form drills, and overspeed training drills

4. Which of the following drills is most specific to increasing an athlete's backpedalling ability?
   a. Sprints with a chute
   b. "Butt kickers"
   c. Cariocas
   d. T-drill

5. Repeated sprints of 200 yd with 2-minute rest intervals in between repetitions are most specific to increasing:
   a. Reaction time
   b. Quickness
   c. Acceleration
   d. Speed endurance

6. The Z-pattern drill is an example of a(n) _____ drill.
   a. Agility training
   b. Resistance training
   c. Speed endurance training
   d. Overspeed training

7. Sprint speed is the product of stride length and stride frequency.   T F

8. The support phase of sprinting describes motion of the leg that is not in contact with the ground.   T F

9. Overspeed training allows the athlete to attain a speed that is greater than the athlete's maximal effort.   T F

10. A 1:1 work:relief ratio is used to specifically target the ATP-PC system during sprint and agility training.   T F

11. Agility is the ability to move rapidly while changing direction.   T F

12. Towing is a mode of overspeed training where the athlete is assisted to attain a supramaximal sprint speed.   T F

References

1. Alcaraz PE, Palao JM, Elvira JL, Linthorne NP. Effects of three types of resisted sprint training devices on the kinematics of sprinting at maximum velocity. *J Strength Cond Res.* 2008;22:890–897.
2. Baron B, Deruelle F, Moullan F, et al. The eccentric muscle loading influences the pacing strategies during repeated downhill sprint intervals. *Eur J Appl Physiol.* 2009;105:749–757.
3. Besier TF, Lloyd DG, Ackland TR, Cochrane JL. Anticipatory effects on knee joint loading during running and cutting maneuvers. *Med Sci Sports Exerc.* 2001;33:1176–1181.
4. Besier TF, Lloyd DG, Cochrane JL, Ackland TR. External loading of the knee joint during running and cutting maneuvers. *Med Sci Sports Exerc.* 2001;33:1168–1175.
5. Besier TF, Lloyd DG, Ackland TR. Muscle activation strategies at the knee during running and cutting maneuvers. *Med Sci Sports Exerc.* 2003;35:119–127.
6. Cavagna GA, Komarek L, Mazzoleni S. The mechanics of sprint running. *J Physiol.* 1971;217:709–721.
7. Cissik JM, Barnes M. *Sport Speed and Agility.* Monterey (CA): Coaches Choice; 2004. pp. 15–85.
8. Clark DA, Sabick MB, Pfeiffer RP, et al. Influence of towing force magnitude on the kinematics of supramaximal sprinting. *J Strength Cond Res.* 2009;23:1162–1168.
9. Clark KP, Stearne DJ, Walts CT, Miller AD. The longitudinal effects of resisted sprint training using weighted sleds vs. weighted vests. *J Strength Cond Res.* 2010;24(12):3287–3295.
10. Corn RJ, Knudson D. Effect of elastic-cord towing on the kinematics of the acceleration phase of sprinting. *J Strength Cond Res.* 2003; 17:72–75.
11. Cronin J, Hansen K, Kawamori N, McNair P. Effects of weighted vests and sled towing on sprint kinematics. *Sports Biomech.* 2008; 7:160–172.
12. Davis DS, Barnette BJ, Kiger JT, Mirasola JJ, Young SM. Physical characteristics that predict functional performance in division I college football players. *J Strength Cond Res.* 2004;18:115–120.

13. Delecluse C. Influence of strength training on sprint running performance: current findings and implications for training. *Sports Med*. 1997;24:147–156.

14. Dintiman GB. Acceleration and speed. In: Foran B, editor. *High-Performance Sports Conditioning*. Champaign (IL): Human Kinetics; 2001. pp. 167–192.

15. Dintiman G, Ward B, Tellez T. *Sports Speed*. 2nd ed. Champaign (IL): Human Kinetics; 1998. pp. 191–220.

16. Ebben WP, Davies JA, Clewien RW. Effect of the degree of hill slope on acute downhill running velocity and acceleration. *J Strength Cond Res*. 2008;22:898–902.

17. Fry AC, Kraemer WJ, Weseman CA, et al. The effects of an off-season strength and conditioning program on starters and non-starters in women's intercollegiate volleyball. *J Appl Sport Sci Res*. 1991;5:174–181.

18. Gottschall AS, Kram R. Ground reaction forces during downhill and uphill running. *J Biomech*. 2005;38:445–452.

19. Graham J, Ferrigno V. Agility and balance training. In: Brown LE, Ferrigno VA, editors. *Training for Speed, Agility, and Quickness*. 2nd ed. Champaign (IL): Human Kinetics; 2005. pp. 71–222.

20. Hoffman J. *Physiological Aspects of Sport Training and Performance*. Champaign (IL): Human Kinetics; 2002. pp. 93–108.

21. Hoffman JR, Maresh CM, Armstrong LE, Kraemer WJ. Effects of off-season and in-season resistance training programs on a collegiate male basketball team. *J Hum Muscle Perf*. 1991;1:48–55.

22. Hoffman JR, Kang J, Ratamess NA, Hoffman MW, Tranchina CP, Faigenbaum AD. Examination of a pre-exercise, high energy supplement on exercise performance. *J Int Soc Sports Nutr*. 2009;6:1–8.

23. Kristensen GO, Van Den Tillaar R, Ettema GJC. Velocity specificity in early-phase sprint training. *J Strength Cond Res*. 2006;20: 833–837.

24. Kraemer WJ, Ratamess NA, Volek JS, Mazzetti SA, Gomez AL. The effect of the Meridian shoe on vertical jump and sprint performances following short-term combined plyometric/sprint and resistance training. *J Strength Cond Res*. 2000;14:228–238.

25. Lejeune TM, Willems PA, Heglund NC. Mechanics and energetics of human locomotion on sand. *J Exp Biol*. 1998;210:2071–2080.

26. Lentz D, Hardyk A. Speed training. In: Brown LE, Ferrigno VA, editors. *Training for Speed, Agility, and Quickness*. 2nd ed. Champaign (IL): Human Kinetics; 2005. pp. 17–70.

27. Lockie RG, Murphy AJ, Spinks CD. Effects of resisted sled towing on sprint kinematics in field-sport athletes. *J Strength Cond Res*. 2003; 17:760–767.

28. Marcovic G. Poor relationship between strength and power qualities and agility performance. *J Sports Med Phys Fitness*. 2007;47:276–283.

29. Marcovic G, Jukic I, Milanovic D, Metikos D. Effects of sprint and plyometric training on muscle function and athletic performance. *J Strength Cond Res*. 2007;21:543–549.

30. Marcovic G, Sekulic D, Marcovic M. Is agility related to strength qualities?—Analysis in latent space. *Coll Anthropol*. 2007;31:787–793.

31. Maulder PS, Bradshaw EJ, Keogh JW. Kinematic alterations due to different loading schemes in early acceleration sprint performance from starting blocks. *J Strength Cond Res*. 2008;22:1992–2002.

32. McHenry P, Raether J. *101 Agility Drills*. Monterey (CA): Coaches Choice; 2004. pp. 51–133.

33. Mero A. Force-time characteristics and running velocity of male sprinters during the acceleration phase of sprinting. *Res Q*. 1988;59:94–98.

34. Mero A, Komi PV. Electromyographic activity in sprinting at speeds ranging from sub-maximal to supra-maximal. *Med Sci Sports Exerc*. 1987;19:266–274.

35. Mero A, Komi PV, Gregor RJ. Biomechanics of sprint running. *Sports Med*. 1992;13:376–392.

36. Miller MG, Herniman JJ, Ricard MD, Cheatham CC, Michael TJ. The effects of a 6-week plyometric training program on agility. *J Sports Sci Med*. 2006;5:459–465.

37. Myer GD, Ford KR, Brent JL, Divine JG, Hewett TE. Predictors of sprint start speed: the effects of resistive ground-based vs. inclined treadmill training. *J Strength Cond Res*. 2007;21:831–836.

38. Ostrander EA, Huson HJ, Ostrander GK. Genetics of athletic performance. *Ann Rev Genomics Hum Genet*. 2009;10:407–429.

39. Paradisis GP, Cooke CB. The effects of sprint running training on sloping surfaces. *J Strength Cond Res*. 2006;20:767–777.

40. Plisk SS. Speed, agility, and speed-endurance development. In: Baechle TR, Earle RW, editors. *Essentials of Strength Training and Conditioning*. 3rd ed. Champaign (IL): Human Kinetics; 2008. pp. 455–485.

41. Ratamess NA, Kraemer WJ, Volek JS, et al. The effects of ten weeks of resistance and combined plyometric/sprint training with the Meridian Elyte athletic shoe on muscular performance in women. *J Strength Cond Res*. 2007;21:882–887.

42. Ross RE, Ratamess NA, Hoffman JR, Faigenbaum AD, Kang J, Chilakos A. The effects of treadmill sprint training and resistance training on maximal running velocity and power. *J Strength Cond Res*. 2009;23:385–394.

43. Sheppard JM, Young WB. Agility literature review: classifications, training and testing. *J Sports Sci*. 2006;24:919–932.

44. Smythe R. *Acceleration: An Illustrated Guide*. Portland (OR): Speed City, Inc; 1988. pp. 50–108.

45. Spinks CD, Murphy AJ, Spinks WL, Lockie RG. The effects of resisted sprint training on acceleration performance and kinematics in soccer, rugby union, and Australian football players. *J Strength Cond Res*. 2007;21:77–85.

46. Verstegen M, Williams P. *Core Performance*. Emmaus (PA): Rodale Books; 2004. pp. 38–68.

47. Verstegen M, Marcello B. Agility and coordination. In: Foran B, editor. *High-Performance Sports Conditioning*. Champaign (IL): Human Kinetics; 2001. pp. 139–165.

48. Weyand PG, Sternlight DB, Bellizzi MJ, Wright S. Faster top running speeds are achieved with greater ground forces not more rapid leg movements. *J Appl Physiol*. 2000;89:1991–1999.

49. Weyand PG, Davis JA. Running performance has a structural basis. *J Exp Biol*. 2005;208:2625–2631.

50. Wisloff U, Castagna C, Helgerud J, Jones R, Hoff J. Strong correlation of maximal squat strength with sprint performance and vertical jump height in elite soccer players. *Br J Sports Med*. 2004;38:285–288.

51. Young WB, Farrow D. A review of agility: practical applications for strength and conditioning. *Strength Cond J*. 2006;28:24–29.

52. Young WB, James R, Montgomery I. Is muscle power related to running speed with changes of direction? *J Sports Med Phys Fitness*. 2002;42:282–288.

53. Young W, McLean B, Ardagna J. Relationship between strength qualities and sprinting performance. *J Sports Med Phys Fitness*. 1995;35:13–19.

54. Zafeiridis A, Saraslanidis P, Manou V, Ioakimidis P, Dipla K, Kellis S. The effects of resisted sled-pulling sprint training on acceleration and maximum speed performance. *J Sports Med Phys Fitness*. 2005;45:284–290.

55. Zatsiorsky VM, Kraemer WJ. *Science and Practice of Strength Training*. 2nd ed. Champaign (IL): Human Kinetics; 2006. pp. 30–33.

16

Aerobic Training

objectives

After completing this chapter, you will be able to:

- Discuss factors that affect aerobic endurance performance
- Discuss aerobic endurance training program design and how to manipulate exercise mode, intensity, volume, rest intervals, and frequency to increase Vo_{2max} and performance
- Discuss how to include different forms of aerobic training into the program
- Discuss aerobic training for endurance and anaerobic athletes
- Discuss the impact altitude has on human performance
- Discuss compatibility issues with concurrent high-intensity aerobic and strength/power training
- Discuss the impact hot and cold environments have on aerobic endurance exercise performance

Aerobic training (AT) comprises several modes of activities that primarily stress the aerobic energy system and produce a number of cardiovascular (CV) and respiratory adaptations that increase endurance. High levels of aerobic fitness are mandatory for endurance athletes such as cyclists, distance runners, triathletes, and swimmers. Increases in aerobic capacity allow the marathon runner to maintain a better pace and reduce event times, allow the cyclist to become more efficient and improve trial times, and allow the swimmer to reduce times during distance events in the pool. However, other groups of athletes benefit from AT for their sports which not only require strength and power but require the athlete to possess sufficient muscular and CV endurance, *i.e.*, boxers, wrestlers, hockey, soccer, and basketball players. A high aerobic capacity allows the athlete to recover faster from workouts and competitions.

Several physiological adaptations accompany AT including increases in cardiac output (Q_c), stroke volume (SV), plasma volume, blood flow, angiogenesis, and hemoglobin concentrations. At the muscle level, AT increases mitochondrial and capillary density, oxidative enzyme activity, myoglobin content, fat utilization during exercise and at rest, buffer capacity, and fiber-type transitions (favoring oxidative fibers). Collectively, these changes lead to increases in maximal oxygen uptake (Vo_{2max}) resulting from increased Q_c and arterio-venous (A-VO_2) difference. The purpose of this chapter is to discuss AT program design, environmental considerations, and the effects of high-intensity AT performed concurrently with resistance training (RT).

FACTORS RELATED TO AEROBIC EXERCISE PERFORMANCE

Aerobic exercise endurance performance depends on several factors including VO_2. A higher Vo_{2max} indicates greater aerobic fitness. Elite male distance runners have Vo_{2max} values ranging from 70 to 85 mL kg^{-1} min^{-1} (50). Elite distance runners can maintain an average of 94% of their Vo_{2max} for a 5-km race and 82% of their Vo_{2max} for a marathon (50). Studies show high correlations between Vo_{2max} and performance in endurance events (69). However, athletes with similar Vo_{2max} values may have largely different endurance performances. As Noakes (50) pointed out, two elite runners (Steve Prefontaine and Frank Shorter), whose best 1-mile run times were less than 8 seconds different from each other, had a Vo_{2max} difference of 16%. In these cases, other factors are stronger predictors of endurance performance. However, Vo_{2max} has been used to predict race times and vice versa. For example, Mercier et al. (46) developed a nomogram that predicts running times (from 3- to 42-km distances) from Vo_{2max} values (Fig. 16.1).

In conjunction with a high Vo_{2max}, endurance athletes have greater fuel use efficiency, *e.g.*, preferential metabolism of fat during exercise. An athlete with a high Vo_{2max} has better oxygen intake, delivery, and utilization. Therefore, the endurance athlete essentially becomes a fat-burning machine. When fat is a preferred fuel, glycogen is spared, less lactic acid is formed, and there are fewer pH disturbances. The lactate threshold (LT) increases and enables exercise in a less acidic environment. The

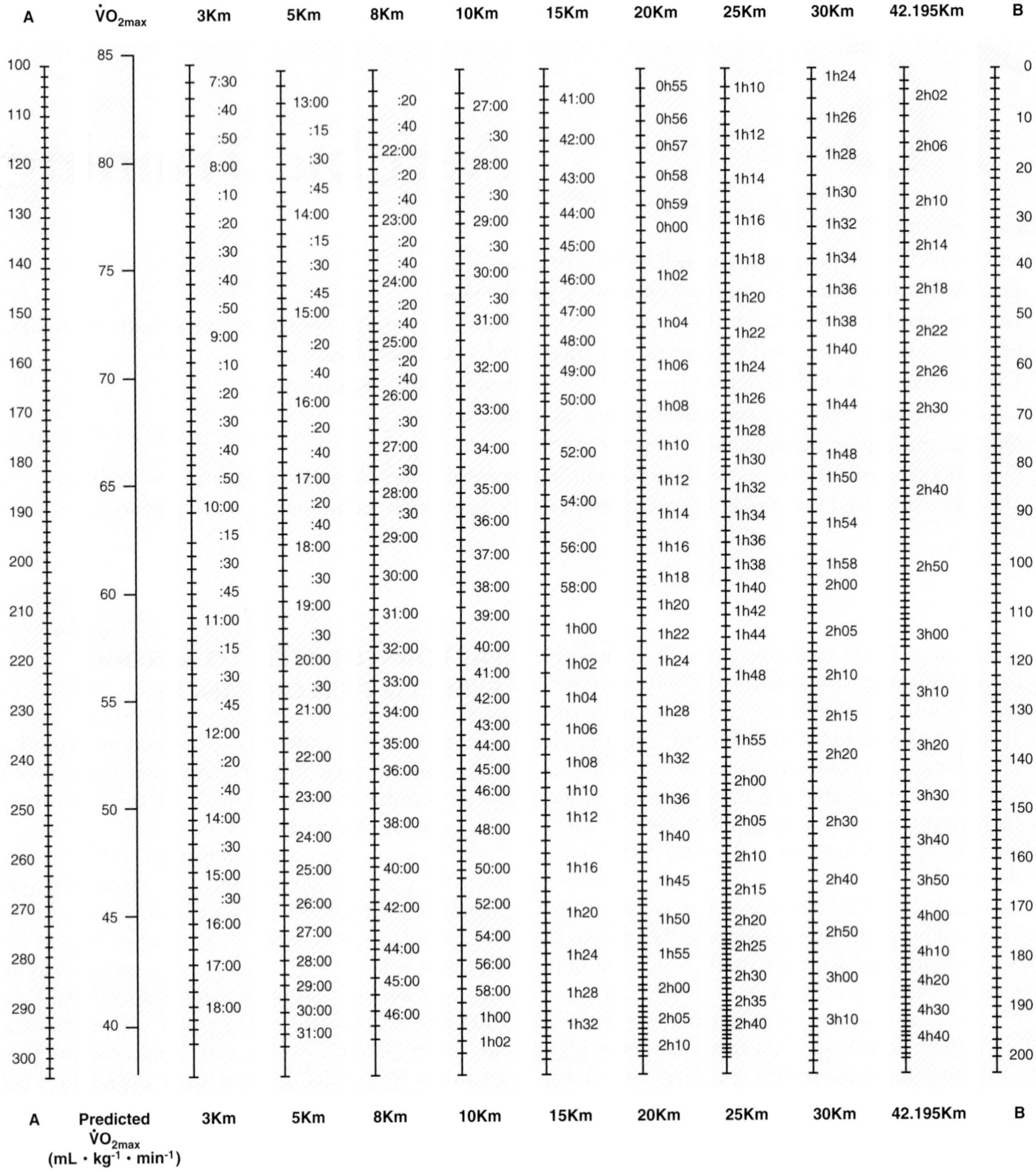

A	$\dot{V}O_{2max}$	3Km	5Km	8Km	10Km	15Km	20Km	25Km	30Km	42.195Km	B

(Nomogram scales — values listed top to bottom per column)

A (Predicted $\dot{V}O_{2max}$, mL·kg⁻¹·min⁻¹): 100, 110, 120, 130, 140, 150, 160, 170, 180, 190, 200, 210, 220, 230, 240, 250, 260, 270, 280, 290, 300

$\dot{V}O_{2max}$: 85, 80, 75, 70, 65, 60, 55, 50, 45, 40

3Km: 7:30, :40, :50, 8:00, :10, :20, :30, :40, :50, 9:00, :10, :20, :30, :40, :50, 10:00, :15, :30, :45, 11:00, :15, :30, :45, 12:00, :20, :40, 14:00, :30, 15:00, :30, 16:00, 17:00, 18:00

5Km: 13:00, :15, :30, :45, 14:00, :15, :30, :45, 15:00, :20, 16:00, :20, :40, 17:00, 18:00, :30, 19:00, :30, 20:00, :30, 21:00, :45, 22:00, 23:00, 24:00, 25:00, 26:00, 27:00, 28:00, 29:00, 30:00, 31:00

8Km: :20, :40, 22:00, :20, :40, 23:00, :20, :40, 24:00, :20, :40, 25:00, :20, :40, 26:00, :30, 27:00, :30, 28:00, :30, 29:00, :30, 30:00, 31:00, 32:00, 33:00, 34:00, 35:00, 36:00, 38:00, 40:00, 42:00, 44:00, 45:00, 46:00

10Km: 27:00, :30, 28:00, :30, 29:00, :30, 30:00, :30, 31:00, 32:00, 33:00, 34:00, 35:00, 36:00, 37:00, 38:00, 39:00, 40:00, 41:00, 42:00, 43:00, 44:00, 45:00, 46:00, 48:00, 50:00, 52:00, 54:00, 56:00, 58:00, 1h00, 1h02

15Km: 41:00, 42:00, 43:00, 44:00, 45:00, 46:00, 47:00, 48:00, 49:00, 50:00, 52:00, 54:00, 56:00, 58:00, 1h00, 1h02, 1h04, 1h06, 1h08, 1h10, 1h12, 1h16, 1h20, 1h24, 1h28, 1h32

20Km: 0h55, 0h56, 0h57, 0h58, 0h59, 0h00, 1h02, 1h04, 1h06, 1h08, 1h10, 1h12, 1h14, 1h16, 1h18, 1h20, 1h22, 1h24, 1h28, 1h32, 1h36, 1h40, 1h45, 1h50, 1h55, 2h00, 2h05, 2h10

25Km: 1h10, 1h12, 1h14, 1h16, 1h18, 1h20, 1h22, 1h24, 1h26, 1h28, 1h30, 1h32, 1h34, 1h36, 1h38, 1h40, 1h42, 1h44, 1h48, 1h55, 2h00, 2h05, 2h10, 2h15, 2h20, 2h25, 2h30, 2h35, 2h40

30Km: 1h24, 1h26, 1h28, 1h30, 1h32, 1h34, 1h36, 1h38, 1h40, 1h44, 1h48, 1h50, 1h54, 1h58, 2h00, 2h05, 2h10, 2h15, 2h20, 2h30, 2h40, 2h50, 3h00, 3h10

42.195Km: 2h02, 2h06, 2h10, 2h14, 2h18, 2h22, 2h26, 2h30, 2h40, 2h50, 3h00, 3h10, 3h20, 3h30, 3h40, 3h50, 4h00, 4h10, 4h20, 4h30, 4h40

B: 0, 10, 20, 30, 40, 50, 60, 70, 80, 90, 100, 110, 120, 130, 140, 150, 160, 170, 180, 190, 200

■ **FIGURE 16.1.** Prediction of running performance from Vo_{2max} data. (Reprinted with permission from Mercier D, Leger L, Desjardins M. Nomogram to predict performance equivalence for distance runners. *Track Technique*. 1986;94:3004–3009.)

LT is the first major inflection point where blood lactate abruptly increases beyond resting levels. It occurs at a higher percentage of Vo_{2max} with training and allows the athlete to exercise at a higher intensity. Some coaches use the second major lactate inflection point (onset of blood lactate accumulation or ~4 mmol of lactate) as the threshold intensity. Interestingly, some studies have shown LT to be a better indicator of maximal endurance performance than Vo_{2max} (52,70). *Maximal lactate steady state* is the intensity where maximal lactate production equals lactate clearance and may be used as a predictor of aerobic endurance performance. Athletes predisposed to high endurance performances have a higher proportion of type I muscle fibers. Type I fibers are highly oxidative (resulting in less lactate formation) and are fatigue-resistant. Endurance athletes have higher proportions of type I fibers than anaerobic athletes and sedentary individuals (10).

Athletes with high exercise economy have a distinct advantage in endurance sports. **Exercise economy** refers

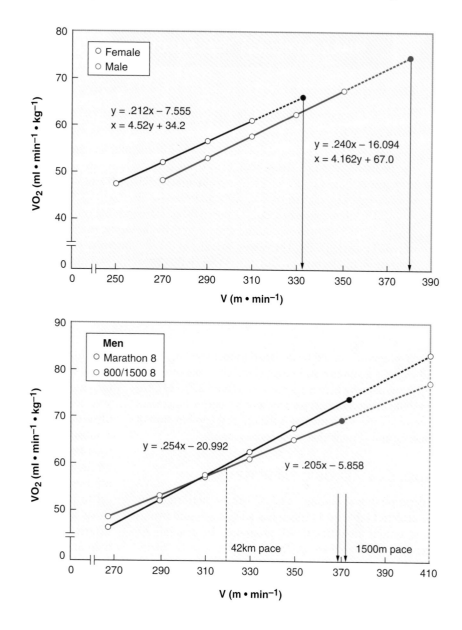

FIGURE 16.2. Running economy. (Reprinted with permission from Daniels J, Daniels N. Running economy of elite male and elite female runners. *Med Sci Sports Exerc*. 1992;24:483–489.)

to the energy cost of exercise at a given velocity. Less energy is expended per exercise velocity. When athletes with similar VO_{2max} values are compared, exercise economy becomes a stronger predictor of aerobic endurance performance (18). Several factors affect exercise economy including age, training status, stride length and rate (for running), the stretch-shortening cycle (SSC) and muscular stiffness, footwear, and wind resistance (18,54). Exercise economy increases when RT and AT are performed concurrently. In a review of the literature, Yamamoto et al. (69) showed that concurrent training in highly trained runners improved 3K and 5K times by 2.9% and running economy by 4.6% (range, 3%–8.1%). Figure 16.2 depicts data from Daniels and Daniels (18). In the first graph, male and female runners were compared. At a given velocity, men were able to perform at a lower VO_2 than women, indicating greater running economy. Although women may have lower running

economy than men, the majority of data show that AT program guidelines are similar between genders. In the second graph, male distance runners were compared to male runners who competed in 800- to 1,500-m events. At higher velocities, the 800- to 1,500-m runners showed greater running economy than the marathon runners. Other studies have shown experienced runners have better running economy than untrained subjects (49). In addition, training at altitude and RT enhance running economy (55).

AEROBIC TRAINING

Developing an aerobic endurance training program has similar characteristics as other modalities. Manipulation of exercise selection, intensity, volume, rest intervals (for interval training), and frequency can target specific goals of

Interpreting Research

The Importance of Lactate Threshold Differences in Endurance Athletes

Coyle EF, Coggan AR, Hopper MK, Walters TJ. Determinants of endurance in well-trained cyclists. *J Appl Physiol.* 1988;64:2622–2630.

Vo_{2max} is critical to endurance performance but is one of a few factors which highly affects performance (exercise economy and LT). Coyle et al. (16) studied 14 cyclists with similar levels of Vo_{2max}. They were subdivided into groups based on LT where one group reached their LT at lower exercise intensity (~65% of Vo_{2max}) and the other group reached their LT at higher exercise intensity (~82% of Vo_{2max}). Subjects were tested at 88% of Vo_{2max}. The high-intensity group's time to fatigue was double the low-intensity group (~61 vs. 29 min). Both groups had similar mitochondrial enzyme activity; however, the high-intensity group had a higher percentage of type I muscle fibers. The vastus lateralis of the low-intensity group showed much higher rates of glycogen utilization and lactate production. More than 92% of the variance in performance was explained by LT and muscle capillary density. The results of this study showed that at similar levels of Vo_{2max} other factors such as muscle fiber type and LT play critical roles in aerobic endurance performance.

AT. AT programs should be designed to increase Vo_{2max}, LT, and exercise economy, and target some elements of speed. Vo_{2max} can improve between a range of 5% and 25% (43). No threshold duration exists per workout for optimal increases in aerobic capacity. Rather, it is the optimal combination of intensity and volume that achieves best results.

MODES OF AEROBIC EXERCISE

Several modes of aerobic exercise can be performed by the athlete (Table 16.1). Each has advantages and brings some unique qualities to AT programs. In general, AT exercises are classified as: (a) those that can be maintained at a constant intensity, (b) those where energy expenditure is related to skill, and (c) those modes where skill and intensity are variable (games, sports). The vital elements to aerobic modes of training are its level of continuity and the magnitude of muscle mass involvement. Continuous exercise that stresses large muscle groups produces greater increases in aerobic capacity. *Fitness walking* and *hiking* are aerobic modalities that tend to be lower in intensity and are performed for longer durations. Intensity for each can increase by adding an incline (hill) or using hand weights or backpacks

(for hiking). *Jogging* and *running* are excellent forms of AT for athletes. Athletes may jog for short distances (at higher speeds), moderate distances (5–10 km), and long distances (half-marathons, marathons, and ultra-marathons). Running is excellent as it produces a substantial increase in heart rate (HR) and requires a total-body effort. Jogging and running place greater stress on the musculoskeletal system so the chances of overuse injuries increase. Proper volume and frequency are critical to prevent overuse injuries. A good pair of running shoes assists in shock absorption. A firm heel counter, external stabilizer, Achilles pad, midsole, and outsole help protect the body against the rigors of repetitive foot contacts. Athletes who frequently run for distance should change/replace their athletic shoes every 500 miles.

Stair climbing is an excellent form of AT. Raising the body against gravity (while maintaining an upright posture) requires additional muscle mass involvement. Stair climbing may be performed on cardio machines or steps (although it may be difficult to find an area with enough steps to climb continuously). On machines, the athlete should not rely on the use of hand rails for support as this makes the exercise easier. This could result from weak quadriceps and gluteal muscles or poor endurance. Stair

TABLE 16.1 MODES OF AEROBIC TRAINING

Walking	Stair climbing
Hiking	Cycling/spinning
Jogging/running	Aquatics
Aerobic dance	Swimming
Step aerobics	Rope skipping
Cross-country skiing	Rowing
Skating	Sports

climbing is weight-bearing and can create high levels of fatigue in lower-body musculature. It is effective for increasing muscular endurance but in some lesser aerobically trained athletes, leg fatigue may limit the maximal CV effect.

Cycling is non-weight-bearing and can cause a substantial amount of lower-body fatigue. It is more difficult to attain a higher HR for cycling as it is mostly a lower-body activity (unless arm ergometry is used). Cycling is an effective mode of exercise to increase muscular and aerobic endurance. Hills and faster speeds increase the intensity during outdoor cycling. Intensity is easy to control on indoor cycle ergometers. Spinning classes have become popular and is a good way to add variety to cycle training. Outdoor cycling equipment has changed over the years. The tapered helmets and tight clothing help minimize wind resistance, enable greater cycling speeds to be attained, and increase metabolic efficiency. When cycling outdoors, the athlete should wear a protective helmet and adhere to safety/traffic rules. Arm cycle ergometry may be used primarily to increase upper body endurance and poses less of a CV stimulus compared to lower-body cycling. Arm exercise generally lowers the oxygen consumption requirement by 30% and max HR by 10–15 bpm compared to lower-body cycling and running of similar workload (43).

Aerobic dance classes have increased in popularity since their inception in the early 1970s by Jacki Sorensen. Aerobics classes integrate many types of movements (walking, stepping, jogging, skipping, kicking, and arm swinging) into a routine to music that varies in length. Aerobics classes may be low-, moderate-, and high-impact. The difference is that in low-impact classes one foot usually remains on the floor to support body weight whereas in high-impact classes exercises are used that require elevation of both feet off the floor leading to greater musculoskeletal loading. Complexity increases with the addition of more challenging movements. *Step aerobics* is popular and increases the intensity by the height of steps used. Steps (usually around 4–12 in.) increase the activity of the SSC. In recent times, other modalities have been added to aerobics classes. RT (dumbbells, bands), core/stability, plyometrics, and balance-type movements have been incorporated into classes to add greater variety and train other components of fitness. For example, some "boot camp" classes have incorporated speed, agility, plyometric, calisthenic, weight training, pilates, and military-type (army crawls) drills into circuits within each class. The continuity of each class can be a potent stimulus for increasing aerobic and muscular endurance. Other components of fitness can be trained with different exercises incorporated into the class.

Swimming and *aquatic exercise* provide little orthopedic stress. The buoyancy of the water adds resistance to movement but reduces weight-bearing requirements. More resistance can be added to aquatic exercise by increasing the depth of the water or by using aqua dumbbells, fins, and paddles. Swimming is a form of RT and is a total-body exercise which can increase muscle and aerobic endurance. One limitation is that HRs do not reach as high a level as they do during land-based exercises, *e.g.*, on average 10–13 beats $\cdot$ min^{-1} less in the water (43). Water cools the body, lessens the effects of gravity on the CV system, and applies compressive force to the body which results in less CV demand and a lower HR. An athlete must know how to swim to reap the CV benefits. Different strokes (breast stroke, side stroke, back stroke, butterfly, freestyle) can be used to increase variety and muscle activation. Aquatic exercise is similar to aerobics classes (different types including low-impact, toning, deep water running, and kickboxing) or weight training workouts with the exception that they take place in the water. Impact is minimal and there is less thermal stress to the individuals. Swimming skill may not be required for an aquatics class in the shallow end of the pool.

Cross-country skiing recruits all major muscles of the body and the CV demand is very high. As a result, cross-country skiers have high Vo$_{2max}$ values, similar to or sometimes greater than marathon runners, cyclists, and triathletes (43). A limitation may be the outdoor conditions, but cardio machines that replicate the motions can be used indoors.

Rowing and *skating* can increase aerobic capacity. Rowing involves a total-body effort and can lead to high levels of muscle fatigue which makes it effective for increasing muscle endurance. Skating can provide a CV effect but it is important to minimize gliding, or the metabolic demands will be lower. *Rope skipping* requires skill to increase the continuity. Rope skipping is also used to train for agility and foot speed. Aerobic rope skipping workouts include basic foot movements so the duration can be expanded.

Playing sports (independent of the athlete's main sport) can be viewed as AT to some degree. For example, playing tennis, racquetball, and pick-up games of basketball poses a sufficient aerobic stimulus. However, continuous play is needed to maximize the benefits. The flow of the game and the skill level of the participants are critical. These sports provide a good CV workout when skill level is high, competitive, and continuous play is seen for the majority of the activity. However, an athlete will experience only a small effect if there are constant stoppages due to a lack of skill of the participant, a lack of skill by other players/opponents, or other factors that stop games temporarily (fouls in basketball, retrieving the ball, pauses between points scored and serving in tennis, etc.). The benefit is that sports are competitive and fun to play, which increase motivation and participation. The benefits from sports participation may be augmented when other modes of AT are included in the training program.

The athlete and coach need to decide which modes of training will be included. Each mode has advantages and disadvantages. The pros and cons are compared and modes are selected based on this. Modes that are similar to the demands of the athlete's major sport should be selected. A running program is specific to many sports that require sufficient aerobic conditioning such as basketball, boxing, and wrestling. Modes that are challenging, yet perhaps not specific, can be integrated in the workout to add variety as they may be used for total conditioning purposes.

Cross-Training

Cross-training refers to including different modes of exercise into the training program. Cross-training exposes the athlete to many stimuli. As a result, aerobic and anaerobic conditioning improves. Cross-training has the advantage of adding variety and is thought to reduce the likelihood of overuse injuries. It is an effective way to train past plateaus. For example, the advanced runner who has peaked performance with little progression may be best served by including some other modes of training. The increase in fitness from the other modes can have a transfer effect to running and allows the athlete to have mental relief while still training intensely. An athlete can integrate multiple modes of AT in a weekly training program. For example, in a 3-day-per-week program, the athlete can run on Monday, cycle on Wednesday, and stair climb on Friday. Progression can take place on a biweekly basis where either the intensity or volume is increased. If two modalities are used, the athlete can run on Monday, cycle on Wednesday, run on Friday, cycle on Monday, etc. Numerous possibilities exist when cross-training. Most athletes include multiple training modes in their own programs.

INTENSITY

Intensity selection during AT is critical to changes in aerobic capacity. Intensity prescription must match the goals of the program for that day. Intensity and volume/duration are inversely related. A delicate balance is needed to maximize the CV response yet provide enough duration to be a potent stimulus to increase aerobic capacity. Multiple strategies are used and intensity prescription matches the goals for that workout. LT and exercise economy (in addition to Vo_{2max}) increase endurance performance and these are often trained at moderately high to high intensities. Some researchers have postulated that training at a higher intensity for lower mileage may be more effective for enhancing distance running performance (38). Low-intensity, long-duration workouts are good for weight control and increasing submaximal muscle endurance. Aerobic capacity may increase but it depends on the athlete's training status. Athletes with high levels of aerobic fitness may not improve their aerobic capacity with low-intensity workouts. High-intensity workouts increase aerobic capacity, economy, and LT.

Hill training (at 85%–90% effort for 30-s to 5-min periods) in runners increases intensity and is associated with faster endurance run times (38). Increasing intensity increases muscle fiber recruitment and CV demands, which have a more profound effect on increasing aerobic and muscle endurance.

There are three general ways to monitor or prescribe AT intensity: (a) HR, (b) percentage of Vo_{2max} or reserve, and (c) ratings of perceived exertion (RPE). The most common method used to prescribe intensity is to use HR. There is a very close relationship between HR and oxygen consumption. The first step in intensity prescription is to determine the athlete's maximal HR. This is calculated by taking 220–the athlete's age (HR is in beats per minute [bpm]). For example, a 20-year-old athlete's max predicted HR is 200 bpm. For older adults, a revised formula: $HR_{max} = 207-0.7(age)$ has been recommended (43,59). At this point two methods may be used. The first is to multiply the max HR by the desired training percentage. For example, the 20-year-old athlete desiring to train at 70% intensity would attain an exercise HR of 140 bpm (200 bpm × 0.70). This is known as the HR_{max} method. However, the second method, the *heart rate reserve (HRR) method*, is preferred. The HRR method, also known as the Karvonen formula (36), takes into account the athlete's resting HR which is a measure of aerobic fitness. The HRR value obtained aligns almost identically to a percentage of Vo_{2max} between 50% and 100% intensities whereas using the straight percentage of max HR may yield values of $\%Vo_{2max}$ that differ by a range of 3%–14% (52). The Karvonen, or HRR formula is:

$$\text{target HR} = \%INT\,(HR_{max} - HR_{rest}) + HR_{rest}.$$

If our athlete has a resting HR of 68 bpm, then his/her target HR (based on the Karvonen formula) would be: THR = 0.70 (200 bpm – 68 bpm) + 68 bpm = 174 bpm. Compared to the standard percentage formula, the HRR method does take into consideration one's fitness level (via the resting HR) and provides a better indication of target HR for AT. Figure 16.3 depicts an intensity training zone based on targeted HRs. Many times a targeted zone is calculated rather than one specific HR. Using the Karvonen formula, a HR zone of 121–180 bpm is shown based on 40%–85% of HRR. Low-, moderate-, and high-intensity AT zones are identified. Age only explains ~75% of the variability of HR so other variables such as training status and exercise mode are critical (52). *The ACSM has recommended 40%–85% of HRR and 50%–90% of HR_{max} for intensity prescription during AT* (1). The wide range of values takes into consideration fitness level such that unfit populations begin at the lower end of the spectrum and fit athletes benefit from training at the opposite end. It is important to point out that HR is a self-correcting variable (changes with improved fitness) for intensity prescription. Submaximal exercise HR is reduced as a CV

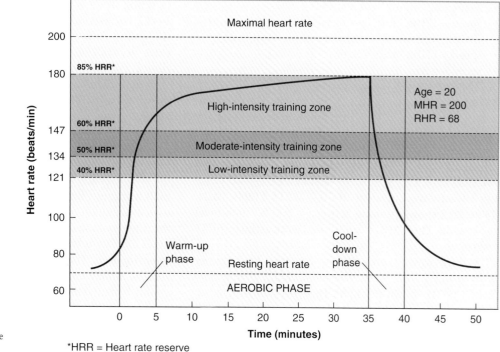

■ **FIGURE 16.3.** Intensity zone based on heart rate.

*HRR = Heart rate reserve

adaptation. It takes greater effort to reach a target HR as aerobic capacity improves. Thus, maintaining a targeted HR percentage as an intensity guide can still be progressive because the athlete will have to work harder in order to reach the targeted level. The use of HR monitors makes it easy to monitor HR. For example, an athlete can be given a 12-week AT program with intensity prescription of 60% of HRR for the first 4 weeks, 65% of HRR for the second 4 weeks, and 70% of HRR for the last 4 weeks. Although the athlete maintains the same target HRR value for 4-week periods, progression takes place within each cycle as it becomes more difficult to reach the desired HR as conditioning improves. Thus, the athlete is forced to continually work harder to maintain the target HRR value.

The second way to prescribe intensity is based on a percentage of Vo_{2max} or reserve. Selecting a percentage of Vo_{2max} use the following equation:

$$\text{Target } VO_2 = \%INT(Vo_{2max}).$$

However, the VO_2 reserve (VO_2R) method can be used where

$$VO_2R = \%INT(Vo_{2max} - 3.5) + 3.5.$$

The VO_2R method takes into consideration the difference between Vo_{2max} and resting VO_2 ($3.5\,mL \cdot kg^{-1} \cdot min^{-1}$) and correlates highly to the HRR method [59]. Let's view a 20-year-old athlete with a Vo_{2max} of $52\,mL \cdot kg^{-1} \cdot min^{-1}$. Using the first method, if the target intensity is 70% then

the target VO_2 equals $36.4\,mL \cdot kg^{-1} \cdot min^{-1}$ ($52 \times 0.70 = 36.4\,mL \cdot kg^{-1} \cdot min^{-1}$). Using the VO_2R method, the target VO_2 equals $37.5\,mL \cdot kg^{-1} \cdot min^{-1}$ ($0.70[52 - 3.5] + 3.5$). *The ACSM recommends 50%–85% VO_2R for AT when the VO_2R method is used* [1]. A limitation of this method is that true VO_2 data are not readily available (outside of the laboratory setting) so estimation is used.

The ACSM metabolic equations can be used in calculation [5]. Variables used in the regression equations include speed, percent grade, work rate, and step height (for those equations used for walking, running, cycling [arm and leg], and stepping). These equations are:

- *Walking:* VO_2 ($mL \cdot kg^{-1} \cdot min^{-1}$) = 0.1(speed in $m \cdot min^{-1}$) + 1.8(speed in $m \cdot min^{-1}$)(% grade) + $3.5\,mL \cdot kg^{-1} \cdot min^{-1}$
- *Running:* VO_2 ($mL \cdot kg^{-1} \cdot min^{-1}$) = 0.2(speed in $m \cdot min^{-1}$) + 0.9(speed in $m \cdot min^{-1}$)(% grade) + $3.5\,mL \cdot kg^{-1} \cdot min^{-1}$
- *Leg Cycling:* VO_2 ($mL \cdot kg^{-1} \cdot min^{-1}$) = 1.8(work rate in $kg \cdot m \cdot min^{-1}$)/body mass (kg) + $7.0\,mL \cdot kg^{-1} \cdot min^{-1}$
- *Arm Cycling:* VO_2 ($mL \cdot kg^{-1} \cdot min^{-1}$) = 3.0(work rate in $kg \cdot m \cdot min^{-1}$)/body mass (kg) + $3.5\,mL \cdot kg^{-1} \cdot min^{-1}$
- *Stepping:* VO_2 ($mL \cdot kg^{-1} \cdot min^{-1}$) = 0.2(step rate in $steps \cdot min^{-1}$) + 2.394(step rate in $steps \cdot min^{-1}$) (step height in meters) + $3.5\,mL \cdot kg^{-1} \cdot min^{-1}$

In our previous example, substituting the target VO_2 in the equation for running is calculated:

- VO_2 ($mL \cdot kg^{-1} \cdot min^{-1}$) = 0.2(speed in $m \cdot min^{-1}$) + 0.9(speed in $m \cdot min^{-1}$)(% grade) + $3.5\,mL \cdot kg^{-1} \cdot min^{-1}$
- $37.5\,mL \cdot kg^{-1} \cdot min^{-1} = 3.5\,mL \cdot kg^{-1} \cdot min^{-1} + 0.2$ (speed) — note: assuming % grade is 0 this latter part is not needed

- $34\,mL \cdot kg^{-1} \cdot min^{-1} = 0.2(speed)$
- Speed = 170 m · min⁻¹ — speed units are in $m \cdot min^{-1}$
- Conversion: speed (mph) = speed $(m \cdot min^{-1})/26.8$
- Speed = $170\,m \cdot min^{-1}/26.8$
- Speed = 6.3 mph

In our example, the athlete needs to run at 6.3 mph to achieve the target VO_2R value. Without performing the calculation, another estimate may be used via metabolic equivalents (METS). 1 MET = $3.5\,mL \cdot kg^{-1} \cdot min^{-1}$. Our targeted VO_2 of $37.5\,mL \cdot kg^{-1} \cdot min^{-1}$ is equivalent to 10.7 METS (VO_2 = 35.7/3.5). A conversion table is used yielding an activity equivalent of 10.7 METS (Table 16.2). Table 16.2 shows running between 6 and 6.7 mph meet the criteria. Thus, METS can be used as an estimate of AT intensity.

A third way to prescribe or monitor AT intensity is by using a RPE scale. The most common, the *Borg Scale* (13), is shown in Figure 16.4. It is constructed to increase linearly with workload in conjunction with HR and oxygen consumption during aerobic exercise. The Borg Scale consists of a continuum of intensity anchors ranging from 6 to 20, *e.g.*, very, very light (*i.e.*, 6–8) to very, very hard (*i.e.*, 19–20). A zero is added to the rating

(a rating of 14 = 140 bpm) to estimate HR. A value of 14–17 corresponds to 60%–85% of HRR, 86%–92% of HR_{max}, and 76%–85% of VO_{2max} (43). The Borg Scale provides accurate estimates in recreational, athletic, and clinical populations.

Some athletes aerobically train without direct monitoring of intensity. They may not assess HR but train based on performance variables. Intensity can be estimated by the pattern of progression used during AT. Many athletes have a designated distance used in training. For example, the athlete may be prescribed a 5-mile run. In week 1, the athlete/coach times the run and establishes a base. In each workout (5 miles is the desired length), the athlete tries to maintain or improve upon that time. The shorter the time completed, the faster the running. Reduced times indicate better performance but do not quantify the intensity used. The use of time trials can be motivational and the athlete (when training on a similar course) may establish mental markers within the event which provides a guide to where they should be. For example, the athlete may acknowledge that reaching a certain landmark in the course means he/she should be exercising under a certain time. If not, then the athlete needs to increase speed to reach the desired pace. This is seen in many modes such

TABLE 16.2 EXERCISE AND METABOLIC EQUIVALENTS (METS)

METS	EXERCISE	METS	EXERCISE
1.0	Lying/sitting quietly	8.0	Calisthenics — vigorous
2.0	Walking flat — <2 mph	8.0	Circuit training
2.5	Walking flat — 2 mph	8.0	Outdoor cycling — 12–13.9 mph
3.0	Light RT	8.0	Walking flat — 5.0 mph
3.0	Stationary cycling — 50 W	8.5	Step aerobics — 6–8 in. steps
3.0	Walking flat — 2.5 mph	9.0	Running flat — 5.2 mph
3.3	Walking flat — 3 mph	9.0	Stair stepping — 12-in. steps, 30 steps · min⁻¹
3.5	Light calisthenics	10.0	Outdoor cycling — 14–15.9 mph
3.5	Stair stepping — 20 steps · min⁻¹, 4-in. steps	10.0	Running — 6.0 mph
3.8	Walking flat — 3.5 mph	10.0	Step aerobics — 10–12 in. steps
4.0	Water aerobics	10.0	Swimming laps — freestyle, vigorous
4.8	Stair stepping — 30 steps · min⁻¹	10.5	Stationary cycling — 200 W
5.0	Low-impact aerobic dance	11.0	Running — 6.7 mph
5.0	Walking flat — 4.0 mph	11.5	Running — 7.0 mph
5.5	Stationary cycling — 100 W	12.0	Outdoor cycling — 16–19 mph
6.0	Outdoor cycling — 10–11.9 mph	12.5	Running — 7.5 mph
6.0	Vigorous RT	12.5	Stationary cycling — 250 W
6.3	Stair stepping, 12-in. steps, 20 steps · min⁻¹	13.5	Running — 8.0 mph
6.3	Walking flat — 4.0 mph	14.0	Running — 8.5 mph
6.9	Stair stepping, 8-in. steps, 30 steps · min⁻¹	15.0	Running — 9.0 mph
7.0	High-impact aerobic dance	16.0	Outdoor cycling — >20 mph
7.0	Stationary cycling — 150 W	16.0	Running — 10 mph
7.0	Swimming laps — slow, mod effort		

Adapted with permission from Reuter BH, Hagerman PS. Aerobic endurance exercise training. In: Baechle TR, Earle RW, editors. *Essentials of Strength Training and Conditioning*. 3rd ed. Champaign (IL): Human Kinetics; 2008. pp. 489–503.

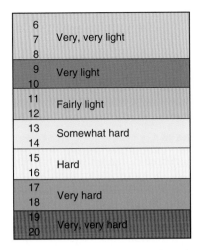

6	
7	Very, very light
8	
9	Very light
10	
11	Fairly light
12	
13	Somewhat hard
14	
15	Hard
16	
17	Very hard
18	
19	Very, very hard
20	

■ **FIGURE 16.4.** Borg scale of perceived exertion. The scale with correct instructions can be obtained from Borg Perception, see the home page: *www.borgperception.se/index.html*. (Reprinted with permission from Borg G. *Borg's Perceived Exertion and Pain Scales*. Champaign [IL]: Human Kinetics; 1998.)

as running, cycling, cross-country skiing, and swimming. In viewing swimming competitions, *e.g.*, the Olympics, on television, often the pace times are shown. These serve as valuable guides to influence coaching strategies. Although not a direct measure of intensity, time trials are commonly used by athletes as a form of overload or progression. In addition, the athlete may be prescribed a fixed workout duration. For example, the athlete may be prescribed a 30-minute run, 2 days per week, for 6 weeks. In each workout the athlete attempts to cover a larger distance in the same period of time. Greater effort and speed are needed to train farther in the same time period.

FREQUENCY

The frequency of AT has been a topic of debate as it is affected by other variables such as intensity, duration, mode, training status, and recovery of the athlete. Frequency will vary depending on whether the athlete is in off-, pre-, or in-season training. High-intensity and/ or long-duration workouts may necessitate a reduction in frequency to reduce the risk of overuse injuries and overtraining. Highly trained athletes have greater tolerance for volume and can handle a higher frequency. Endurance athletes may train 5 days per week in the off-season and incorporate some anaerobic training to improve overall conditioning. However, during the preseason the athlete may increase volume and frequency greatly for endurance events and may have multiple workouts in a day. Studies have shown that Vo_{2max} increases similarly between 2- and 5-day frequencies (33,43). However, the intensity may be the critical variable and not the frequency per se. Other physiological

Myths & Misconceptions

Low-Intensity AT is the Best Way to Increase VO$_{2max}$

It has been suggested that low-to-moderate intensity, long-duration AT is the best way to increase Vo_{2max}. However, a threshold training intensity is needed to increase endurance capacity and, in many cases, the higher the intensity the larger the Vo_{2max} improvement. The threshold is based on training status and only surpassing a threshold intensity will lead to improvement. Likewise, a smaller window of adaptation is evident for athletes with a high Vo_{2max}. In a review of the literature by Swain and Franklin (60), it was shown that individuals with a Vo_{2max} below 40 mL kg^{-1} min^{-1} always increased their aerobic capacity even at intensities as low as 30% of VO_2R but individuals with Vo_{2max} values between 41 and 51 mL kg^{-1} min^{-1} showed a threshold (~45% of VO_2R) where training only above the threshold led to aerobic capacity improvements (60). The majority of studies cited in their review found greater increases in Vo_{2max} with higher-intensity AT than lower-intensity training (using constant total volume) (60). Figure 16.5 depicts data generated from Swain (58) showing a continuum of adaptations in Vo_{2max} based on training intensity and initial training status. Gormley et al. (26) had subjects train at 50%, 75%, and 95% of VO_2R (with equal training volumes) and found that a continuum of increases (20.6%, 14.3%, and 10% increases, respectively) were seen for the 95%, 75%, and 50% groups, respectively. Interestingly, Helgerud et al. (30) showed increases in Vo_{2max} after 8 weeks of interval training at 90%–95% of HR_{max} but failed to observe an increase in Vo_{2max} with continuous AT at 70% and 85% of HR_{max}. These data demonstrate the utility of interval training in the training of aerobic athletes and show interval training at high intensities may elicit greater improvements in aerobic capacity than lower-intensity training at a similar volume (59). Based on the available data, the threshold training intensity needed to increase aerobic capacity increases as one's level of aerobic fitness increases and higher-intensity AT leads to greater improvement. Table 16.3 depicts current threshold intensities and subsequent recommendations for AT where progression is the goal (59).

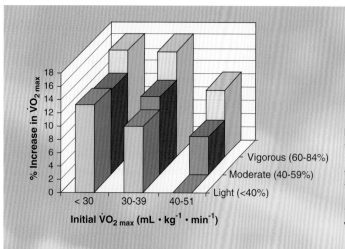

FIGURE 16.5. Increases in Vo_{2max} at different intensities of training for individuals with various levels of aerobic fitness. Data show greater improvements in Vo_{2max} with higher intensities of aerobic endurance training. (Reprinted with permission from Swain DP. Cardiorespiratory exercise prescription. In: Ehrman JK, ed. *ACSM's Resource Manual for Guidelines for Exercise Testing and Prescription*. 6th ed. Philadelphia, PA: Lippincott Williams & Wilkins; 2010. pp. 448–462.)

TABLE 16.3 THRESHOLD INTENSITIES OF AEROBIC TRAINING NEEDED TO INCREASE AEROBIC CAPACITY (59)

FITNESS LEVEL	VO_{2MAX} (ML · KG^{-1} · MIN^{-1})	RECOMMENDED MINIMUM INTENSITY
Low to moderate	<40	30% VO_2R or HRR
Average to good	40–51	45% VO_2R or HRR
High	52–59	75% VO_2R or HRR
Very high	≥60	90%–100% VO_2R or HRR

adaptations in addition to Vo_{2max} changes are sought so a higher frequency can be used to target these components (economy, LT, muscle endurance). *The ACSM has recommended 3–5 days of AT per week* (1). For greater specificity, *the ACSM has recommended: 5 days per week for moderate-intensity training, 3 days per week for high-intensity training, and 3–5 days per week when combination moderate- and high-intensity workouts are used* (59).

For low- to moderate-intensity AT, frequencies of 5–7 days per week can be used (59). Table 16.4 depicts some different workout strategies relative to AT frequency. However, advanced-to-elite aerobic athletes may train with a higher frequency in preparation for a competition. A high frequency is seen by those individuals who AT for weight loss where low-intensity, long-duration workouts are often used.

TABLE 16.4 EXAMPLES OF INTENSITY PRESCRIPTION STRATEGIES BASED ON AEROBIC TRAINING FREQUENCIES OF 3–6 DAYS PER WEEK

FRQ	MON.	TUES.	WED.	THURS.	FRI.	SAT.	SUN.
3	H	—	H	—	H	—	—
3	H	—	LM	—	H	—	—
3[a]	LM	—	LM	—	LM	—	—
4	H	LM	—	H	LM	—	—
4	LM	—	H	—	LM	—	H
4[a]	LM	LM	—	LM	LM	—	—
4	H	—	H	—	H	—	LM
5	H	LM	—	H	LM	—	LM
5	H	LM	H	LM	H	—	—
5[a]	LM	LM	LM	LM	LM	—	—
6	H	LM	H	LM	H	LM	—
6[a]	LM	LM	LM	LM	LM	LM	—

[a]LM weeks used for body weight control.
H, high-intensity workout; LM, low-to-moderate-intensity workout.

VOLUME AND DURATION

Duration refers to the length of time a workout lasts whereas *volume* refers to the total number of foot contacts, repetitions, or distances covered. Both are highly related to each other and depend on the intensity, frequency, and training status of the athlete. AT workouts of low-to-moderate intensity are often moderate to long in duration. Athletes training for endurance events have been known to exercise at high volumes. High-intensity workouts involve shorter durations and are of low-to-moderate training volumes. *The ACSM has recommended 20–60 minutes of continuous or intermittent aerobic exercise for healthy adults* (1), although the volume of athletes training for endurance sports exceeds this range frequently. Table 16.5 depicts an example 8-week intermediate AT program based on ACSM guidelines. It is designed to establish an aerobic base for subsequent higher-intensity training. The goals are to increase duration on the lower-intensity workouts and increase intensity on the higher-intensity workout.

There is no optimal volume of training for everyone. Rather, volume (and intensity) relates to the type of training activity. For example, the volume of AT for a marathon runner will be much higher than the volume for a basketball player as the runner must compete for 26 miles whereas the basketball player must continuously play for two halves but will take frequent breaks due to time-outs, substitutions, and breaks in the action (more anaerobic activity). Volume should be carefully prescribed. Fluctuations in weekly training volumes are common. Many athletes alternate between high-intensity, moderate-volume and moderate-intensity, and high-volume workouts during a training week. Ultra-endurance athletes typically have one very long duration workout per week. Progression in volume may entail the athlete covering a greater distance in a specific or general period of time, adding distance and time, or adding more repetitions or increasing the distance of each repetition (for interval training).

TYPES OF AEROBIC ENDURANCE TRAINING WORKOUTS

AT programs can vary greatly in structure, *e.g.*, prolonged low-to-moderate intensity workouts (long slow duration) to higher-intensity workouts intermittent in structure. This section describes some common types of workouts used by endurance athletes.

Continuous Workouts: Long Slow Distance

Long slow distance training consists of low-to-moderate-intensity exercise performed for moderate-to-long durations. It may be referred to as *steady-pace training*. It is designed to increase Vo_{2max} and muscle endurance. Long slow distance training is typically performed between 30 minutes and 2 hours at a slower-than-race pace (60%–80% of Vo_{2max}). Many endurance athletes perform long slow distance training 1–2 days per week (52). For a marathon runner who uses a 2-day-per-week, frequency of long slow distance training, the athlete can structure his/her workout by placing these workouts in between higher-intensity days to facilitate recovery. Because of the lower intensity, long slow distance runs may spare muscle glycogen to some degree by a preferential increase in fat utilization. These workouts may be used in nonathletic populations for weight control. However, the intensity used for long slow distance training is below the endurance athlete's normal competition pace so this could be a disadvantage if performed too frequently in ultra-endurance athletes. The use of long slow distance training for other athletes with the goal of improving aerobic capacity is common.

Pace/Tempo

Pace/tempo training requires the athlete to workout at an intensity similar to or slightly higher than the normal race intensity. The intensity corresponds to the LT. Pace/tempo training can be continuous (20–30 min) or intermittent where short bouts are followed by a recovery period (52). The purpose is to develop a race type of

TABLE 16.5 SAMPLE 8-WEEK BASE 3-DAY PER WEEK BASE INTERMEDIATE AEROBIC RUNNING PROGRAM

WEEK	MON.	TUES.	WED.	THURS.	FRI.	SAT.	SUN.
1	60% HRR 30 min	—	70% HRR 20 min	—	60% HRR 30 min	—	—
2	60% HRR 30 min	—	70% HRR 20 min	—	60% HRR 30 min	—	—
3	60% HRR 35 min	—	70% HRR 20 min	—	60% HRR 35 min	—	—
4	60% HRR 35 min	—	70% HRR 20 min	—	60% HRR 35 min	—	—
5	60% HRR 40 min	—	75% HRR 20 min	—	60% HRR 40 min	—	—
6	60% HRR 40 min	—	75% HRR 20 min	—	60% HRR 40 min	—	—
7	60% HRR 45 min	—	75% HRR 20 min	—	60% HRR 45 min	—	—
8	60% HRR 45 min	—	75% HRR 20 min	—	60% HRR 45 min	—	—

pace for the athlete. Thus, the intensity should not be increased too much; rather, the distance can be increased when appropriate (52). Athletes typically include race/tempo training 1–2 days per week.

Fartlek Training

Fartlek (a Swedish word meaning speed play) **training** was introduced in the United States in the 1940s and is comprised of loosely structured exercise (usually runs but can apply to cycling and swimming) performed at various intensities and lengths with mixed periods of hard and easy runs (38,43). They are combinations of other training types. For example, the athlete may run at a moderate pace (~70% of Vo_{2max}) for a period of time and then run at a high intensity for a short time period, and repeat the process for the desired length, *i.e.*, the athlete may run at a steady pace for a period of time (6 min) and then run at 30–60 second bursts. Fartlek training is typically performed 1–2 days per week for 20–60 minute workout and can be placed in between lower-intensity workouts (pace/tempo and/or long slow distance training). Because of the intensity fluctuations, Fartlek training has the potential to increase Vo_{2max}, LT, and running economy (52). Because of the fluctuations, it is more difficult to prescribe training HRs. Fartlek training is useful to preparing the athlete to adjusting to competition pace shifts (29).

Interval Training

Interval training refers to repeated bouts of intense exercise followed by recovery periods of at least the length of the exercise bout (depending on the work:relief ratio). Intervals can be applied to aerobic (in addition to anaerobic) training. For AT, the bouts of exercise typically last 2–5 minutes (although they can be shorter) and 1:1 or 1:1.5 work:relief ratios are commonly used for 4–6 intervals. The intensity selected is similar to the athlete's Vo_{2max} (or at least 95% of Vo_{2max}) (52). The work or interval segment can be manipulated in a couple of ways. If a certain distance is to be covered, the coach should time each interval and keep records for each set. With each successive set the athlete tries to achieve that time. Time is the critical factor for monitoring the set. As sets progress, the coach can account for fatigue by granting the athlete some additional time for completion. The second way is to prescribe a specific time and record the distance the athlete covers during that time. With progression, the athlete covers greater distance in the same period of time. The coach records the distance per set and uses it as a set marker. Interval training workouts are typically performed 1–2 days per week and may cover up to 8% of the weekly total mileage in 3,000- to 10,000-m runners (29). They are stressful and are commonly placed in between lower-intensity workouts. Many coaches believe interval training to be a critical (and perhaps most beneficial method) for improving distance running performance (38). Some studies have shown interval training to be more effective for increasing aerobic capacity in trained individuals than continuous training (30,59).

Repetition Training

Repetition training comprises a series of runs that are faster than current race pace with complete recovery (38). The intensity is greater than the athlete's Vo_{2max} and last 30–90 seconds (52). Longer recovery periods in between repetitions are used as the intensity is higher, *i.e.*, work:relief ratios of 1:4–1:6 (29,52). There is a potent anaerobic component to repetition training. Thus, speed, economy, and buffer capacity can increase. Some have recommended that, for middle-distance runners, repetition training comprising a total volume between 2/3 and 1½ times the length of the racing distance (3.3–7.5 km for a 5-km runner) (14). For long-distance runners, repetition training comprising $\frac{1}{10}$, $\frac{1}{5}$, and $\frac{1}{3}$ of the total race distance be used with recovery periods of 5–30 minutes have been recommended (14).

TRAINING FOR ENDURANCE SPORTS

Training for endurance and ultra-endurance sports entails a multifactorial strategy. It is important for athletes to have already developed an aerobic base. Base AT (off-season training) to increase Vo_{2max} is critical and consists mostly of moderate-intensity training 5–6 days per week. Specific training can ensue. Periodized training consisting of high-intensity AT coupled or alternated with moderate-intensity, long-duration workouts form the foundation of training. Supplemental strength training and some speed (or perhaps plyometrics) training is included at a lower frequency. For example, a 6-day training routine may comprise one long endurance workout, two to three high-intensity, short-to-moderate-duration workouts (intervals, Fartleks, repetitions, tempos, hills, strides/technique), and two to three low-to-moderate-intensity, moderate-duration workouts used for base training (and facilitate recovery in between high-intensity workouts). Speed work can be incorporated into the high-intensity days and total-body RT can be performed separately. RT is an important and sometimes overlooked component for the endurance athlete. The goal is not to maximize increases in lean body mass. Mass increase adds weight to the athlete and potentially leads to greater wind resistance encountered both of which can have a negative effect on race speed. Although endurance athletes possess a predominance of ST muscle fibers, strength and power gains do occur and these can help with race performance. Flexibility training is performed at the end of workouts as part of a cool-down.

Training for the event begins several months in advance. General preparation training consists of increasing Vo_{2max}. Long, continuous training workouts predominate. Special preparation begins a few months before the season or competition. Training volume increases and greater specificity is added to the training weeks. Higher-intensity workouts are added to improve other facets of race performance, *i.e.*, LT, economy, and speed. Precompetition training is most specialized. Frequency (6–7 days per week) and volume increase. The mileage for long-duration workouts increases and more interval training is added. Brief lower-volume/intensity workouts are included during transitional phases. These equate to unloading weeks in a periodized scheme. For example, a runner preparing for a marathon may use the following pattern for his/her single long-duration workout of the week:

Week 1 → 12 miles: Week 2 → 14 miles: Week 3 → 16 miles: Week 4 → 10 miles: Week 5 → 16 miles: Week 6 → 18 miles: Week 7 → 20 miles: Week 8 → 12 miles: Week 9 → 20 miles: Week 10 → 22 miles: Week 11 → 24 miles: Week 12 → 15 miles followed by a 1- to 2-week taper period.

In each workout the volume increases by 2 miles over a 3-week period. The fourth week corresponds to a lower-volume unloading week to allow recovery from the previous weeks of training and transition to another phase of training. Volume progressively increases over time (with the exception of the lower-volume weeks). A tapering period is used 1–2 weeks before competition as tapering enhances performance. The athlete may overreach (increase volume/frequency in short term) prior to the tapering period which could result in some plateau. Tapering comprises a decrease in volume and perhaps frequency to maximize recovery and performance. Final technical points are addressed and race strategies are developed. The taper period corresponds to final nutritional preparations, *i.e.*, carbohydrate loading and increased fluid intake, and final race preparations. By the end of this phase the athlete is ready for competition.

Endurance athletes from different sports have adopted many training strategies. A triathlon is an ultra-endurance sport, which consists of swimming, cycling, and running. The distances may vary depending on the race. An Ironman triathlon is most rigorous and consists of 3.8-km swim, 180-km cycling, and 42-km run (9). The sequence of events is swimming, cycling, and running. The initial swim reduces optimal cycling power and subsequent cycling may produce a reduction in running efficiency (9). The triathlete must be proficient in all three modalities. Vlecks et al. (63) studied British Olympic and Ironman distance triathletes and showed that Olympic distance triathletes trained 15.6 ± 3.7 hours per week (5.6 ± 2.6-h swimming, 6.3 ± 3.0-h biking, and 3.7 ± 1.4-h running) and Ironman triathletes trained 19.5 ± 7.6 hours per week (6.1 ± 4.5-h swimming, 8.8 ± 4.5-h biking, and 3.9 ± 1.7-h running). Olympic distance triathletes trained 12.0 ± 3.0 times per week (4.0 ± 1.1 workouts swimming, 3.8 ± 1.7 workouts biking, and 4.17 ± 2.0 workouts running) and Ironman triathletes trained 14.3 ± 3.2 times per week (5.1 ± 1.9 workouts swimming, 4.0 ± 2.2 workouts biking, and 4.6 ± 2.0 workouts running) (63). The training consisted mostly of long low-to-moderate-intensity bike rides (>1.5 h) and runs (>1 h), 20–60-minute cycling time trials and

20–30 minute continuous or interval runs, and hill work (63). Gulbin and Gaffney (27) showed that Ironman triathletes spent 21.5 ± 10.8 weeks training for the event and their training distances per week for swimming, cycling, and running were 8.8 ± 4.3 km, 270 ± 107 km, and 58.2 ± 21.9 km at paces of 18.1 min $\cdot$ km^{-1}, 31.8 km $\cdot$ h^{-1}, and 4.55 min $\cdot$ km^{-1}, respectively. Triathletes many times have multiworkout days specifically training two of the three competition modalities.

Distance runners use multiple training strategies to enhance performance. The volume depends on the type of competitive race, *e.g.*, 5 km, 10 km, half-marathon (21.1 km), marathon (42.195 km), and ultra-marathons (50 and 100 km). Some elite distance runners train twice a day and run between 100 and 150 miles a week (43). Distance training comprises base-building, light, high-quality work, high-intensity intervals, and LT training (38). In fact, elite runners typically alternate between high- and low-to-moderate-intensity workouts and include a substantial amount of speed training to increase LT and running economy (50). Table 16.6 presents data from Kurz et al. (38) who studied several Division I collegiate cross-country runners. The data show shifts in training volume and modes of training over each of the three training phases. They showed the use of speed work, Fartlek training, mileage, and practicing twice per day was associated with slower team times (possibly due to overtraining) during the transition phase. Intervals and tempo training were associated with better running performance. In addition, hill training was related to faster run times during the transition phase. Table 16.7 depicts a sample weekly training program designed for an athlete preparing for a 5-km race. The program is setup so that the longest run of the week takes place on Sunday followed by a day of rest. The rest of training days alternate between high- and moderate-intensity workouts.

Cyclist use multiple training strategies. Professional cyclists may ride 30,000–35,000 km per year and may compete for up to 90 days (21). Typical road races and off-road cross-country cycling events may last between 1 and 5 hours whereas multistage races consist of several back-to-back days of racing and may total more than 3,800 km as is the case for the Tour de France (21). Similar to other endurance sports, cycling performance is related to Vo_{2max}, peak power output and power output at the LT, LT and blood lactate concentrations, efficiency, and breathing pattern (21). Cyclists have high Vo_{2max}; ranges of 66–85 mL $\cdot$ kg^{-1} min^{-1} have been reported in male cyclists and 58–68 $\cdot$ mL $\cdot$ kg^{-1} $\cdot$ min^{-1} in female cyclists (21). In cyclists with a similar Vo_{2max}, LT and lactate values at peak cycling power are strong predictors of endurance performance (11,17). Some have suggested a power:body mass ratio of >5.5 W $\cdot$ kg^{-1} is a necessary prerequisite for elite cycling (21). Cycling efficiency is related to type I muscle fiber percentages. Cycling programs consist of base training at moderate intensities for long durations (several hours) and progress to higher-intensity interval training as the

TABLE 16.6 TRAINING CHARACTERISTICS OF DIVISION I CROSS-COUNTRY RUNNERS (38)

VARIABLE	TRANSITION PHASE	COMPETITION PHASE	PEAKING PHASE
Total miles per week	59.5 ± 10.6	72.4 ± 9.1	58.9 ± 10.3
Longest run (miles)	11.5 ± 2.1	13.4 ± 2.2	10.9 ± 1.3
Average number of days per week of:			
Tempo	11.1 ± 0.8	1.6 ± 1.4	2.3 ± 2.0
Short/easy runs	1.9 ± 2.1	2.1 ± 1.8	11.2 ± 7.1
Repetitions	0.1 ± 0.3	0.7 ± 0.6	2.4 ± 2.4
Intervals	0.1 ± 0.3	0.8 ± 0.6	2.7 ± 2.0
Hills	0.6 ± 0.7	0.6 ± 0.7	1.2 ± 4.2
Fartlek	0.5 ± 0.5	0.7 ± 0.5	0.6 ± 0.9
Cross-training	0.5 ± 1.6	0.3 ± 0.6	0.7 ± 1.9
Drills	1.3 ± 2.0	1.6 ± 1.3	5.3 ± 5.9
Weights	1.5 ± 1.4	1.8 ± 0.9	3.6 ± 3.3
Rest	0.5 ± 0.5	0.3 ± 0.5	2.8 ± 1.6
Practice (2× per day)	1.5 ± 1.9	3.5 ± 1.5	7.1 ± 5.4

competitions approach (21). Interval training is effective to enhance aerobic capacity and muscle endurance when volume increases are no longer augmenting performance (21). In fact, Tabata et al. (61) have shown that high-intensity interval training produced greater gains in Vo_{2max} and anaerobic capacity than moderate intensity cycling at 70% of Vo_{2max}.

TRAINING AT ALTITUDE

The effects of altitude on human performance became evident at the 1968 Olympic games (55). Since then, it has been well documented that altitude (typically ~2,000–3,000 m) poses a physiological stress to the athlete via **hypoxia** (oxygen deprivation) and training at altitude is frequently used to improve performance at sea level. The original altitude training began as athletes lived and trained at altitudes of 1,500–4,000 m (67). Although still practiced currently especially by those athletes who live at altitude, more common method is to "live high, train low (LHTL)" or some type of simulated variation. A third variation is to "live low, train high (LLTH)." Although some research shows slight benefits, many studies have shown it to be an inferior mode of altitude training (67).

The benefits of altitude training derive from acclimatization, physiological adaptations to hypoxic exercise, or a combination of both. As altitude increases, barometric pressure and partial pressure of oxygen (PO_2) decrease. Table 16.8 depicts the relationship between altitude,

Case Study 16.1

Angela is a relatively new cross-country runner who is preparing for an upcoming 10-km race. She has some base AT and her Vo_{2max} was estimated at 48 mL · kg⁻¹ · min⁻¹. She has continued to run recreationally but would now like to try competing. The race is in 15 weeks and she approaches you to help develop a program to peak her performance at race time.

Question for Consideration: **What type of AT program would you prescribe?**

TABLE 16.7 SAMPLE PRECOMPETITION TRAINING WEEK FOR ATHLETE PREPARING FOR 5-KM RACE

DAY	WORKOUT
Monday	Rest
Tuesday	Fartlek runs — 4 miles — fast 30-s, moderate 5 min, repeat…
Wednesday	Easy pace — 3 miles
Thursday	Interval training — 8 × 400 m with 1:1 ratio
Friday	Easy pace — 4 miles
Saturday	Interval training — 6 × 400 m with 1:1 ratio
	3 × 100 m strides — 1:1.5 ratio
Sunday	Long run — 5–7 miles

TABLE 16.8 RELATIONSHIP BETWEEN ALTITUDE, BAROMETRIC PRESSURE, AND PO_2

ALTITUDE (m)	ALTITUDE (ft)	BAROMETRIC PRESSURE (mm Hg)	PO_2 (mm Hg)
0	0	760	159
1,000	3,280	674	141
1,500	4,920	634	133
2,000	6,560	596	125
3,000	9,840	526	110
4,000	13,120	462	97
5,000	16,400	405	85
6,000	19,690	354	74
7,000	22,970	308	64
8,000	26,250	267	56
9,000	29,530	230	48

Adapted with permission from McArdle WD, Katch FI, Katch VL. *Exercise Physiology: Energy, Nutrition, and Human Performance.* 6th ed. Philadelphia, PA: Lippincott Williams and Wilkins; 2007. pp. 489–502, 615–650.

barometric pressure, and PO_2. Acclimatization to chronically reduced inspired PO_2 invokes a series of central and peripheral adaptations that serve to maintain adequate tissue oxygenation. Factors such as elevation, exposure duration, training intensity/volume, and training duration affect the magnitude of adaptation. The most rapid physiological responses to altitude occur during the first few weeks of exposure. It generally takes about 2 weeks (depending on the altitude) to adapt to hypoxia up to 2,300 m, and may take an additional week for every additional 610-m increase up to 4,600 m (43). Altitude acclimatization can increase blood hemoglobin concentrations, hematocrit, buffering capacity, and improve structural and biochemical properties of skeletal muscle within several weeks (6,35). Acclimatization to altitude often limits the cardiorespiratory distress from acute or chronic hypoxia (35). However, this positive effect may not improve Vo_{2max} because the positive effects (increased hematocrit, right shift of the oxyhemoglobin dissociation curve, and increased diffusion capacity within the lungs) may be negated by reduced blood flow to the thorax and periphery, decreased muscle mass, and decreased oxidative enzyme activity (31,35,64). Other effects that may negate the positive effects of training at altitude are decreased plasma volume, depression of hematopoesis and increased hemolysis, suppressed immune function (increasing the risk of illness), increased tissue damage via oxidative stress, greater glycogen depletion (via greater sympathetic stimulation), and increased respiratory muscle work upon return to sea level (6). Table 16.9 depicts immediate and chronic responses/adaptations to altitude exposure.

Altitude exposure can atrophy skeletal muscle, particularly at heights above 6,000 m (64). Continuous hypoxia can decrease muscle CSA by 10%–22% (34,42). The changes in mitochondrial and capillary density may reflect a loss of muscle size and not a change in absolute number per se although new capillary formation may occur (43). Atrophy occurs in FT and ST fibers to a similar magnitude.

SUBMAXIMAL AND MAXIMAL AEROBIC EXERCISE PERFORMANCE AT ALTITUDE

Submaximal VO_2 for a specific exercise and power output is similar at altitude and at sea level. However, because of the progressive decline in Vo_{2max} with increasing altitude, the relative difficulty associated with each workload increases. The impairment is most evident during activities in which a given distance must be traversed in the least amount of time. This decrement increases as the aerobic energy requirements for the activity increase, as high-intensity, anaerobic exercise of short duration may not be affected up to an altitude of 5,200 m (15). At sea level, events lasting 2–5 minutes, 20–30 minutes, and 2–3 hours will be ~2%, 7%, and 17% longer, respectively, at 2,300 m (22). The threshold altitude appears to be ~1,600 m for events 2–5 minutes and 600 m for events longer than 20 minutes (43). With continued altitude exposure, acclimatization occurs and the additional difficulty of exercise is reduced.

Acute exposure to altitude increases the blood lactate response to exercise. However, several weeks of exposure to hypoxia unexpectedly reduces the lactate response to exercise, a phenomenon known as the *lactate paradox* (43). The lactate paradox has been controversial and puzzling to physiologists over the years as high-altitude natives, or those individuals acclimated to hypoxic conditions, have shown attenuated blood lactate responses to maximal aerobic exercise in some studies (32). The attenuation becomes more apparent as altitude increases (32). Although the precise mechanisms are still unclear and debatable, the lactate paradox during maximal aerobic exercise appears to be related to reduced lactate

TABLE 16.9 IMMEDIATE AND CHRONIC RESPONSES/ADAPTATIONS TO ALTITUDE EXPOSURE

IMMEDIATE	CHRONIC
Plasma volume ↓ (up to 25%)	Acid/base shifts
Acid/base shifts	Hyperventilation
Hyperventilation	Submax HR ↑
Submax HR and cardiac output ↑	Cardiac output and stroke volume ↓
Stroke volume ↔	Catecholamines ↑
Blood pressure ↑	Plasma volume ↓
Catecholamines ↑	Hematocrit, RBC count, 2,3-DPG, and hemoglobin ↑
Blood lactate ↑ — submax exercise	Capillary and mitochondrial density ↑
	Aerobic enzyme content ↑ **or** ↓
	Glycolytic enzymes ↑ **or** ↓
	Body weight and lean tissue mass ↓
	Vo_{2max} ↓
	Myoglobin ↑
	Immune function ↓
	Glycogen depletion and tissue damage ↑
	↓ blood lactate — max and submax exercise

production (rather than clearance from the blood) possibly from upregulated ATP-coupling pathways decreasing the contribution of fast glycolysis to meet the energy demand (32). However, some evidence indicates the lactate paradox may be transient and dissipate after chronic (>6 weeks) exposure to hypoxia (41).

Maximal aerobic capacity is impaired at barometric pressures below 400 mm Hg (above 4,500 m) (35). A loss of 1%–3.2% in Vo_{2max} for every 305 m of ascent above 1,600 m may be seen (35). Terrados (60) showed that Vo_{2max} decreased significantly at 1,200 m in sedentary individuals and at 900 m for elite athletes. The Vo_{2max} decline begins at 600–700 m with a linear reduction of 8% for every additional 1,000 m up to 6,300 m and is more rapid and curvilinear beyond this point (with largest reductions seen in men). Aerobic capacity at 4,000 m may be 75% of sea-level value (43). A-VO$_2$ difference is lower at altitude. AT prior to altitude exposure offers little protection against the reductions observed (43). The inability to achieve sea level Vo_{2max} at altitude makes it difficult for highly trained endurance athletes to perform well. Interestingly, detraining could take place if an athlete trains at altitude at a much lower workload (67,68). The decrease in Vo_{2max} occurs because barometric pressure decreases and PO_2 drops such that alveolar oxygen tension and arterial blood saturation are impaired (oxygen availability decreases). The initial response is to increase pulmonary ventilation in order to counteract the low PO_2. Fitness level is critical as highly fit individuals (>63 mL · kg^{-1} · min^{-1}) generally have larger decrements in Vo_{2max} at altitude than less fit individuals (22). Gore et al. (25) showed a 3.6% decrease in Vo_{2max} at 580 m in untrained individuals and a 7% decline in endurance

athletes. However, at higher altitudes (>7,000 m) this difference due to fitness level diminishes.

ALTITUDE TRAINING AND SEA LEVEL PERFORMANCE

Sea level performance (Vo_{2max}) may not change as a result of just living at altitude for a period of time (43). Training at altitude may not improve aerobic exercise performance at sea level albeit the scientific literature has been inconsistent in studying this training phenomenon. One would think performance would increase with this live high, train high (LHTH) approach. However, some flaws in study design make it difficult to accurately interpret the results of some studies. Bailey and Davies (6) examined 34 studies. Twelve of these studies showed increased endurance performance capacity with altitude training, although only four of these included a control group. Twenty-seven studies did not report a potentiating effect and fifteen of these included a control group. Overall, Vo_{2max} increases of up to 17.5% were shown (for altitude exposures of 7–70 days at 1,250–5,700 m) with most not statistically significant. A problem with training at altitude is that the lower absolute workloads and intensity athletes are forced to adopt. For example, training at 78% of Vo_{2max} at 300 m would only yield an intensity of 60% at 2,300 m (43). When training at altitude, some have recommended at least 7 weeks of sea level training in between altitude cycles to maximize intensity and volume (19). Proper diet, fluid replacement (at least one extra liter of water or carbohydrate-containing beverage), and vitamin/mineral supplementation is important when training at altitude (19).

LIVE HIGH, TRAIN LOW

It has been suggested that Vo_{2max} may be improved the most when athletes live high (acclimatization) but train low (at higher intensity). This is accomplished by spending several hours per day at high altitude but traveling to a lower altitude for the workouts, or by living and training at sea level but using an altitude simulation device during the nonexercise hours. This mode of altitude training began in the early 1990s and studies have shown the LHTL approach to be more effective than other approaches including LHTH (12). Although Vo_{2max} increases were shown in elite and subelite athletes, studies have shown performance increases (aerobic endurance power, running economy) independent of changes in Vo_{2max} (6,12). The acute acclimatization can increase RBC production, hemoglobin, and erythropoietin, which allow the athlete to train harder at a lower altitude or sea level (43,65). An altitude of 2,200–2,500 m is effective for increasing erythropoiesis during living high and ~3,100 m may be most effective for increasing nonhematological parameters (48). The optimal duration appears to be ~4 weeks for accelerating erythropoiesis but <3 weeks can increase exercise economy and buffer capacity (48). Daily doses of 20–22 h·d⁻¹ at 2,500 m appear sufficient to increase performance and erythropoiesis, whereas the minimum dose for stimulating erythropoiesis is ~12 h·d⁻¹ (48). Wilber et al. (68) recommend the following guidelines for living high and training low: *an altitude of 2,000–2,500 m for a minimum of 4 weeks for 22 hours per day.* Stray-Gundersen and Levine (58) have shown living for 4 weeks at 2,500 m increased sea level performance by ~1.5% (with a range of 0%–6%). The benefits lasted for *at least 3 weeks upon return to sea level.* A recent study showed elite middle distance runners improved their race times by 1.9% following a period of 44 ± 7 days at a simulated altitude of 2,846 m and training at an altitude of 1,700–2,200 m (56). Schmitt et al. (57) studied elite runners, cross-country skiers, and swimmers and showed that 13–18 days of training at 1,200 m coupled with sleeping at 2,500–3,500 m in hypoxic rooms produced greater changes in Vo_{2max} (7.8% vs. 3.3%) and peak power (4.1% vs. 1.9%) than living and training low while both groups increased exercise efficiency. Although after 15 days at lower altitude Vo_{2max} decreased in both groups, peak power was still augmented in the LHTL group. Wehrlin et al. (65) had elite athletes live at 2,500 m for 18 h⁻¹ and train at 1,000–1,800 m for 24 days and showed increased serum erythropoietin, hemoglobin, RBC, and hematocrit, and these changes were associated with an increase in Vo_{2max} and improved 5,000-m running times. Thus, most studies support the concept that LHTL is the most effective mode of altitude training. Athletes may simulate altitude via a number of products on the market including hypobaric chambers, hypoxic masks/systems, nitrogen dilution, and altitude tents (see Fig. 16.6). In addition,

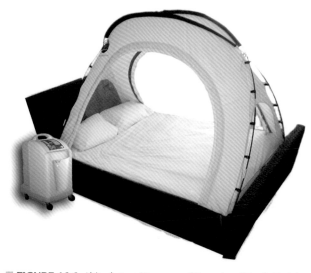

FIGURE 16.6. Altitude tent (Courtesy of Hypoxico Altitude Training Systems, New York, NY).

athletes who live at altitudes can train at sea level (while still at an altitude) by supplemental oxygen to simulate a sea level environment (67).

COMPATIBILITY BETWEEN HIGH-INTENSITY AEROBIC AND ANAEROBIC TRAINING

One topic of interest in the S&C field is the effects of concurrent high-intensity strength/power and AT. The training effects of each may antagonize one another. Although strength, power, and endurance will improve through concurrent training, one or the other may be attenuated if both are trained intensely with high volume. In most cases, power and strength gains may be mostly attenuated. Concurrent training may not attenuate aerobic endurance performance as long as the frequency of AT is not sufficiently reduced to accommodate strength and power training (33), although one study has shown that the addition of strength training can hinder Vo_{2max} improvements (24). The simultaneous effects on strength and power development have been variable. Maximal strength may be compromised (concurrent aerobic endurance and strength training produced less of a strength increase than strength training alone) whereas no incompatibility may occur based on program design.

Key programming issues include whether or not high-intensity aerobic endurance and strength training are performed in the same session, the sequence of each, volume and intensity, and training status of the subjects when examining potential incompatibility. Some factors identified to lead to an incompatibility include:

- *Inadequate recovery between workouts* — too high a frequency with reference to the volume/intensity of concurrent training leading to overtraining. This

Myths & Misconceptions

Training High is the Most Effective Mode of Altitude Training

Some have suggested that training high is the best way for the athlete to use altitude to his/her advantage. However, recent studies have shown superior performance enhancement when the athlete lives high but trains low to maintain a sufficient training intensity. Bonetti and Hopkins (12) performed a meta-analysis on altitude/hypoxia endurance training. They classified altitude/hypoxia training studies into six categories and calculated the effects for Vo_{2max} and other variables. Artificial hypoxia was provided by nitrogen houses, hypobaric chambers, inhalers, and altitude tents.

- LHTH — 14 studies (1,640–2,690 m, 12–30 days)
- LHTL — 6 studies (1,780–2,805 m, 13–28 days)
- Artificial LHTL (8–18 hours of long, continuous daily exposure to hypoxia) — 12 studies (2,000–3,500 m, 12–30 days)
- Artificial LHTL (1.5–5 hours of brief continuous daily exposure to hypoxia) — 5 studies (3,650–5,500 m, 6–19 days)
- Artificial LHTL (<1.5 hours of brief intermittent daily exposure to hypoxia) — 6 studies (3,400–6,000 m, 15–26 days)
- Artificial LLTH — 8 studies (2,500–4,500 m, 9–47 days)

For maximal endurance power output, substantial improvements in subelite athletes were seen with artificial brief intermittent LHTL (1%–4%), LHTL, and artificial, long, and continuous LHTL. In elite athletes, LHTL scored most favorably. For Vo_{2max}, increases were likely with LHTH in subelite athletes but LHTH produced decreases in elite athletes. Other mediators were unclear as to their effects. The authors concluded that naturally LHTL provided the best training strategy for enhancing endurance performance in elite and subelite athletes.

may be particularly true for lower-body training. For example, if an athlete is strength training the lower body 2–3 days per week and performs high-intensity AT on the days in between, it can be argued that a lack of full recovery may occur in between workouts.

- *Residual fatigue*—if high-intensity AT is performed prior to strength and power training, then suboptimal effort will be applied during strength training due to fatigue and could limit the progression of strength and power development.
- *Altered neuromuscular recruitment patterns/adaptations* —based on the antagonistic neuromuscular adaptations of each modality, greater fast-to-slow fiber-type transitions and attenuated type I muscle fiber hypertrophy may occur with concurrent training (37,51). Antagonistic effects on motor unit recruitment (as strength training relies upon type II motor units and AT has high reliance on type I motor units) may be seen. AT could limit muscle hypertrophy which may attenuate potential strength/power gains.

Several studies that have shown an incompatibility have examined 3 d · wk^{-1} of RT + 3 d · wk^{-1} of AT on alternating days (training on 6 consecutive days) or 4–6 d · wk^{-1} of combined high-intensity strength training and AT (8,20,37). When both aerobic and strength training are performed during the same session (yielding 3 d · wk^{-1} frequency with at least 1 day off in between workouts), the incompatibility has not been shown as frequently (40,44,45) with the exception of Sale et al. (53) who showed that 4 individual days per week of training was better than 2 concurrent days for increasing leg press 1 RM (25% vs. 13%). These studies show that increasing the recovery period between workouts may minimize the incompatibility.

Power development may be more limited than strength. Although power training and AT performed simultaneously in endurance athletes can lead to both power and endurance improvements (47), the magnitude of power development may be slightly less than power training alone. Häkkinen et al. (28) showed similar strength increases following 21 weeks of concurrent training or strength training only; however, strength training only resulted in improvements in rate of force development (RFD) whereas concurrent training did not.

The sequence of training may play a role in the adaptation. Leveritt and Abernethy (39) studied lifting performance 30 minutes following a 25-minute aerobic exercise workout and found the number of repetitions performed during the squat was reduced by 13%–36% over 3 sets. Bell et al. (7) compared endurance training before RT and vice versa and found that both increased Vo_{2max} similarly regardless of the sequence; however, the group that performed RT first attained greater strength gains. At least lower-body exercise performance could be reduced when AT is performed first. Less is known about high-intensity AT preceding high-intensity upper-body RT. Strength and endurance training can be performed simultaneously providing adequate recovery is allowed between workouts, strength training is performed initially, and the volume and intensity of aerobic exercise are not too high. It is recommended that specific training phases be used to target each one for those athletes that require both aerobic and anaerobic conditioning. Low-to-moderate intensity base AT could be performed during strength training phases and maintenance RT can be used if aerobic endurance is the goal of the training phase.

AEROBIC ENDURANCE TRAINING FOR ANAEROBIC ATHLETES

Several sports rely heavily upon aerobic and anaerobic energy sources (wrestling, boxing, soccer, hockey, basketball). AT is vital for these athletes as improving CV fitness is important for weight control, enhanced recovery during and between workouts, and stamina. It is important to accurately time aerobic and anaerobic workouts and place them in proper sequence to minimize antagonizing effects. Training periodization is the key. Off-season training should focus on strength and power training with a small amount of AT for base conditioning purposes. The end of the off-season is marked by preseason strength/power testing. Strength and power correlate well with performance of anaerobic sports and need to be emphasized during off-season training. Strength maintenance likely will become the goal during the preseason period as sprint/agility/plyometric workouts increase in frequency to peak power performance. The intensity of AT increases at this time to peak for the beginning of the season. Anaerobic conditioning drills are incorporated to increase buffering capacity and acid-base balance. Maintenance strength training and high-intensity AT can coexist. In-season training is characterized by maintenance programs for most components. Sport participation can maintain and improve conditioning. Specific conditioning may be trained a few days per week depending on the competition schedule. The amount depends on the athlete's playing status. For example, bench players receive less quality practice time and may be less conditioned than starters (33). The S&C coach must increase the amount of non-sport-training to keep their conditioning ready for play. It can be difficult for the coach to balance the rigors of sport practice/competition with training but successful coaches with quality programs will minimize injuries, maximize performance, and prevent end-of-season detraining.

AEROBIC ENDURANCE TRAINING IN HOT AND COLD ENVIRONMENTS

The external environment plays a key role in the response to aerobic endurance exercise. Thermoregulation is critical to environmental adaptations during exercise. The hypothalamus is the center of thermoregulation and acts like a thermostat to maintain thermal balance. Thermoregulatory systems work to balance heat gain (exercise, basal metabolic rate [BMR], hormonal control, environment, thermic effect of food) with heat loss (radiation, conduction, convection, and evaporation) (Fig. 16.7) (43). At rest, radiation, conduction, and convection predominate for maintaining thermal balance. **Conduction** is the heat exchange between two solid surfaces in direct contact with one another which accounts for less than 2% of heat loss during most situations (33). **Radiation** involves the transfer of energy waves from one body and is absorbed by another. **Convection** is the heat exchange that occurs between the surface of the body and a fluid medium, i.e., air (33). **Evaporation** is most critical for heat dissipation during exercise in the heat. Evaporation of water results from perspiration and quickly cools the body. The human body surface contains ~2–4 million sweat glands to aid in cooling the athlete (43). The cooled skin assists in cooling blood near the body's surface. Water loss from respiratory tracts and sweat collectively prevents excessive increases in core temperature. As temperature outdoors increases, conduction, convection, and radiation lose efficacy in facilitating heat loss, so perspiration becomes critical to cool the body during exercise in the heat. Perspiration evaporation becomes more difficult when the **relative humidity** is high. *Relative humidity* refers to the ratio of water in the air at a particular temperature to the total quantity of moisture that the air could contain (43). A high relative humidity percentage forces the sweat to bead and drip on the athlete rather than evaporate. As a result, cooling mechanisms are reduced, so exercise in hot, humid weather poses a greater risk to fatigue and heat injury than exercise at normal ambient temperature. Blood flow toward the skin increases as a mechanism of body cooling. Greater blood flow to the body's surface increases heat loss via radiation and provides some control over increases in core temperature during exercise. At rest muscle temperature ranges from 33°C to 35°C (66). As muscle temperature increases during exercise, heat transfer shifts from muscle to arterial blood which travels to the skin. The rate of transfer of heat from the core to the skin is determined by the temperature gradient and the conductance of skin (66).

AEROBIC EXERCISE IN THE HEAT

A paradox exists for the human body during exercise in the heat. Skeletal muscle requires greater blood flow for

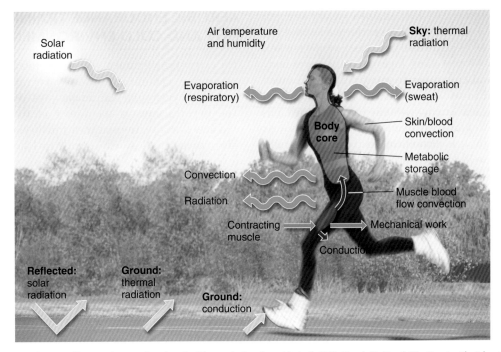

■ **FIGURE 16.7.** Regulation of heat exchange. (Reprinted with permission from McArdle WD, Katch FI, Katch VL. *Exercise Physiology:Nutrition, Energy, and Human Performance.* 7th ed. Philadelphia, PA: Lippincott Williams & Wilkins; 2010. pp. 615.)

oxygen and nutrient delivery during exercise. Under normal ambient conditions, up to 80% of Q_c may be diverted to muscle to meet the physical demands of exercise. However, the surface of the skin requires greater blood flow for heat dissipation. Cardiac output must be partitioned and this can result in a rise in the body's core temperature and can make aerobic exercise more challenging, *e.g.*, the reduced blood flow makes the workout more anaerobic and can lead to higher elevations of blood lactate, greater muscle glycogen breakdown, lost electrolytes, and fatigue. The reduced blood flow to the skin is seen, in part, to compensate for plasma volume reductions that accompany sweat loss in order to maintain Q_c (43). Circulatory and muscle blood flow supersede thermal regulation in Q_c distribution during exercise in the heat. Thus, core temperature will increase in proportion to intensity. Some studies indicate that aerobic athletes may show no ill effects of exercise in the heat up to ~105.0°F. Athletes with high aerobic capacity have greater thermoregulatory compensation and therefore have better tolerance to exercise in the heat than lesser-trained or untrained individuals (43). Heat acclimation typically takes around 7–14 days of strenuous exercise where 1.5–2 hours per day of exercise (every third day) >50% of Vo_{2max} is recommended (66). The ACSM has recommended 10–14 days of exercise training in the heat to increase heat acclimatization (4). Fatigue coincides with core temperatures of 38–40°C (43). Some studies have shown core temperature to rise to 37.3°C when exercising at 50% of Vo_{2max} and 38.5°C at 75% of Vo_{2max} (43).

Core temperatures above 40°C define *exertional hyperthermia*, where heat production from increased skeletal muscle activity accumulates faster than heat dissipation (4). Heat production during intense exercise is 15–20 times greater than at rest (4). Brain temperature is higher than core temperature such that at high temperatures the athlete could experience signs of exhaustion and can potentially collapse. Negative effects of exercising in the heat are exacerbated by obesity, low fitness levels, lack of acclimatization, sleep deprivation, sweat gland dysfunction, some infections, and use of certain medications (4).

The effects of exercise in the heat are exacerbated by dehydration. Dehydration is most prominent with reductions in body mass of >2% (23) and results in an increased plasma (>290 mOsmol) and urine osmolality (>700 mOsmol) and urine specific gravity (>1.020) (3). Fluid loss due to dehydration results in reduced plasma volume, Q_c, heat dissipation, skin blood flow, sweat rates, and increased core temperature and perceived exertion (3,43). As dehydration increases, thermoregulation becomes more difficult. Dehydration of 3%–5% leads to reduced sweat production and skin blood flow thereby reducing heat dissipation (3). For example, 1 hour of exercise produces approximately 0.5–1.0 L loss of sweat and rates as high as 3.7 L · h^{-1} have been shown during high-intensity aerobic exercise in athletes while football players may lose up to 8.8 L · d^{-1} (due to large size and equipment) (3,33,43,66). Athletes have shown sweat rates of 1–2.5 L · h^{-1} on average (64) and women typically have lower sweat rates and electrolyte losses than men (3). Greater sweat can be lost with higher intensities and/or durations of aerobic exercise. An elite marathon runner may experience up to 5 L of fluid loss (or ~6%–10% of body mass) during competition (43). The concentration of sweat contains an average of 35 mEq · L⁻¹ of sodium, 5 mEq · L⁻¹ of potassium, 1 mEq · L⁻¹ of calcium, 0.8 mEq · L⁻¹ of magnesium, and 30 mEq · L⁻¹ of chloride and varies depending on genetics, diet, sweat rate, and level of heat acclimatization (3). The risks of heat illness increase greatly if the athlete begins the workout in a dehydrated state. Dehydration negatively affects CV function, increases heat storage, decreases the time to exhaustion, and reduces endurance exercise performance (3). For each liter of sweat loss, exercise HR increases by ~ 8 bpm with a concomitant decrease in Q_c of 1 L · min⁻¹ (43). Dehydration of 4.3% loss of body mass can reduce walking performance by 48% and decrease Vo_{2max} by up to 22% (43).

Proper hydration before, during, and after aerobic endurance exercise is critical to optimal CV, thermoregulation, and exercise performance. Thirst often lags behind so the athlete must drink at intervals to minimize thermal strain. The following recommendations regarding fluid balance may assist athletes during exercise in the heat (3,23,43,66):

- At least 500 mL of water/sports drink should be consumed the night prior to anticipated aerobic exercise in the heat.
- 500 mL of water/sports drink should be consumed upon wakening on the morning of exercise in the heat. Some athletes have prehydrated themselves with a mixture of water (1–2 L) and glycerol (43) although the use of glycerol has not been recommended (3). The ACSM recommends ~5–7 mL · kg⁻¹ of body mass at least 4 hours before exercise (3). The fluid (water or sports drink) should taste good and be between 15°C and 21°C.
- 400–600 mL of water should be consumed ~20 minutes before the workout.
- During exercise in the heat (especially prolonged exercise <3 hours), fluid intake (if possible) should match or be close to sweat rate. Sweat rates typically range from 0.4 to 1.8 L · h⁻¹ (3). In general, water/sports drink can be consumed as needed at a rate of 0.4–0.9 L · h⁻¹ (or 0.15–0.3 L every 10–20 min) (3).
- After exercise, ~1.5 L of water/sports drink should be consumed per kilogram of body mass lost (3).
- In lieu of water, beverages containing a mixture of carbohydrates (5%–8%), amino acids, and vitamins and minerals (sodium, potassium, chloride, magnesium, etc.) can be used to rehydrate, replace lost electrolytes, and provide nutrients for energy during exercise. The ACSM has recommended a sport beverage contain 20–30 mEq · L⁻¹ of sodium chloride and 2–5 mEq · L⁻¹ of potassium per liter of fluid consumed (3).

AEROBIC EXERCISE IN COLD TEMPERATURES

Cold temperatures pose a stress to the athlete during exercise but typically do not limit aerobic performance. Cold environments can increase energy expenditure and may result in some additional fluid loss (2). Higher levels of aerobic fitness have only a small effect on cold tolerance. Precautions need to be taken in order to prevent cold-related injuries such as hypothermia, frostbite, and cold-induced asthma. Cold exposure leads to peripheral vasoconstriction which decreases peripheral blood flow and convection between the core and outer shell and results in greater insulation and maintenance of core temperature. Heat is lost from the body at a faster rate than it is replaced. Vasoconstriction begins when skin temperature drops to 34–35°C and becomes maximal at skin temperatures of 31°C or less in water or 26–28°C under local conditions (2). Exposure to cold increases metabolic heat production (*cold-induced thermogenesis*) via shivering. Acclimatizing helps reduce the stress associated with cold temperatures. Chronic exposure to cold temperatures helps the athlete adjust via habituation (less-pronounced cold responses), exaggerated shivering, and greater heat conservation (2). Several factors affect the acute response to cold exposure. Rain and water immersion augment the effects of cold temperatures. Water has a higher thermal capacity for convection than air resulting in greater heat loss. Athletes with higher levels of subcutaneous body fat have greater insulation capacity and a higher level of vasoconstriction to limit heat loss (2). Gender differences exist where women may experience greater heat loss due to lower levels of muscle mass (despite having higher levels of body fat). Cold tolerance decreases with aging due to decreased vasoconstriction and heat conservation and becomes more prominent when the athlete has low blood sugar (which impairs the shivering response) (2).

Precautions need to be taken when exercising in the cold. The temperature, windchill, precipitation, immersion depth (for water), and altitude (colder temperatures with a rise in elevation) need to be monitored and addressed accordingly. Cold temperatures with a high windchill factor require the athlete to prepare accordingly perhaps by adjusting clothing. Proper clothing insulates the athlete, allows for sweat dissipation, and helps maintain core temperature in a cold environment. The ACSM (2) has recommended three layers of clothing: (a) an inner layer in contact with the skin which does not readily absorb moisture but moves it to other layers (lightweight polyester or polypropylene); (b) a middle layer which provides primary insulation (polyester fleece or wool); and (c) an outer layer which maximizes moisture transfer to the environment. The outer layer may not be necessary unless it is raining or very windy (2,5). The level of insulation is modulated based on exercise intensity and duration. Clothing insulation (CLO) should be

TABLE 16.10 CLOTHING INSULATION UNITS

CLOTHING	CLO UNIT
Shirt, lightweight pants, socks, shoes, underwear briefs	0.6
Shirt, pants, jacket, socks, shoes, underwear briefs	1.0
Wind/waterproof jogging suit, T-shirt, briefs, running shorts, socks, athletic shoes	1.03
Fleece long-sleeve shirt, fleece pants, athletic socks and shoes	1.19
Lightweight jacket, thermal long underwear tops and bottoms, briefs, shell pants, athletic shoes and socks	1.24
Lightweight jacket, long-sleeve fleece shirt, fleece pants, underwear briefs, shell pants, athletic shoes and socks	1.67
Ski jacket, thermal long underwear bottoms, knit turtleneck, sweater, ski pants, knit hat, goggles, gloves, ski socks, and boots	2.3
Parka with hood, shell pants, fiber fill pant liners, thermal long underwear tops and bottoms, sweat shirt, gloves, thick socks, and boots	3.28
Cold weather expedition suit, thermal long underwear tops and bottoms, sweat shirt, gloves, thick socks, and boots	3.67

Adapted with permission from American College of Sports Medicine. American College of Sports Medicine Position Stand: Prevention of cold injuries during exercise. *Med Sci Sports Exerc.* 2006;38: 2012-2029.

adjusted to minimize sweating. CLO units can serve as a guide. Table 16.10 depicts various clothing insulation units. Figure 16.8 depicts clothing insulation needs based on aerobic exercise intensity (in MET). The colder the weather the higher the CLO unit (as evidenced by the down slope of each line). As exercise intensity increases, the CLO unit decreases. Less-insulative clothing is needed as the athlete exercises at progressively higher intensities. Clothing selection must match the potential exercise stimulus. One should not overdress initially to match the cold temperatures at rest but should dress according to the potential clothing insulation needed during exercise. Overdressing can cause too great of heat maintenance (leading to more sweating) and add weight to the athlete. Wet weather increases the insulation requirement. Up to 50% of heat loss occurs through the head at rest while

wearing winter clothing, so knit caps provide needed insulation (2). CLO requirements during exercise are a function of temperature and metabolic rate. Layering is recommended for greater flexibility in balancing insulation needs with heat production (2).

Summary Points

✔ AT elicits a number of beneficial CV, respiratory, metabolic, and neuromuscular adaptations that allow the athlete to improve endurance and performance.
✔ Aerobic endurance performance is correlated to Vo_{2max}, exercise economy, LT, and muscle fiber types.
✔ Several modes of aerobic exercise can be used in training. Variation is important to keep motivation high and provide the body with different stimuli.

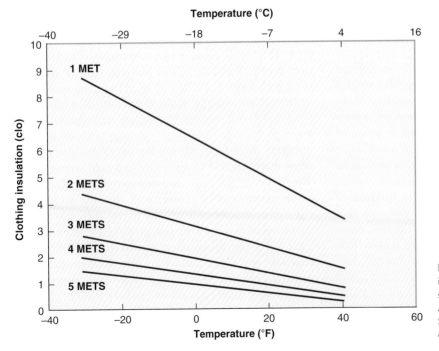

FIGURE 16.8. CLO units for various intensities of exercise. (Reprinted with permission from American College of Sports Medicine. American College of Sports Medicine Position Stand: Prevention of cold injuries during exercise. *Med Sci Sports Exerc.* 2006;38:2012–2029)

✔ Training intensity can be prescribed in three general ways via Vo_{2max}, HR, or RPE. In addition, monitoring of performance (distance covered in a specific amount of time or time to cover a specific distance) can also be used.

✔ Aerobic endurance training should be performed 2–5 days per week for at least 20–60 minutes based on ACSM guidelines. These guidelines are extended significantly for athletes training for endurance sports.

✔ Continuous, long duration, pace/tempo, Fartlek, interval, hills, and repetition training are methods used to enhance AT.

✔ Altitude poses a physiological stress to athletes. Current research suggests that "living high, training low" is more effective than "living high, training high" and "living low, training high" for increasing sea-level Vo_{2max} and endurance performance.

✔ High-intensity AT can impede strength and power gains if performed simultaneously with strength training at a high volume and frequency. This incompatibility can be prevented by allowing more recovery in between workouts and by performing strength training before AT in sequence when they are performed during the same workout.

✔ Hot and cold environments pose a stress to athletes during AT. Special precautions need to be made to enhance safety and maximize performance.

Review Questions

1. A mode of AT known for "speed play" is:
   a. Interval training
   b. Fartlek training
   c. Repetition training
   d. Hill training

2. Endurance training entails training targeting increases in:
   a. Vo_{2max}
   b. Exercise economy
   c. Lactate threshold
   d. All of the above

3. The most recommended means of altitude training currently involves:
   a. Live high, train high
   b. Live low, train low
   c. Live high, train low
   d. Live low, train high

4. When using the Borg RPE scale to monitor aerobic exercise intensity, which of the following ranges provides the best stimulus for increasing Vo_{2max} in a healthy, trained individual?
   a. 6–9
   b. 9–12
   c. 12–14
   d. 14–17

5. The most critical method of heat loss during exercise in the heat is:
   a. Evaporation
   b. Convection
   c. Conduction
   d. Radiation

6. Running at 7 mph can elicit an energy expenditure value of _____ MET.
   a. 9
   b. 10
   c. 11.5
   d. 14

7. Aerobic exercise in water generally yields higher HRs compared to land-based activities because the cool water temperature facilitates greater cardiac output. T F

8. Hill training can be used to increase the intensity of AT workouts. T F

9. The ACSM recommends consumption of a fluid (water or sports drink) with a volume of ~5–7 mL · kg^{-1} of body mass at least 4 hours preexercise hydration. T F

10. The heart rate max (HR_{max}) method of aerobic exercise intensity prescription is calculated by multiplying the target intensity (decimal form) by the difference of the max predicted HR and resting HR and then adding the resting HR to the total. T F

11. *Exercise economy* refers to the energy cost of exercise at a given velocity. T F

12. The ACSM recommends 20–60 minutes of continuous or intermittent aerobic exercise for increasing aerobic capacity in healthy adults. T F

References

1. American College of Sports Medicine. American College of Sports Medicine Position Stand: The recommended quantity and quality of exercise for developing and maintaining cardiorespiratory and muscular fitness, and flexibility in healthy adults. *Med Sci Sports Exerc.* 1998;30:975–991.

2. American College of Sports Medicine. American College of Sports Medicine Position Stand: Prevention of cold injuries during exercise. *Med Sci Sports Exerc.* 2006;38:2012–2029.

3. American College of Sports Medicine. American College of Sports Medicine Position Stand: Exercise and fluid replacement. *Med Sci Sports Exerc.* 2007;39:377–390.

4. American College of Sports Medicine. American College of Sports Medicine Position Stand: Exertional heat illness during training and competition. *Med Sci Sports Exerc.* 2007;39:556–572.

5. American College of Sports Medicine. *ACSM's Guidelines for Exercise Testing and Prescription.* 8th ed. Philadelphia (PA): Lippincott Williams & Wilkins; 2010. pp. 198–200.

6. Bailey DM, Davies B. Physiological implications of altitude training for endurance performance at sea level: a review. *Br J Sports Med.* 1997;31:183–190.

7. Bell GJ, Petersen SR, Quinney HA, Wenger HA. Sequencing of endurance and high-velocity strength training. *Can J Sport Sci.* 1988;13:214–219.

8. Bell GJ, Syrotuik D, Martin TP, Burnham R, Quinney HA. Effect of concurrent strength and endurance training on skeletal muscle properties and hormone concentrations in humans. *Eur J Appl Physiol.* 2000;81:418–427.

9. Bentley DJ, Millet GP, Vleck VE, McNaughton LR. Specificity aspects of contemporary triathlon: implications for physiological analysis and performance. *Sports Med.* 2002;32:345–359.

10. Bergh U, Thorstensson A, Sjodin B, et al. Maximal oxygen uptake and muscle fiber types in trained and untrained humans. *Med Sci Sports.* 1978;10:151–154.

11. Bishop D, Jenkins DG, Mackinnon LT. The relationship between plasma lactate parameters, W_{peak} and 1-h cycling performance in women. *Med Sci Sports Exerc.* 1998;30:1270–1275.

12. Bonetti DL, Hopkins WG. Sea-level exercise performance following adaptation to hypoxia: a meta-analysis. *Sports Med.* 2009;39:107–127.

13. Borg GA. Psychophysical bases of perceived exertion. *Med Sci Sports Exerc.* 1982;14:377–381.

14. Cissik JM. Improving aerobic performance. In: Chandler TJ, Brown LE, editors. *Conditioning for Strength and Human Performance.* Philadelphia (PA): Lippincott Williams & Wilkins; 2008. pp. 292–305.

15. Coudert J. Anaerobic performance at altitude. *Int J Sports Med.* 1992;13(suppl):S82–S85.

16. Coyle EF, Coggan AR, Hopper MK, Walters TJ. Determinants of endurance in well-trained cyclists. *J Appl Physiol.* 1988;64:2622–2630.

17. Coyle EF, Feltner ME, Kautz SA, et al. Physiological and biomechanical factors associated with elite endurance cycling performance. *Med Sci Sports Exerc.* 1991;23:93–107.

18. Daniels J, Daniels N. Running economy of elite male and elite female runners. *Med Sci Sports Exerc.* 1992;24:483–489.

19. Dick FW. Training at altitude in practice. *Int J Sports Med.* 1992;13(suppl):S203–S205.

20. Dudley GA, Djamil R. Incompatibility of endurance- and strength-training modes of exercise. *J Appl Physiol.* 1985;59:1446–1451.

21. Faria EW, Parker DL, Faria IE. The science of cycling: physiology and training—part 1. *Sports Med.* 2005;35:285–312.

22. Fulco CS, Rock PB, Cymerman A. Maximal and submaximal exercise performance at altitude. *Aviat Space Environ Med.* 1998;69:793–801.

23. Ganio MS, Casa DJ, Armstrong LE, Maresh CM. Evidence-based approach to lingering hydration questions. *Clin Sports Med.* 2007;26:1–16.

24. Glowacki SP, Martin SE, Maurer A, et al. Effects of resistance, endurance, and concurrent exercise on training outcomes in men. *Med Sci Sports Exerc.* 2004;36:2119–2127.

25. Gore CJ, Hahn AG, Scroop GS. Increased arterial desaturation in trained cyclists during maximal exercise at 580 m altitude. *J Appl Physiol.* 1996;80:2204–2210.

26. Gormley SE, Swain DP, High R, et al. Effect of intensity of aerobic training on Vo_{2max}. *Med Sci Sports Exerc.* 2008;40:1336–1343.

27. Gulbin JP, Gaffney PT. Ultraendurance triathlon participation: typical race preparation of lower level triathletes. *J Sports Med Phys Fitness.* 1999;39:12–15.

28. Häkkinen K, Alen M, Kraemer WJ, et al. Neuromuscular adaptations during concurrent strength and endurance training versus strength training. *Eur J Appl Physiol.* 2003;89:42–52.

29. Harter L, Groves H. 3000–10,000 Meters. In: *USA Track and Field Coaching Manual.* Champaign (IL): Human Kinetics; 1999. pp. 109–122.

30. Helgerud J, Hoydal K, Wang E, et al. Aerobic high-intensity intervals improve Vo_{2max} more than moderate training. *Med Sci Sports Exerc.* 2007;39:665–671.

31. Hochachka PW. Muscle enzymatic composition and metabolic regulation in high altitude adapted natives. *Int J Sports Med.* 1992;13(suppl):S89–S91.

32. Hochachka PW, Beatty CL, Burelle Y, Trump ME, McKenzie DC, Matheson GO. The lactate paradox in human high-altitude physiological performance. *News Physiol Sci.* 2002;17:122–126.

33. Hoffman J. *Physiological Aspects of Sport Training and Performance.* Champaign (IL): Human Kinetics; 2002. pp. 109–119.

34. Hoppeler H, Desplanches D. Muscle structural modifications in hypoxia. *Int J Sports Med.* 1992;13(suppl):S166–S168.

35. Jackson CG, Sharkey BJ. Altitude, training and human performance. *Sports Med.* 1988;6:279–284.

36. Karvonen M, Kentala K, Musta O. The effects of training on heart rate: a longitudinal study. *Ann Med Exp Biol Fenn.* 1957;35:307–315.

37. Kraemer WJ, Patton JF, Gordon SE, et al. Compatibility of high-intensity strength and endurance training on hormonal and skeletal muscle adaptations. *J Appl Physiol.* 1995;78:976–989.

38. Kurz MJ, Berg K, Latin R, DeGraw W. The relationship of training methods in NCAA Division I cross-country runners and 10,000-meter performance. *J Strength Cond Res.* 2000;14:196–201.

39. Leveritt M, Abernethy PJ. Acute effects of high-intensity endurance exercise on subsequent resistance activity. *J Strength Cond Res.* 1999;13:47–51.

40. Leveritt M, Abernethy PJ, Barry B, Logan PA. Concurrent strength and endurance training: the influence of dependent variable selection. *J Strength Cond Res.* 2003;17:503–508.

41. Lundby C, Saltin B, van Hall G. The "lactate paradox", evidence for a transient change in the course of acclimatization to severe hypoxia in lowlanders. *Acta Physiol Scand.* 2000;170:265–269.

42. MacDougall JD, Green HJ, Sutton JR, et al. Operation Everest II: structural adaptations in skeletal muscle in response to extreme simulated altitude. *Acta Physiol Scand.* 1991;142:421–427.

43. McArdle WD, Katch FI, Katch VL. *Exercise Physiology: Energy, Nutrition, and Human Performance.* 6th ed. Philadelphia (PA): Lippincott Williams & Wilkins; 2007. pp. 489–502, 615–650.

44. McCarthy JP, Agre JC, Graf BK, Pozniak MA, Vailas AC. Compatibility of adaptive responses with combining strength and endurance training. *Med Sci Sports Exerc.* 1995;27:429–436.

45. McCarthy JP, Pozniak MA, Agre JC. Neuromuscular adaptations to concurrent strength and endurance training. *Med Sci Sports Exerc.* 2002;34:511–519.

46. Mercier D, Leger L, Desjardins M. Nomogram to predict performance equivalence for distance runners. *Track Technique*. 1986;94:3004–3009.

47. Mikkola JS, Rusko HK, Nummela AT, Paavolainen LM, Häkkinen K. Concurrent endurance and explosive type strength training increases activation and fast force production of leg extensor muscles in endurance athletes. *J Strength Cond Res*. 2007;21: 613–620.

48. Millet GP, Roels B, Schmitt L, Woorons X, Richalet JP. Combining hypoxic methods for peak performance. *Sports Med*. 2010; 40:1–25.

49. Morgan DW, Bransford DR, Costill DL, Daniels JT, Howley ET, Krahenbuhl GS. Variation in the aerobic demand of running among trained and untrained subjects. *Med Sci Sports Exerc*. 1995;27:404–409.

50. Noakes T. *Lore of Running*. 4th ed. Champaign (IL): Human Kinetics; 2003. pp. 39–105.

51. Putman CT, Xu X, Gillies E, MacLean IM, Bell GJ. Effects of strength, endurance and combined training on myosin heavy chain content and fibre-type distribution in humans. *Eur J Appl Physiol*. 2004;92:376–384.

52. Reuter BH, Hagerman PS. Aerobic endurance exercise training. In: Baechle TR, Earle RW, editors. *Essentials of Strength Training and Conditioning*. 3rd ed. Champaign (IL): Human Kinetics; 2008. pp. 489–503.

53. Sale DG, Jacobs I, MacDougall JD, Garner S. Comparison of two regimens of concurrent strength and endurance training. *Med Sci Sports Exerc*. 1990;22:348–356.

54. Saunders PU, Pyne DB, Telford RD, Hawley JA. Factors affecting running economy in trained distance runners. *Sports Med*. 2004;34:465–485.

55. Saunders PU, Pyne DB, Gore CJ. Endurance training at altitude. *High Alt Med Biol*. 2009;10:135–148.

56. Saunders PU, Telford RD, Pyne DB, Gore CJ, Hahn AG. Improved race performance in elite middle-distance runners after cumulative altitude exposure. *Int J Sports Physiol Perform*. 2009;4:134–138.

57. Schmitt L, Millet G, Robach P, et al. Influence of "living high-training low" on aerobic performance and economy of work in elite athletes. *Eur J Appl Physiol*. 2006;97:627–636.

58. Stray-Gundersen J, Levine BD. Live high, train low at natural altitude. *Scand J Med Sci Sport*. 2008;18(suppl):21–28.

59. Swain DP. Cardiorespiratory exercise prescription. In: Ehrman JK, editor. *ACSM's Resource Manual for Guidelines for Exercise Testing and Prescription*. 6th ed. Philadelphia (PA): Lippincott Williams & Wilkins; 2010. pp. 448–462.

60. Swain DP, Franklin BA. VO_2 reserve and the minimal intensity for improving cardiorespiratory fitness. *Med Sci Sports Exerc*. 2002;34:152–157.

61. Tabata I, Nishimura K, Kouzaki M, et al. Effects of moderate-intensity endurance and high-intensity intermittent training on anaerobic capacity and Vo_{2max}. *Med Sci Sports Exerc*. 1996;28:1327–1330.

62. Terrados N. Altitude training and muscular metabolism. *Int J Sports Med*. 1992;13(suppl):S206–S209.

63. Vleck VE, Bentley DJ, Millet GP, Cochrane T. Triathlon event distance specialization: training and injury effects. *J Strength Cond Res*. 2010;24:30–36.

64. Wagenmakers AJM. Amino acid metabolism, muscular fatigue and muscle wasting: speculations on adaptations at high altitude. *Int J Sports Med*. 1992;13(suppl):S10–S113.

65. Wehrlin JP, Zuest P, Hallen J, Marti B. Live high-train low for 24 days increases hemoglobin mass and red cell volume in elite endurance athletes. *J Appl Physiol*. 2006;100:1938–1945.

66. Wendt D, van Loon LJC, van Marken Lichtenbelt WD. Thermoregulation during exercise in the heat: strategies for maintaining health and performance. *Sports Med*. 2007;37:669–682.

67. Wilber RL. Application of altitude/hypoxic training by elite athletes. *Med Sci Sports Exerc*. 2007;39:1610–1624.

68. Wilber RL, Stray-Gundersen J, Levine BD. Effect of hypoxic "dose" on physiological responses and sea-level performance. *Med Sci Sports Exerc*. 2007;39:1590–1599.

69. Yamamoto LM, Lopez RM, Klau JF, et al. The effects of resistance training on endurance distance running performance among highly trained runners: a systematic review. *J Strength Cond Res*. 2008;22:2036–2044.

70. Yoshida T, Udo M, Iwai K, Yamaguchi T. Physiological characteristics related to endurance running performance in female distance runners. *J Sports Sci*. 1993;11:57–62.

17

Training Periodization and Tapering

After completing this chapter, you will be able to:

- Define periodization and understand the benefits of dividing a training year into smaller phases
- Define General Adaptation Syndrome and discuss its application to periodized training
- Discuss how tapering can be useful for optimizing performance for single competitions
- Discuss different models of periodization and how volume and intensity can be manipulated to achieve a targeted goal
- Identify ways in which macrocycles can be developed in athletes during different types of competitive seasons

Periodization is the process of manipulating acute training program variables in order to bring the athlete to maximal performance at the appropriate time of the year, and to reduce the risk of overtraining (45). Periodization is based upon manipulating intensity and volume throughout the training year, although other program variables are altered as well. Periodization divides training into smaller units corresponding to specific goals and has long been used as a method of organizing training. The concept of periodization dates back to the ancient Olympic Games (776 BC–393 AD) where *Philostratus* was thought to have developed a simplified system where Greek Olympians trained during a preparatory phase prior to the Olympics (3). Articles on periodization strategies were seen in the Eastern European sport science literature during the 1920s and 1930s. In Russia, texts were published between 1917 and 1925 by authors such as Kotov, Gorinewsky, and Birsin describing training phases and organization (47). Sport-specific texts describing periodization principles for training in track and field, skiing, boxing, gymnastics, and water sports were published in Russia circa 1938 (47). Programs became more sophisticated as evidenced by the 4-year German training program which was used in preparation for the 1936 Olympic Games (3). In England circa 1946, Dyson published a text delineating training into noncompetitive, precompetitive, initial competition, main competition, and postcompetitive periods (47). Revisions, adaptations, and application of periodization techniques and methodology continued through the 1950s and 1960s. In 1965 a model of a periodized training program that separated the training year into different phases and cycles was published by Russian sport scientist Leonid Matveyev. He developed the model based on questionnaires concerning the training practices obtained from Russian athletes preparing for the 1952 Olympic Games (3,31). He borrowed the term *periodization* and based this model on a schedule where there was one major competition per year (3). Variations developed to cater to athletes who had multiple competitions per year or a competitive season. Periodized training principles were not commonly seen in North America during the first half of the 20th century. European success prompted scientists and coaches from the United States to study Eastern European training methods and develop models based on the work of Matveyev and his predecessors (44). Nevertheless, the underlying goal of periodization was to optimize the training stress and recovery.

Matveyev divided the training year into three distinct phases; *preparatory*, *competitive*, and *transition* (Figs. 17.1 and 17.2). Each training phase relates to a change in volume and intensity. In addition, Matveyev quantified technical training during each phase where appropriation to technique increased in proportion to training intensity. The preparatory phase comprises two subphases known as *general* and *specific preparation*. In general preparation training, volume is high and intensity is low. The primary purpose is to prepare the athlete for more intense and sport-specific training in the latter phases. A physiological base is trained during the preparatory phase to prepare the body adequately for the competition phase. Because intensity is low to moderate, the athlete may experience less stress which helps prepare the athlete for subsequent phases while

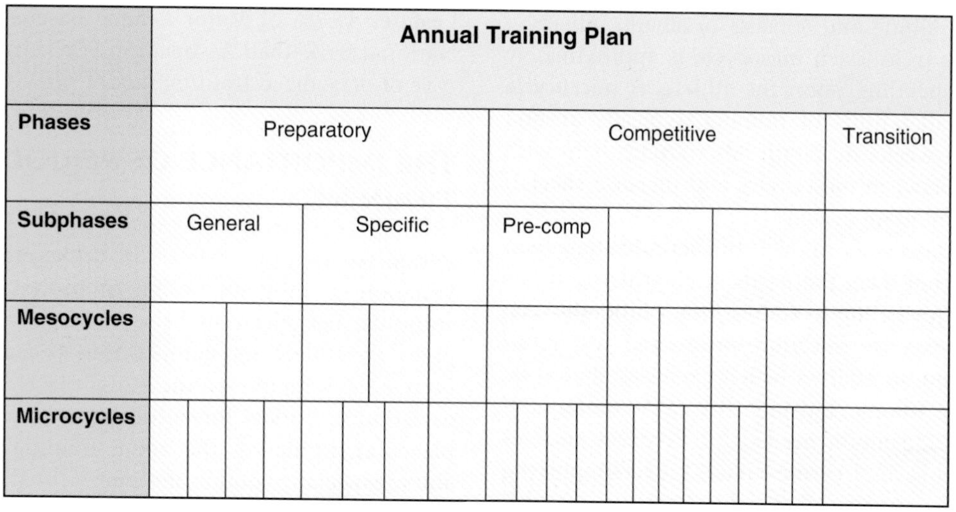

Annual Training Plan							
Phases	Preparatory			Competitive			Transition
Subphases	General	Specific	Pre-comp				
Mesocycles							
Microcycles							

■ **FIGURE 17.1.** Annual training plan proposed by Matveyev. (Reprinted with permission from Bompa TO, Haff GG. *Periodization: Theory and Methodology of Training*. 5th ed. Champaign (IL): Human Kinetics; 2009. pp. 125–256.)

reducing the risk of overtraining. The second part of the preparatory phase consists of more time devoted to exercises that mimic sport-specific movements in which exercise intensity is increased and volume is reduced. The competitive phase is divided into two phases, precompetition and main competition. The *precompetition* phase consists of the exhibition contests, *e.g.*, preseason games or scrimmages in a sport like American football, while the primary or most important competitions are considered part of the *main competition* phase. The difference is how volume and intensity are manipulated. During the precompetition phase, volume of training is reduced while intensity of training is increased further. As the main competition phase nears, training intensity reaches its peak while training volume is reduced. A stabilization phase coincides with the main

competition phase where fitness improvements derived from off-season training are maintained during the season (47). The final phase is the *transition phase* in which a period of active rest is used to recover from the previous training phases. The transition phase is restorative and assists in removing fatigue from the athlete from the previous competition phase. During active rest, both training volume and intensity are reduced and other forms of exercise may be introduced.

With periodization, training plans are subdivided into smaller segments called *cycles*. The **macrocycle** refers to an extended training period (usually a training year) and can be broken into different mesocycles. In some cases, the term **monocycle** has been used to describe a yearly periodization macrocycle based on peaking for one major competition (3). A **mesocycle** refers to several weeks

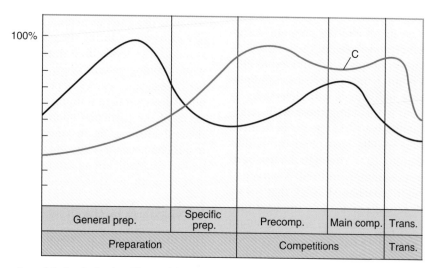

■ **FIGURE 17.2.** Matveyev's model of periodization. The *purple line* indicates volume and the *blue line* indicates intensity. (Reprinted with permission from Bompa TO, Haff GG. *Periodization: Theory and Methodology of Training*. 5th ed. Champaign (IL): Human Kinetics; 2009. pp. 125–256.)

to months of training and consists of smaller microcycles. The duration for each mesocycle is approximately 1–4 months depending upon the athlete. A **microcycle** consists of smaller units of training, typically around 5–10 days to 4 weeks in length. Microcycles help with the transition between mesocycles and increase specialization within program design.

Although Matveyev's model of periodization was novel, it could not meet the needs of all athletes. It has been criticized for failing to address other program variables such as exercise selection, order, and rest interval length, failing to address which exercises should be included in the volume and intensity calculations (and the level of periodization needed for exercises such as single-joint and several core exercises), oversimplifying the volume and intensity relationship between microcycles, failing to address the integration of other modalities of training in addition to resistance training (RT), and for lacking appropriate focus on technical training at all phases, *e.g.*, during low- and moderate-intensity phases in addition to high-intensity phases (47). The model was based on training for one major competition per year excluding athletes with multiple competition seasons or an extended competition season. Often a macrocycle is based on a competition season rather than a single competition. The structure is based on Matveyev's periodization model. However, the competitive season is expanded. The athlete peaks right at the beginning of the competitive season and maintains their performance gains throughout the season. The maintenance phase is characterized by high intensity training. However, the volume is greatly reduced.

Matveyev's periodization model culminated in peak strength and power. Thus, endurance goals could not be maximized (3). Limitations demonstrated the need for other models and forms of periodization to exist to meet the needs of all athletes. Other models and integrated approaches have since been developed thereby meeting the needs of a larger number of athletes. Periodized training is used as a means of altering program design to optimize performance and recovery (14). However, the use of periodization concepts is not limited to elite athletes or advanced training but is used successfully as the basis of training for individuals with diverse backgrounds and fitness levels including those with recreational (16) and rehabilitative (7,13) goals. Periodized training is effective for middle-aged populations during general weight training (22). Among athletes, periodized training is most commonly utilized. A survey of 137 Division I strength coaches showed that ~93% of the coaches used periodized models in their programs (9). Approximately 95% of high school strength and conditioning (S&C) coaches surveyed reported using periodized training for their athletes (8). Ebben et al. (10–12) and Simenz et al. (43) showed that ~69% of National Football League, 91.3% of National Hockey League, 85.7% of Major League Baseball, and 85% of National Basketball Association S&C coaches use some type of periodized training model.

THE IMPORTANCE OF PERIODIZED TRAINING

Periodized training enables the athlete to have planned variation in program design to optimize the training stimulus. Periodization helps manage fatigue and prepares an athlete for competition. Because the human body adapts rapidly to the stress placed on it, planned variation is critical for subsequent adaptations to take place. Manipulating the acute training program variables (especially volume and intensity) allows the athlete to make the necessary physiological adaptations while reaching their peak condition at the appropriate time. In addition to intensity and volume, it is important to note that other variables are manipulated, *e.g.*, rest intervals, exercise selection, and order. For example, exercises can be added and removed periodically. This provides the athlete different training stimuli and allows the athlete to train at higher intensities without as great a risk of overtraining. Integrated periodization approaches are common and involve manipulating several variables to meet the needs of the athletes. Altering training volume and intensity in conjunction with appropriately timed short unloading phases (periods of low-intensity, low-volume training) minimizes the risk of **overtraining syndrome**. Several models of periodization are sequential owing to the fact that it is very difficult if not impossible to maintain maximal performance over an extended period of time. Thus, peaking at the right times is essential. Many athletes participate in sports that place importance on an entire season of competition. For these sports, peak condition needs to be achieved by the onset of the competitive year, and maintained throughout the competitive season. A *maintenance* (or stabilization) phase ensues, which is designed to maintain the strength, power, and size gains made during the off-season. Exercise intensity is reduced to levels used during the strength mesocycle while training volume is lowered by reducing the number of assistance exercises performed during each workout. Adjustments to training programs are specific to the needs of the particular sport that the athlete plays and the individual's goals. In contrast, athletes who focus on a major competition occurring toward the end of the competitive year will attempt to reach peak condition at that specific point in the season.

GENERAL ADAPTATION SYNDROME

Periodized training is rooted in the work of renowned endocrinologist Dr. Hans Selye (42). Selye discussed a *General Adaptation Syndrome* which has great application to the training of athletes. Selye recognized that stress

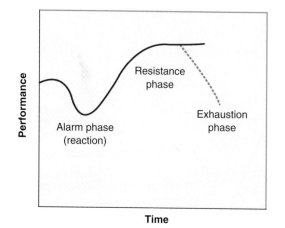

FIGURE 17.3. Selye's general adaptation syndrome. (Reprinted with permission from Selye H. *The Stress of Life*. New York, NY: McGraw-Hill; 1956.)

plays a role in disease development and an application has been made to training. General Adaptation Syndrome (Fig. 17.3) comprises three response phases to stressful demands. The initial phase is the *alarm phase* (sometimes referred to as the *shock phase*) and consists of both shock and soreness. Performance during this phase will decrease. This would be synonymous to the initial effects a workout has on the athlete. The second phase is physiological *adaptation* to this new stimulus. The body adapts to the new training stimulus and an improvement in performance ensues. Once the body has adapted, no further adaptations will take place unless the stimulus is altered. The third phase is *exhaustion* (sometimes referred to as *staleness* or *mal-adaptation*) where constant increases in the exercise stimulus are not accompanied by appropriate rest and/or recovery periods. The body is unable to make any further adaptation, and unless this stimulus is reduced, overtraining could occur. If sufficient recovery is allowed, the body can properly adapt and performance may increase further. Periodization is used to avoid or minimize periods of exhaustion and to maintain an effective exercise stimulus that leads to maximizing athletic potential (18).

TAPERING AND PERFORMANCE

A **taper** period is one where there is a reduction in workload prior to a major competition to maximize performance (34). Tapering is used when an athlete is peaking for a single competition as opposed to a competitive season. It is common for athletes to overreach near the end of precompetition training and reduce volume and/or frequency (while maintaining intensity) to induce a rebound in performance (3). Reductions in intensity are counterproductive; thus, it is recommended that tapering be performed at a similar intensity to the peaking phase (3,34). Volume reductions of 50%–90% are effective and correlate positively to performance gains

in endurance athletes (33,34). Volume is reduced by shortening workouts and decreasing frequency although volume reductions are preferred while maintaining a similar or slightly reduced frequency (3). Decreasing frequency can enhance short-term performance yet maintain performance over a 2–4-week period (3). High-frequency (at least 80% of normal frequency) tapering produces better performance than low-frequency tapering (every third day) and may be necessary for advanced to elite athletes (3,34).

Most studies have shown tapering can augment performance. For example, Vo_{2max} and endurance performance improvements of 1.2%–22% in runners, swimmers, triathletes, and cyclists have been shown during short-term taper periods, *e.g.*, 1–3 weeks (35). Bosquet et al. (5) performed a meta-analysis primarily focused on running, swimming, and cycling endurance performance and showed that optimal tapering involved a 2-week duration where volume was exponentially reduced by 41%–60% without modification of intensity or frequency. Studies failing to show improvements mostly used longer tapering periods of 3–4 weeks (35). Strength and power increases of 2%–27% have been shown following tapering periods of 7–35 days (21,35,38,48). A tapering period of 4–8 days increases muscle glycogen content by 15%–34% (35). Thus, aerobic and anaerobic performance improvements of ~0.5%–6% (3% average) can be expected from a proper taper (34).

Part of the challenge is to select an appropriate taper type and length. Figure 17.4 depicts data presented by Bosquet et al. (4) showing that the optimal taper length tends to be ~8–14 days for endurance performance. Figure 17.5 depicts types of tapers used (34). A nonprogressive, or *step taper*, embellishes a standard reduction in training load. For example, a 40% reduction in load would occur immediately and then is maintained for the duration of the taper period. Although it is effective for enhancing performance, it may be inferior to progressive tapers (3,34). A progressive taper involves a systematic reduction in training load (volume). It can be linear or exponential. A *linear taper* involves a gradual reduction in training load throughout the taper period. For example, the athlete could reduce training load by 3%–5% for each workout until the desired load reduction has been attained. A *slow exponential taper* has a slower reduction in training load compared to a *fast exponential taper*. For example, a fast exponential taper may result in a nonlinear load reduction where load may be reduced 45% during the first 1–2 workouts, an additional 10% the next 1–2 workouts, 10% the next 1–2 workouts, and 5% the last 1–2 workouts for a 1.5-week taper. A slow exponential taper may result in a nonlinear load reduction where load may be reduced 25% during the first 1–2 workouts, an additional 15% the next 1–2 workouts, 10% the next 1–2 workouts, and 5% the last 1–2 workouts for a 1.5-week taper. Fast exponential tapers produce greater improvements in performance than linear or slow exponential tapers and have been recommended to peak athletic performance (3,34).

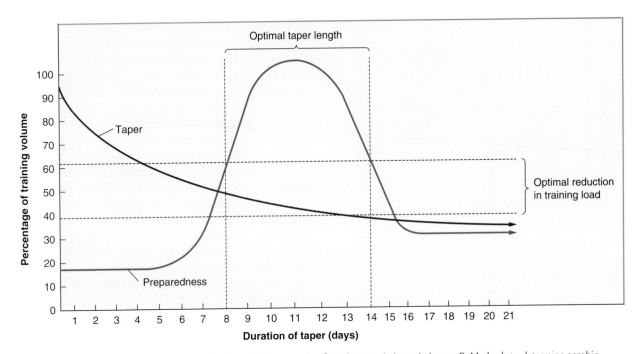

■ **FIGURE 17.4.** Tapering and performance. (Reprinted with permission from Bosquet L, Leger L, Legros P. Methods to determine aerobic endurance. *Sports Med.* 2002;32:675–700.)

BASIC MODELS OF PERIODIZATION

Although there are many ways in which a coach or athlete can vary a training program, three basic models of periodization have been studied mostly in regard to RT although periodization can be applied to aerobic endurance, sprint/agility, and plyometric training programs as well. The three basic models include the classic (linear), undulating, and reverse linear periodization models.

CLASSICAL MODEL OF PERIODIZATION

The *classical model of periodization* was one of the first used and developed from the work of Matveyev (31). Although sometimes referred to as *linear periodization*, a closer examination shows that this model is not truly linear throughout but intensity and volume can fluctuate at various intervals. In fact, intensity and/or volume fluctuation can take place within a designated microcycle. For example,

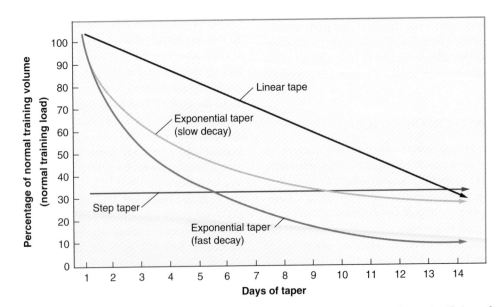

■ **FIGURE 17.5.** Common types of tapers used by athletes. (Reprinted with permission from Mujika I, Padilla S. Scientific bases for precompetition tapering strategies. *Med Sci Sports Exerc.* 2003;35:1182–1187.)

over a 4-week period, 1 week may comprise more than 35% of the total monthly volume load whereas the other 3 weeks may comprise between 15% and 25% of the total volume load per week (47). The term *linear* implies a constant volume and intensity progression and this is not usually the case. Thus, the term *linear periodization* is somewhat misleading. This model is characterized by high training volume initially and a reduction in volume (with subsequent increase in intensity) with each phase in succession (44) (Table 17.1). The classical model is designed to maximize strength and power, or peak anaerobic performance. Each training phase is designed to emphasize a particular fitness component. The initial phase is the *hypertrophy phase* (or strength endurance phase) where muscle growth and endurance improvements are emphasized. A secondary objective is to build a foundation and better prepare the athlete for higher intensities of training later in the cycle. Structural multiple-joint exercises are performed for 3–5 sets per exercise for 8–20 repetitions for 50%–75% of 1 RM. This phase may last 4–6 weeks but can be longer (9–12 weeks) in those athletes with a limited training background. The next phase is a *strength phase* where intensity is increased and volume is decreased (structural multiple-joint exercises performed for 3–5 sets of 4–6 repetitions [80%–85% of 1 RM] with heavier weights). This phase may last from 1 to 3 months. The subsequent phases include *strength/power* and *peaking phases* that extend upon strength training with high-intensity structural exercise performance and repetitions decrease. The goal is to maximize strength and power by the end of the cycle. More power exercises are included. It has been recommended that power training be emphasized after a strength training phase as strength is the foundation for power development and power may be better developed following appropriate strength training (3). The strength/power phase consists of higher intensity and lower volume (3–5 sets of 2–5 repetitions). The strength/power phase is critical to translate developed strength into higher power development. The peaking phase occurs prior to the most important competitions of the year. In between phases unloading weeks are performed where the athlete decreases volume and intensity to facilitate recovery and prepare for the next higher-intensity training phase. Maintenance takes place in-season where lower volume and frequency are seen (1–3 sets of 1–3 repetitions for structural exercises using a wide range of intensities).

NONLINEAR (UNDULATING) MODEL OF PERIODIZATION

A second periodization model is the *undulating (nonlinear)* model. The undulating model enables variation in intensity and volume within each 7–10-day cycle by rotating different protocols (14,25). Nonlinear methods attempt to train the various components of the neuromuscular system within the same 7 to 10-day cycle. During a single workout only one characteristic is trained in a given day per structural exercise, *e.g.*, strength, power, muscular endurance, and hypertrophy. For example, in loading schemes for structural exercises in the workout, the use of heavy, moderate, and lighter resistances may be randomly rotated over a week (Monday, Wednesday, Friday), *e.g.*, 3–5 repetitions (with loads ≤3–5 RM), 8–10 repetitions (with loads ≤8–10 RM), and 12–15 repetitions (with loads ≤12–15 RM) may be used in the rotation. This model may be appropriate for athletes who play a varied schedule such as basketball, hockey, baseball, or soccer players that may have several games or competitions in a given week or the schedule of games and travel does not permit a regularly scheduled in-season strength maintenance program. Each exercise needs to be considered independently where structural exercises follow a similar periodization scheme. However, assistance exercises may follow a different periodized scheme depending on program objectives. Thus, each exercise can be periodized within a desired time frame as the goal of each exercise can differ.

Another undulating model that has been studied is the *weekly undulated periodized model*. In this model, intensity and volume vary on a weekly basis as opposed to a daily basis. For example, for structural exercises an athlete may train at 70% of his/her 1 RM week 1, 80% of his/her 1 RM week 2, and 90% of his/her 1 RM week 3. Volume decreases as intensity increases. The athlete then repeats this cycle for weeks 4–6 and so on. This model has produced similar increases in maximal strength as classical and daily undulated models (6).

REVERSE LINEAR PERIODIZATION MODEL

Up to this point, models that targeted peak strength and power were discussed. However, models structured in the opposite manner are used to target cardiovascular and muscular endurance improvements. *Reverse linear periodization* is the opposite of the classical model where

TABLE 17.1 CLASSICAL MODEL OF PERIODIZATION IN A STRENGTH/POWER ATHLETE

	MESOCYCLE			
	HYPERTROPHY	STRENGTH	STRENGTH/POWER	PEAKING
Sets	3–5	3–5	3–5	3–5
Repetitions	8–20	4–6	2–5	1–3
Intensity (% 1 RM)	50%–75%	80%–85%	85%–90%	>90%

Myths & Misconceptions

Periodized and Nonperiodized Training are Equally Effective for Increasing Long-Term Athletic Performance

Some have suggested that training variation is not necessary for progression. Periodized RT increases muscle size, strength, endurance, and power in athletes with a variety of training backgrounds (17,18,26). The effects are most prominent over long-term training periods where the planned variation is effective for reducing plateaus. Several studies compared various periodized models to nonperiodized multiple- and single-set models of training and have shown periodized training is superior for increasing maximal strength, cycling power, motor performance, and jumping ability (14,17,24,27–30,32,36,44–46,50,51) with the exception of a short-term study, which showed similar performance improvements between periodized and multiple-set nonperiodized models (2). It is thought that longer training periods (at least 4 wk) are necessary to underscore the benefits of periodized training compared with nonperiodized training (50). Periodization has been shown superior via a meta-analytical review of the literature to nonperiodized RT (41). Thus, periodization is necessary for progression. *Periodized RT (classical, reverse linear, undulating, and integrated models) is recommended by the ACSM for progression for strength, power, hypertrophy, and endurance training* (1).

moderate-to-high intensity, low-volume training is used initially. Intensity decreases and volume increases with each successive phase. Some strength enhancement may be targeted early in training. However, the primary goal is to peak muscle endurance or size at the end of the cycle. By the end of the cycle the athlete will be training with higher sets and repetitions, with shorter rest intervals, which are effective for enhancing muscular endurance. This model is commonly used by endurance athletes and bodybuilders preparing for competitions and has been shown to be superior for enhancing muscle endurance to other periodization models when volume and intensity were equated (40). However, strength improvements following this model are inferior compared to linear and undulating models (40).

PERIODIZED TRAINING STUDIES

Few studies have compared different periodization models. Most often, the classical model is compared to an undulating model. The daily undulating model has compared favorably with the classical model (4). Several studies examining 9–15 weeks of training showed similar strength, lifting velocity, power, and vertical jump increases in athletes and fit individuals using undulating and classical models (6,15,20,23). In contrast, the undulating model has been shown to be more effective for increasing 1 RM bench press, arm curl, and leg press strength following 12 weeks of training than the classic model (32,37,39). Interestingly, Buford et al. (6) showed that 9 weeks of linear, daily, and weekly undulating models produced similar increases in 1 RM leg press (79%–100%) and bench press (18%–25%) although daily undulating training produced consistent lower percentage gains. Lastly, the undulating model was shown to be inferior

to the classic model for enhancing in-season strength in freshman college football players (19). Although it is clear that all types of periodized training are effective for increasing performance, studies have either shown similar strength increases or one model favoring another. The classic and undulating models both appear equally effective for maximizing strength and power performance (6,15,20,23). For endurance enhancement, the reverse linear model is superior for maximal improvement (40).

Case Study 17.1

Shawn is an Olympic weightlifter preparing for a competition. The competition is 8 months away and will be the only competition Shawn will be competing in this year. Shawn has been competing for 7 years and was coming off a competition 1 month ago. He is now in transition and seeks your guidance for developing an 8-month periodized macrocycle to get him ready for the competition.

Question for Consideration: **What training advice would you give Shawn?**

PERIODIZATION FOR AN ATHLETE WITH MULTIPLE MAJOR COMPETITIONS

Some sports like track and field require two major competitive seasons, *e.g.*, indoor and outdoor. Thus, periodization involves two major training cycles (sometimes known as *bicycles*). Ultimately, the monocycle is divided into two macrocycles similar in structure. Each macrocycle is characterized by classic periodization marked by an increase in intensity and decrease in volume until peaking occurs precompetition. In some programs the last competition may be most important. Thus, the highest volume may be seen during the first preparatory phase. The preparatory phases of the second macrocycle would be relatively short in duration compared to the first. Changes in intensity are similar during each cycle. The challenge of multicycle training is the reduction in the preparatory phase. It is recommended that bi-cycle periodized programs be limited to more advanced athletes. In other cases, athletes compete in three or more major competitions (tennis, boxing, mixed martial arts) in a single year these training plans are referred to as *tricycles* or *multicycles*.

PERIODIZATION FOR A STRENGTH/POWER ATHLETE IN A TEAM SPORT

Power training entails the integration of resistance (heavy RT for strength, ballistic RT to enhance velocity), plyometric, sprint, and agility training. A sample periodized program for a football player is shown in Figure 17.6. This model follows the classic periodization design (17,18). The preparatory phase's primary objective is to prepare the athlete for more strenuous training and to increase muscle hypertrophy (muscle hypertrophy is desirable in a collision sport like football). This mesocycle may last ~6–8 weeks and some endurance activities may be performed. The 6 to 8-week strength mesocycle is characterized by an increase in intensity and a reduction in volume. The subsequent strength/power phase incorporates more sport-specific exercises. During this 6 to 8-week mesocycle, training intensity will be further elevated while training volume is reduced. The use of ballistic and plyometric exercises may be included during this phase. Sport-specific conditioning, agility, and speed training may be included 2–3 days per week. The peaking phase precedes training camp. It is shorter in duration (4–6 weeks) and is designed to peak strength and power performance for the start of the season. Training intensity is increased while training volume is reduced. This is often accomplished by reducing the number of assistance exercises in the program. The onset of training camp initiates the beginning of the preseason period where RT is reduced to 2 days per week maintenance phase (structural

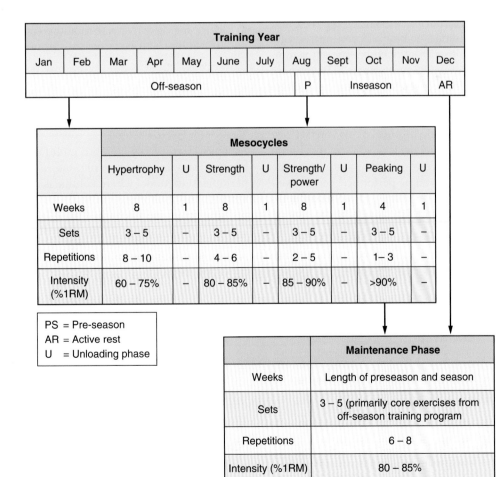

FIGURE 17.6. Periodization for a football player. (Reprinted with permission from Hoffman JR, Ratamess NA. *A Practical Guide to Developing Resistance Training Programs*. 2nd ed. Monterey (CA): Coaches Choice Books; 2008.)

exercises with several assistance exercises). Training intensity is similar while repetition number increases. Anaerobic training (sprints or intervals) is continued 2–3 days per week in order to maintain the athletes' sport-specific conditioning level.

PERIODIZATION OF SPRINT, AGILITY, AND PLYOMETRIC TRAINING

Periodization of sprint, agility, and plyometric training follows a pattern common to peaking for strength and power (Table 17.2). However, the logistical progression occurs from base training to speed-specific training to sport-specific speed and agility training. Plyometric training follows a basic pattern of low-to-moderate-intensity drills to high-intensity drills over time along with a slight increase in volume, *e.g.*, foot contacts. Training during the early preparation phase involves base anaerobic conditioning. The preparatory phase could last 3–6 months for athletes involved in one or two major competitions and 2–3 months for team sports athletes (3). General preparation includes anaerobic conditioning. Volume tends to be somewhat high with moderate intensity of drills. Plyometric drills are low to moderate in intensity initially and linear sprint drills stress technique and base building. Interval training is common. Sprinting intensity may range from 70% to 85% of maximal speed for multiple repetitions for 50 to 200-m distances. The purpose is to develop a base for subsequent high-intensity training. Some speed endurance training can be introduced here for those athletes whose sports involve repeated sprints of at least moderate distance. Short interset rest intervals with high-intensity drills (>90%) of maximum for 50–150 m are effective (3). Some low-to-moderate intensity aerobic training can be performed here as well for those athletes who have a mild-to-moderate aerobic component in their sport. The length of the general preparatory phase may be longer in novice athletes and less for advanced to elite athletes.

Specific preparatory training involves a transition to more specific training. Volume can remain similar but may start to decrease near the end of the phase as intensity increases. Resisted sprint running and overspeed drills can be incorporated here in addition to linear sprints of varying distance. More complex plyometric drills and agility drills are included. The agility drills may be of moderate complexity and work toward increasing complexity and become more reactive as the phase progresses. Precompetition training marks the time where the athlete has peaked strength and power (by the end) and is refining speed and agility by sport-specific training. Speed and agility training is highly sport-specific and in its highest complexity of the macrocycle. The intensity remains high and volume is gradually reduced. The competitive season is marked mostly by maintenance training. Participation in sport practice and games/competitions assists in maintaining peak performance. However, a 1 to 2-day-per-week (if allowed by the competition schedule) maintenance program (low volume, high intensity) can be valuable for the athlete to maintain performance and reduces the likelihood of mid- to late-season detraining. The transition period marks a time of active rest to allow complete recovery and restoration of body/psyche following a stressful competitive season.

PERIODIZATION OF AEROBIC ENDURANCE TRAINING

Athletes maximizing aerobic endurance performance benefit from following variations of a reverse linear periodization model where volume is moderate initially and intensity is moderate to high (40) (Table 17.3). The preparatory phase is characterized by aerobic training

TABLE 17.2 SAMPLE ANNUAL TRAINING PLAN FOR STRENGTH/POWER ATHLETE

MO	1	2	3	4	5	6	7	8	9	10	11	12
	PREPARATORY						COMPETITIVE				TRANSITION	
Speed	General prep Anaerobic base Technique Speed endurance		Specific prep Max speed Overspeed/resisted Speed endurance Technique				Precomp Max speed Supramax. Sport spec.		Competitions Maintenance High int, low vol Low freq Sport practice			Active rest Other training modalities
Agility			Moderate/high int Reactive drills				Sport spec. Reactive		Maintenance High int, low vol Low freq Sport practice			
Plyometrics	Low-to-moderate		Moderate-to-high Sport spec.				High int Sport spec.		Sport practice			
Strength	Hyper.	Strength	Str/pow	Peak			Maintenance		Maintenance			

Adapted with permission from Bompa TO, Haff GG. *Periodization: Theory and Methodology of Training.* 5th ed. Champaign, IL: Human Kinetics; 2009. pp. 125–256.

TABLE 17.3 SAMPLE ANNUAL TRAINING PLAN FOR AN ENDURANCE ATHLETE WITH ONE MAJOR COMPETITION

MO	1	2	3	4	5	6	7	8	9	10	11	12
	PREPARATORY					COMPETITIVE						TRANSITION
	General		Specific			Precompetition					T C	Active rest
Endurance	Base aerobic		Base aerobic intervals, pace			Base aerobic – LSD						
						Progressive distance increase						
						intervals, fartleks, pace, hill. Repetitions						
						Increase intensity, Moderate volume						
Speed			Base			Base						
			Technique			Technique						
Strength	Strength		Str/End			Endurance			Maintenance			

T, taper; C, competition; LSD, long slow duration.

(AT) to increase Vo_{2max}. Resistance training targeting some strength improvements is critical to help increase exercise economy. By the end of the specific preparatory phase, volume increases and intensity matches the type of aerobic activities performed. During precompetition, combination strategies are employed. The athlete may have 1–3 workouts per week that are longer in duration and of moderate intensity. One workout may be dedicated to longer distance/duration than the other workouts. Throughout the precompetition training phase, the duration of the long run gradually increases with the exception of unloading weeks where volume is reduced. The remaining moderate-to-high distance/duration workouts only increase gradually. The remaining workouts during precompetition are dedicated to higher-intensity AT. Steady-state AT can only take the endurance athlete so far. Interval training (or training targeting lactate threshold and exercise economy improvements) is necessary to provide additional endurance improvements in trained athletes (17). Thus, the athlete during precompetition may train 2–3 days per week at higher intensity and lower volume. Specialized workouts including Fartlek training, hills, intervals, pace/tempo work, and repetition training are performed for greater specialization. Technique work is included and speed drills can be added. While the intensity may remain constant and duration increases with long slow distance workouts, the intensity can increase and volume can remain constant for specialized AT drills. Strength training can continue during precompetition but at a lower frequency and volume, *i.e.*, maintenance training. In some cases, the intensity of strength training can decrease, volume can increase, and rest intervals may decrease to target muscle endurance improvements which may benefit race performance. By the end of the precompetition phase, the athlete is ready for competition and may have partially overreached at this level. A tapering period can be used in the last week where volume is reduced producing a rebound effect to maximize performance during competition.

PERIODIZATION OF AEROBIC AND ANAEROBIC TRAINING COMPONENTS

Some sports require high muscular strength, power, speed, agility, sufficient levels of muscle endurance, and a sufficient aerobic conditioning level, *e.g.*, wrestling, mixed martial arts, soccer, basketball, and boxing. For these athletes, the general preparatory phase is marked by a classic periodization scheme for RT and a few days per week AT (low intensity, moderate duration) not to impede anaerobic fitness development. During the specific preparatory phase, progressive RT continues (and peaks by the end of the phase) and a 2 to 3-day-per-week sprint, agility, and plyometric program is initiated. During the precompetition phase, RT is reduced to maintenance training (1–3 days per week, high intensity, and low volume) whereas the intensity (complexity) and volume of sprint, plyometric, and agility training increase modestly. Aerobic endurance training increases in intensity and is performed 2–3 days per week. Aerobic training can be performed on a separate day or following an anaerobic training workout. By the end of the precompetition phase, the athlete's aerobic endurance increases, anaerobic conditioning is improved and/or maintained, and the athlete is ready for the competition season.

SAMPLE PERIODIZED STRENGTH TRAINING PROGRAMS

The coach and athlete can separate the year into basic segments and apply the training principles to each phase of training. Tables 17.4–17.6 provide some examples

TABLE 17.4 SAMPLE PERIODIZED PROGRAM FOR A WRESTLER

MONDAY	SETS × REPS (WEEK NOS)
Hang clean[a]	3 × 6 (1–4); 5 (5–8); 4 × 5 (9–12); 5 × 3 (13–15)
Bench press	3 × 10–12 (1–4); 8–10 (5–8); 6–8 (9–12); 3–5 (13–15)
Close-grip bench press	3 × 10–12 (1–4); 8–10 (5–8); 6–8 (9–12); 3–5 (13–15)
Shoulder press	3 × 10–12 (1–4); 8–10 (5–12); 6–8 (13–15)
Pull-up progressions	
Wide-grip pull-ups	3 × 10–25 (1–5)
Towel pull-ups	3 × 10–15 (6–10)
Weighted pull-ups or unilateral pull-ups	3 × 8–10 (11–15)
Internal/external rotations	3 × 10
MB Russian twist	3 × 25–50
Stability ball crunches	3 × 25–50
Manual resistance — neck	2 × 10

WEDNESDAY	SETS × REPS (WEEK NOS)
Back squat	3 × 10–12 (1–4); 8–10 (5–8); 4 × 6–8 (9–12); 5 × 3–5 (13–15)
Overhead squat	3 × 6–8 (1–7)
Front squat	3 × 6–8 (8–15)
Unilateral leg press	3 × 8–10 (1–7)
Split squat/lunge	3 × 8–10 (8–15)
Stiff-leg deadlift	3 × 10–12 (1–6); 8–10 (7–12); 6–8 (13–15)
Back extensions	3 × 15–20
Calf raise	3 × 15–20
Thick bar deadlift	3 × 10
Plyometric leg raise	3 × 15–25
Trunk stabilization ("plank")	3 × 1 min

FRIDAY	SETS × REPS (WEEK NOS)
Power snatch	3 × 6 (1–4); 5 (5–8); 4 × 5 (9–12); 5 × 3 (13–15)
Bent-over barbell row	3 × 10–12 (1–4); 8–10 (5–8); 6–8 (9–12); 3–5 (13–15)
Close-grip lat pull-down	3 × 10–12 (1–5); 8–10 (6–10); 6–8 (11–15)
Weighted dips	3 × 12–15 (1–4); 10–12 (5–8); 8–10 (9–15)
Pullovers	3 × 8–10
Push-up progressions	
Basic	3 × 25–50 (1–5)
Stability ball	3 × 15–30 (6–10)
MB plyo push-ups	3 × 10 (11–15)
Partner plate pass	3 × 25
Weighted curl-ups	3 × 25
Wrist and reverse wrist curls	3 × 10

Intensity — 60%–85% of 1 RM periodized.

Rest intervals — 2–3 min for core exercises; 1–2 min for assistance exercises; 30 s–1 min for abs.

[a]Progress to power clean.

Reprinted with permission from Hoffman JR, Ratamess NA. *A Practical Guide to Developing Resistance Training Programs.* 2nd ed. Monterey (CA): Coaches Choice Books; 2008.

of periodized strength training programs for athletes. Table 17.4 depicts a sample wrestling strength training program. The program is 15 weeks in length but can be adapted to be longer when unloading weeks are used in between phases. Key qualities include periodized intensity and volume of structural exercises. Loading is increased and volume is decreased (the numbers in parentheses indicate training week numbers). In addition, periodized exercise selection was used where pull-up and push-up progressions were included. Table 17.5 depicts a periodized program for a strength competition athlete. The program initiates from strength/power phases and progresses to sport specific and peak power endurance phases. The program includes several sport-specific exercises the athlete may perform in competition. Table 17.6 depicts a sample program for a boxer.

This program consists of periodized intensity and volume for structural exercises as well as inclusion of a variety of sport-specific exercises. All programs depicted are consecutive. That is, unloading weeks are not shown. It is recommended that the coach and athlete include periodic unloading weeks to help the athlete recover from the previous phase and prepare the body for the upcoming training phase.

TABLE 17.5 15-WEEK PERIODIZED PROGRAM FOR A STRENGTH COMPETITION ATHLETE

WEEKS 1–4: STRENGTH/POWER

MONDAY	TUESDAY	THURSDAY	FRIDAY
Power clean 5 × 5	Squat 5 × 5-6	Power clean 5 × 5	Deadlift 4 × 5
Bench press 5 × 5-6	Front squat 4 × 5-6	Push press 4 × 5	Box squat 4 × 6
Incline barbell press 4 × 6	Bent-over rows 3 × 6-8	Close-grip bench press 4 × 6	Zercher squat 3 × 5-6
Shoulder press 4 × 6	Power shrugs 3 × 8	Triceps push-downs 3 × 6-8	Reverse hyperext. 3 × 6-8
Sit-ups 3 × 10-15	Good mornings 3 × 8	Barbell curls 3 × 6-8	Glute-ham raise 3 × 10

WEEKS 5–8: STRENGTH/POWER

MONDAY	TUESDAY	THURSDAY	FRIDAY
Power clean 5 × 3-5	Squat 5 × 3-5	Power clean 5 × 3-5	Deadlift 5 × 3-5
Bench press 5 × 3-5	Half rack squats 4 × 3-5	Push press 4 × 3-5	DL rack pulls 4 × 3-5
Incline barbell press 4 × 5	Bent-over rows 3 × 5-6	Close-grip bench press 4 × 5	Front squats 4 × 3-5
Shoulder press 4 × 5	Power shrugs 3 × 6	Triceps push-downs 3 × 6-8	Reverse hyperext. 3 × 6-8
Torso rotations 3 × 10-15	Good mornings 3 × 8	Barbell curls 3 × 5-6	Glute-ham raise 3 × 8

WEEKS 9–12: PEAK STRENGTH/POWER — SPORT SPECIFIC

MONDAY	TUESDAY	THURSDAY	FRIDAY
Power clean 5 × 1-3	Squat 5 × 1-3	Mastiff log clean & press 4 × 3-5	Deadlift 5 × 1-3
Bench press 5 × 1-3[a]	Quarter rack squats 4 × 3-5	Incline bench press 4 × 3	DL rack pulls 4 × 3-5
Mastiff log clean and press 4 × 3-5	KB swings 3 × 5	Close-grip bench press 4 × 5	Super yoke SQ walks 3 × 20y
ISOM lat raise (T-hold) 3 × 20-30s	Power shrugs 4 × 5	Farmer's walk 2 × 30 y	Reverse hypers 4 × 5
Torso rotations 3 × 10-12	Thick bar DL 4 × 5	Barbell curls 3 × 5(+ISOM holds)	One-arm DB rows 3 × 6

WEEKS 13–15: SPORT SPECIFIC — PEAK POWER/ ENDURANCE[c]

MONDAY	TUESDAY	THURSDAY	FRIDAY
Power clean 5 × 1-3	Squat 5 × 1-3	Bench press 5 × 1-3[a]	Deadlift 5 × 1-3
Mastiff log clean and press 4 × 3-5[b]	Mastiff stone medley 2-4 × 5 stones	ISOM T-holds 3 × 30-40 s	Super yoke SQ walks 3 × 20 y
Tire flips 2-4 × 8-10	Truck pulls (with harness) 2-4 × 30 y	Farmer's walk 2-4 × 40 y	Loading medley 2-4 times

Periodized core intensity — 70%-100%.

Rest intervals — 3-5 min for cores; 2-3 min for assistance exercises.

Off days — 1 d/week for base cardiovascular exercise; 1 d/wk for interval training/plyometrics.

[a] Switch to incline bench press if competition includes inclines for max reps — in this case, higher repetitions are performed.

[b] Exercises may change based on specific competitions; sport-specifics are timed so each set is completed as rapidly as possible.

KB, kettle bells.

[c] More reps performed if the competition includes this event for max reps; distances for sport-specific events depend upon competition length.

Reprinted with permission from Hoffman JR, Ratamess NA. *A Practical Guide to Developing Resistance Training Programs*. 2nd ed. Monterey (CA): Coaches Choice Books; 2008.

TABLE 17.6 12-WEEK BOXING STRENGTH TRAINING PROGRAM[a]

WEEKS 1–4

MONDAY	WEDNESDAY	FRIDAY
Hang clean 4 × 6	Power snatch 4 × 6	Hang clean 4 × 6
Squat 4 × 8–10	Bench press 4 × 8–10	Deadlift 4 × 8–10
DB jump squat 3 × 6	Incline bench press 3 × 8–10	One-arm rows 3 × 8–10
Box step-ups 3 × 10	Dips 3 × 10–15	Weighted pull-ups 3 × 10–15
Good mornings 3 × 8–10	Side lateral raise 3 × 10	Curls 3 × 10
MB side throws 3 × 8–10	Lying triceps ext. 3 × 10	Wrist/reverse curls 3 × 10
Sit-ups 3 × 25–50	Internal/external rotations 3 × 10	Torso rotations 3 × 25
Four-way neck 2 × 10	Scapula stabilizer circuit 2 × 10	Stability ball crunches 3 × 50

WEEKS 5–8

MONDAY	WEDNESDAY	FRIDAY
Hang clean 4 × 5	Power snatch 4 × 5	Hang clean 4 × 5
Squat 4 × 6–8	Bench press 4 × 6–8	Deadlift 4 × 6–8
DB jump squat 3 × 6	Alternate DB incline press 3 × 8–10	Bent-over rows 3 × 8–10
Box step-ups 3 × 10	DB jabs, uppercuts, hooks 3 ×15–20	Weighted pull-ups 3 × 10–15
Back extensions 3 × 8–10	SB push-ups 3 × 15–20	Curls 3 × 10
MB side throws 3 × 8–10	Lying triceps ext. 3 × 10	Wrist/reverse curls 3 × 10
Sit-ups 3 × 25–50	Internal/external rotations 3 × 10	Barbell twists 3 × 15
Four-way neck 2 × 10	Scapula stabilizer circuit 2 × 10	KB rotation swings 3 × 15–20

WEEKS 9–12

MONDAY	WEDNESDAY	FRIDAY
Hang clean 5 × 3	Power snatch 5 × 3	Hang clean 5 × 3
Squat 4 × 5	Bench press 4 × 5	Deadlift 4 × 5
DB jump squat 3 × 6	Alternate DB incline press 3 × 8–10	Bent-over rows 3 × 6–8
Lunges 3 × 8–10	DB jabs, uppercuts, hooks 3 ×15–20	Weighted pull-ups 3 × 10–15
Back extensions 3 × 8–10	Push-ups (on fists) 3 × 20–25	Curls 3 × 10
Russian twists 3 × 25–50	Triceps push-down 3 × 10	Wrist/reverse curls 3 × 10
Sit-ups 3 × 25–50	Internal/external rotations 3 × 10	Barbell twists 3 × 20
Four-way neck 2 × 10	Scapula stabilizer circuit 2 × 10	KB rotation swings 3 × 15–20

Intensity — 60%–90% of 1 RM periodized.

Rest Intervals – 2–3 min for core exercises; 1–2 min for assistance exercises; 30 s–1 min for abs.

[a]Only includes resistance training workouts; aerobic training, road work, plyometrics/agility, and boxing specific workouts (*i.e.*, heavy bag work, speed bag work, sparring, shadow boxing, etc.) performed separately.

KB, kettle bells; SB, stability ball; MB, medicine ball; DB, dumbbell.

Reprinted with permission from Hoffman JR, Ratamess NA. *A Practical Guide to Developing Resistance Training Programs*. 2nd ed. Monterey (CA): Coaches Choice Books; 2008.

Myths & Misconceptions

Only Athletes Can Benefit from Periodized Training

Some individuals have suggested that periodized training programs are most suitable for athletes with little applicability to other populations. However, studies show that essentially all populations can benefit from periodized training when it has been suitably adapted to meet the needs of those individuals (26). A recent study has shown that a 4-week undulating periodized strength training program produced substantial work-related improvements in patients rehabilitating from lumbar fusion surgery (7). Part of the misconception may develop from the perception among some that all periodized training programs involve some combination of high-intensity resistance, sprint, agility, aerobic endurance, and/or plyometric training. Although that may be the case for athletes, the acute program variables can be manipulated to meet the needs of any population. Periodization simply involves planned variation that can accommodate training at all levels. Several studies have examined periodized programs in untrained populations and showed strength gains and high rates of adherence (26). The key element is that periodized training includes planned variation, and a training program can be varied in numerous ways to meet the needs of a population. There are infinite ways to develop variations of periodization models by manipulating the exercises, order of exercise performance, intensity, volume, rest intervals, and frequency. For example, variations of classic and undulating models can be developed to target intensity and volume ranges that are more appealing to the general population (8–15 repetitions). A periodized program does not have to culminate in a peaking phase where some exercises are performed for 1–3 repetitions of heavy weights of more than 95% of 1 RM. Rather, a target zone of low-to-moderate intensities can be used if that meets the goals of the individual. Periodization implies variation and all individuals who exercise need to vary the training stimulus to avoid plateaus and boredom. The keys to improvement are progressive overload, variation, and training specificity (26) and periodized programs include elements of all of these to improve performance and various parameters of health. *The ACSM recommends training periodization for healthy adults and older adults when development of optimal fitness is the goal* (1).

Summary Points

✔ Periodization is the process of manipulating training program variables to bring the athlete to maximal performance at the appropriate time of the year, and to reduce the risk of overtraining. It is superior to non-periodized training for progression in strength and power.

✔ Several models of periodization are based on the work of Matveyev who divided training into preparatory, competition, and transition phases. The yearly macrocycle can be divided into mesocycles and microcycles to target specific goals.

✔ Periodized training is rooted in the work of Dr. Hans Selye who characterized adaptation into three segments: alarm, resistance, and exhaustion.

✔ Tapering for single-competition athletes enhances performance. Although several tapers are used successfully, it is recommended that a 2-week fast exponential taper be used at high intensity with similar frequency and 41%–60% reduction in volume.

✔ Three often-studied models of periodization include the classic, undulating, and reverse linear models. All are successful for increasing performance. Some studies show similar improvements between classic and undulating models whereas some studies show undulating or the classic model superior. Reverse linear periodization is most effective for endurance improvements.

✔ Periodized programs can be designed for all components of fitness including strength, power, speed, agility, aerobic endurance, muscle endurance, and plyometric training.

Review Questions

1. A short 1-week cycle that makes up part of a larger cycle is a:
   a. Monocycle
   b. Macrocycle
   c. Mesocycle
   d. Microcycle

2. A standard reduction in training volume load after a period of high-intensity training or overreaching (peaking cycle) is known as a:
   a. Step taper
   b. Linear taper
   c. Fast exponential taper
   d. Slow exponential taper

3. A progressive rise in intensity with concomitant decrease in volume with each training phase is characteristic of the _____ model of periodization.
   a. Reverse linear
   b. Classic
   c. Daily undulating
   d. Weekly undulating

4. When planning a taper phase, a reduction in training _____ is most recommended.
   a. Intensity
   b. Frequency
   c. Rest intervals
   d. Volume

5. The preparatory phase of training for a soccer player is characterized by:
   a. Low volume, low intensity
   b. Low volume, high intensity
   c. High volume, low intensity
   d. High volume, high intensity

6. The first phase of General Adaptation Syndrome characterized by the magnitude of the training stimulus is the:
   a. Alarm phase
   b. Adaptation phase
   c. Maladaptation phase
   d. Exhaustion phase

7. Periodization is the process of manipulating acute training program variables to maximize performance and reduce the risk of overtraining.　T　F

8. Periodization of training can only benefit elite athletes and has no application to recreational exercise.　T　F

9. The general preparatory phase consists of high volume, low intensity, and is used to prepare athletes for sport-specific training phases.　T　F

10. Tapering consists a nonlinear reduction in workload prior to a major competition.　T　F

11. Athletes attempting to maximize aerobic endurance performance benefit the most from use of a classical periodization model.　T　F

12. Periodization of sprint, agility, and plyometric training may follow a pattern similar to resistance training when peaking for strength and power.　T　F

References

1. American College of Sports Medicine. American College of Sports Medicine Position Stand. Progression models in resistance training for healthy adults. *Med Sci Sports Exerc*. 2009;41:687–708.
2. Baker D, Wilson G, Carlyon R. Periodization: the effect on strength of manipulating volume and intensity. *J Strength Cond Res*. 1994;8:235–242.
3. Bompa TO, Haff GG. *Periodization: Theory and Methodology of Training*. 5th ed. Champaign (IL): Human Kinetics; 2009. p. 125–256.
4. Bosquet L, Leger L, Legros P. Methods to determine aerobic endurance. *Sports Med*. 2002;32:675–700.
5. Bosquet L, Montpetit J, Arvisais D, Mujika I. Effects of tapering on performance: a meta-analysis. *Med Sci Sports Exerc*. 2007;39:1358–1365.
6. Buford TW, Rossi SJ, Smith DB, Warren AJ. A comparison of periodization models during nine weeks with equated volume and intensity for strength. *J Strength Cond Res*. 2007;21:1245–1250.
7. Cole K, Kruger M, Bates D, Steil G, Zbreski M. Physical demand levels in individuals completing a sports performance-based work conditioning/hardening program after lumbar fusion. *Spine J*. 2009;9:39–46.
8. Duehring MD, Feldmann CR, Ebben WP. Strength and conditioning practices of United States high school strength and conditioning coaches. *J Strength Cond Res*. 2009;23:2188–2203.
9. Durrell DL, Pujol TJ, Barnes JT. A survey of the scientific data and training methods utilized by collegiate strength and conditioning coaches. *J Strength Cond Res*. 2003;17:368–373.
10. Ebben WP, Blackard DO. Strength and conditioning practices of National Football League strength and conditioning coaches. *J Strength Cond Res*. 2001;15:48–58.
11. Ebben WP, Carroll RM, Simenz CJ. Strength and conditioning practices of National Hockey League strength and conditioning coaches. *J Strength Cond Res*. 2004;18:889–897.
12. Ebben WP, Hintz MJ, Simenz CJ. Strength and conditioning practices of Major League Baseball strength and conditioning coaches. *J Strength Cond Res*. 2005;19:538–546.
13. Fees M, Decker T, Snyder-Mackler L, Axe MJ. Upper extremity weight-training modifications for the injured athlete: a clinical perspective. *Am J Sports Med*. 1998;26:732–742.
14. Fleck SJ. Periodized strength training: a critical review. *J Strength Cond Res*. 1999;13:82–89.
15. Hartmann H, Bob A, Wirth K, Schmidtbleicher D. Effects of different periodization models on rate of force development and power ability of the upper extremity. *J Strength Cond Res*. 2009;23:1921–1932.
16. Herrick AB, Stone WJ. The effects of periodization versus progressive resistance exercise on upper and lower body strength in women. *J Strength Cond Res*. 1996;10:72–76.
17. Hoffman J. *Physiological Aspects of Sport Training and Performance*. Champaign (IL): Human Kinetics; 2002. p. 109–119.
18. Hoffman JR, Ratamess NA. *A Practical Guide to Developing Resistance Training Programs*. 2nd ed. Monterey (CA): Coaches Choice Books; 2008.
19. Hoffman JR, Wendell M, Cooper J, Kang J. Comparison between linear and nonlinear in-season training programs in freshman football players. *J Strength Cond Res*. 2003;17:561–565.
20. Hoffman JR, Ratamess NA, Klatt M, et al. Comparison between different off-season resistance training programs in Division III American college football players. *J Strength Cond Res*. 2009;23:11–19.
21. Izquierdo M, Ibanez J, Gonzalez-Badillo JJ, et al. Detraining and tapering effects on hormonal responses and strength performance. *J Strength Cond Res*. 2007;21:768–775.
22. Kerksick CM, Wilborn CD, Campbell BL, et al. Early-phase adaptations to a split-body, linear periodization resistance training program in college-aged and middle-aged men. *J Strength Cond Res*. 2009;23:962–971.
23. Kok LY, Hamer PW, Bishop DJ. Enhancing muscular qualities in untrained women: linear versus undulating periodization. *Med Sci Sports Exerc*. 2009;41:1797–1807.
24. Kraemer WJ. A series of studies—the physiological basis for strength training in American football: fact over philosophy. *J Strength Cond Res*. 1997;11:131–142.
25. Kraemer WJ, Fleck SJ. *Optimizing Strength Training: Designing Nonlinear Periodization Workouts*. Champaign (IL): Human Kinetics; 2007. p. 1–256.
26. Kraemer WJ, Ratamess NA. Fundamentals of resistance training: progression and exercise prescription. *Med Sci Sports Exerc*. 2004;36:674–688.
27. Kraemer WJ, Ratamess N, Fry AC, et al. Influence of resistance training volume and periodization on physiological and

performance adaptations in college women tennis players. *Am J Sports Med*. 2000;28:626–633.

28. Kraemer WJ, Häkkinen K, Triplett-McBride NT, et al. Physiological changes with periodized resistance training in women tennis players. *Med Sci Sports Exerc*. 2003;35:157–168.

29. Kraemer WJ, Nindl BC, Ratamess NA, et al. Changes in muscle hypertrophy in women with periodized resistance training. *Med Sci Sports Exerc*. 2004;36:697–708.

30. Marx JO, Ratamess NA, Nindl BC, et al. The effects of single-set vs. periodized multiple-set resistance training on muscular performance and hormonal concentrations in women. *Med Sci Sports Exerc*. 2001;33:635–643.

31. Matveyev L. *Fundamentals of Sports Training*. Moscow: Progress; 1981.

32. Monteiro AG, Aoki MS, Evangelista AL, et al. Nonlinear periodization maximizes strength gains in split resistance training routines. *J Strength Cond Res*. 2009;23:1321–1326.

33. Mujika I, Goya A, Padilla S, et al. Physiological responses to a 6-d taper in middle-distance runners: influence of training intensity and volume. *Med Sci Sports Exerc*. 2000;32:511–517.

34. Mujika I, Padilla S. Scientific bases for precompetition tapering strategies. *Med Sci Sports Exerc*. 2003;35:1182–1187.

35. Mujika I, Padilla S, Pyne D, Busso T. Physiological changes associated with the pre-event taper in athletes. *Sports Med*. 2004;34:891–927.

36. O'Bryant HS, Byrd R, Stone MH. Cycle ergometer performance and maximum leg and hip strength adaptations to two different methods of weight-training. *J Appl Sport Sci Res*. 1988;2:27–30.

37. Prestes J, Frollini AB, de Lima C, et al. Comparison between linear and daily undulating periodized resistance training to increase strength. *J Strength Cond Res*. 2009;23:2437–2442.

38. Ratamess NA, Kraemer WJ, Volek JS, et al. The effects of amino acid supplementation on muscular performance during resistance training overreaching. *J Strength Cond Res*. 2003;17:250–258.

39. Rhea MR, Ball SD, Phillips WT, Burkett LN. A comparison of linear and daily undulating periodized programs with equated volume and intensity for strength. *J Strength Cond Res*. 2002;16:250–255.

40. Rhea MR, Phillips WT, Burkett LN, et al. A comparison of linear and daily undulating periodized programs with equated volume and intensity for local muscular endurance. *J Strength Cond Res*. 2003;17:82–87.

41. Rhea MR, Alderman BL. A meta-analysis of periodized versus nonperiodized strength and power training programs. *Res Q Exerc Sport*. 2004;75:413–422.

42. Selye H. *The Stress of Life*. New York (NY): McGraw-Hill; 1956.

43. Simenz CJ, Dugan CA, Ebben WP. Strength and conditioning practices of National Basketball Association strength and conditioning coaches. *J Strength Cond Res*. 2005;19:495–504.

44. Stone MH, O'Bryant H, Garhammer J. A hypothetical model for strength training. *J Sports Med*. 1981;21:342–351.

45. Stone MH, O'Bryant HS, Schilling BK, et al. Periodization: effects of manipulating volume and intensity. Part 1. *Strength Cond J*. 1999; 21:56–62.

46. Stone MH, Potteiger JA, Pierce KC, et al. Comparison of the effects of three different weight-training programs on the one repetition maximum squat. *J Strength Cond Res*. 2000;14:332–337.

47. Verkhoshansky Y, Siff M. *Supertraining*. 6th ed. Ultimate Athlete Concepts; 2009. pp. 313–336.

48. Volek JS, Ratamess NA, Rubin MR, et al. The effects of creatine supplementation on muscular performance and body composition responses to short-term resistance training overreaching. *Eur J Appl Physiol*. 2004;91:628–637.

49. Wathen D, Baechle TR, Earle RW. Periodization. In: Baecle TR, Earle RW, editors. *Essentials of Strength Training and Conditioning*. 3rd ed. Champaign (IL): Human Kinetics; 2008. pp. 507–522.

50. Willoughby DS. A comparison of three selected weight training programs on the upper and lower body strength of trained males. *Ann J Appl Res Coaching Athletics* 1992;March:124–146.

51. Willoughby DS. The effects of meso-cycle-length weight training programs involving periodization and partially equated volumes on upper and lower body strength. *J Strength Cond Res*.1993;7:2–8

Part Four

Assessment

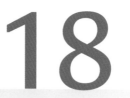

Assessment and Evaluation

After completing this chapter, you will be able to:

- Discuss the importance of testing and evaluation of athletes
- Discuss the importance of selecting tests that are valid and reliable
- Discuss the importance of selecting assessments which measure the health-related fitness components of body composition, muscle strength and endurance, cardiovascular endurance, and flexibility
- Discuss the importance of selecting assessments which measure the skill-related fitness components of power, speed, agility, and balance/coordination

Testing and evaluation of athletes are critical components of sports training. Testing serves many functions that benefit the athlete and coach:

- *Testing can identify athletic strengths and weaknesses:* training programs are designed, in part, to correct weaknesses. "A chain is only as strong as its weakest link" is a common expression used in sports. The results of testing allow the coach and athlete to recognize strengths and weaknesses. For example, if the athlete scores well (top 95%) on various strength measures but is lower on power measures, then it is wise for the coach to cap, or limit, strength training (maintenance). The necessary time needed to increase strength further may impede potential time for the athlete to focus on weaknesses. Power training could take precedence in this athlete. Although strength is a precursor to power development, some athletes have high levels of strength (based on slow-velocity assessments) but do not move at a high enough velocity needed for their sport. Testing results reveal a potential weakness and direct the coach to include more high-velocity exercises to produce balanced athletic development.
- *Evaluation of progress:* testing is critical to evaluating progress from the athletes' training programs. Although a coach can get a sense of progress from training logs, specific assessments evaluate the efficacy of the training program and serve as a motivational factor for improvement. A regular testing schedule gives the athlete a target date to peak fitness performance.
- *Identifying training loads:* the results of strength assessments serve a basis for intensity prescription for

structural exercises during resistance training (RT). For example, one microcycle of the yearly periodized scheme may entail the athlete perform an exercise at 70% of his/her 1 RM. The coach needs to know the 1 RM in order to accurately prescribe the training load. Thus, strength testing results can be used for load prescription. This also applies to aerobic exercise prescription when intensity is prescribed as a percentage of Vo_{2max} (or VO_2R).

- *Assessment of athletic talent:* the results of testing can help the coach properly identify athletes participating in certain sports. This may be particularly true for younger athletes. An athlete who scores low on strength and power assessments but high on an aerobic capacity assessment can be directed by a coach to participate in endurance-based sports. Testing can be used as a form of athletic identification for specific sports. The earlier an athlete identifies the qualities needed for success in certain sports, the sooner training can begin to maximize that athlete's potential.

TEST SELECTION AND ADMINISTRATION

Tests should be valid, reliable, and used with stringent standards. **Validity** refers to the degree which a test measures what it is supposed to measure (25). Different types of validity can be seen. *Construct validity* is the ability of a test to represent the underlying theory or construct. It is of particular interest to the athlete or coach as it is a primary source of validity for the test. For example, the 225-lb bench press test is extensively used at National Football League (NFL) combines. Its ability to assess

451

strength is highly questionable unless the athlete's 1 RM is near 225 lb. An athlete who performs 25 repetitions for the test is truly being assessed on muscular endurance therefore the validity of this test is poor for most athletes. *Face validity* gives the appearance to the athlete and other observers that the test is measuring what it is supposed to. Face validity increases the athlete's motivation and response to the test. *Content validity* refers to the observations of experts regarding a test or a testing battery. A coach can ensure high content validity by performing a needs analysis along with metabolic, kinesiological, and biomechanical breakdowns of the sport to develop a specific test battery. *Criterion-referenced validity* (the extent test scores correlate to sports performance skills) is critical to test selection. For example, 1 RM squat correlates to vertical jump performance. Thus, tests with high criterion-referenced validity relate highly to sport-specific performance and should be included in the testing battery.

Reliability is a measure of the magnitude of repeatability or consistency a test exhibits (25). Tests selected must provide reliable measures of athletic performance. For example, an athlete who scores a peak power output of 4,600 W during a jump squat on 1 day and 5,850 W just 3 days later will not be given reliable results. Clearly some alterations in testing conditions were evident to explain such large variation (it is not possible for an athlete to increase power this much in 3 days if testing was conducted properly). Reliability depends upon the accuracy of the tester, equipment, and dietary and environmental conditions. Having different coaches perform similar tests (skinfold test, 40-yd dash) can reduce reliability (*intertester reliability*). Everyone has differences in technique and these differences are reflected by variations in scores. Standardization of testing procedures is mandatory for reliable results. Determination of **test-retest reliability** (correlation between multiple testing

days) is mandatory for research purposes but can serve useful to the coach as well. A test cannot be valid if it is not reliable. Reliability is maximized when standard principles of test selection and administration are strictly adhered to.

The tests selected should be as specific to the sport as possible and should be valid for the fitness component being measured. Figure 18.1 outlines several important testing considerations. Tests should be selected that are metabolically (energy system) and biomechanically (movement pattern) specific to the athlete's sport. The training status of the athlete is important. A well-trained athlete may have very good technique and will be able to apply 100% effort in each trial. A lesser-skilled athlete may have technical difficulties which could limit his/her level of effort. Thus, test complexity must match the skill set of the athletes. Familiarization and practice are critical to test selection and administration. A lack of familiarization/practice will result in poor performances that could have been better, provided the athlete had at least 1–2 practice sessions. For example, untrained older women need ~3 times as many familiarization sessions before strength testing than young women (57). Familiarization affects effort and maximal effort can only be applied when the athlete is familiar with the test. In research, a lack of familiarization is evidenced by very large increases in strength over short-term training periods. Experienced athletes require little familiarization but a short practice session could be beneficial. If athletes are not being tested on drills they routinely perform in training, at least 1–2 practice sessions should be given and possibly more depending on individual responses.

The age and gender of the athletes could play a role in test selection and administration. Older individuals need more preparation time for maximal testing. Young (children and adolescents) athletes may require more familiarization as

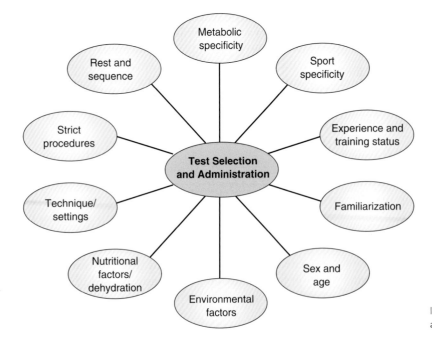

■ FIGURE 18.1. Factors affecting test selection and administration.

well. Although most tests can be applied similarly for both genders, performance will vary and some caution may be necessary. For example, a pull-up test in men can be used as an assessment of muscle endurance. However, in women (due to upper-body strength differences) it may be viewed more as a strength test as opposed to an endurance test.

Environmental (temperature, humidity, altitude, precipitation, terrain) factors can affect testing results. Temperature (hot and cold) plays a role indoors and outdoors. For example, testing an athlete's aerobic capacity one day in 98°F (with high humidity) weather versus 77°F (with low humidity) has a substantial effect on performance. Greater health risks are prevalent in hot and humid weather. Hot and humid weather can negatively affect aerobic more than anaerobic performance (2,3). Temperature plays a role indoors but it is controllable by the coach. It is important to test the athlete at a similar altitude. Changing altitudes can alter aerobic endurance performance. The level of precipitation is critical. Any moisture or wetness on the surface can affect athletic performance to some degree especially if the athlete is being tested in rainy conditions versus a nonprecipitous day. Lastly, the terrain is important. Maximal athletic performance can vary depending on the surface (grass vs. sand vs. hills vs. concrete). The coach should test athletes in the most ideal ways as possible, and attempting to control environmental factors is an important consideration. This includes standardizing footwear, as a new pair of athletic shoes can reduce sprint and agility times compared to an older pair of shoes.

Nutritional factors play considerable roles during testing. An athlete who is nutrient deficient or dehydrated may not perform up to task especially during aerobic endurance assessments. Body composition analyses can be compromised by altered hydration and nutrient status. Adequate fluid, carbohydrate, protein, and micronutrient intake is needed to maximize performance (59). Standardization is important. Standardization includes sports supplements, *e.g.*, creatine monohydrate which enhances performance (59,72). Testing an athlete on one occasion where nutrient intake is superior to testing on another occasion can affect the results especially if supplements are not accounted for. Coaches need to be cognizant of athlete's nutritional habits and should encourage a high-quality, nutrient-dense meal the evening before testing as well as adequate food and beverage intake up to ~1–2 hours before testing.

Test administration plays a critical role in measuring athletic performance including the procedures used, settings, equipment, or techniques used during each exercise, range of motion (ROM) used per exercise, sequence of testing, and rest intervals between trials. The coach and staff must ensure that strict procedural standardization is employed or results will be affected by testing errors.

Several administration factors should be addressed prior to testing. The testing staff should be carefully considered and well trained. Everyone needs to function

similarly and use standardized procedures. Technique should be synchronized so all testers use similar criteria especially when a large group of athletes are being tested simultaneously. All testers should be highly familiar with the tests and protocols used. If possible, one tester should oversee the testing of a single component. For example, one tester should perform all skinfold tests for body composition and one tester should time all sprint and agility tests for consistency. Multiple testers of the same assessment increases variability. Tests should be well organized and administered efficiently. Athletes should be carefully instructed on test performance and should be encouraged during performance. Fatigue should be minimized so the sequence of tests is critical. Testing can be made more efficient when it occurs on multiple days. However, some tests can be performed in the same day while minimizing fatigue from previous tests. Figure 18.2 depicts a general recommended testing sequence when multiple tests are

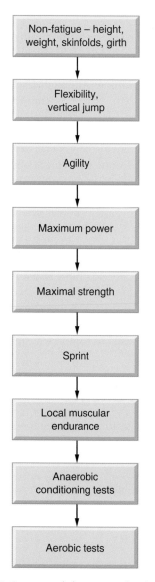

FIGURE 18.2. Recommended sequence of testing.

Myths & Misconceptions

Testing Must Be Performed Frequently to Be Useful

Some have advocated frequent testing of athletes. However, testing can be a useful tool if it is performed at a lower frequency as well. The type of test is important. Some tests (body weight, percent body fat, and flexibility) can be performed frequently (daily) because they are not strenuous on the athlete's body. For example, frequent body weight, percent fat, and hydration status (urine-specific gravity) testing for a wrestler is advantageous based on the needs of the sport for constant monitoring. However, some assessments are more suited for less frequent testing (1 RM strength). Maximal strength testing may occur only a few times in a year. A coach can get a sense of whether the athlete is progressing or not by closely monitoring training logs. A coach can indirectly ascertain if the athlete is improving when his/her training weights/repetitions have increased. The need for testing decreases when the coach can gain valuable information from training logs. The critical component is that testing should not interfere with the athlete's training schedule.

performed. These tests can be separated into multiple testing days when needed. The sequence involves low-fatigue assessments initially and progresses to more challenging and fatiguing tests.

All steps should be taken by the testing staff to ensure maximal safety of the athletes. This includes the decision to test or not test an athlete with a predisposing injury, illness, or medical condition. Although testing can be beneficial, it is not worth the risk of causing potential damage to an injured athlete. Close monitoring is necessary and constant communication with the athletic training and medical staffs is essential to properly screen athletes at risk for injury. Environmental conditions must be factored. Hot and humid conditions pose a threat to athletes, so caution must be used when planning a testing session on a hot/humid day. Lastly, proper data management is important. All data forms should be designed and prepared prior to testing. Data can be stored in a database for record keeping. Spreadsheets are recommended as they allow the coach not only the ability to monitor testing performance over time but can be used to develop norms and standards. They allow the coach to easily calculate means, standard deviations, or perform some general statistical procedures that are used to compare means over time.

ASSESSMENT OF HEALTH-RELATED FITNESS COMPONENTS

Testing of several health-related components of fitness is paramount to a comprehensive testing battery for athletes. These include body composition and anthropometry, muscle strength and endurance, cardiovascular (CV) endurance, and flexibility.

BODY COMPOSITION AND ANTHROPOMETRY

Body composition describes the relative proportions of fat, bone, and muscle mass in the human body.

Anthropometry is a term describing measurement of the human body in terms of dimensions such as height, weight, circumferences, girths, and skinfolds. Body composition and anthropometric assessments are standard practice for coaches and athletes. Valuable information regarding percent body fat, fat distribution, lean body mass, limb lengths, and circumferences are gained through body composition assessment. There are several ways to measure body composition in athletes including skinfold tests, bioelectrical impedance, dual X-ray absorptiometry (DEXA), underwater weighing, computed tomography (CT) and magnetic resonance imaging (MRI) scans, air displacement plethysmography (BOD POD), and near-infrared interactance (60). Although DEXA use has increased over the several years, underwater weighing is still considered the "gold standard" of body composition assessment and is the preferred method of comparison when validating and developing prediction equations for skinfold analysis. Skinfold assessment is very practical and is the only method described in this section.

Height and Body Weight

Height and body weight are basic measurements. Height is assessed with a *stadiometer* (a vertical ruler mounted on a wall with a wide horizontal headboard). Height can vary slightly throughout the day where values are higher in the morning. When measuring height, the athlete needs to remove shoes, stand as straight as possible with heels together, take a deep breath, hold it, and stand with head level. Body weight is best measured on a calibrated physician's scale with a beam and moveable weights. Clothing is a major issue and should be standardized (shoes removed, minimal clothing, items removed from pockets). Body weight changes at various times of day due to meal/beverage consumption, urination, defecation, and potential dehydration/water loss. A standard time (early in the morning) is recommended.

Skinfold Assessment

Skinfold assessments are one of the most popular and practical methods to estimate percent body fat. Skinfold assessment can be relatively accurate provided that a trained coach or technician is performing the measurement with high-quality calipers. Skinfold analysis is based on the principle that the amount of subcutaneous fat (fat immediately below the skin) is directly proportional to the total amount of body fat, and regression analysis is used to estimate total percent body fat. Variability in percent body fat prediction from skinfold analysis is ~±3%–5% assuming that appropriate techniques and equations are used. Body fat varies with gender, age, race or ethnicity, training status, and other factors so numerous regression equations have been developed to predict body density and percent fat from skinfold measurements. Skinfold assessment for athletes is most accurate when prediction equations are used that closely match the population. The number of sites range from 3 to 7. Prediction equations are used to estimate body density, and body density calculation is used to estimate percent body fat. **Body density** is described as the ratio of body mass to body volume.

The procedures for skinfold assessment include:

- The number of sites and equation are first selected (Fig. 18.3).
- A fold of skin is firmly grasped between the thumb and index finger of the left hand (about 8 cm apart) while the subject is relaxed. A larger grasping area (>8 cm) may be needed for large individuals who could max out the measurement capacity of the caliper.
- The jaws of the caliper are placed over the skinfold 1 cm below the fingers of the tester, released, and the measurement is taken within 2–3 seconds.
- All measurements are taken on the right side of the body 2–3 times for consistency to the nearest 0.5 mm. It is important to rotate through all of the sites first as opposed to taking two or three measurements sequentially from the same site.
- For several tests each site is averaged and summed to estimate body density and percent body fat via a regression equation or prediction table.

Table 18.1 depicts several equations used to estimate percent body fat from body density estimates. Those equations most appropriate to use will be selected based on gender, age, ethnicity, and activity level. Those appropriate equations should have been cross-validated, and general equations have been shown to produce accurate estimates across all segments of the population. Percent body fat can be calculated once body density has been determined. Most often, the Siri (66) or Brozek (7) equations are used although other population-specific equations (Table 18.2) have been developed. Table 18.3 depicts classifications based on percent body fat.

$$Siri\ Equation:\ (4.95/B_d - 4.50) \times 100$$
$$Brozek\ Equation:\ (4.57/B_d - 4.142) \times 100$$

Girth Measurements

Girth measurements provide useful information regarding changes in muscle size and body composition. The advantages of taking circumference measurements is that it is easy, inexpensive, does not require specialized equipment (other than a tape measure), and quick to administer. The procedures for girth measurements include (60):

1. The tape measure is applied in a horizontal plane to the site so it is taut and the circumference is read to the nearest half of a centimeter. Minimal clothing should be worn.
2. Duplicate measures should be taken at each site and the average is used. If readings differ by more than 5–10 mm then an additional measurement is taken.
3. Athletes should remain relaxed while measurements are taken.
4. A large source of error is a lack of standardization of the measurement site. The correct placement of the tape measure per site is as follows:
   a. *Chest* — tape is placed around the chest at level of the fourth ribs after subject abducts arms. Measurement is taken when athlete adducts arms back to starting position and at the end of respiration.
   b. *Shoulder* — tape is placed horizontally at the maximal circumference of the shoulders while athlete is standing relaxed.
   c. *Abdominal* — tape is placed over the abdomen at the level of the greatest circumference (often near the umbilicus) while athlete is standing relaxed.
   d. *Right thigh* — tape is placed horizontally over the thigh below the gluteal level at the largest circumference (upper thigh) while athlete is standing.
   e. *Right calf* — tape is placed horizontally over the largest circumference of the calf midway between the knee and ankle while athlete is standing relaxed.
   f. *Waist* — tape is placed around smallest area of the waist, ~1 in. above the navel.
   g. *Hip* — tape is placed around largest area of the buttocks (with minimal clothing).
   h. *Right upper arm* — tape is placed horizontally over the midpoint of the upper arm between the shoulder and elbow while athlete is standing, relaxed, and elbow is extended.
   i. *Right forearm* — tape is placed horizontally over the proximal area of the forearm where circumference is the largest while athlete is standing relaxed.

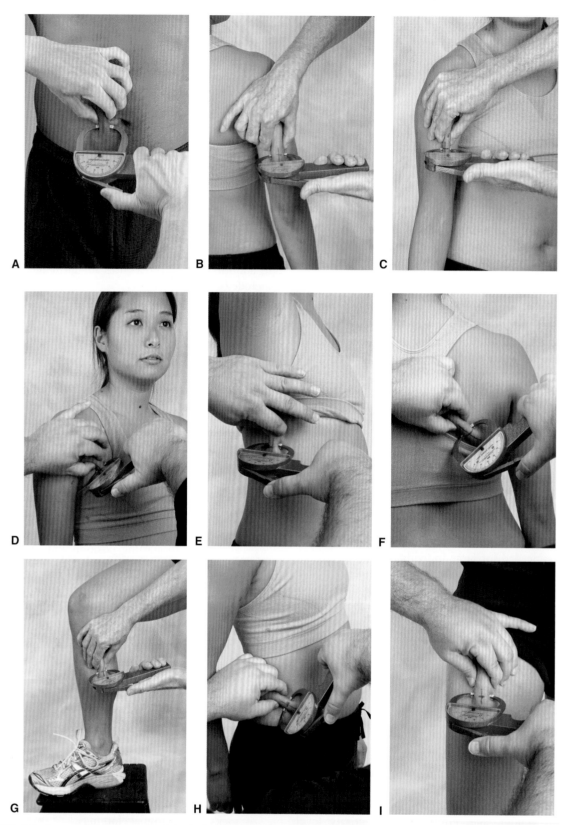

■ **FIGURE 18.3.** Common skinfold sites. **A.** Abdominal: vertical fold, 2 cm to the right side of the umbilicus. **B.** Triceps: vertical fold on the posterior midline of the upper arm, halfway between the acromion and olecranon processes, with the arm held freely to the side of the body. **C.** Biceps: vertical fold on the anterior aspect of the arm over the belly of the biceps muscle, 1 cm above the level used to mark the triceps site. **D.** Chest: diagonal fold, one-half the distance between the anterior axillary line and the nipple (men), or one-third of the distance between the anterior axillary line and the nipple (women). **E.** Midaxillary: vertical fold on the midaxillary line at the level of the xiphoid process of the sternum. An alternate method is a horizontal fold taken at the level of the xiphoid/sternal border in the midaxillary line. **F.** Subscapular: diagonal fold (at a 45° angle), 1–2 cm below the inferior angle of the scapula. **G.** Medial calf: vertical fold at the maximum circumference of the calf on the midline of its medial border. **H.** Suprailium: diagonal fold in line with the natural angle of the iliac crest taken in the anterior axillary line immediately superior to the iliac crest. **I.** Thigh: vertical fold; on the anterior midline of the thigh, midway between the proximal border of the patella and the inguinal crease (hip). (From Thompson W, ed. *ACSM's Resources for the Personal Trainer*. 3rd ed. Baltimore (MD): Lippincott Williams & Wilkins; 2010.)

TABLE 18.1 BODY DENSITY PREDICTION EQUATIONS FROM SKINFOLD MEASUREMENTS

SITES	POPULATION	GENDER	EQUATION	REFERENCE
2: thigh, subscapular	Athletes	Male	$D_b = 1.1043 - (0.00133 \times \text{thigh}) - (0.00131 \times \text{subscapular})$	Sloan and Weir (67)
2: suprailiac, triceps	Athletes	Female	$D_b = 1.0764 - (0.00081 \times \text{suprailiac}) - (0.00088 \times \text{triceps})$	Sloan and Weir (67)
3: chest, abdomen, thigh	General	Male	$D_b = 1.10938 - 0.0008267(\text{sum of 3 sites}) + 0.0000016(\text{sum of 3 sites})^2 - 0.0002574(\text{age})$	Jackson and Pollock (38)
3: triceps, suprailiac, thigh	General	Female	$D_b = 1.099421 - 0.0009929(\text{sum of 3 sites}) + 0.0000023(\text{sum of 3 sites})^2 - 0.0001392(\text{age})$	Jackson et al. (40)
3: chest, triceps, subscapular	General	Male	$D_b = 1.1125025 - 0.0013125(\text{sum of 3 sites}) + 0.0000055(\text{sum of 3 sites})^2 - 0.000244(\text{age})$	Pollock et al. (56)
3: triceps, suprailiac, abdomen	General	Female	$D_b = 1.089733 - 0.0009245(\text{sum of 3 sites}) + 0.0000025(\text{sum of 3 sites})^2 - 0.0000979(\text{age})$	Jackson and Pollock (39)
4: biceps, triceps, subscapular, suprailiac	General	Male Female 20–29 yr	$D_b = 1.1631 - 0.0632(\text{log sum of 4 sites})$	Durnin and Womersley (20)
4: biceps, triceps, subscapular, suprailiac	General	Male Female 30–39 yr	$D_b = 1.1422 - 0.0544(\text{log sum of 4 sites})$	Durnin and Womersley (20)
7: thigh, subscapular, suprailiac, triceps, chest, abdomen, axillary	General	Female	$D_b = 1.0970 - 0.00046971(\text{sum of 7 sites}) + 0.00000056(\text{sum of 7 sites})^2 - 0.00012828(\text{age})$	Jackson et al. (40)
7: thigh, subscapular, suprailiac, triceps, chest, abdomen, axillary	General	Male	$D_b = 1.112 - 0.00043499(\text{sum of 7 sites}) + 0.00000055(\text{sum of 7 sites})^2 - 0.00028826(\text{age})$	Jackson and Pollock (38)

MUSCLE STRENGTH

The most important reason to assess muscle strength is to evaluate strength training programs. Strength testing comes in various forms depending on the type of strength measured, *e.g.*, dynamic concentric (CON) and eccentric (ECC), isometric (ISOM), or isokinetic (ISOK). The gold standard of dynamic strength testing is the 1 RM which is performed with free weights and machines. Although other RMs can be used, the 1 RM provides the most accurate strength assessment when performed properly. The 1 RM is the maximal amount of weight that can be lifted once for a specific exercise. High test-retest reliabilities

TABLE 18.2 POPULATION-SPECIFIC EQUATIONS TO CALCULATE PERCENT BODY FAT FROM BODY DENSITY

POPULATION	AGE	SEX	EQUATION
White	7–12	Male	$(5.30/D_b - 4.89) \times 100$
		Female	$(5.35/D_b - 4.95) \times 100$
	13–16	Male	$(5.07/D_b - 4.64) \times 100$
		Female	$(5.10/D_b - 4.66) \times 100$
	17–19	Male	$(4.99/D_b - 4.55) \times 100$
		Female	$(5.05/D_b - 4.62) \times 100$
	20–80	Male	$(4.95/D_b - 4.50) \times 100$
		Female	$(5.01/D_b - 4.57) \times 100$
African-American	18–32	Male	$(4.37/D_b - 3.93) \times 100$
	24–79	Female	$(4.85/D_b - 4.39) \times 100$
American Indian	18–60	Female	$(4.81/D_b - 4.34) \times 100$
Hispanic	20–40	Female	$(4.87/D_b - 4.41) \times 100$
Japanese	18–48	Male	$(4.97/D_b - 4.52) \times 100$
		Female	$(4.76/D_b - 4.28) \times 100$
	61–78	Male	$(4.87/D_b - 4.41) \times 100$
		Female	$(4.95/D_b - 4.50) \times 100$

Adapted with permission from (26) and (27).

TABLE 18.3 PERCENT BODY FAT CLASSIFICATIONS

	AGE (YR)						
RATING (MALE)	**<17**	**18–25**	**26–35**	**36–45**	**46–55**	**56–65**	**>66**
Very lean	5	4–7	8–12	10–14	12–16	15–18	15–18
Lean	5–10	8–10	13–15	16–18	18–20	19–21	19–21
Leaner than avg	—	11–13	16–18	19–21	21–23	22–24	22–23
Average	11–25	14–16	19–21	22–24	24–25	24–26	24–25
Slightly high	—	18–20	22–24	25–26	26–28	26–28	25–27
High	26–31	22–26	25–28	27–29	29–31	29–31	28–30
Obese	>31	>28	>30	>30	>32	>32	>31
RATING (FEMALE)	**<17**	**18–25**	**26–35**	**36–45**	**46–55**	**56–65**	**>66**
Very lean	12	13–17	13–18	15–19	18–22	18–23	16–18
Lean	12–15	18–20	19–21	20–23	23–25	24–26	22–25
Leaner than avg	—	21–23	22–23	24–26	26–28	28–30	27–29
Average	16–30	24–25	24–26	27–29	29–31	31–33	30–32
Slightly high	—	26–28	27–30	30–32	32–34	34–36	33–35
High	31–36	29–31	31–35	33–36	36–38	36–38	36–38
Obese	>36	>33	>36	>39	>39	>39	>39

YMCA Fitness Testing and Assessment Manual, 4ᵗʰ edition, 2000.

have been shown for 1 RM testing (intraclass correlations ranging from 0.79 to 0.99) (43). 1 RM testing can be performed with many exercises. However, multiple-joint exercises like the squat, bench press, deadlift, and power clean are most commonly used. The 1 RM power clean may be viewed as a power assessment as well. Although several protocols for strength testing can be effective, the following is a sample of one (43):

1. A light warm-up of 5–10 repetitions at 40%–60% of perceived max is performed.
2. After a 1-minute rest, 3–5 repetitions at 60%–80% of perceived maximum is performed.
3. Step 2 will take the athlete close to the 1 RM. A conservative increase in weight is made, and a 1 RM lift is attempted. If the lift is successful, a rest period of ~3 minutes is allowed. It is important to allow enough rest before the next maximal attempt. A 1 RM should be obtained within 3–5 sets to avoid excessive fatigue. The process of increasing the weight up to a true 1 RM can be enhanced by the prior familiarization and expertise of the coaches in evaluating performance. This process continues until a failed attempt occurs then weight is adjusted accordingly.
4. The 1 RM value is recorded as the weight of the last successfully completed lift.

It is very important that communication takes place between the athlete and testing staff. A trained staff can recognize an athlete's capacity and determine a proper progression pattern of loading. Feedback from the athlete is critical to determine the loading progressions especially if the lifter has experience and a general idea of the perceived 1 RM. A trial and error approach is seen with athletes with limited experience although an experienced coach may be able to view an athlete and have a certain loading in mind. "How do you feel?" "Are you ready to go?" "How close to your 1 RM do you think you are?" "Can you lift 5 more pounds?" These types of questions and others are vital to the interaction with the athletes as they attempt to exert maximal force. Lastly, rest period length and the number of preliminary repetitions (warm-up) are important. It is essential that the number of repetitions be adequate for proper warm-up but be few enough to not fatigue the athlete. These factors need to be individualized as athletes lifting very heavy weights will require more warm-up sets and longer rest intervals than those lifting lighter weights. Some individuals may require at least 5-minute rest between attempts whereas some individuals need only 1–2 minutes of rest depending on the loading. If a greater number of repetitions are performed (5–10 RM) it is suggested that fewer warm-up sets be used. Figure 18.4 presents a checklist for strength training (43). This list can provide a guide for coaches and athletes as it reminds all testers of specific considerations needed prior to and during strength testing. The following protocol is suggested for testing a 6 RM and could be modified to test other RMs (43).

1. Athlete warms up with 5–10 repetitions with 50% of estimated 6 RM.
2. After 1 minute of rest, the athlete performs 6 repetitions at 70% of the estimated 6 RM.

Strength-Testing Checklist

- ☐ Has the individual been medically cleared to weight train, and can this individual safety perform strength or endurance testing?

- ☐ Does this individual require any special accommodations?

- ☐ Is the time of day similar between multiple testing sessions?

- ☐ Is muscle strength or endurance to be tested?

- ☐ Is a 1 RM or multiple RM to be used?

- ☐ What is the age and gender of the individual?

- ☐ Was the individual thoroughly familiarized with the testing protocol? How many familiarization sessions were performed?

- ☐ Was proper technique explained and demonstrated (including range of motion, grips, stances, body position, and so on)?

- ☐ Was test-retest reliability of the equipment and protocol performed?

- ☐ What is the individual's training history?

- ☐ Was adequate nutrition intake (and hydration) consumed before testing?

- ☐ Was ambient temperature controlled for?

- ☐ If the individual is experienced, what is his or her perceived or expected RM?

- ☐ What type of muscle action is to be tested?

  - ☐ Concentric?

  - ☐ Eccentric?

  - ☐ Isometric?

- ☐ What type of resistance is to be used?

  - ☐ Dynamic constant external resistance?

  - ☐ Variable resistance?

  - ☐ Isokinetic?

  - ☐ Isometric?

- ☐ For machine-based exercise, what are the appropriate machine settings and starting position of the resistance?

- ☐ Was the individual properly positioned, and does the equipment accurately accommodate the individual?

- ☐ For isometric training, what joint angles will be examined?

- ☐ What is the velocity of movement?

- ☐ Are knowledgeable spotters present?

- ☐ Was the equipment calibrated according to manufacture's guidelines?

- ☐ Test specificity:

  - ☐ Were the movement patterns tested similar to those performed during training?

  - ☐ Is there metabolic (energy system) specificity?

- ☐ Were adequate instructions given?

- ☐ Was a proper warm-up performed? Did it include submaximal practice repetitions for testing exercises?

- ☐ Did the individual use proper technique, and did spotters assist in lifting the weight?

- ☐ Was proper breathing patterns used?

- ☐ Was the lifter verbally encouraged throughout the testing protocol, and was a proper lifting environment set for testing?

- ☐ Was visual feedback given for isokinetic testing?

- ☐ Were the proper units of measurement used?

- ☐ What was the individual's 1RM or multiple RM score?

- ☐ Were ergogenics controlled for? What types (if any) were used?

  - ☐ Lifting accessories and apparel?

  - ☐ Nutrition supplements?

  - ☐ Drugs?

- ☐ Did the individual give 100% effort?

- ☐ Were there any other factors that may have affected the test (e.g., illness, injury)?

■ **FIGURE 18.4.** Strength testing checklist. (Reprinted with permission from Kraemer WJ, Fry AC, Ratamess NA, French DN. Strength testing: development and evaluation of methodology. In: Maud PJ, Foster C, ed. *Physiological Assessments of Human Performance*. 2nd ed. Champaign (IL): Human Kinetics; 2006. pp. 119–150.)

3. Step 2 is repeated at 90% of the estimated 6 RM for 3–6 repetitions.

4. After at least 2–3 minutes of rest, depending on the effort required for the previous set, 6 repetitions are performed with 100%–105% of the estimated 6 RM.

5. After at least 3–5 minutes of rest, if Step 4 is successful, increase the resistance by 2.5%–5% for another 6 RM attempt. If six repetitions were not completed in Step 4, subtract 2.5%–5% of the resistance used in Step 4 and attempt another 6 RM.

6. If weight was removed for Step 5 and 6 repetitions were performed, this is the athlete's 6 RM. If the athlete was not successful with this reduced resistance, retesting should occur after 24 hours of rest.

Proper spotting is mandatory for free weight strength testing. Spotters, who are experienced and have a sufficient level of strength and knowledge of correct exercise execution, should be used. The spotter must be able to recognize poor exercise technique and identify hazardous situations. The procedures for proper spotting are exercise-specific. Although not all exercises require a spotter, it is recommended that a spotter be present during strength testing for those exercises that involve lifting the weight over head (shoulder press), lying supine on a bench and lifting the weight over the face or trunk (bench press), or placing the bar on the rear or posterior aspects of the shoulders (back squat). Spotters are not necessary for Olympic lifts or for exercises involving lifting the weight off of the floor. The major difference between spotting for strength training compared to testing is the amount of assistance

given to the lifter. It is recommended that a spotter apply minimal force to keep the bar moving during training. However, this is not ideal for strength testing. It is important that fatigue be kept to a minimum. The spotter may provide substantial assistance to spare the lifter unwanted fatigue. The spotter should not touch the bar until failure has occurred. Even the slightest touch gives assistance to the lifter and can overinflate the 1 RM value. Tables 18.4 and 18.5 provide some strength norms and data of various athletic populations.

Isometric Strength Testing

ISOM tests are performed at a static position. The evaluation angle, standardization between athletes, feedback, and motivation all make ISOM testing demanding. Force/torque varies throughout joint ROM; therefore careful consideration is needed for standardizing joint angles. Some devices used include the hip and back dynamometer, handgrip dynamometer, and ISOK devices. A calibrated force plate can be used with an immovable

TABLE 18.4 NORMATIVE VALUES FOR RELATIVE LEG PRESS AND BENCH PRESS STRENGTH (1 RM/BODY MASS) IN A GENERAL POPULATION

| | RELATIVE LEG PRESS STRENGTH | | | | | | | | | |
| | 20–29 Y | | 30–39 Y | | 40–49 Y | | 50–59 Y | | 60+ Y | |
% RANK	M	F	M	F	M	F	M	F	M	F
90	2.27	2.05	2.07	1.73	1.92	1.63	1.80	1.51	1.73	1.40
80	2.13	1.66	1.93	1.50	1.82	1.46	1.71	1.30	1.62	1.25
70	2.05	1.42	1.85	1.47	1.74	1.35	1.64	1.24	1.56	1.18
60	1.97	1.36	1.77	1.32	1.68	1.26	1.58	1.18	1.49	1.15
50	1.91	1.32	1.71	1.26	1.62	1.19	1.52	1.09	1.43	1.08
40	1.83	1.25	1.65	1.21	1.57	1.12	1.46	1.03	1.38	1.04
30	1.74	1.23	1.59	1.16	1.51	1.03	1.39	0.95	1.30	0.98
20	1.63	1.13	1.52	1.09	1.44	0.94	1.32	0.86	1.25	0.94
10	1.51	1.02	1.43	0.94	1.35	0.76	1.22	0.75	1.16	0.84

| | RELATIVE BENCH PRESS STRENGTH | | | | | | | | | |
| | 20–29 Y | | 30–39 Y | | 40–49 Y | | 50–59 Y | | 60+ Y | |
% RANK	M	F	M	F	M	F	M	F	M	F
90	1.48	0.54	1.24	0.49	1.10	0.46	0.97	0.40	0.89	0.41
80	1.32	0.49	1.12	0.45	1.00	0.40	0.90	0.37	0.82	0.38
70	1.22	0.42	1.04	0.42	0.93	0.38	0.84	0.35	0.77	0.36
60	1.14	0.41	0.98	0.41	0.88	0.37	0.79	0.33	0.72	0.32
50	1.06	0.40	0.93	0.38	0.84	0.34	0.75	0.31	0.68	0.30
40	0.99	0.37	0.88	0.37	0.80	0.32	0.71	0.28	0.66	0.29
30	0.93	0.35	0.83	0.34	0.76	0.30	0.68	0.26	0.63	0.28
20	0.88	0.33	0.78	0.32	0.72	0.27	0.63	0.23	0.57	0.26
10	0.80	0.30	0.71	0.27	0.65	0.23	0.57	0.19	0.53	0.25

Reprinted with permission from Hoffman J. *Norms for Fitness, Performance, and Health*. Champaign (IL): Human Kinetics; 2006: pp. 1–113.

TABLE 18.5 PERCENTILES FOR THE BENCH PRESS AND THE PREDICTED 1 RM FOR PLAYERS IN THE NFL COMBINE

	DB			DL			LB		
		PRED 1 RM			PRED 1 RM			PRED 1 RM	
% RANK	REPS	LB	KG	REPS	LB	KG	REPS	LB	KG
90	18.0	345	157	28.1	416	189	29.3	423	192
80	17.0	340	155	26.0	400	182	27.0	405	184
70	15.0	325	148	25.0	395	180	26.0	400	182
60	14.0	320	145	24.0	385	175	25.2	396	180
50	13.0	315	143	23.0	380	173	22.5	378	172
40	12.0	305	139	21.6	371	169	21.6	372	169
30	10.0	295	134	20.0	360	164	19.1	356	162
20	10.0	295	134	18.8	353	160	15.4	329	150
10	8.0	280	127	17.0	340	155	13.7	319	145
$\overline{X}$	13.2	315	143	22.8	378	172	22.2	375	170
SD	4.1	28	13	4.4	29	13	5.7	38	17
n		62			68			26	

	OL			RB			TE		
		PRED 1 RM			PRED 1 RM			PRED 1 RM	
% RANK	REPS	LB	KG	REPS	LB	KG	REPS	LB	KG
90	30.0	430	195	23.0	380	173	27.4	411	187
80	27.0	405	184	20.0	360	164	24.2	389	177
70	25.6	398	181	19.0	355	161	22.4	377	171
60	24.0	385	175	18.0	345	157	20.4	363	165
50	23.0	380	173	18.0	345	157	19.0	355	161
40	22.0	375	170	17.0	340	155	18.0	345	157
30	21.0	365	166	16.0	335	152	18.0	345	157
20	20.0	360	164	15.0	325	148	17.4	342	155
10	17.0	340	155	14.0	320	145	13.8	320	145
X	23.3	382	174	17.9	346	157	20.1	361	164
SD	5.1	35	16	3.3	22	10	4.2	28	13
n		97			67			11	

Pred 1 RM, predicted 1 RM; DB, defensive back; DL, defensive line; LB, linebacker; OL, offensive line; RB, running back; TE, fight end.
Reprinted with permission from Hoffman J. *Norms for Fitness, Performance, and Health*. Champaign, (IL): Human Kinetics; 2006: pp. 1–113.

resistance for several free weight/Smith machine exercises (43). Although peak force/torque assessment is often the primary purpose, rate of ISOM force development can be measured. Fatigue tests (muscle endurance) can be performed with ISOM devices. These tests involve maintaining a certain level of muscular tension over a specified period of time. Many protocols can be used for ISOM testing. All athletes should warm up with low-intensity exercises before testing. Following the warm-up, some practice trials may be performed with submaximal effort (50%–60% of maximal voluntary contraction). The actual test requires only 2–3 maximal voluntary efforts. Additional trials may be necessary if, in fact, it appears the athlete is still improving. The peak force for the highest trial is recorded. Table 18.6 provides some norms for maximal grip strength.

Isokinetic Strength Testing

ISOK testing is performed with a dynamometer that maintains the lever arm at a constant angular velocity. This type of strength evaluation accounts for CON and ECC velocity of movement that is uncontrolled with free weights and machines. The cost of an ISOK dynamometer can be prohibitive, but many laboratories, training rooms, and clinical facilities use them extensively. Although many units enable single-joint movements, there are some devices on the market that utilize multiple-joint movements that have shown high test-retest reliability (43). Due to the complex nature of ISOK testing, there are a number of considerations including the selection of:

1. velocity and order;
2. number of repetitions to be performed;

TABLE 18.6 NORMATIVE VALUES OF DOMINANT GRIP STRENGTH (KG) IN ADULTS

	20–29 Y		30–39 Y		40–49 Y		50–59 Y		60–69 Y	
	M	**F**	**M**	**F**	**M**	**F**	**M**	**F**	**M**	**F**
Excellent	>54	>36	>53	>36	>51	>35	>49	>33	>49	>33
Good	51–54	33–36	50–53	34–36	48–51	33–35	46–49	31–33	46–49	31–33
Average	43–50	26–32	43–49	28–33	41–47	27–32	39–45	25–30	39–45	25–30
Fair	39–42	22–25	39–42	25–27	37–40	24–26	35–38	22–24	35–38	22–24
Poor	<39	<22	<39	<25	<37	<24	<35	<22	<35	<22

Reprinted with permission from Hoffman J. *Norms for Fitness, Performance, and Health.* Champaign (IL): Human Kinetics; 2006. pp. 1–113.

3. rest intervals;
4. CON and/or ECC muscle action(s);
5. a standardized ROM;
6. standardized test position and proper postural stabilization;
7. equipment calibration and test-retest reliability;
8. feedback, instruction, and familiarization; and
9. gravity compensation.

Studies examining ISOK training have shown velocity-specific strength increases with some spillover above (up to 210° s^{-1}) and below (up to 180° s^{-1}) the training velocity (43). Training at moderate velocity (180–240° s^{-1}) produces the greatest strength increases across all testing velocities (43). Testing should match the training velocity, or a spectrum of slow, moderate, and fast velocities can be selected. Three to five repetitions are recommended with rest intervals of 1–3 minutes in between sets to attain peak torque (43). Test-retest reliability for ISOK testing is generally high when position is standardized, equipment is calibrated, and maximal effort is given by the athletes. Optimal ISOK testing allows the athletes to observe their performance via visual feedback as they actually perform the test. In fact, torque may be 3%–19% higher when visual feedback is used (43).

Estimating Repetition Maximums

In some cases, estimating a 1 RM or multiple RM may be preferred. Table 18.7 depicts some popular prediction equations used by athletes, men and women with little experience, and older adults (43). The load selection ranged from 55%–95% of 1 RM (for 2–20 repetitions) with mean ~68%–80% of 1 RM. Prediction is attractive from an administrative standpoint, but its validity is questionable as these equations can underestimate and overestimate 1 RM in certain populations in cross-validation studies (43). Accuracy is greater when <10 repetitions are performed using nonlinear equations. In fact, accuracy improves as repetition number decreases. There is greater accuracy the closer to the 1 RM is performed (2 or 3 repetitions). Many studies have used the bench press, thus the accuracy appears greater with this exercise. The error rate increases when these equations are applied to other exercises such as the squat and deadlift. For field settings involving large numbers of athletes and limited time or athletes with little RT experience, a case may be made for 1 RM estimation. However, most accurate results are obtained from true RM testing. Lastly, the number of repetitions performed relative to the 1 RM for different exercises is highly variable. Hoeger et al. (28)

TABLE 18.7 FORMULAS USED TO ESTIMATE 1 RM LIFTING PERFORMANCE (43)

REFERENCE	EQUATION
Brzycki (8)	1 RM = Wt./1.0278 − 0.0278(# reps) %1 RM = 102.78 − 2.78(# reps)
Epley (21)	1 RM = [0.033(Wt.)(# reps) + Wt.]
Lander (44)	1 RM = Wt./1.013 − 0.02671(# reps) %1 RM = 101.3 − 2.67123(# reps)
Mayhew et al. (50)	1 RM (lb) = 226.7 + 7.1(#reps w/ 225) (used in college football players)
Cummings and Finn (16)	1 RM = Wt.(1.149) + 0.7119 1 RM = Wt.(1.175) + # reps (0.839) − 4.2978 (used in untrained women)
Mayhew et al (49)	1 RM = Wt./{[52.2 + 41.9e$^{-0.055(\# reps)}$]/100} %1 RM = 52.2 + 41.9e$^{-0.055(\# reps)}$
O'Connor et al. (53)	1 RM = Wt. (1 + 0.025 × # reps)
Wathen (73)	1 RM = 100 × Wt./[48.8 + 53.8e$^{-0.075(\# reps)}$]
Abadie et al. (1)	1 RM = 8.8147 + 1.1828(7–10 RM)

Myths & Misconceptions

Maximal Strength Testing is Dangerous and Should Only Be Used Sparingly

In some cases there is a general fear of injuring athletes with maximal strength testing. Some coaches prefer prediction of 1 RM strength or using multiple RMs in lieu of maximal strength testing. However, research has consistently shown strength testing to be safe. In fact, strength testing is safe in clinical populations as well. Very few injuries have occurred during strength testing and the major reasons for injury include a lack of supervision or proper spotting, accident, or perhaps the athlete was overtrained or already injured and prone to joint/muscle injuries or worsening a preinjury. Therefore, strength testing is not dangerous when performed correctly and serves as a valuable asset to the athlete. The decision of how and when to strength test athletes belongs to the coach and should fit within the periodized annual training plan. Although safe, strength testing should not be overused either. Frequent strength testing can disrupt the training plan and forces the athlete into heavy lifting during nonmaximal strength or power training phases. Rather, strength testing should be included at strategic periods where the athlete is in peak condition, *e.g.*, the end of off-season training.

showed that at 80% of 1 RM, double the number of repetitions could be performed for the leg press compared to the leg curl. The amount of muscle mass used and the selection of a free weight or machine for the same exercise affect the accuracy.

MUSCLE ENDURANCE

Local muscle endurance tests involve measuring the ability of a selected muscles to perform repeated contractions over time. The contractions can be low to moderate in intensity (*submaximal endurance*) or high in intensity (*high-intensity endurance*). Muscle endurance tests typically come in three categories: (a) performing body weight exercises for a maximal number of repetitions or maximal number of repetitions in a specified time; (b) repetitions for a weight training exercise at an absolute percentage of 1 RM; and (c) sustained maximal duration trials.

Body Weight Exercises

The most common exercises assessed are the partial curl-up, push-up, sit-up, and pull-up. Other exercises such as dips and body weight squats have been used. For the partial curl-up test:

- The athlete lies flat on a mat with arms at the side and knees flexed to 90°. An index card can be placed horizontally at the finger tips. The index card is used to standardize ROM.
- With a metronome set to 50 beats · min^{-1} (to allow 25 curl-ups), the athlete performs curl-ups in a slow manner to the metronome. Shoulder blades are lifted off of the mat (~30°) and the finger tips must surpass the edge of the index card in order for a repetition to count. The athlete performs as many repetitions as possible without pausing. Failure to maintain the pace or ROM are criteria to end the test.

- A variation is to perform this test using conventional sit-ups. The athlete can perform as many sit-ups as possible in 1 minute (although some assessments allow 2 minutes). Here, the athlete gently keeps hands behind his/her head while a partner supports his/her ankles.

The push-up test is performed in a similar manner:

- For men, a standard push-up position is used for the test. For women, a modified push-up used where knees are placed on the ground and the ankles are crossed.
- Athletes then proceed to perform as many push-ups as possible in good form. Some tests may pose a time limit on the athlete (2 minutes for the Army standard test). A repetition only counts when full ROM is attained (nearly touching the chest to the ground at the bottom position). An object can be placed low to mark the touching point, *i.e.*, rolled up towel or a tester's fist when assessing male athletes.

Pull-ups can be performed where the athlete must pull his/her body high enough to where the chin surpasses the bar.

Tables 18.8 and 18.9 present norms for the partial curl-up and push-up tests, respectively. Table 18.10 depicts norms for pull-ups in college men. Table 18.11 depicts norms for traditional sit-up performance.

Absolute Repetition Number

Weight training exercises can be performed for a maximal number of repetitions with a standard load. An important consideration is the resistance to use. Relative loading is based on a percentage of the individual's RM capability, whereas absolute loading has the same resistance for all athletes and all tests (the 225-lb max rep bench press performed at NFL combines for football prospects). For pre- to posttesting, relative muscle endurance performance does not change. Thus, absolute loading is recommended as an increase in the number of repetitions performed is

TABLE 18.8 PERCENTILES FOR PARTIAL CURL-UPS BY AGE GROUPS AND SEX

| | AGE AND SEX | | | | | | | | | |
| | 20–29 | | 30–39 | | 40–49 | | 50–59 | | 60–69 | |
PERCENTILE[a]	M	F	M	F	M	F	M	F	M	F
90	75	70	75	55	75	50	74	48	53	50
80	56	45	69	43	75	42	60	30	33	30
70	41	37	46	34	67	33	45	23	26	24
60	31	32	36	28	51	28	35	16	19	19
50	27	27	31	21	39	25	27	9	16	13
40	24	21	26	15	31	20	23	2	9	9
30	20	17	19	12	26	14	19	0	6	3
20	13	12	13	0	21	5	13	0	0	0
10	4	5	0	0	13	0	0	0	0	0

[a]Descriptors for percentile rankings: 90, well above average; 70, above average; 50, average; 30, below average; 10, well below average.
Reprinted with permission from Thompson W, editor. *ACSM's Guidelines for Exercise Testing and Prescription.* 8th ed. Baltimore, (MD): Lippincott Williams & Wilkins; 2010

TABLE 18.9 FITNESS CATEGORIES FOR PUSH-UPS BY AGE GROUPS AND SEX

| | AGE AND SEX | | | | | | | | | |
| | 20–29 | | 30–39 | | 40–49 | | 50–59 | | 60–69 | |
CATEGORY	M	F	M	F	M	F	M	F	M	F
Excellent	36	30	30	27	25	24	21	21	18	17
Very good	35	29	29	26	24	23	20	20	17	16
	29	21	22	20	17	15	13	11	11	12
Good	28	20	21	19	16	14	12	10	10	11
	22	15	17	13	13	11	10	7	8	5
Fair	21	14	16	12	12	10	9	6	7	4
	17	10	12	8	10	5	7	2	5	2
Needs improvement	16	9	11	7	9	4	6	1	4	1

Reprinted with permission from Thompson W, editor. *ACSM's Guidelines for Exercise Testing and Prescription.* 8th ed. Baltimore, (MD): Lippincott Williams & Wilkins; 2010.

TABLE 18.10 PULL-UP NORMS FOR COLLEGE MEN

CLASSIFICATION	NUMBER OF PULL-UPS
Excellent	15+
Good	12–14
Average	8–11
Fair	5–7
Poor	0–4

Reprinted with permission from Hoffman J. *Norms for Fitness, Performance, and Health.* Champaign (IL): Human Kinetics; 2006. pp. 1–113.

TABLE 18.11 YMCA NORMS FOR THE SIT-UP TEST IN ADULTS

PERCENTILE	18–25 Y		26–35 Y		36–45 Y		46–55 Y		56–65 Y		>65 Y	
	M	*F*	*M*	*F*	*M*	*F*	*M*	*F*	*M*	*F*	*M*	*F*
90	77	68	62	54	60	54	61	48	56	44	50	34
80	66	61	56	46	52	44	53	40	49	38	40	32
70	57	57	52	41	45	38	51	36	46	32	35	29
60	52	51	44	37	43	35	44	33	41	27	31	26
50	46	44	38	34	36	31	39	31	36	24	27	22
40	41	38	36	32	32	28	33	28	32	22	24	20
30	37	34	33	28	29	23	29	25	28	18	22	16
20	33	32	30	24	25	20	24	21	24	12	19	11
10	27	25	21	20	21	16	16	13	20	8	12	9

Reprinted with permission from Hoffman J. *Norms for Fitness, Performance, and Health.* Champaign (IL): Human Kinetics; 2006. pp. 1–113.

seen with training. For most individuals, the relationship between strength and absolute muscular endurance is positive, whereas the relationship between strength and relative endurance is negative (43). Any exercise can be used for endurance testing. A specific load needs to be applied among all athletes and test performance is predicated upon the maximal number of repetitions performed with that load. This could be a certain percentage of the athlete's pretesting max or a specific load. Norms can be developed with a large number of athletes performing the test over time. One example is the YMCA Bench Press test (Table 18.12):

- The loading for the bench press is 80 lb for men and 35 lb for women. A metronome is set at 60 beats · min⁻¹ to yield ~30 reps per minute.
- The athlete performs as many repetitions as possible with proper form and ROM (touching the bar to chest). Failing to perform the repetitions in proper ROM, fatigue, and inability to maintain cadence are criteria to terminate the test.

Sustained Maximal Duration Trials

Sustained maximal duration trials usually involve an ISOM muscle action held for maximal time. Many variations can be performed but there are few norms published in athletes. We have used endurance tests including maximal ISOM elbow flexion (90°) against a standard load and grip endurance test where individuals hold or maintain a position against a load for maximal time. One sustained maximal duration test is the *flexed-arm hang.* The flexed-arm hang (Table 18.13) measures the amount of time an athlete can maintain the final ISOM pull-up position. That is, the athlete maintains his/her position with chin above the bar for as long as possible. Failure to maintain position is criteria for test termination. This test is greatly affected by the athlete's body weight and level of strength.

FLEXIBILITY

Flexibility depends on several factors including tendon and ligament stiffness, muscle viscosity and bulk, distensibility of the joint capsule, and muscle temperature. Flexibility is joint specific so no single test can measure total-body flexibility (4). Flexibility can be assessed by goniometers, electrogoniometers, a Leighton flexometer, inclinometer, and a tape measure. Goniometers (Fig. 18.5) are most practical as a plastic goniometer is inexpensive and easy to use to assess static flexibility. It acts similar to a protractor. The center of the goniometer is placed at the joint axis of rotation and the arms are aligned with the bony segments. The Leighton flexometer is a type of gravity-based

TABLE 18.12 YMCA BENCH PRESS NORMS

% RANK	18–25 Y		26–35 Y		36–45 Y		46–55 Y		56–65 Y		>65 Y	
	M	F	M	F	M	F	M	F	M	F	M	F
95	42	42	40	40	34	32	28	30	24	30	20	22
75	30	28	26	25	24	21	20	20	14	16	10	12
50	22	20	20	17	17	13	12	11	8	9	6	6
25	13	12	12	9	10	8	6	5	4	3	2	2
5	2	2	2	1	2	1	1	0	0	0	0	0

Number of repetitions in 1 min using 80 lb (36.3 kg) for men and 35 lb (15.9 kg) for women.

TABLE 18.13 FLEXED-ARM HANG STANDARDS FOR YOUTH

PERCENTILE	AGE (Y)											
	6	7	8	9	10	11	12	13	14	15	16	17+
Boys												
90	16	23	28	28	38	37	36	37	61	62	61	56
80	12	17	18	20	25	26	25	29	40	49	46	45
70	9	13	15	16	20	19	19	22	31	40	39	39
60	8	10	12	12	15	15	15	18	25	35	33	35
50	6	8	10	10	12	11	12	14	20	30	28	30
40	5	6	8	8	8	9	9	10	15	25	22	26
30	3	4	5	5	6	6	6	8	11	20	18	20
20	2	3	3	3	3	4	4	5	8	14	12	15
10	1	1	1	2	1	1	1	2	3	8	7	8
Girls												
90	15	21	21	23	29	25	27	28	31	34	30	29
80	11	14	15	16	19	16	16	19	21	23	21	20
70	9	11	11	12	14	13	13	14	16	15	16	15
60	6	8	10	10	11	9	10	10	11	10	10	11
50	5	6	8	8	8	7	7	8	9	7	7	7
40	4	5	6	6	6	5	5	5	6	5	5	5
30	3	4	4	4	4	4	3	4	4	4	3	4
20	1	2	3	2	2	2	1	1	2	2	2	2
10	0	0	0	0	0	0	0	0	0	1	0	1

Note: Time listed in seconds.

Adapted by permission from Presidents Council for Physical Fitness, Presidents Challenge Normative Data Spreadsheet (online). Available at www.presidentschallenge.org.

goniometer used to measure flexibility Inclinometers measure the angles of slope and therefore can be used to assess joint ROM. Both inclinometers and flexometers can be strapped to the athlete or held by hand and the ROM is recorded. Electrogoniometers are attached to body segments and can measure static and dynamic ROM. These are used in laboratory settings. Joint ROM can be assessed in angular motion terms (degrees or

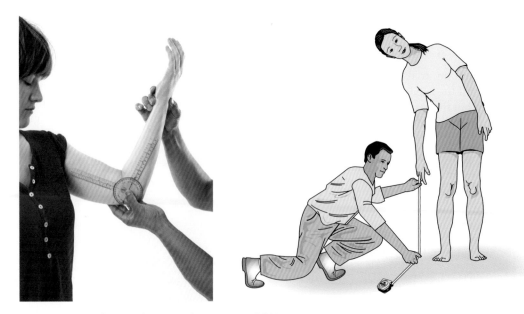

FIGURE 18.5. Plastic goniometer and tape measure ROM measurement.

TABLE 18.14 AVERAGE RANGES OF JOINT MOTION

JOINT	JOINT MOTION	ROM (DEGREES)
Hip	Flexion	90–125
	Hyperextension	10–30
	Abduction	40–45
	Adduction	10–30
	Internal rotation	35–45
	External rotation	45–50
Knee	Flexion	120–150
	Rotation (when flexed)	40–50
Ankle	Plantar flexion	20–45
	Dorsiflexion	15–30
Shoulder	Flexion	130–180
	Hyperextension	30–80
	Abduction	170–180
	Adduction	50
	Internal rotation	60–90
	External rotation	70–90
	Horizontal flexion	135
	Horizontal extension*	45
Elbow	Flexion	140–160
Radioulnar	Forearm pronation (from midposition)	80–90
	Forearm supination (from midposition)	80–90
Cervical spine	Flexion	40–60
	Hyperextension	40–75
	Lateral flexion	40–45
	Rotation	50–80
Thoracolumbar spine	Flexion	45–75
	Hyperextension	20–35
	Lateral flexion	25–35
	Rotation	30–45

Reprinted with permission from Hoffman J. *Norms for Fitness, Performance, and Health*. Champaign, (IL): Human Kinetics; 2006: pp. 1–113.

radians) and linear terms (inches, centimeters) with use of a tape measure (Fig. 18.5). Table 18.14 presents normal joint ROM for eight major joints in the human body.

Perhaps the most common indirect assessment of flexibility is the *sit-and-reach test*. It is used to assess lower back, gluteal, and hamstring muscle flexibility (mostly hamstring flexibility) (4). This test is not only affected by flexibility but may also rely upon abdominal girth and limb/torso lengths. Thus, a *modified sit-and-reach test* is used which establishes a zero point based on limb/torso lengths (Fig. 18.6). The procedures for the modified sit-and-reach are:

- A sit-and-reach box or tape measure/stick is needed. Following a proper warm-up, the athlete sits shoeless with feet against the sit-and-reach box. The athlete's starting position is determined by having the athlete place arms together with right hand over left hand, feet flat against the box with knees fully extended, and back against the wall. The athlete reaches forward by protracting only the shoulder girdle to determine the starting position. This calibrates the starting point and limits limb/torso length bias.

- While keeping the knees extended, the athlete slowly bends at the waist forward as far as possible (without bouncing) and pushes the sliding device maximally to achieve the greatest ROM possible. This final position is held momentarily. It is important to make sure the athlete keeps feet flat against box, does not bend knees, and does not ballistically reach when performing the test. The score is recorded.

- The best of three trials is recorded. If the best trial is the third trial, then additional 1–2 trials can be given. This may occur if the warm-up is insufficient. Table 18.15

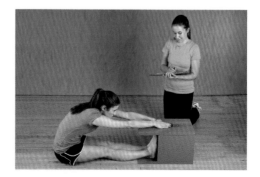

■ **FIGURE 18.6.** The sit-and-reach test.

TABLE 18.15 SIT-AND-REACH TEST SCORES

	SIT AND REACH TEST SCORES							
	MEN				WOMEN			
PERCENTILE RANK	20–29 YR		30–39 YR		20–29 YR		30–39 YR	
	IN.	CM	IN.	CM	IN.	CM	IN.	CM
99	>23.0	>58	>22.0	>56	>24.0	>61	>24.0	>61
90	21.75	55	21.0	53	23.75	60	22.5	57
80	20.5	52	19.5	50	22.5	57	21.5	55
70	19.5	50	18.5	47	21.5	55	20.5	52
60	18.5	47	17.5	44	20.5	52	20.0	51
50	17.5	44	16.5	42	20.0	51	19.0	48
40	16.5	42	15.5	39	19.25	49	18.25	46
30	15.5	39	14.5	37	18.25	46	17.25	44
20	14.5	37	13.0	33	17.0	43	16.5	42
10	12.25	31	11.0	28	15.5	39	14.5	37
01	<10.5	<27	<9.25	<23	<14.0	<36	<12.0	<30

Reprinted with permission from Thompson W, editor. *ACSM's Guidelines for Exercise Testing and Prescription.* 8th ed. Baltimore (MD): Lippincott Williams & Wilkins; 2010.

depicts percentile rank norms for modified sit-and-reach performance data for men and women.

Another test is the *trunk rotation test.* This can be performed with essentially no equipment or a specialized device (an Acuflex rotation tester). The procedures are:

- A vertical line is marked on a wall. The athlete stands with his/her back to the wall (with a shoulder width stance) at approximately arms length away.
- The athlete rotates to the right as far as possible (with arms straight in front and parallel to floor), touches the wall, and this position is marked. The athlete then rotates to the left, touches the wall, and the position is marked. Feet must remain stationary while trunk, shoulders, and knees are free to move.
- The distance from the line is measured. A positive score is one where the mark exceeds the vertical line and a mark before the vertical line indicates a negative score.
- *Scoring:* >20 cm = excellent; 15–20 cm = very good; 10–15 cm = good; 5–10 cm = fair; 0–5 cm (or a negative score) = poor.

AEROBIC CAPACITY

Aerobic capacity assessments estimate Vo_{2max}. Because most athletes and coaches will not have access to metabolic carts to directly assess maximal aerobic capacity, prediction from field tests is most practical. These tests have been validated and typically require variables such as heart rate (HR) or test time to predict Vo_{2max}. Estimates of Vo_{2max} from the HR response to exercise are based on the assumptions that a steady-state HR is

obtained for each work rate, a linear relationship exists between HR and work rate, the max work load achieved is indicative of the Vo_{2max}, max HR for a given age is uniform, and mechanical efficiency is similar between athletes (4). In some cases (1.5-mile run) several athletes can be tested simultaneously. Critical to the accuracy of these estimates is the effort level put forth by the athlete. Aerobic capacity can be underestimated if the athlete does not perform with maximal effort. The most common modes include field tests, cycle ergometer/treadmill, and step tests.

Field Tests

Field tests include running and walking assessments of fixed length or a specified time. Three common running field tests are the 1.5-mile run, 12-minute run, and the multistage 20-m shuttle run tests. The procedures are as follows:

- *1.5-Mile Run* — this test is commonly performed on a quarter-mile track. Following a proper warm-up, the athlete(s) begin at the starting line and runs as rapidly as possible (at a steady pace) for 6 laps (1.5 miles) until crossing the finish line. The coach (with a stopwatch) begins timing on "go" and stops timing when the athlete crosses the finish line. The time is recorded. Vo_{2max} can be estimated by the following equation:

$$(Vo_{2max} \text{ of } (mL \cdot kg^{-1} \cdot min^{-1}) = 3.5 + (483/\text{run time in minutes})$$

Or can be estimated with gender-specific equations (34):

Men: Vo_{2max} (mL · kg^{-1} · min^{-1}) = 91.736
− (0.1656 × body mass in kilograms) − (2.767
× run time in min)

Women: Vo_{2max} (mL · kg^{-1} · min^{-1}) = 88.020
− (0.1656 × body mass in kilograms) − (2.767
× run time in minutes)

- *Cooper 12-Minute Run* — this test is performed on a track with markings at each 100-m interval. The athletes begin at the starting line and upon the signal "go," run as rapidly as possible (at a steady pace) for 12 minutes. Upon the signal to "stop," the distance the athlete successfully completed is measured. For example, 6.5 laps = 2,600 m. The distance is recorded. Vo_{2max} can be estimated by the following equation:

$$(Vo_{2max} \text{ of (mL · kg}^{-1} \text{ · min}^{-1}) = 0.0268 \text{ (distance covered)} - 11.3$$

- *Multistage 20-m Shuttle Run* — has variations and is known as the *beep test* or Progressive Aerobic CV Endurance Run (PACER) test as it has been adapted to other segments of the population (children and adolescents) since its development in the early 1980s (45). A flat, nonslippery area marked with parallel lines or cones separated by exactly 20 m and the beep test CD/multimedia package are needed for this field test. A shorter 15-m variation can be used if athletes are tested in a small facility (which requires a conversion chart). A scorekeeper is used to record completed laps/shuttles. The CD provides audio cues (beeps) that allow the athlete to set a pace during running. The athlete continuously runs between the two lines or cones (touching the line each time) at a pace based on the stage or level of the test. For example, a beep starts the test, the athlete runs 20 m, and returns 20 m upon the next beep. Sufficient pacing is important to ensure that athletes do not overwork during initial stages. The test is progressive where the beeps are closer together with each successive stage thereby forcing the athlete to run at a faster pace until the athlete can no longer maintain the pace. There are ~21 levels each lasting a minute with most athletes completing between 6 and 15. An additional sound or triple beep may be used to indicate completion of a level. The test ends when athletes can no longer keep pace with the beeps on two successive trials. Athletes should be allowed multiple practice sessions before testing to familiarize themselves to the beep cadence. The final score is the level (indicated by the number or corresponding velocity) or number of laps attained before athlete cannot maintain pace for successive shuttles. There are different variations of the test. The original version developed by Leger and Lambert (45) begins with a starting velocity of 8.0 km · h^{-1} and progresses 0.5 km · h^{-1} with each stage (every 2 min) of the test. Another variation using adults and children begins with a starting velocity of 8.5 km · h^{-1} and progresses 0.5 km · h^{-1} with each minute (stage) of the test (46). Other studies were conducted that allowed prediction of Vo_{2max} from the number of levels completed (58) and number of laps/shuttles completed (55). Validity and test-retest reliability of the test are good (45,55,58) with reliability being greater in adults than children (46). Research shows that men (Vo_{2max} of ~58–59 mL · kg^{-1} · min^{-1}) complete an average of 11.4–12.6 levels with 105–121 total shuttles (laps) and women (Vo_{2max} of ~47.4 mL · kg^{-1} · min^{-1}) complete an average of 9.6 levels with 85 total shuttles (55,58). Vo_{2max} can be estimated using the following equations:

Adults (mean age of 26 yr): (Vo_{2max} of (mL · kg^{-1} · min^{-1}) = 5.857(speed in km · h^{-1}) −19.458 (45)

Adults and children (8–19 yr): Vo_{2max} (mL · kg^{-1} · min^{-1}) = 31.025 + 3.238 (speed in km h^{-1})− 3.248(age in years) + 0.1536 (age in years × speed in km · h^{-1}) where speed begins at 8.0 + 0.5(stage number) (46)

Adults (19–36 yr): Vo_{2max} (mL · kg^{-1} · min^{-1}) = 14.4 + 3.48(level completed) where level completed (number) is the last fully completed stage of the test (58)

Men (26–47 yr): Vo_{2max} (mL · kg^{-1} · min^{-1}) = 18 + 0.39(laps or shuttles completed) (55) —Note: this equation is based on a small number (9) of subjects.

Norms for the 1.5-mile run and 12-minute run tests are presented in Table 18.16 and Vo_{2max} norms are presented in Table 18.17.

Cycle Ergometer Tests

Cycle ergometer tests are single- or multistage submaximal tests where Vo_{2max} is predicted from exercise HR. Accurate assessment of HR is mandatory. A HR monitor is preferred. Palpation can be used but introduces a large magnitude of error. Factors that affect HR (hot/humid temperature, caffeine, stress) must be controlled for greater accuracy. Two common cycle ergometer tests are the Astrand-Rhyming and YMCA tests.

- *Astrand-Rhyming Test* — is a single-stage submaximal test lasting 6 minutes in duration. The pedal rate is standardized at 50 rpm. HR is measured after the first 2 minutes. If HR ≥120 bpm the athlete continues at the initial work rate. If HR ≤120 bpm the athlete increases work rate to the next increment level. HR is measured during the fifth and sixth minutes of the exercise and averaged to be used in the nomogram

TABLE 18.16. PERCENTILE RANKS FOR DISTANCE RUN DURING 12-MIN RUN (*TOP*) AND FOR 1.5-MILE (2.41-KM) RUN TIME (MIN:S) (*BOTTOM*)

DISTANCE RUN DURING 12-MIN RUN

	AGE (Y)									
PERCENTILE	20–29		30–39		40–49		50–59		60+	
MEN	N = 1,675		N = 7,095		N = 6,837		N = 3,808		N = 1,005	
	ML	KM	ML	KM	ML	KM	ML	KM	ML	KM
90	1.74	2.78	1.71	2.74	1.65	2.64	1.57	2.51	1.49	2.38
80	1.65	2.64	1.61	2.58	1.54	2.46	1.45	2.32	1.37	2.19
70	1.61	2.58	1.55	2.48	1.47	2.35	1.38	2.21	1.29	2.06
60	1.54	2.46	1.49	2.38	1.42	2.27	1.33	2.13	1.24	1.98
50	1.50	2.40	1.45	2.32	1.37	2.19	1.29	2.06	1.19	1.90
40	1.45	2.32	1.39	2.22	1.33	2.13	1.25	2.00	1.15	1.84
30	1.41	2.26	1.35	2.16	1.29	2.06	1.21	1.94	1.11	1.78
20	1.34	2.14	1.29	2.06	1.23	1.97	1.15	1.84	1.05	1.68
10	1.27	2.03	1.21	1.94	1.17	1.87	1.09	1.74	0.95	1.52
WOMEN	N = 764		N = 2,049		N = 1,630		N = 878		N = 202	
90	1.54	2.46	1.45	2.32	1.41	2.26	1.29	2.06	1.29	2.06
80	1.45	2.32	1.38	2.21	1.32	2.11	1.21	1.94	1.18	1.89
70	1.37	2.19	1.33	2.13	1.25	2.00	1.17	1.87	1.13	1.81
60	1.33	2.13	1.27	2.03	1.21	1.94	1.13	1.81	1.07	1.71
50	1.29	2.06	1.25	2.00	1.17	1.87	1.10	1.76	1.03	1.65
40	1.25	2.00	1.21	1.94	1.13	1.81	1.06	1.70	0.99	1.58
30	1.21	1.94	1.16	1.86	1.10	1.76	1.02	1.63	0.97	1.55
20	1.16	1.86	1.11	1.78	1.05	1.68	0.98	1.57	0.94	1.50
10	1.10	1.76	1.05	1.68	1.01	1.62	0.93	1.49	0.89	1.42

1.5 MI (2.41 KM) RUN TIME (MIN:S)

| | AGE (Y) | | | | |
| PERCENTILE | 20–29 | 30–39 | 40–49 | 50–59 | 60+ |
MEN	N = 1,675	N = 7,095	N = 6,837	N = 3,808	N = 1,005
90	9:09	9:30	10:16	11:18	12:20
80	10:16	10:47	11:44	12:51	13:53
70	10:47	11:34	12:34	13:45	14:53
60	11:41	12:20	13:14	14:24	15:29
50	12:18	12:51	13:53	14:55	16:07
40	12:51	13:36	14:29	15:26	16:43
30	13:22	14:08	14:56	15:57	17:14
20	14:13	14:52	15:41	16:43	18:00
10	15:10	15:52	16:28	17:29	19:15
WOMEN	N = 764	N = 2,049	N = 1,630	N = 878	N = 202
90	11:43	12:51	13:22	14:55	14:55
80	12:51	13:43	14:31	15:57	16:20
70	13:53	14:24	15:16	16:27	16:58
60	14:24	15:08	15:57	16:58	17:46
50	14:55	15:26	16:27	17:24	18:16
40	15:26	15:57	16:58	17:55	18:44
30	15:57	16:35	17:24	18:23	18:59
20	16:33	17:14	18:00	18:49	19:21
10	17:21	18:00	18:31	19:30	20:04

Reprinted with permission from Hoffman J. *Norms for Fitness, Performance, and Health*. Champaign (IL): Human Kinetics; 2006. pp. 1–113.

TABLE 18.17 PERCENTILE VALUES FOR MAXIMAL AEROBIC POWER (ML · KG · MIN⁻¹)

PERCENTILE	AGE (Y)				
	20–29	30–39	40–49	50–59	60+
MEN					
90	51.4	50.4	48.2	45.3	42.5
80	48.2	46.8	44.1	41.0	38.1
70	46.8	44.6	41.8	38.5	35.3
60	44.2	42.4	39.9	36.7	33.6
50	42.5	41.0	38.1	35.2	31.8
40	41.0	38.9	36.7	33.8	30.2
30	39.5	37.4	35.1	32.3	28.7
20	37.1	35.4	33.0	30.2	26.5
10	34.5	32.5	30.9	28.0	23.1
WOMEN					
90	44.2	41.0	39.5	35.2	35.2
80	41.0	38.6	36.3	32.3	31.2
70	38.1	36.7	33.8	30.9	29.4
60	36.7	34.6	32.3	29.4	27.2
50	35.2	33.8	30.9	28.2	25.8
40	33.8	32.3	29.5	26.9	24.5
30	32.3	30.5	28.3	25.5	23.8
20	30.6	28.7	26.5	24.3	22.8
10	28.4	26.5	25.1	22.3	20.8

Reprinted with permission from Hoffman J. *Norms for Fitness, Performance, and Health.* Champaign (IL): Human Kinetics; 2006. pp. 1–113.

(Fig. 18.7). Vo_{2max} data must then be corrected for age using the nomogram in Table 18.18 (4). The workload varies in the following manner:

- Untrained men: 300 or 600 kg · m · min⁻¹ (50 or 100 W)
- Trained men: 600 or 900 kg · m · min⁻¹ (100 or 150 W)
- Untrained women: 300 or 450 kg · m · min⁻¹ (50 or 75 W)
- Trained women: 450 or 600 kg · m · min⁻¹ (75 or 100 W)
- *YMCA Submaximal Cycle Ergometer Test* — this test consists of 2–4 stages that last 3 minutes each. The initial workload is set at 150 kg · m · min⁻¹ (Fig. 18.8). The workload for the second stage depends on the HR measured in the last minute of the first stage. The HR measured during the last minute of each stage is plotted against work rate. The line is then extrapolated to the athlete's age-predicted maximal HR and a perpendicular line (b) is dropped to the axis to determine work rate (29,30) (Fig. 18.9). The work rate in kg m min⁻¹ is converted to watts using the following formula:

$$Work \ rate \ (W) = work \ rate \ (kg \cdot m \cdot min^{-1})/6.12$$

Using the athlete's body mass (kg) Vo_{2max} is calculated via the following equation:

$$Vo_{2max} - ([10.8 \times work \ rate]/body \ mass) + 7$$

Step Tests

Several step tests have been developed over the years. These involve different step heights, rates, and stage durations. Heart rate is typically used in the prediction of Vo_{2max}. One example is the Queens College step test developed by McArdle et al. (51):

- *Queens College Step Test* — males and females use step height of 16.25 in. However, the step rate in men is 24 steps min⁻¹ and women is 22 steps min⁻¹ set to a metronome. The duration of the test is 3 minutes and HR is taken at the conclusion of the test. Vo_{2max} is calculated via the following equations:

$$Vo_{2max} \ (men) = 111.33 - (0.42 \times HR)$$

$$Vo_{2max} \ (women) = 65.81 - (0.1847 \times HR)$$

ASSESSMENT OF SKILL-RELATED FITNESS COMPONENTS

Testing of several skill-related components of fitness is paramount to a comprehensive testing battery for athletes. These include peak power, anaerobic capacity, speed, agility, balance, and functional performance.

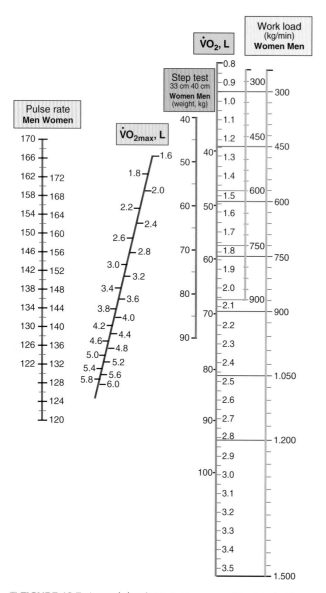

POWER

Power testing is critical to assessing anaerobic athletes. Power is the rate of performing work and is the product of force and velocity. Tests of peak power are explosive and short in duration (a few seconds) and predominantly stress the ATP-PC system. Some of these peak power tests include 1 RM Olympic lifts, jump tests, jump squats on force plate or transducer, medicine ball throws, Margaria-Kalamen test, and rate of force development (RFD) tests. Other tests measure power endurance, *i.e., anaerobic capacity* tests. These track power over time (Wingate test) or measure the amount of time it takes to complete a pattern of movement (300-yd shuttle and line drill). Because these tests are longer in duration (15–90 s), they stress the glycolytic energy system so the maintenance of power is most critical.

Vertical and Broad Jumps

Jump tests are predicated upon the correlation between power and jump height or distance. They are easy to administer and provide valuable information relating to athletic success. This section discusses two jump tests, the vertical and broad jumps although other types of jumps can be assessed.

Vertical Jump

- A tape measure, chalk, or special device like the *Vertec* is needed.
- When using a wall (*Sargent jump test*) the athlete stands against a wall with dominant arm flexed vertically as high as possible. The athlete has chalk on his/her fingers. Thus, the initial step is to determine the starting height as the athlete reaches high, touches the wall, and sets the starting height. Using a countermovement, the athlete jumps as high as possible and touches the highest possible point on the wall (marking it with chalk on the fingertips). The distance between marks is measured. The best of three trials is recorded.

FIGURE 18.7. Astrand-rhyming test nomogram. (Reprinted with permission from Astrand PO, Ryhming I. A nomogram for calculation of aerobic capacity [physical fitness] from pulse rate during submaximal work. *J Appl Physiol*. 1954;7:218–221.)

TABLE 18.18 AGE CORRECTION FACTOR FOR THE ASTRAND-RHYMING CYCLE ERGOMETER TEST

AGE	CORRECTION FACTOR
15	1.10
25	1.00
35	0.87
40	0.83
45	0.78
50	0.75
55	0.71
60	0.68
65	0.65

1st stage	150 kgm/min (0.5 kg)		
	HR: <80	**HR: 80–89**	**HR: 90–100**	**HR: >100**

	HR: <80	**HR: 80–89**	**HR: 90–100**	**HR: >100**
2nd stage	750 kgm/min (2.5 kg)*	600 kgm/min (2.0 kg)	450 kgm/min (1.5 kg)	300 kgm/min (1.0 kg)
3rd stage	900 kgm/min (3.0 kg)	750 kgm/min (2.5 kg)	600 kgm/min (2.0 kg)	450 kgm/min (1.5 kg)
4th stage	1050 kgm/min (3.5 kg)	900 kgm/min (3.0 kg)	750 kgm/min (2.5 kg)	600 kgm/min (2.0 kg)

Directions:

1 Set the 1st work rate at 150 kgm/min (0.5 kg at 50 rpm)

2 If the HR in the third minute of the stage is:
    <80, set the 2nd stage at 750 kgm/min (2.5 kg at 50 rpm)
    80–89, set the 2nd stage at 600 kgm/min (2.0 kg at 50 rpm)
    90–100, set the 2nd stage at 450 kgm/min (1.5 kg at 50 rpm)
    >100, set the 2nd stage at 300 kgm/min (1.0 kg at 50 rpm)

3 Set the 3rd and 4th (if required) according to the work rates in the columns below the 2nd loads

FIGURE 18.8. YMCA cycle ergometer test workload stages. (Reprinted with permission from Thompson W, ed. *ACSM's Guidelines for Exercise Testing and Prescription*. 8th ed. Baltimore (MD): Lippincott Williams & Wilkins; 2010.)

- When using a Vertec, the athlete sets the starting position. The Vertec is adjustable and has color-coded vanes (Fig. 18.10). The very first vane marks the reading on the Vertec. A red vane is placed every 6 in., and blue and white vanes are 1 in. apart, marking whole and half inch measures, respectively. The athlete stands erect with the dominant arm flexed vertically as high as possible and touches (and moves) the corresponding vanes. This demarcates the starting height. For testers, it is important to make sure the athlete extends the body as far as possible (without rising on the toes) or the vertical jump height can be overexaggerated. The height of the Vertec is adjusted (raised) so that the athlete will touch and move a vane (and not the top one) when jumping maximally. Using a countermovement, the athlete jumps as high as possible touching the highest possible vanes. The highest vane touched demarcates the finish height. For subsequent jump trials, it is advantageous for the coach to leave 1–2 vanes (0.5–1.0 in.) under the highest one attained in place. This gives the athlete a target height to shoot for when jumping maximally. Starting height is subtracted from the finish height and the difference is the vertical jump height. The best of three trials is recorded. If the third trial is the best, then a fourth (or fifth) trial should be used.

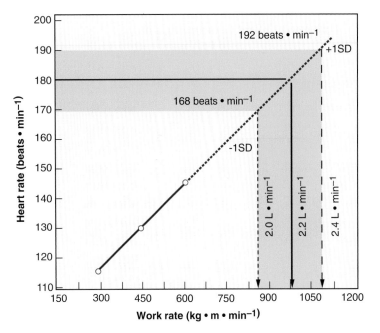

FIGURE 18.9. Relationship between HR and work rate in relation to max aerobic capacity; b = extrapolated work rate. (Reprinted with permission from Thompson W, ed. *ACSM's Guidelines for Exercise Testing and Prescription*. 8th ed. Baltimore (MD): Lippincott Williams & Wilkins; 2010.)

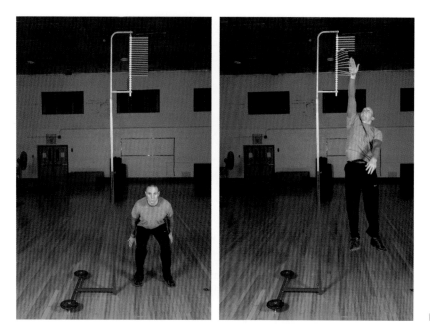

FIGURE 18.10. Vertical jump with a Vertec.

- Power can be calculated from vertical jump height. This can be useful for differentiating between two athletes with similar vertical jump heights. Originally, the *Lewis formula* was used to estimate peak power from vertical jump height using the following equation:

$$Power\ (W) = [\sqrt{4.9} \times body\ mass\ (kg) \times 9.807] \times [\sqrt{jump\ height\ (m)}]$$

However, cross-validation against jumps from a force plate showed that the Lewis formula underestimated mean and peak power by up to 70% (30). Since, other equations have been developed. Harman et al. (24) developed the following accurate regression equations for estimating peak and mean power during the vertical jump:

$$Peak\ power\ (W) = 61.9(jump\ height\ in\ cm) + 36(body\ mass\ in\ kg) + 1,822$$

$$Mean\ power\ (W) = 21.1(jump\ height\ in\ cm) + 23(body\ mass\ in\ kg) + 1,393$$

Johnson and Bahamonde (41) developed the following equations:

$$Peak\ power\ (W) = 78.6(jump\ height\ in\ cm) + 60.3(mass\ in\ kg) + 15.3(ht\ in\ cm) - 15.3(ht\ in\ cm) - 1,308$$

$$Mean\ power\ (W) = 43.8(jump\ height\ in\ cm) + 32.7(mass\ in\ kg) - 16.8(ht\ in\ cm) + 431$$

Sayers et al. (64) developed the following equation:

$$Peak\ power\ (W) = 60.7(jump\ height\ in\ cm) + 45.3(mass\ in\ kg) - 2,055$$

Norms for vertical jump performance in athletes are presented in Table 18.19.

TABLE 18.19 VERTICAL JUMP NORMS FOR ATHLETES

% RANK	MEN (CM)	WOMEN (CM)
91–100	86.35–91.45	76.20–81.30
81–90	81.30–86.34	71.11–76.19
71–80	76.20–81.29	66.05–71.10
61–70	71.10–76.19	60.95–66.04
51–60	66.05–71.09	55.90–60.94
41–50	60.95–66.04	50.80–55.89
31–40	55.90–60.94	45.70–50.79
21–30	50.80–55.89	40.65–45.70
11–20	45.70–50.79	35.55–40.64
1–10	40.65–45.69	30.50–35.54

Reprinted with permission from Chu DA. *Explosive Power and Strength*. Champaign (IL): Human Kinetics; 1996. pp. 167–180.

TABLE 18.20 BROAD JUMP NORMS FOR ATHLETES

% RANK	MEN (M)	WOMEN (M)
91–100	3.40–3.75	2.94–3.15
81–90	3.10–3.39	2.80–2.94
71–80	2.95–09	2.65–2.79
61–70	2.80–2.95	2.50–2.64
51–60	2.65–2.79	2.35–2.49
41–50	2.50–2.64	2.20–2.34
31–40	2.35–2.49	2.05–2.19
21–30	2.20–2.34	1.90–2.04
11–20	2.05–2.19	1.75–1.89
1–10	1.90–2.04	1.60–1.74

Reprinted with permission from Chu DA. *Explosive Power and Strength*. Champaign (IL): Human Kinetics; 1996. pp. 167–180.

Broad Jump (Standing Long Jump)

- A flat area (at least 15 ft in length) (grass field, gym floor, etc.), a tape measure, and a masking tape are needed. Tape serves as a start marker and can be used to secure the tape measure lengthwise. The athlete starts with his/her toes just behind the starting line.
- Using a countermovement with arm swing, the athlete jumps forward as far as possible. The athlete should land on both feet for the trial to count. The athlete should land with feet straddled over the tape measure. A point at the athlete's rearmost heel is marked and the distance is measured. The best of three trials is recorded.
- Table 18.20 presents norms for the broad jump in athletes.

Force Plate and Transducer Assessments

Jump squats performed on a force plate (Fig. 18.11) or with a position transducer attached to the bar can provide power data for the coach. Force plates contain strain gauges or load cells that directly measure ground reaction

force from the athlete. Force output (and moments) can be measured in three planes of motion. Force-time data are generated such that impulse, momentum, and flight time can be determined, as well as velocity-time data. RFD data can be generated directly from the force-time curves or from software calculation. Considering that power is the product of force and velocity, power curves can be generated yielding peak and mean power output data. Power endurance can be calculated. For example, we have used a 20-repetition squat jump test (with 30% of pretraining squat 1 RM) to generate power-time curves and to calculate fatigue rates (highest power output — lowest power output/highest power output × 100) in athletes and have seen fatigue index rates of 13%–21% (61). Some types of force plates can be set in the floor and some are portable and can be used in various locations. Several unilateral and bilateral exercises can be performed on force plates from running to jumps to various ground-based weight training, plyometric, and sport-specific exercises. Unilateral tests can be used to assess potential imbalances. For example, right-to-left differences of more than 15% may indicate some type of injury or may be seen as increasing the risk of injury (52). Thus, comparison of single-leg movements via force, power, velocity, and flight time data can be used to assess the athlete's unilateral kinetic performance (52). Athletes can be assessed on force plates under sport-specific conditions, *e.g.*, jumping to spike a volleyball or rebound in basketball, and pushing off during pitching in baseball. Depth jumps have been used where the athlete steps off of boxes of various heights, lands on the plate, and jumps as explosively as possible. Flight time can be divided by contact time with the plate during landing to calculate the *reactive strength index* which is a measure of the athlete's explosive ability (52). Power data can be expressed in absolute or relative terms. Normalized power data (to body weight) can provide the coach additional data especially for those athletes who require a high strength/

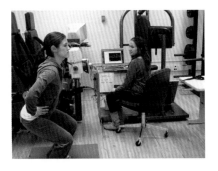

FIGURE 18.11. Force plate testing of a vertical jump. Here, an athlete is preparing to perform a vertical jump test consisting of three successive jumps on the force plate. Power-time curves from the previous set-off jumps can be seen on the monitor screen (Photo courtesy of The College of New Jersey Human Performance Lab.)

power-to-mass ratio like a high jumper who is competing against gravity versus a football player where absolute total-body power is essential (52). Relative power measures allow for comparisons among athletes of different body weights.

The technology used in designing a force plate can be incorporated into sport-specific equipment. Force transducers can be systematically placed in sport-specific training equipment to measure force and power. Placing force transducers into a blocking sled can measure sport-specific force and power in a football player. Force/pressure transducers can be placed into footwear to measure forces produced during various tasks. They have been placed within treadmills (Woodway 3.0) to measure force and velocity during sprinting (62). Special boxing dynamometers have been developed to measure force during straight punches in boxers (68). Critical is the placement of transducers, the planes of detection, and the potential for damage and movement as a result of striking. Thus, reliability is of concern. However, these pieces of equipment appear to provide meaningful data to researchers and coaches when used over time as a tool in the athletic assessment box. The most critical element is that sport-specific tests can be used to truly measure athletic performance during direct motor skill applications.

Although force plates are typically found in biomechanics or exercise physiology laboratories, position and velocity transducers are more practical and affordable for coaches to use. Transducers are applied to bars or the body and measure displacement during movement. Studies have shown them to be valid and reliable during kinetic testing (15). For example, the Tendo (Tendo Sports Machines, Slovak Republic) unit has been used successfully to measure power in athletes (Fig. 18.12). It consists of a position transducer that is applied to one end of the bar and is interfaced with a computer for data collection. It measures bar displacement and time thereby allowing bar velocity to be calculated for each repetition. The weight on the bar is input (to compute force) and power (peak and average) is calculated for each repetition. Instant feedback is provided so athletes can be made aware of their subsequent effort for each repetition. Transducers enable power assessment for any resistance exercise, traditional or ballistic, although ballistic exercises are preferred, e.g., jump squats, bench press throw, and Olympic lifts. The best systems combine transducer data with force plate data in calculation of power. Tendo transducers are reliable ($R = 0.87$–0.94) measures of power during standardized performance of bench press and barbell back squat (22,32).

Although several exercises can be used for assessment, the jump squat is used most primarily because it is a ballistic exercise that yields high-power outputs. Loaded and unloaded jump squats are used for power assessment. When used as an assessment, jump squats that yield the highest power outputs are recommended. Earlier studies showed loaded jump squats (30%–60% of 1 RM) yielded highest values whereas some recent studies have indicated jump squats with body weight only yield highest values (13,42,52). Nevertheless, the coach should select an absolute loading scheme and use that with successive power assessments. Power improvements are greater when the same pre-loading is used for power testing. Because power-loading curves are bell-shaped, changing the loading assesses power on a different segment of the curve which can skew power measurements erroneously. A change in power can reflect a different segment of the curve rather than an adaptation to training.

Power output generated from jump squat assessments is variable when comparing data from one study to another. It is very difficult to compare power outputs from athletes in one study to athletes from another study as there has been little consistency in power data obtained. It is difficult to establish norms for jump squat power as each plate or transducer yields values different from other laboratory's measurements. It is necessary for the coach or staff to generate their own norms based on power data generated from one device.

RFD assessments can be used. There are several ways to measure RFD as force plates generate RFD data during tests such as jump squats or any exercise performed on the plate. A common RFD assessment involves ISOM testing. An ISOM squat (performed on top of a force plate) or leg press (when a force plate or strain gauge is built into the sled) can be used. The bar or sled is fixed at a specific joint angle where it cannot move, e.g., with stoppers, pins in a rack, or ultra-heavy weights added to the bar or sled. The athlete is instructed to produce as much force as possible in the shortest amount of time. From the data generated, several variables of interest can be used. For example, if the athlete's peak force was 4,000 N pretesting, variables such as time to produce 4,000 N (100% of

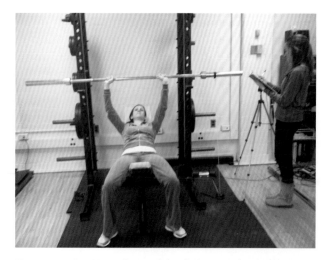

FIGURE 18.12. Use of a transducer during an incline bench press. (Photo courtesy of The College of New Jersey Human Performance Lab.)

peak force) or time to a specific force output, *e.g.*, 60%, 70%, 80%, and 90% of peak force, can be determined. This test can be applied after several weeks or months of training. A reduction in the time to produce these various levels of force indicates an increase in RFD. Thus, RFD tests measure how fast an athlete can produce submaximal or maximal force and can be a valuable tool in athletic assessments. However, because force plates, strain gauges, load cells, and transducers are needed, the cost may be high and prohibitive for some athletic settings.

Margaria-Kalamen Test

The Margaria-Kalamen test measures power by assessing the athlete's ability to ascend stairs as rapidly as possible. It has been used, albeit sparingly, to assess an athlete since its inception in the 1960s (26). The procedures are:

- A staircase with nine or more steps (at least 7-in. high and a lead-up area of ~20 ft) and an electronic timing device are needed. The height of each step needs to be measured and the elevation from the third to the ninth step needs to be calculated (6 × step height) *a priori*. The electronic timer start switch is placed on step 3 and the stop switch is placed on step 9.
- The athlete sprints 20 ft toward the stairs and then rapidly ascends the stairs three steps at a time. Timing begins when the athlete touches the third step and ends upon touching the ninth step. This time is used for calculation.
- Power is calculated via the following formula:

  Power (W) = [Body mass (kg) × vertical height from steps 3 to 9 (m)]/time (s)] × 9.81

- Norms for the Margaria-Kalamen test are shown in Table 18.21.

Upper-Body Power Assessments

Several tests can be used to assess upper-body power. The ballistic bench press is common. This test involves explosively throwing the bar upward. A linear position transducer is used to measure power. Transducers can be used for other upper-body exercises as well. The plyo push-up on a force plate can be used. Several different MB throws (side throws, overhead throws, and underhand throws) can be used. The distance the ball is thrown relates highly to upper-body (or total-body) power. Studies have shown MB tests to be valid and reliable indicators of power. Stockbrugger and Haennel (69) showed that the backward MB toss was a reliable test of power and correlated highly to vertical jump performance. Values of 12–15.4 m have been shown using 3-kg MBs in athletes (34). Cowley and Swensen (14) showed front and side MB throws to provide reliable power data. Ikeda et al. (37) found the side MB throw reliable in men but less reliable in women for predicting trunk rotation power. Thus, several throws can be useful to the coach when developing an upper-body power protocol. Backward throws have a greater lower-body component whereas side throws test rotational power. Direct upper-body power has been assessed using the MB chest pass.

Medicine Ball Chest Pass

- This test can be performed from a standing or seated position. A seated position isolates the upper body to a greater extent. Medicine balls vary, but one standard size can be used ~2%–5% of the athlete's body weight. When standing, a shoulder width stance is used. When seated, a back support is helpful as the athlete needs to keep contact with the support during the throw (a belt can be used). The athlete could sit against a wall as well. The toes should be aligned with a tape marker to set the starting line.
- The athlete passes or puts the MB as far as possible at an angle <45°. Upon landing, the center of the ball is marked and the distance from the starting line is measured. Some coaches prefer to chalk the ball for accuracy. Thus, the chalk will mark the landing spot and will make it easier to identify the correct location.
- The best of three throws is recorded. Norms are difficult for this test because coaches use different

TABLE 18.21 NORMATIVE VALUES (IN W) FOR THE MARGARIA-KALMEN STAIR SPRINT TEST

CATEGORY	15–20 Y		20–30 Y		30–40 Y		40–50 Y		50+ Y	
	M	F	M	F	M	F	M	F	M	F
Excellent	2,197	1,789	2,059	1,648	1,648	1,226	1,226	961	961	736
Good	1,840	1,487	1,722	1,379	1,379	1,036	1,036	810	809	604
Average	1,839	1,486	1,721	1,378	1,378	1,035	1,035	809	808	603
Fair	1,466	1,182	1,368	1,094	1,094	829	829	642	641	476
Poor	1,108	902	1,040	834	834	637	637	490	490	373

Adapted from Fox E, Bowers R, Foss M. *The physiological basis for exercise and sport*, 5th ed. (Dubuque, IA: Wm C. Brown), 676. with permission of The McGraw-Hill Companies: based on data from J. Kalamen, 1968, *Measurement of maximum muscular power in man*. Doctoral Dissertation. The Ohio State University, and R. Margaria, I. Aghemo and E. Rovelli, 1966, "Measurement of muscular power (anaerobic) in man," *J Appl Physiol*, 1993; 21:1662–1664.

size MBs, and standing versus seated will produce different results. Adolescent athletes using the seated pass have been shown to pass a 3-kg MB ~3.8–4.3 m (63) whereas Division III college football players have shown 3-kg MB pass values of 5.3–5.8 m (33). It is recommended that each coach store data and produce his/her own norms when standardized procedures are used.

Anaerobic Capacity Tests

Anaerobic capacity tests measure power endurance. They typically last 15–90 seconds in duration. Three common tests of anaerobic capacity are the Wingate anaerobic power, 300-yd shuttle, and line drill tests.

Wingate Anaerobic Power Test

The Wingate anaerobic power test is an all-out maximal cycle ergometry test lasting 30 seconds (although shorter and longer variations have been used). Cycling is performed against a resistance relative to the athlete's body mass, *e.g.*, 0.075 kg per kilogram of body mass on a Monark cycle ergometer. Although it is mostly used in laboratory settings, the Wingate test has been used to a lesser extent in the testing of athletes since its development in the early 1970s at the Wingate Institute in Israel (5). It is a reliable measure of anaerobic power (5). Several useful variables can be determined including absolute and relative peak power, average power, minimum power, time to peak power, total work, and the fatigue index. A mechanically braked cycle ergometer is needed with a sensor attached to the frame, which can measure flywheel revolutions per minute. Most units are interfaced with a computer and software program that performs all of the calculations for the athletes and coaches. The Wingate test can be applied to measure upper-body anaerobic power as an arm cycle ergometer can be used (29,30). The procedures for the Wingate test are as follows:

- Athlete sits comfortably on the cycle and warms up for ~5 minutes at a comfortable pace (60–70 rpm) against a light resistance or ~20% of the test resistance. A couple of short sprints are performed as part of the warm-up.
- Upon the signal "go," the athlete pedals as fast as possible (against zero resistance to overcome inertia) and the resistance is applied to the flywheel at the onset (0.075 kg per kg of body mass). The athlete pedals as fast as possible throughout the 30-second test duration. It is important to monitor technique and prevent standing during pedaling.
- Norms for men and women are presented in Table 18.22.

300-Yard Shuttle

- For this test, two parallel lines 25 yd apart (on a flat surface) and a stopwatch are needed. When possible, multiple athletes can be tested at once with additional testing personnel.
- The athlete assumes a starting position at one line (after a proper warm-up). Upon the signal "go," the athlete sprints as fast as possible to other line (25 yd away) making foot contact with it. The athlete immediately sprints back to the starting line and this process is repeated for six continuous round trips. Each roundtrip is 50 yd therefore six roundtrips totals 300 yd (23) (Fig. 18.13).
- Time is kept from the "go" signal until the athlete touches the final line at the 300-yd mark. After the first trial, 5 minutes of rest is given and a second trial is performed. The average of both trials is calculated and recorded. Norms for the 300-yd shuttle run are presented in Table 18.23.

TABLE 18.22 NORMS FOR THE WINGATE ANAEROBIC POWER TEST

% RANK	PEAK POWER MEN (W)	(W/KG)	MEAN POWER MEN (W)	(W/KG)	PEAK POWER WOMEN (W)	(W/KG)	MEAN POWER WOMEN (W)	(W/KG)
90	822	10.89	662	8.2	560	9.02	470	7.3
80	777	10.39	618	8.0	527	8.83	419	7.0
70	757	10.20	600	7.9	505	8.53	410	6.8
60	721	9.80	577	7.6	480	8.14	391	6.6
50	689	9.22	565	7.4	449	7.65	381	6.4
40	671	8.92	548	7.1	432	6.96	367	6.1
30	656	8.53	530	7.0	399	6.86	353	6.0
20	618	8.24	496	6.6	376	6.57	337	5.7
10	570	7.06	471	6.0	353	5.98	306	5.3

Reprinted with permission from Maud PJ, Schultz BB. Norms for the Wingate anaerobic test with comparison to another similar test. *Res Q Exerc Sport*. 1989;60:144–151.

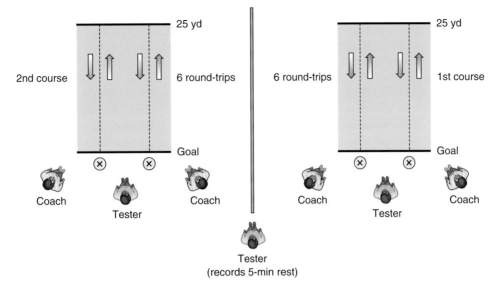

FIGURE 18.13. The 300-yd shuttle run.

Line Drill

- Often referred to as a *suicide drill*, the line drill is performed on a basketball court although it can be modified for other areas. It involves four back-and-forth sprints to all lines on a basketball court.
- The athlete begins from a starting position at the baseline and sprints to the foul line and back. The athlete then sprints from the baseline to the half-court line and back. The athlete then sprints from the baseline to the far foul line and back. Lastly, the athlete sprints from the baseline to the far baseline and back. The athlete must touch each line upon arrival, or the test is terminated and repeated.
- The stopwatch begins upon "go" and stops when the athlete touches the final baseline. The total run is ~470 ft for college and 420 ft for high school athletes (65).
- Two minutes of rest is given in between trials and the athlete may run four in total and may take the average for his/her final score (65).

- There are limitations in the literature regarding norms for the line drill test. Times of 26–31 seconds (mean of 28.5) have been shown in male basketball players (31) and means of 30–32 seconds have been shown in female basketball players (18).

SPEED

Assessments of speed involve maximal linear locomotion. Short sprint tests assess maximal speed and acceleration ability whereas long sprint tests assess speed endurance. Two sprint assessments discussed in this chapter are the 40-yd dash and 120-yd sprint.

40-Yard Dash

- A 40-yd marked area (with room for deceleration) and a stopwatch or electronic timing device are needed for this assessment. Other distances have been used to assess athletes, *e.g.*, 60 and 100 m, however, the 40-yd dash is most commonly used.

TABLE 18.23 NORMS FOR THE 300-YD SHUTTLE RUN

% RANK	BASEBALL	MEN'S BASKETBALL	WOMEN'S BASKETBALL	SOFTBALL
90	56.7	54.1	58.4	63.3
80	58.9	55.1	61.8	65.1
70	59.9	55.6	63.6	66.5
60	61.3	56.3	64.7	67.9
50	62.0	56.7	65.2	69.2
40	63.2	57.2	65.9	71.3
30	63.9	58.1	66.8	72.4
20	65.3	58.9	68.1	74.6
10	67.7	60.2	68.9	78.0

Reprinted with permission from Hoffman J. *Norms for Fitness, Performance, and Health*. Champaign (IL): Human Kinetics; 2006. pp. 1–113.

- Following a proper warm-up, the athlete assumes a starting position using either a 3- or 4-point stance at the starting line. Upon the "go" signal, the athlete sprints as fast as possible through the 40-yd marker. A coach begins the stopwatch on "go" and stops timing once the first segment of the athlete's body crosses the finish line. It is important that the same coach time each athlete for better accuracy and consistency. If an electronic timer is used, infrared sensors are placed at the finish line to stop timing. A start switch is used at the starting line where timing begins once the athlete lifts off during acceleration and stops once the athlete crosses the infrared beam.
- Following a rest period of at least 3 minutes, a second trial is run and the average of the two can be taken. Norms are presented in Table 18.24.

- Repeated 40-yd dashes can be run to assess speed endurance. One test used by the National Association of Speed and Explosion (NASE) is the NASE Repeated 40-s test (19). It involves running ten 40-yd sprints. The rest interval in between varies from sport to sport but may range from 15 to 30 seconds. The best and worst sprint should not deviate by more than 0.2–0.3 second (19). If so, the athlete may need to focus on specific speed endurance training to improve.

120-Yard Dash

- This assessment is conducted similarly to the 40-yd dash with the exception it is three times the distance. However, more relevant information can be determined by the coach. Each 40-yd interval is measured

TABLE 18.24 PERCENTILE RANKS FOR 40-YD (36.6 M) SPRINT TIMES (SEC) AMONG AMERICAN FOOTBALL PLAYERS (*TOP*) AND COLLEGE FOOTBALL PLAYERS PARTICIPATING IN THE NFL COMBINE (*BOTTOM*)

			AMERICAN FOOTBALL PLAYERS				
% RANK	HIGH SCHOOL (14–15Y)	HIGH SCHOOL (16–18Y)	HIGH SCHOOL (14–15Y) E	HIGH SCHOOL (16–18Y) E	NCAA DIII	NCAA DI	NCAA DI E
90	4.86	4.70	5.08	4.98	4.59	4.58	4.75
80	5.00	4.80	5.17	5.10	4.70	4.67	4.84
70	5.10	4.89	5.28	5.21	4.77	4.73	4.92
60	5.20	4.96	5.31	5.30	4.85	4.80	5.01
50	5.28	5.08	5.43	5.40	4.95	4.87	5.10
40	5.38	5.17	5.52	5.46	5.02	4.93	5.18
30	5.50	5.30	5.63	5.63	5.12	5.02	5.32
20	5.84	5.45	5.84	5.73	5.26	5.18	5.48
10	6.16	5.73	6.22	5.84	5.47	5.33	5.70
$\overline{X}$	5.40	5.15	5.54	5.41	4.99	4.92	5.17
SD	0.53	0.45	0.52	0.35	0.35	0.32	0.37
n	113	205	94	151	538	757	608

		COLLEGE FOOTBALL PLAYERS PARTICIPATING IN THE NFL COMBINE					
% RANK	DB	DL	LB	OL	QB	RB	TE	WR
90	4.41	4.72	4.57	5.07	4.60	4.44	4.66	4.42
80	4.45	4.80	4.62	5.15	4.70	4.50	4.78	4.46
70	4.48	4.87	4.66	5.21	4.75	4.55	4.80	4.50
60	4.51	4.90	4.72	5.25	4.79	4.58	4.83	4.52
50	4.54	4.90	4.76	5.30	4.81	4.62	4.90	4.55
40	4.57	4.96	4.78	5.33	4.86	4.65	4.96	4.57
30	4.59	5.03	4.81	5.40	4.91	4.69	4.99	4.61
20	4.62	5.09	4.86	5.47	4.99	4.74	5.02	4.65
10	4.67	5.15	4.92	5.56	5.10	4.82	5.07	4.68
$\overline{X}$	4.54	4.97	4.75	5.31	4.84	4.62	4.89	4.55
SD	0.11	0.19	0.13	0.20	0.17	0.16	0.15	0.10
n	111	100	62	155	41	67	42	98

E = electronic timing device; other measurements were from handheld stopwatches.

DB = defensive backs; DL = defensive linemen; LB = linebackers; OL = offensive linemen; QB = quarterbacks; RB = running backs; TE = tight ends; WR = wide receivers.

Data collected from 1999 NFL combine.

Reprinted with permission from Hoffman J. *Norms for Fitness, Performance, and Health.* Champaign (IL): Human Kinetics; 2006. pp. 1–113.

separately. This gives coaches information on all three phases of sprinting (19).

- Three timers are needed: one to start the test and conclude at the 40-yd mark, one to begin timing at the 40-yd mark and conclude at the 80-yd mark, and one to begin at the 80-yd mark and conclude at the 120-yd mark. A variation is to have all three timers begin timing on "go" and stop upon completion of the 40-, 80-, and 120-yd mark, respectively. The interval times are determined via subtraction of the 40-yd time from the 80-yd time and 80-yd time from the 120-yd time. An electronic timing device can be used and is preferred but three sets of infrared sensors would be needed for each 40-yd interval.
- The athlete begins in a 3- or 4-point stance and sprints as fast as possible throughout the 120-yd distance.
- The initial 40 yd is known as the *stationary 40-yd dash* and times recorded relate similarly to the performance of a normal 40-yd dash. Norms for 40-yd dash times can apply for this segment.
- The second segment is known as the *flying 40-yd dash* because it begins with the athlete already at full speed. Acceleration can be assessed by subtracting the flying 40 time from the static 40 time. Acceleration is good if the athlete's difference is less than 0.7 second (19).
- The third segment is known as the *speed endurance 40 segment* because it measures the athlete's ability to maintain maximal speed. It is determined by subtracting the speed endurance 40 time from the flying 40 time. Speed endurance is good if the difference is less than 0.2 second (19).

AGILITY

Agility tests assess the athlete's ability to rapidly accelerate, decelerate, and change direction in a controlled manner using forward, backward, and/or side shuffling types of movements. Cones and stopwatches are used for agility testing. Tape and tape measures are needed to measure and mark off appropriate distances. Similar to sprint testing, it is important that the same coach or tester measure all tests for each athlete to increase consistency and reduce human-related errors in timing. Although a multitude of drills can be used for assessment, the T-test, hexagon test, pro agility, three-cone drill, Edgren side step, and Davies tests are discussed.

T-Test

- Four cones and a stopwatch are needed. Three cones are aligned in a straight line 5 yd apart and a fourth cone is aligned with the second cone 10 yd apart forming a "T" shape.
- Following a warm-up, the athlete sprints forward 10 yd, shuffles to the left 5 yd to the cone, shuffles back right 10 yd to other cone, shuffles left to the middle cone, and back pedals back to the starting cone. The

athlete faces forward at all times and does not cross his/her feet. Cones are touched at each marker.

- The athlete begins on "go" and timing stops when the athlete backpedals past the starting cone at the completion of the drill. T-test times <9.5 and 10.5 seconds in men and women athletes, respectively, are excellent; 9.5–10.5 seconds (men) and 10.5–11.5 seconds (women) are good; and 10.5–11.5 seconds (men) and 11.5–12.5 seconds (women) are average.

Hexagon Test

- This test requires adhesive tape, a tape measure, and a stopwatch. A hexagon is formed with each side measuring 24 in. to form angles of 120° (26).
- Following a proper warm-up, the athlete begins by standing in the middle of the hexagon. Upon the signal "go," the athlete begins double-leg hopping from the center of the hexagon to each side and back to the center. The athlete starts with the side directly in front and continues clockwise until the drill is complete (which requires three revolutions). Thus, the athlete will jump 18 times and back to the center in a clockwise direction (Fig. 18.14).
- The trial is stopped for violations including landing on the line (rather than over it), loss of balance, or taking extra steps. The best of three trials is recorded.
- Norms for this drill are limited. Studies have shown values of ~12.3 seconds in male athletes, ~14.2 seconds in college men, 12.9–13.2 seconds in female athletes, and 14.3 seconds in college women (26,30).

Pro-Agility Test (20-Yard Shuttle Run)

- This drill can be performed on a football field with parallel lines 5 yd apart. A stopwatch is needed.
- The athlete begins straddling the center line in a 3-point stance. Upon the signal "go," the athlete sprints 5 yd to the line on the left, then sprints right for 10 yd to the furthest line, then sprints left for 5 yd to the center

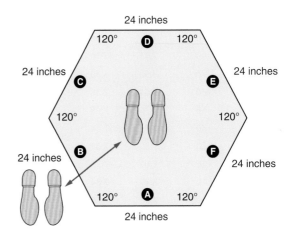

FIGURE 18.14. The hexagon test.

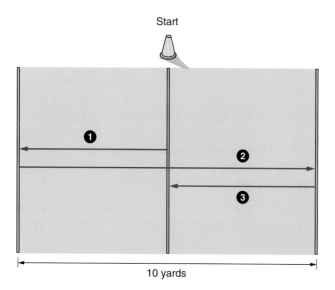

FIGURE 18.15. Pro-agility test.

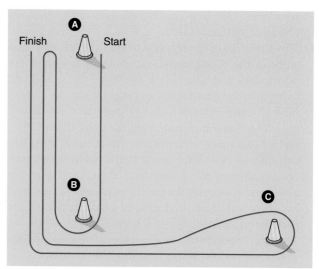

FIGURE 18.16. Three-cone drill.

line (Fig. 18.15). Foot contact must be made with the lines. Timing ends when the athlete passes the center line. The best time of two trials is recorded.

3-Cone Drill

* For this drill, three cones (A, B, and C) are placed in an upside-down "L" configuration with each cone separated by 5 yd (Fig. 18.16). A stopwatch is needed for timing.
* The athlete begins behind the starting line at cone A, sprints to cone B and back to cone A, then sprints to the outside of cone B, rounds cone B and sprints to cone C, rounds cone C, sprints back to cone B, and then sprints back to cone A at the finish point.
* Timing begins on "go" and finishes when the athlete crosses the finish point. The best of three trials is recorded. Few norms are available for this test.

Table 18.25 presents some data obtained from the 1999 NFL combine (30).

Edgren Side-Step Test

* A 12-ft area is needed where lines (tape) are placed 3 ft apart. Five taped lines are needed altogether. A gymnasium floor is recommended.
* Following a proper warm-up, the athlete begins the test by straddling the center line. On "go," the athlete side steps to the right to the outside line, side steps left to the furthest line, and repeats side shuffling back and forth for 10 seconds (Fig. 18.17). A tester counts the number of lines crossed during the 10-second period.

Davies Test

* This is an upper-body agility/strength test (10). Two pieces of tape are placed 36 in. apart. Athlete assumes

TABLE 18.25 THREE-CONE DRILL SCORES (S) FROM THE 1999 NFL COMBINE								
% RANK	DL	LB	DB	OL	QB	RB	TE	WR
90	7.22	7.05	6.87	7.66	7.06	7.17	7.12	6.85
80	7.45	7.16	6.97	7.82	7.13	7.29	7.16	7.01
70	7.52	7.30	7.07	7.98	7.19	7.32	7.27	7.10
60	7.64	7.38	7.09	8.07	7.31	7.36	7.38	7.19
50	7.71	7.49	7.14	8.15	7.36	7.47	7.42	7.28
40	7.78	7.54	7.22	8.28	7.40	7.53	7.48	7.35
30	7.89	7.61	7.29	8.38	7.54	7.60	7.57	7.41
20	8.07	7.70	7.39	8.51	7.59	7.71	7.71	7.49
10	8.47	7.84	7.47	8.66	7.70	7.82	8.04	7.58
Avg	7.75	7.46	7.17	8.18	7.29	7.48	7.47	7.26
SD	0.43	0.30	0.22	0.43	0.57	0.27	0.34	0.30

Reprinted with permission from Hoffman J. *Norms for Fitness, Performance, and Health.* Champaign (IL): Human Kinetics; 2006. pp. 1–113.

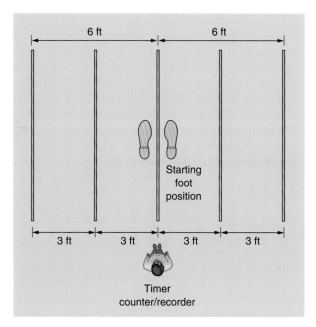

FIGURE 18.17. Edgren side step test.

a push-up position with each hand placed over one piece of tape.

- The athlete moves the right hand to touch the left (while maintaining correct posture) and returns to the starting position. The athlete then moves the left hand to touch the right hand and returns to the starting position while maintaining proper core position throughout. The athlete repeats these alternating movements as rapidly as possible for 15 seconds. The test can be adapted to be performed for a longer duration, *e.g.*, 60 seconds.
- The number of touches is recorded. The athlete is given three trials and the highest number is recorded. Better performance is seen with higher numbers of touches.

POSTURE AND FUNCTIONAL PERFORMANCE

Posture relates to the alignment and function of all segments of the human body at rest and during motion. Proper posture is important for optimal alignment, proper length-tension relationships of skeletal muscle during contraction, and optimal force transmission and absorption throughout the kinetic chain (10). The control of posture during exercise is critical to optimal performance and relates highly to having good core stability and strength. Postural assessment allows the coach to determine potential muscle imbalances (length and strength), weakness, and can be applied to target specific areas with the training program. Although posture can be critiqued during any type of exercise or motor skill, some postural assessments can be performed early which can be used to detect issues that can manifest later during more complex exercise performance.

Functional performance relates to the ability to perform basic athletic skills with stability, mobility, bodily control, and balance (11,12). Basic movements form the base necessary to build upon to perform more complex athletic skills. Functional qualities critical to sports performance include good mobility (especially in the hips and shoulders), ability to shift weight from one foot to the other to maintain balance, transfer power from the core to the limbs, and learn to control posture and bodily movement (11,12). Poor technique and mobility lead to poor posture and subsequent compensation that can place the athlete at greater risk for injury. Thus, testing of basic functional skills may be seen as a precursor to more advanced training.

Postural and performance screening can be done by viewing the athlete's performance in training or during sport practice. However, some screening protocols have been developed. One protocol developed by Gray Cook is known as the *Functional Movement Screen* (11,12). It consists of applying a 0–3 score (0 = pain during movement, 1 = unable to perform prescribed movement, 2 = can perform movement but needs to compensate and has difficulty, and 3 = good performance of skill) to selected movements such as squatting, stepping, lunging, reaching, striding, kicking, pushing, and rotation. The movements assessed include:

- *The Overhead Squat* — a broomstick or dowel is held in an overhead position while the athlete squats as deep as possible. The ideal technique involves heels flat on the ground, knees aligned over toes, the stick or dowel aligned over the feet, and torso upright at a position parallel to the tibias (minimal forward lean). Deviations result in a lower score and can indicate limited mobility of the shoulders, spine, hips, and ankles.
- *Hurdle Step* — assess mobility of the lower body. A mini hurdle is used and is set to a height of the athlete's tibial tuberosity. The athlete takes a hip width stance with toes aligned directly beneath the hurdle. The dowel or broomstick is placed on the rear shoulders with both hands supporting it in place. The athlete steps over the hurdle and touches the heel to the floor while keeping the opposite (support) leg extended and supporting body weight and then returns to the starting position. Optimal performance involves the hips, knees, and ankles remaining aligned within the sagittal plane, minimal to no movement of the lumbar spine, head focusing straight ahead, balance control, dowel or stick remains parallel to the hurdle, and no contact between the foot and hurdle. The athlete performs the test on the opposite side next. Deviations result in a lower score and could indicate poor stability of the support leg or poor mobility of the stepping leg.
- *In-Line Lunge* — a 2 × 6 board is needed. The tester measures the length of the athlete's tibia with a yardstick and marks this length on the board (from the athlete's toes) as the athlete steps on the board with one foot. A dowel is held behind the back with right arm up and

left arm down so that it touches the head, spine, and sacrum. The athlete lunges and places the heel of the lead leg on the mark and lowers the back knee until it touches the board. The athlete performs the test on the opposite side next. Optimal performance involves no torso movement, feet remain in a sagittal plane, knee touches the board behind the lead heel, and balance is maintained throughout. Deviations result in a lower score and could indicate poor hip mobility, balance, low stability in the knee and ankle, and an imbalance between adductor weakness and abductor tightness.

- *Shoulder Mobility* — the athlete makes a fist with each hand, placing the thumb inside the fist, and assumes a maximally adducted/internally rotated position with one arm and an abducted and externally rotated position with the other arm. The tester measures the distance between both of the athlete's fist along the back with a tape measure. Optimal performance involves attaining a ROM with both arms, *i.e.*, within one hand's length when measured. The athlete performs the test using the opposite limb arrangement. Deviations result in a lower score and could indicate poor shoulder ROM, poor scapular and thoracic spine mobility, and excessive development and shortening of the pectoralis minor and latissimus dorsi (leading to rounded shoulders).

- *Active Straight-Leg Raise* — the athlete lies supine with head on the floor and palms up with a 2 × 6 board positioned under the athlete's knees. The athlete lifts the leg with a dorsiflexed ankle position and an extended knee while the opposite leg remains straight (while the lower back remains on the floor). Once the athlete reaches the final position (as far back as the leg will reach before the knee begins to bend), the tester aligns a dowel through the medial malleolus of the ankle perpendicular to the floor. The athlete performs the test using the opposite leg. Optimal performance involves the dowel located between the mid-thigh and hip area of the opposite leg. Deviations result in a lower score and could indicate poor hamstring flexibility and tightness of the hip flexors associated with anterior pelvic tilt.

- *Trunk Stability Push-Up* — the athlete assumes a prone position with hands shoulder width apart and thumbs aligned with top of the head (men) or chin (women). From that position, the athlete performs a push-up with no lag in the lumbar spine. Optimal performance involves being able to do a push-up with proper posture. Poor performance may indicate a lack of strength and/or poor trunk stabilization.

- *Rotary Stability* — a 2 × 6 board is used for alignment while the athlete assumes a quadruped position on the floor. The athlete lifts the arm (flexes the shoulder) and leg (hip extension) on the same side of the body by ~6 in. The athlete then flexes both limbs to where the elbow touches the knee. The athlete performs the same skill with the opposite side. Optimal performance involves the athlete maintaining posture, moving both

limbs in the desired ROM, and not having the limbs cross over the board. Poor performance may indicate poor trunk stabilization and rotational strength. A variation used in functional screening is the *seated rotation test*. The athlete sits upright on the floor with back straight and legs crossed in a doorway. The athlete holds a dowel on the front shoulders with arms crossed on top. The athlete rotates as far as possible to the right and then to the left. A good score is seen when the athlete is able to touch the dowel to the wall (12).

BALANCE

Balance is the ability to maintain static and dynamic equilibrium. The assessment of balance can be of great value to the athlete. Athletes with poor balance or inferior performance on balance tests are at greater risk of ankle and knee injuries (35,71). For unilateral testing, differences in balance ability between dominant and nondominant leg can be assessed and compared. Balance training reduces incidence of recurrent ankle sprains and ACL injuries in soccer and volleyball players (35). Athletes have superior balance compared to nonathletes with gymnasts and soccer players scoring very high among groups of athletes tested (6,17,47,70). It is thought that balance training promotes greater joint stability and stiffness resulting from higher agonist and antagonist muscle activation thereby reducing the risk of injury (35). Thus, balance testing can be used to monitor stability increases during training.

Balance can be tested in different ways. The basic modes to test balance include timed static standing tests (eyes closed or on one leg), dynamic unilateral standing tests that involve a measureable movement with opposite limb or upper extremities, balance tests using unstable surfaces (stabilometers, wobble board, BOSU, pads, foam rollers, stability balls), standing tests on force plates (to measure *postural sway* or total shifts of the center of pressure during a prescribed time), and using specialized balance testing equipment (NeuroCom System, Biodex Stability Systems, Tetrax System). The following are some balance tests used:

- *Single-Leg Squat* — the athlete stands with hands on hips, a shoulder width stance, and eyes focused straight ahead. The athlete squats on one leg while the opposite leg is elevated (knee and hip flexed). The exercise ROM depends on strength level as well as body size so ROM can be adjusted based on the individual athlete. The coach looks at posture (erect torso), hip position, and knee movement. Too great of an inward movement of the knee (valgus stress) is contraindicated. This test is particularly effective in testing female athletes who are much more likely to sustain an ACL injury than their male athlete counterparts. Excessive valgus stress places the knee at greater risk for injury so close monitoring of hip and knee position during this test can identify problems that could adversely affect athletes on the field or court.

- *Anterior Reach* — the athlete begins with feet oriented with a marker located perpendicular to a tape measure. With hands positioned on the hips, the athlete extends a leg out as far as possible (while balancing on the opposite leg) keeping the front foot close to the floor without touching. The induced flexion of the support knee requires some degree of muscle strength and balance to perform. The distance reached with the front leg is measured. The best score of 3–4 trials is recorded for each leg. Balance must be maintained and the reaching leg cannot touch the floor for the trial to count.

- *Single-Leg Balance Test* — the athlete stands on one leg (without shoes) with the opposite leg bent and off of the ground. Hips remain level and head focused straight ahead. The eyes begin open but then are closed for 10 seconds. A negative test indicates good balance whereas a positive test indicates equilibrium issues or a sense of imbalance.

- *Standing Stork Test* — the athlete stands on one leg with the contralateral hip and knee flexed such that the toes are touching the opposite knee. Hands remain on the hips. Upon "go," the athlete plantar flexes onto his/her toes and the coach begins timing with a stopwatch. The athlete remains in this position for as long as possible. Multiple trials can be used and the longest time is recorded. For men, holding this position for >50 seconds is excellent, 40–50 seconds is above average, and <20 seconds is poor. For women, holding this position for >30 seconds is excellent, 20–30 seconds is above average, and <10 seconds is poor. Familiarization is very important for this test as great variability can be seen. Thus, the athlete should be given a few practice sessions prior to testing.

- *Stabilometer Balance Test* — stabilometers consist of platforms that are adjusted to move in all planes of motion relative to horizontal position (5°) (Fig. 18.18). The test involves the athlete's ability to maintain balance for a period of time. Some tests use a maximal time limit of 30 seconds and test the athlete's balance within

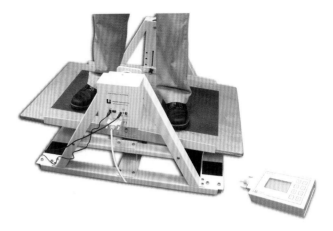

FIGURE 18.18. A stabilometer (Lafayette Instruments Inc., model 16030) used for Balance Testing. It has fully integrated timing functions, electronic angle measurement for increased accuracy, and allows a wide range of testable parameters including variable test times, selectable angle limits, and digital tilt angle readout.

that time frame. The degree of deviation depends on the athlete's ability so an appropriate angular deviation needs to be selected to accurately assess the athlete within the required time period. The time the athlete remains in balance is recorded. Multiple trials can be used and the best time is recorded. Like force plates, stabilometers can be quite costly.

- *Force Plate Tests* — several postural sway tests (which measure the deviation of the center of pressure) can be performed on a force plate. Many tests are unilateral and vary in duration (*i.e.,* 20 s) (36). Some tests involve the athletes closing their eyes as well. Variables such as the total length of path, sway velocity, front-to-back sway, and medial-to-lateral sway can be assessed.

- *Star Excursion Balance Test* — incorporates a single-leg stance on a support leg with maximum reach of the opposite leg. The athlete stands in the center of a grid with eight lines (120 cm) extending out at 45° increments (Fig. 18.19). The eight lines represent

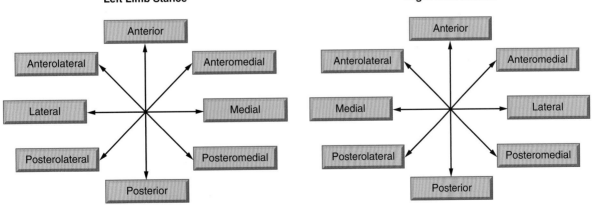

FIGURE 18.19. The star excursion balance test configuration. (Reprinted with permission from Olmsted LC, Carcia CR, Hertel J, Schultz SJ. Efficacy of the star excursion balance tests in detecting reach deficits in subjects with chronic ankle instability. *J Athl Train.* 2002;37:501–506.)

the anterolateral, anterior, anteromedial, medial, posteromedial, posterior, posterolateral, and lateral directions. However, the anterior, medial, and posterior directions may suffice in the testing of athletes (70). The athlete maintains a single-leg stance while reaching with the contralateral leg as far as possible for each taped line lightly touches the furthest point possible (54). The athlete then returns to a bilateral stance and the coach measures the distance from the center of the grid to the touch point with a tape measure. The best (or average) of three trials is recorded and the same is performed for the opposite side. Fifteen seconds of rest is given between reaches. Trials are discarded if the athlete does not touch the line, lifts the stance foot from the center grid, loses balance, or does not maintain start and return positions for one full second.

Case Study 18.1

Darryl is a recent college graduate who is now the official strength and conditioning coach of a collegiate Division II basketball team. In addition to developing the team's yearly strength and conditioning program, Darryl must also design the team's testing battery.

Question for Consideration: **Based on your knowledge of the sport of basketball and the needs of a basketball player, what type of testing battery can Darryl develop for his team to assess the critical health- and skill-related components of fitness paramount to basketball?**

Summary Points

✔ Tests selected should be valid, reliable, and sport specific. The testing battery should include at least one test each for the major health- and skill-related components of fitness specific to the athlete's sport.

✔ The testing staff should be well trained, familiarized to testing procedures and equipment used, aware of each athlete's situation, and should be assigned to specific athletes when multiple testing sessions are planned per year.

✔ Results of tests are compared to norms for the athlete's age-matched means for that sport, or the coach can develop his/her own norms and use that data for comparison.

✔ Testing the health-related fitness components includes assessments for body composition, muscle strength and endurance, cardiovascular endurance, and flexibility.

✔ Testing the skill-related fitness components includes assessments for power, speed, agility, and balance/coordination.

Review Questions

1. In assessing the effectiveness of the program you recently designed, you want to test the athlete's agility. Which one of the following assessments would be most appropriate?
   a. 120-yd dash
   b. 1.5-mile run
   c. Medicine ball chest pass
   d. T-test

2. Which of the following strength tests can also be used as a measure of total-body power?
   a. 1 RM bench press
   b. 1 RM power clean
   c. 1 RM squat
   d. 1 RM deadlift

3. A 21-year-old male athlete performs a grip strength test and records a max value of 68 kg. His grip strength is classified as:
   a. Excellent
   b. Good
   c. Average
   d. Poor

4. The sit-and-reach test mostly assesses flexibility of the:
   a. Shoulder muscles
   b. Low back, gluteal muscles, and hamstrings
   c. Anterior knee muscles
   d. Ankle plantar flexors

5. The Wingate test is a measure of:
   a. Maximal strength
   b. Flexibility
   c. Anaerobic capacity
   d. Aerobic endurance

6. Which of the following is an assessment of maximal sprinting speed?
   a. T-test
   b. 40-yd dash
   c. Stork test
   d. Margaria-Kalamen test

7. The multistage 20-m shuttle run is an assessment of maximal aerobic capacity.   T F

8. Reliability is a measure of repeatability or consistency a test exhibits.   T F

9. Skinfold analysis is considered the "gold standard" of body composition assessment.   T F

10. The hexagon test is an assessment of agility.   T F

11. When selecting a test sequence when multiple assessments are performed during the same session,

a lower-body muscle endurance test should be performed before a maximal agility test.   T F

12. Posture relates to the alignment and function of all segments of the human body at rest and during motion.   T F

References

1. Abadie BR, Altorfer GL, Schuler PB. Does a regression equation to predict maximal strength in untrained lifters remain valid when the subjects are technique trained? *J Strength Cond Res.* 1999;13:259–263.

2. American College of Sports Medicine. American College of Sports Medicine Position Stand: Exercise and fluid replacement. *Med Sci Sports Exerc.* 2007;39:377–390.

3. American College of Sports Medicine. American College of Sports Medicine Position Stand: Exertional heat illness during training and competition. *Med Sci Sports Exerc.* 2007;39:556–572.

4. American College of Sports Medicine. *ACSM's Guidelines for Exercise Testing and Prescription.* 8th ed. Philadelphia (PA): Lippincott Williams & Wilkins; 2010. pp. 70–105.

5. Bar-Or O. The Wingate anaerobic test. An update on methodology, reliability and validity. *Sports Med.* 1987;4:381–394.

6. Bressel E, Yonker JC, Kras J, Heath EM. Comparison of static and dynamic balance in female collegiate soccer, basketball, and gymnastics athletes. *J Athl Train.* 2007;42:42–46.

7. Brozek J, Grande F, Anderson J, et al: Densitometric analysis of body composition: revision of some quantitative assumptions. *Am NY Acad Sci.* 1963;110:113–140.

8. Brzycki M. Strength testing: predicting a one-rep max from reps-to-fatigue. *JOHPERD* 1993;64:88–90.

9. Chu DA. *Explosive Power and Strength.* Champaign (IL): Human Kinetics; 1996. pp. 167–180.

10. Clark MA, Lucett SC, Corn RJ. *NASM Essentials of Personal Fitness Training.* Philadelphia (PA): Lippincott Williams & Wilkins; 2008. pp. 99–138.

11. Cook G. Baseline sports-fitness testing. In: Foran B, editor. *High-Performance Sports Conditioning.* Champaign (IL): Human Kinetics; 2001. pp. 19–48.

12. Cook G. *Athletic Body in Balance.* Champaign (IL): Human Kinetics; 2003. pp. 31–38.

13. Cormie P, McCaulley GO, McBride JM. Power versus strength-power jump squat training: influence on the load-power relationship. *Med Sci Sports Exerc.* 2007;39:996–1003.

14. Cowley PM, Swensen TC. Development and reliability of two core stability field tests. *J Strength Cond Res.* 2008;22:619–624.

15. Cronin JB, Hing RD, McNair PJ. Reliability and validity of a linear position transducer for measuring jump performance. *J Strength Cond Res.* 2004;18:590–593.

16. Cummings B, Finn KJ. Estimation of a one repetition maximum bench press for untrained women. *J Strength Cond Res.* 1998;12:262–265.

17. Davlin CD. Dynamic balance in high level athletes. *Percept Mot Skills.* 2004;98:1171–1176.

18. Delextrat A, Cohen D. Strength, power, speed, and agility of women basketball players according to playing position. *J Strength Cond Res.* 2009;23:1974–1981.

19. Dintiman G, Ward B, Tellez T. *Sports Speed.* 2nd ed. Champaign (IL): Human Kinetics; 1998. pp. 1–44.

20. Durnin JVGA, Womersley J. Body fat assessed from total body density and its estimation from skinfold thickness: measurements on 481 men and women aged from 16 to 72 years. *Br J Nutr.* 1974; 32:77–97.

21. Epley B. Poundage chart. In: *Boyd Epley Workout.* Lincoln (NE); 1985.

22. Faigenbaum AD, Ratamess NA, McFarland J, et al. Effect of rest interval length on bench press performance in boys, teens, and men. *Ped Exerc Sci.* 2008;20:457–469.

23. Gillam GM. 300 yard shuttle run. *NSCA J.* 1983;5:46.

24. Harman EA, Rosenstein MT, Frykman RM, Rosenstein RM, Kraemer WJ. Estimation of human power output from vertical jump. *J Appl Sport Sci Res.* 1991;5:116–120.

25. Harman E. Principles of test selection and administration. In: Baechle TR, Earle RW, editors. *Essentials of Strength Training and Conditioning.* 3rd ed. Champaign (IL): Human Kinetics; 2008. pp. 237–247.

26. Harman E, Garhammer J. Administration, scoring, and interpretation of selected tests. In: Baechle TR, Earle RW, editors. *Essentials of Strength Training and Conditioning.* 3rd ed. Champaign (IL): Human Kinetics; 2008. pp. 249–292.

27. Heyward VH, Stolarczyk LM. *Applied Body Composition Assessment.* Champaign (IL): Human Kinetics; 1996. pp. 82.

28. Hoeger WK, Barette SL, Hale DF, Hopkins DR. Relationship between repetitions and selected percentages of one repetition maximum. *J Appl Sport Sci Res.* 1990;1:11–13.

29. Hoffman J. *Physiological Aspects of Sport Training and Performance.* Champaign (IL): Human Kinetics; 2002. pp. 109–119.

30. Hoffman J. *Norms for Fitness, Performance, and Health.* Champaign (IL): Human Kinetics; 2006. pp. 1–113.

31. Hoffman JR, Epstein S, Einbinder M, Weinstein Y. A comparison between the Wingate anaerobic power test to both vertical jump and line drill tests in basketball players. *J Strength Cond Res.* 2000;14:261–264.

32. Hoffman JR, Ratamess NA, Kang J, Rashti SL, Faigenbaum AD. Effect of Betaine supplementation on power performance and fatigue. *J Int Soc Sports Nutr.* 2009;6:1–10.

33. Hoffman JR, Ratamess NA, Klatt M, et al. Comparison between different off-season resistance training programs in Division III American College football players. *J Strength Cond Res.* 2009; 23:11–19.

34. Housh TJ, Cramer JT, Weir JP, Beck TW, Johnson GO. *Physical Fitness Laboratories on a Budget.* Scottsdale (AZ): Holcomb Hathaway Publishers, Inc.; 2009. pp. 50–162.

35. Hrysomallis C. Relationship between balance ability, training and sports injury risk. *Sports Med.* 2007;37:547–556.

36. Hrysomallis C. Preseason and midseason balance ability of professional Australian footballers. *J Strength Cond Res*. 2008;22: 210–211.

37. Ikeda Y, Kijima K, Kawabata K, Fuchimoto T, Ito A. Relationship between side medicine-ball throw performance and physical ability for male and female athletes. *Eur J Appl Physiol*. 2007;99: 47–55.

38. Jackson AS, Pollock ML. Generalized equations for predicting body density of men. *Br J Nutr*. 1978;40:497–504.

39. Jackson AS, Pollock ML. Practical assessment of body composition. *Phys Sports Med*. 1985;13:76–90.

40. Jackson AS, Pollock ML, Ward A. Generalized equations for predicting body density of women. *Med Sci Sports Exerc*. 1980;12: 175–181.

41. Johnson DL, Bahamonde R. Power output estimate in university athletes. *J Strength Cond Res*. 1996;10:161–166.

42. Kawamori N, Haff GG. The optimal training load for the development of muscular power. *J Strength Cond Res*. 2004;18:675–684.

43. Kraemer WJ, Fry AC, Ratamess NA, French DN. Strength testing: development and evaluation of methodology. In: Maud PJ, Foster C, editors. *Physiological Assessments of Human Performance*. 2nd ed. Champaign (IL): Human Kinetics; 2006. pp. 119–150.

44. Lander J. Maximum based on reps. *NSCA J*. 1985;6:60–61.

45. Leger LA, Lambert J. A maximal multistage 20-m shuttle run test to predict Vo$_{2max}$. *Eur J Appl Physiol Occup Physiol*. 1982;49: 1–12.

46. Leger LA, Mercier D, Gadoury C, Lambert J. The multistage 20 metre shuttle run test for aerobic fitness. *J Sports Sci*. 1988;6: 93–101.

47. Matsuda S, Demura S, Uchiyama M. Centre of pressure sway characteristics during static one-legged stance of athletes from different sports. *J Sports Sci*. 2008;26:775–779.

48. Maud PJ, Schultz BB. Norms for the Wingate anaerobic test with comparison to another similar test. *Res Q Exerc Sport*. 1989; 60:144–151.

49. Mayhew JL, Ball TE, Arnold MD, Bowen JC. Relative muscular endurance performance as a predictor of bench press strength in college men and women. *J Appl Sport Sci Res*. 1992;6:200–206.

50. Mayhew JL, Ware JS, Bemben MG, et al. The NFL-225 test as a measure of bench press strength in college football players. *J Strength Cond Res*. 1999;13:130–134.

51. McArdle WD, Katch FI, Katch VL. *Exercise Physiology: Energy, Nutrition, and Human Performance*. 6th ed. Philadelphia (PA): Lippincott Williams & Wilkins; 2007. pp. 250–251.

52. Newton RU, Kraemer WJ. Power. In: Ackland TR, Elliott BC, Bloomfield J, editors. *Applied Anatomy and Biomechanics in Sport*. 2nd ed. Champaign (IL): Human Kinetics; 2009. p. 155–175.

53. O'Conner B, Simmons J, O'Shea P. *Weight Training Today*. St. Paul (MN): West Publishers; 1989.

54. Olmsted LC, Carcia CR, Hertel J, Schultz SJ. Efficacy of the star excursion balance tests in detecting reach deficits in subjects with chronic ankle instability. *J Athl Train*. 2002;37:501–506.

55. Paliczka VJ, Nichols AK, Boreham CAG. A multi-stage shuttle run as a predictor of running performance and maximal oxygen uptake in adults. *Brit J Sports Med*. 1987;21:163–165.

56. Pollock ML, Schmidt DH, Jackson AS. Measurement of cardiorespiratory fitness and body composition in the clinical setting. *Compr Ther*. 1980;6:12–27.

57. Ploutz-Snyder LL, Giamis EL. Orientation and familiarization to 1RM strength testing in old and young women. *J Strength Cond Res*. 2001;15:519–523.

58. Ramsbottom R, Brewer J, Williams C. A progressive shuttle run test to estimate maximal oxygen uptake. *Brit J Sports Med*. 1988;22:141–144.

59. Ratamess NA. *Coaches Guide to Performance-Enhancing Supplements*. Monterey (CA): Coaches Choice Books; 2006.

60. Ratamess NA. Body composition status and assessment. In: *ACSM's Resource Manual for Guidelines for Exercise Testing and Prescription*. 6th ed. Philadelphia (PA): Lippincott, Williams, & Wilkins; 2009. pp. 264–281.

61. Ratamess NA, Kraemer WJ, Volek JS, et al. The effects of amino acid supplementation on muscular performance during resistance training overreaching. *J Strength Cond Res*. 2003;17:250–258.

62. Ross RE, Ratamess NA, Hoffman JR, Faigenbaum AD, Kang J, Chilakos A. The effects of treadmill sprint training and resistance training on maximal running velocity and power. *J Strength Cond Res*. 2009;23:385–394.

63. Santos EJAM, Janeira MAAS. Effects of reduced training and detraining on upper and lower body explosive strength in adolescent male basketball players. *J Strength Cond Res*. 2009;23:1737–1744.

64. Sayers SP, Harackiewicz DV, Harman EA, Frykman PN, Rosenstein MT. Cross-validation of three jump power equations. *Med Sci Sports Exerc*. 1999;31:572–577.

65. Semenick D. The line drill test. *NSCA Journal*. 1990;12:47–49.

66. Siri WE. The gross composition of the body. *Adv Biol Med Physiol*. 1956;4:239–280.

67. Sloan AW, Weir JB. Nomograms for prediction of body density and total body fat from skinfold measurements. *J Appl Physiol*. 1970;28:221–222.

68. Smith MS, Dyson RJ, Hale T, Janaway L. Development of a boxing dynamometer and its punch force discrimination efficacy. *J Sport Sci*. 2000;18:445–450.

69. Stockbrugger BA, Haennel RG. Validity and reliability of a medicine ball explosive power test. *J Strength Cond Res*. 2001;15:431–438.

70. Thorpe JL, Ebersole KT. Unilateral balance performance in female collegiate soccer athletes. *J Strength Cond Res*. 2008;22:1429–1433.

71. Trojian TH, McKeag DB. Single leg balance test to identify risk of ankle sprains. *Br J Sports Med*. 2006;40:610–613.

72. Volek JS, Ratamess NA, Rubin MR, et al. The effects of creatine supplementation on muscular performance and body composition responses to short-term resistance training overreaching. *Eur J Appl Physiol*. 2004;91:628–637.

73. Wathen D. Load assignment. In: Baechle T, editor. *Essentials of Strength Training and Conditioning*. Champaign (IL): Human Kinetics; 1994. pp. 435–446.

Glossary

A

A-band—the dark band of skeletal muscle occupied primarily by myosin.

Abdominal bracing—cocontraction of all abdominal and lumbar muscles to increase intra-abdominal pressure and reduce risk of low back injuries.

Acceleration—the rate of change of velocity over time.

Accommodation—staleness resulting from a lack in change in the training program.

Actin—a protein involved in muscle contraction.

Action potential—electrical current that allows nerves to communicate with other nerves and tissues.

Adenosine triphosphate—high-energy compound that provides substantial energy for all of the cell's needs from hydrolysis of chemical bonds.

Aerobic training—continuous exercise training targeting improvements in maximal oxygen uptake.

Agility—the ability of an athlete to change direction rapidly without a loss of speed, balance, or bodily control.

Agonist—the primary muscle(s) contracting to perform a specific movement.

Amine hormone—a hormone derived from amino acids.

Anabolic steroids—testosterone-derived drugs that increase muscle strength, power, size, and endurance.

Anatomical position—reference standard for motion analysis where the individual stands erect with joints extended, palms facing forward, and feet parallel.

Angular motion—occurs when all points on a body or object move in circular patterns around the same axis.

Angular specificity—principle stating that isometric strength increases are greatest at the specific training joint angle or range of motion.

Antagonist—the opposing muscle or muscle group during a movement.

Anthropometry—measurement of the human body in terms of dimensions such as height, weight, circumferences, girths, and skinfolds.

Arterio-venous oxygen (A-VO$_2$) difference—the oxygen difference between arterial circulation and the tissues allowing for diffusion of oxygen at the tissue level.

Autocrine—hormonal action where hormone is released and acts upon the releasing tissue or organ.

Autogenic inhibition—reflex relaxation that occurs in an agonist muscle group following fatiguing contraction via Golgi tendon organ activation.

Autonomic nervous system—branch of nervous system consisting of nerves conveying efferent information to smooth muscle, cardiac muscle, and other glands, tissues, and organs.

B

Balance—the ability of an individual to maintain equilibrium.

Ballistic resistance training—an explosive type of resistance training where the load is lifted at maximal speed throughout the range of motion (to limit deceleration).

Ballistic stretching—dynamic stretching involving a bouncing type of motion where the final position is not held.

Barbells—bars of various lengths that can be loaded with weights or plates.

Baroreceptor—a stretch-sensitive sensory receptor located in the walls of blood vessels, which detects blood pressure.

Basal metabolic rate—the minimal level of energy needed to sustain bodily functions.

Beta oxidation—a process leading to the conversion of fatty acids to acetyl CoA.

Bilateral deficit—maximal force produced by both limbs contracting bilaterally is smaller than the sum of the limbs contracting unilaterally.

Bioenergetics—the flow of energy change within the human body from mostly carbohydrates, fats, and proteins.

Biomechanics—the science of applying the principles of mechanics to biological systems.

Blood doping—intravenous infusion of blood or blood products to increase athletic performance.

Blood pressure—the pressure in the arteries following contraction of the left ventricle.

Body composition—the proportion of fat and fat-free mass throughout the body.

Body density—the ratio of body mass to body volume.

Bohr effect—a right and downward shift of the oxy-hemoglobin curve resulting from changes in pH and temperature (named after Christian Bohr).

Bone mineral density—the quantity of mineral deposited in bone, which is used as a common assessment of bone anabolism.

Buoyancy—upward force acting in the opposite direction of gravity in water.

C

Capillary density—number of capillaries expressed relative to muscle cross-sectional area.

Cardiac muscle—type of muscle found in the heart.

Cardiac output—the total volume of blood pumped by the heart per minute.

Cardiocytes—cardiac cells.

Cardiovascular drift—an increase in heart rate during exercise that compensates for a reduction in stroke volume caused by fluid loss.

Cardiovascular endurance—the ability to perform prolonged aerobic exercise at moderate to high exercise intensities.

Catch-up growth—accelerated growth of bone following an injury.

Central nervous system—branch of nervous system that consists of the brain and spinal cord.

Chemiosmotic Hypothesis—hypothesis proposed by Paul Mitchell to explain the electron transport chain. Protons are pumped across the inner mitochondrial membrane into the intermembrane space where proton content is high creating an electrical potential source (proton-motive force) that drives the phosphorylation of ADP to ATP.

Closed-chain kinetic exercise—an exercise where the distal segments are fixed.

Cluster training—training used by Olympic weightlifters that requires inserting intraset rest intervals in between reps.

Collagen—a protein that helps give tissues strength and pliability.

Complex training—a system where plyometric exercises are incorporated in between sets of resistance exercise.

Conditioning—generic term for improving physical fitness and performance.

Conduction—heat exchange between two solid surfaces in direct contact with one another.

Convection—heat exchange that occurs between the surface of the body and a fluid medium.

Cool-down—a postworkout light exercise activity that provides an adjustment period between exercise and rest.

Cross-bridge—attachment formed between actin and myosin.

Cross education—refers to strength and endurance gained in the nontrained limb during unilateral training.

Cross-links—hydrogen bonds formed between chains in collagen.

Cross-reactivity—a molecule similar to a hormone in structure which has the ability to react with the hormone's receptor.

Cross-training—form of training where different modes of exercise are included in the program.

D

Delayed onset muscle soreness—the soreness associated with muscle damage accompanying unaccustomed or high-intensity exercise.

Detraining—the complete cessation of training or substantial reduction in frequency, volume, or intensity that results in performance reductions and a loss of some of the beneficial physiological adaptations associated with training.

Diastolic blood pressure—peripheral resistance to flow during relaxation (diastole).

Dumbbells—small versions of barbells designed mostly for single-arm use.

Dynamic constant external resistance—a series of concentric and eccentric muscle actions where tension produced throughout joint range of motion varies despite a constant load lifted.

Dynamic Stretching—stretching that involves actively moving a joint through its full range of motion without any relaxation or holding of joint positions.

E

Elasticity—property of connective tissue to return to its original length after being stretched.

Electromyography—instrumentation used to measure skeletal muscle activity.

Endergonic—a reaction that results in stored or absorbed energy.

Energy—the ability to perform work.

Energy expenditure—amount of energy an individual burns in the form of kilocalories.

Endocrine—hormonal action where the hormone is released into circulation.

Ergogenic—a substance that can directly enhance performance.

Evaporation—process by which water is converted from liquid to vapor.

Excess postexercise oxygen consumption—the additional oxygen consumed over baseline levels following exercise, formerly known as oxygen debt.

Exercise economy—the energy cost of exercise at a given velocity.

Exercise order—the sequence in which exercises are performed.

Exercise selection—the exercises selected or chosen to be performed during a workout or throughout a training program.

Exergonic—a reaction that results in energy release.

Expiration—a passive process (at rest) where air exits the lungs.

F

Fartlek training—loosely structured exercise performed at various intensities and lengths with mixed periods of hard and easy exercise.

Fascicle—part of skeletal muscle formed from muscle fibers stacked in parallel.

Fast glycolysis—breakdown of glucose for energy resulting in lactate formation.

Fick equation—VO_2 = cardiac output × the arteriovenous difference.

Firing rate—the number of times per second a motor unit discharges.

Fixator—a muscle that contracts to stabilize either the point of origin or insertion for a corresponding muscle.

Flexibility—the ability of a joint to move freely its range of motion.

Flight phase—describes motion of the leg that is not in contact with the ground.

Free weights—weights that the individual must control and move freely in any direction.

Frequency—a term used to describe the number of training sessions per week or day.

Frontal plane—divides the body into anterior and posterior regions.

G

Gluconeogenesis—process of glucose formation.

Glycogen—stored form of glucose in the liver and skeletal muscle.

Glycogenolysis—the breakdown of liver and muscle glycogen to glucose.

Glycolysis—breakdown of carbohydrates to resynthesize ATP in the cytoplasm.

Golgi tendon organs—proprioceptors located at the muscle-tendon junction that conveys information regarding muscle tension to the central nervous system.

Ground reaction force—the reactive force applied by the ground during contact.

Growth plate—cartilaginous area of the epiphyses where longitudinal bone growth takes place.

H

Haldane effect—concept where oxygenated hemoglobin has less ability to bind CO_2 than deoxygenated hemoglobin.

Half-life—the time it takes for half of the hormone secreted to be degraded.

Health-related fitness components—those components that are designated as improving health, wellness, and one's quality of life.

Heart rate—the frequency the heart beats per minute.

Hematocrit—the percent of formed elements relative to total blood volume.

Hemoconcentration—a higher hormone value resulting from fluid volume reduction despite having the same amount of hormone present.

Hemoglobin—iron-containing protein that transports oxygen in the blood.

Homeostasis—normal resting bodily function.

Hook grip—grip used for Olympic lifting where the thumb is wrapped around the bar and the first three fingers are wrapped around the thumb and bar.

Hormone—a chemical messenger released from an endocrine gland that mediates specific functions.

Hydrolysis—process by which water is added to a reaction to break a large molecule down into smaller molecules.

Hyperplasia—longitudinal splitting of fibers resulting in an increased number of cells.

Hypertrophy—scientific term used to describe tissue growth.

Hypervolemia—an increase in blood volume.

Hypoxia—lack of oxygen.

Hysteresis—the amount of energy lost as heat during the elastic recoil.

I

I-band—the light band of skeletal muscle primarily occupied by actin.

Insertion—the distal attachment of a skeletal muscle to bone (via a tendon).

Inspiration—active event that leads to air entering the lungs.

Insulin resistance—a condition where normal amounts of insulin are inadequate to produce a response.

Insulin sensitivity—the ability of insulin to activate its receptor influencing glucose and amino acid transport.

Integrative training—combining several modalities of training to target multiple health- and skill-related components of fitness.

Intensity—describes the magnitude of loading (or weight lifted) during resistance exercise.

Interval training—type of training where high-intensity intermittent exercise is followed by periods of lower-intensity exercise in cyclical manner.

Isoinertial—term used to describe weight training repetitions as it assumes the mass lifted to be constant.

Isokinetic—a velocity-controlled muscle action.

K

Kegs—fluid-filled drums used in resistance training.

Kettle bells—circular weights with handles attached.

Kinematics—the branch of biomechanics that deals with the description of motion.

Kinetics—the branch of biomechanics that deals with the forces that cause motion.

Krebs cycle—energy pathway yielding two ATP and the formation of electron complexes that lead to great energy production.

L

Lactate threshold—the intensity that blood lactate increases beyond resting levels.

Lean body mass—fat-free mass consisting of muscle, water, bones, and organs/tissues.

Leptin resistance—condition where leptin does not activate its receptors to regulate appetite and energy expenditure.

Linear motion—occurs when all points on a body or object move the same distance, at the same time, in the same direction.

Lipolysis—breakdown of fat.

M

Macrocycle—a plan for an extended training period (usually a year).

Maintenance training—reduced training volume, frequency, and sometimes intensity to maintain performance especially during in-season phase in athletes.

Mechanical advantage—the ratio of the moment arm of muscle force (effort arm) to the moment arm of resistance (resistance arm).

Mechanical stress—the internal force observed divided by the cross-sectional area of the connective tissue structure.

Mechanotransduction—transduction of a mechanical force applied to tissue into a local cellular signal.

Medicine balls—weighted rubber or leather balls that vary in size.

Mesocycle—several weeks to months of training.

Metabolism—the sum of all chemical reactions in the human body to sustain life.

Microcycle—consists of smaller units of training, typically around 1 to 4 weeks.

Minimal essential strain—minimal threshold stimulus (volume and intensity) that is needed for new bone formation.

Mitochondria—site of aerobic respiration in a cell.

Mitochondrial density—the number of mitochondria expressed relative to muscle cross-sectional area.

Moment arm—the perpendicular distance between the force's line of action to the fulcrum.

Monocycle—a yearly periodization macrocycle based on peaking for one major competition.

Motor nervous system—branch of peripheral nervous system that consists of the somatic and autonomic nervous systems.

Motor unit—a single alpha motoneuron and all of the muscle fibers it innervates.

Movement-specific training—the use of exercises that train movements rather than muscle groups.

Multiple-joint exercise—exercise that stresses more than one joint or major muscle group.

Muscle action—the type, *e.g.*, eccentric, concentric, and isometric, of muscular contractions.

Muscle fiber—the muscle cell formed from myofibrils stacked in parallel.

Muscle spindle—proprioceptors located within muscle fibers that respond to changes in muscle length.

Muscular endurance—the ability to sustain performance and resist fatigue.

Muscular strength—the maximal amount of force one can generate during a specific movement pattern at a specified velocity of contraction.

Myocardium—muscle of the heart.

Myofibril—formed from sarcomeres stacked in series.

Myogenesis—the process of muscle fiber formation.

Myosin—a protein involved in muscle contraction.

Myosin ATPase—enzyme that breaks down ATP to facilitate muscle contraction.

Myostatin—a protein that inhibits myogenesis.

N

Needs analysis—an element of program design that consists of answering questions based upon goals and desired outcomes, assessments, access to equipment, health, and the demands of the sport.

Negative feedback—A system that will cause the elevation of a substance when it is low or reduce the substance when it is elevated.

Neural drive—the quantity of signaling from motor nerves to skeletal muscles.

Neutralizer—a muscle that contracts to eliminate one movement of a multiarticular muscle.

Nonpennate fiber arrangement—muscles have their fibers run parallel to the muscle's line of pull.

Nucleus—contains the genetic material of the cell.

O

Occlusive resistance exercise—resistance exercise that uses a device to intentionally restrict blood flow and make a workout more anaerobic.

Onset of blood lactate accumulation—intensity where blood lactate values exceed 4 mmol L^{-1}.

Open-chain kinetic exercise—an exercise that enables the distal segments to freely move against loading.

Origin—the proximal attachment of a skeletal muscle to bone (via a tendon).

Osmosis—movement of water across a membrane from a high to low concentration.

Osteoarthritis—a disease marked by articular cartilage degeneration.

Osteoporosis—disease marked by a weakening of bone tissue.

Overspeed training—training technique that allows the athlete to attain supramaximal speed.

Overtraining syndrome—physiological and psychological condition that occurs when athletes consistently train with too high a volume or intensity resulting in performance decrements and other physical symptoms.

Oxygen deficit—the difference between oxygen supply and demand.

P

Paracrine—hormonal action where hormone released acts upon adjacent cells of tissue or organ of release.

Parasympathetic nervous system—branch of autonomic nervous system that returns the body back to homeostasis.

Pennate fiber arrangement—muscle fibers arranged obliquely to the central tendon, or line of pull.

Peptide hormone—a hormone that is a protein that ranges in size.

Periodization—the process of manipulating acute training program variables in order to bring the individual to maximal performance at the appropriate time of the year, and to reduce the risk of overtraining.

Peripheral nervous system—the branch of the nervous system that consists of the sensory and motor divisions.

Phosphocreatine—a high-energy phosphate that provides energy for high-intensity activities lasting up to 5 to 10 seconds.

Plasticity—transient or permanent deformation where the tissue remains at least partially elongated and does not return entirely to its original length following consistent deformation.

Plyometrics—an explosive type of exercise stressing the stretch-shortening cycle consisting of jumps, hops, skips, bounds, and throws.

Poisson's ratio—ratio of strain in the longitudinal direction to strain in the lateral direction.

Postactivation potentiation—principle that states recruitment of type II motor units is easier when an individual performs a moderately high to high-intensity muscle contractions first.

Posture—alignment and function of all segments of the human body at rest and during motion.

Power—rate of performing work.

Preexhaustion—a technique that requires the lifter to perform a single-joint exercise first to fatigue a muscle group.

Prehabilitation—training where the primary goal is to improve conditioning to reduce the risk of injuries.

Progressive overload—gradual increase in stress placed on the human body during training.

Proprioceptive neuromuscular facilitation (PNF)—stretching that incorporates combinations of concentric, eccentric, isometric muscle actions, and passive stretching.

R

Radiation—the transfer of energy waves from one body and is absorbed by another.

Rate of force development—the rate at which various levels of muscular force are attained.

Rate-pressure product—measure of myocardial work (the product of heart rate and systolic blood pressure).

Reaction time—the ability to respond rapidly to a stimulus.

Reactive hyperemia—blood flow increase in response to ischemic anaerobic exercise conditions.

Reciprocal inhibition—involves muscle relaxation resulting from contracting the antagonist muscle group.

Recruitment—the voluntary activation of motor units during effort.

Rehabilitation—training to strengthen a previously injured area of the body.

Relative humidity—the ratio of water in the air at a particular temperature to the total quantity of moisture that the air could contain.

Releasing hormone—a hormone with a primary purpose of releasing another hormone.

Reliability—a measure of the magnitude of repeatability or consistency a test exhibits.

Repetition—a complete movement cycle including an eccentric and concentric muscle action, *e.g.*, lifting the weight up and down. May refer to a single isometric contraction.

Repetition velocity—the velocity at which repetitions are performed.

Resistance training—a grand umbrella term referring to any consistent method or form of exercise requiring one to exert force against a resistance. Characterized by training with free weights and machines, implements, medicine balls, bands/tubing, manual resistance, water, or any object that provides resistance to movement.

Respiration—the transport of oxygen to the tissue level and removal of carbon dioxide.

Respiratory quotient—a measure of carbon dioxide produced per unit of oxygen.

Rest intervals—the amount of rest taken between sets and exercises.

S

Sagittal plane—divides the body into right and left segments.

Sarcolemma—skeletal muscle fiber membrane.

Sarcomere—the functional unit of skeletal muscle.

Sarcoplasm—cytoplasm in skeletal muscle.

Selective androgen receptor modulators—nonsteroidal molecules that can activate the androgen receptor and produce tissue growth.

Selective recruitment—the preferential recruitment of type II motor units that occurs in response to a change in direction of exerted forces and explosive muscle actions.

Set—a specified group or number of repetitions.

Single-joint exercise—an exercise that stresses one joint or major muscle group.

Size principle—property that states motor units are recruited and decruited in an orderly progression based on size.

Skeletal muscle—type of muscle that produces skeletal movement upon contraction.

Skill-related fitness components—components of fitness essential to athletic performance and the ability to perform activities of daily living.

Slow glycolysis—breakdown of glucose for energy resulting in formation of acetyl CoA.

Smooth muscle—type of muscle found in the walls of hollow organs and blood vessels.

Somatic nervous system—branch of the motor nervous system that conveys information from the central nervous system efferently to skeletal muscle.

Specific gravity—ratio of the mass of an object to its mass of water displacement.

Specificity—principle that states all training adaptations are specific to the stimulus applied.

Speed—the capacity of an athlete to perform a motor skill (typically linear sprints) as rapidly as possible.

Speed endurance—the ability to maintain maximal speed over a period of time.

Sports adrenal medulla—the greater potential to secrete catecholamines during exercise in trained individuals as an adaptation to training.

Sprint training—nonassisted and assisted high-speed drills aimed at increasing linear movement speed.

Stability balls—inflatable balls that come in many sizes.

Stabilizer—a muscle that contracts to stabilize either the point of origin or insertion for a corresponding muscle.

Static stretching—stretching that involves holding a joint position (statically) with some level of discomfort for an extended period of time.

Steroid hormone—a hormone made of three 6-carbon rings and one 5-carbon ring that is synthesized from cholesterol.

Sticking region—The area of greatest difficulty of an exercise where the velocity of the weight slows down.

Strain—magnitude of deformation that takes place in proportion to the amount of stress applied.

Strength training—the use of resistance methods to increase one's ability to exert or resist force for the purpose of improving performance (with any form of resistance equipment). The term *strength training* has been adapted to characterize the conditioning programs of athletes.

Strength-to-mass ratio—the ratio of an athlete's muscle strength for a given exercise to their body mass.

Stretch-shortening cycle—the phenomenon whereby concentric muscle force production is enhanced when the concentric muscle's action is preceded by an eccentric muscle action.

Stride length—the length of each stride during sprinting, which is determined by leg length, leg strength and power, and sprinting mechanics.

Stride rate—the number of foot contacts per period of time.

Stroke volume—the volume of blood ejected from the left ventricle each beat.

Summation—the effect of multiple twitches within skeletal muscle.

Support phase—describes motion of the leg that is in contact with the ground.

Sympathetic nervous system—branch of the autonomic nervous system that prepares the body for the stress of exercise.

Synchronization—occurs when two or more motor units fire at fixed time intervals.

Systolic blood pressure—the pressure in the left ventricle during systole.

T

Taper—period where there is a nonlinear reduction in workload prior to a major competition.

Tendon stiffness—force transmitted per unit of strain.

Terminal cisternae—sac that stores calcium in sarcoplasmic reticulum.

Test-retest reliability—the correlation coefficient determined from multiple testing days.

Tetanus—maximal force production when summation is peaked.

Torque—the turning effect produced by a force and is the product of force and moment arm length.

Transfer exercises—exercises that stress a segment of an Olympic lift used to enhance (transfer) performance of the entire lift.

Transport protein—proteins that protect a hormone from metabolism and help deliver the hormone to its receptor.

Transverse plane—divides the body into upper and lower regions.

T-tubule (transverse tubule)—extensions of the sarcolemma that transmit signal deep into muscle fiber.

Twitch—the contraction of muscle in response to a stimulus.

V

Valgus stress—a stress in which abduction is seen in a joint where abduction is not a prescribed movement.

Validity—the degree that a test measures what it is supposed to measure.

Valsalva maneuver—an increase in intrathoracic and intra-abdominal pressure brought about by holding one's breath.

Variation—the alteration in one or more program variables over time to keep the training stimulus optimal.

Ventilatory threshold—the point where minute ventilation increases exponentially.

Vibrations—mechanical oscillations that are defined by their frequency and amplitude.

Volume—the total amount of work performed during a workout. Represented by the total number of sets, resistance, and repetitions performed.

Volume load—calculated by multiplying the load lifted (in kilograms) by the number of sets and repetitions.

W

Warm-up—performing low-intensity exercise to prepare the body for more intense physical activity.

Weightlifting—the act of lifting weights to enhance performance and health (not the sport!).

Weight training—exercise training performed using free weights, machines, or similar equipment for the purposes of increasing muscle strength, power, size, endurance, or any other goals associated with training.

Index

Note: Page number in *Italics* indicate figures and page numbers followed by t indicate the tables.